Liver Cells and Drugs

Cellules Hépatiques et Médicaments

Colloques INSERM
ISSN 0768-3154

Other *Colloques* published as co-editions by John Libbey Eurotext and INSERM

147 Modern Trends in Aging Research. *Nouvelles Perspectives de la Recherche sur le Vieillissement.*
Edited by Y. Courtois, B. Faucheux, B. Forette, D.L. Knook and J.A. Tréton.
ISBN : John Libbey Eurotext 0 86196 125 0X
INSERM 2 85598 340 1

149 Binding Proteins of Steroid Hormones. *Protéines de liaison des Hormones Stéroïdes.*
Edited by M.G. Forest and M. Pugeat.
ISBN : John Libbey Eurotext 0 86196 125 0
INSERM 2 85598 340 1X

151 Control and Management of Parturition. *La Maîtrise de la Parturition.*
Edited by C. Sureau, P. Blot, D. Cabrol, F. Cavaillé and G. Germain.
ISBN : John Libbey Eurotext 0 86196 125 0
INSERM 2 85598 340 1

153 Hormones and Cell Regulation (11th European Symposium). *Hormones et Régulation Cellulaire (11ᵉ Symposium Européen).*
Edited by J. Nunez and J.E. Dumont
ISBN : John Libbey Eurotext 0 86196 104 8
INSERM 2 85598 324 X

158 Biochemistry and Physiopathology of Platelet Membrane. *Biochimie et Physiopathologie de la Membrane Plaquettaire.*
Edited by G. Marguerie and R.F.A. Zwaal
ISBN : John Libbey Eurotext 0 86196 114 5
INSERM 2 85598 345 2

162 The Inhibitors of Hematopoiesis. *Les Inhibiteurs de l'Hématopoïèse.*
Edited by A. Najman, M. Guigon, N.-C. Gorin, and J.-Y. Mary
ISBN : John Libbey Eurotext 0 86196 125 0
INSERM 2 85598 340 1

165 Hormones and Cell Regulation (12th European Symposium). *Hormones et Régulation Cellulaire (12ᵉ Symposium Européen).*
Edited by J. Nunez, J.E. Dumont and E. Carafoli
ISBN : John Libbey Eurotext 0 86196 133 1
INSERM 2 85598 347 9

167 Sleep Disorders and Respiration. *Les Evénements Respiratoires du Sommeil.*
Edited by P. Lévi-Valensi and B. Duron
ISBN : John Libbey Eurotext 0 86196 127 7
INSERM 2 85598 344 4

Liver Cells and Drugs

Cellules Hépatiques et Médicaments

Proceedings of the International Symposium on « Liver cells and drugs »
held in Rennes on July 7-10, 1987

Sponsored by the Institut National de la Santé
et de la Recherche Médicale (INSERM)

Edited by
André Guillouzo

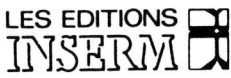

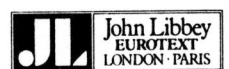

British Library Cataloguing in Publication Data

International Symposium on Liver Cells and Drugs (*1987 : Rennes, France*)
Liver cells and drugs.
1. Man. Liver. Drug therapy
I. Title   II. Guillouzo, Andre   III. Series 616.3'62061

ISBN 0 86196 128 5
ISSN 0768-3154

First published in 1988 by

John Libbey & Company Ltd
80/84 Bondway, London SW8 1SF, England. (01) 582 5266
John Libbey Eurotext Ltd
6 rue Blanche, 92120 Montrouge, France. (1) 47 35 85 52
ISBN 0 86196 128 5

Institut National de la Santé et de la Recherche Médicale
101 rue de Tolbiac, 75654 Paris Cedex 13, France.
(1) 45 84 14 41
ISBN 2 85598 341 X

ISSN 0768-3154
© 1988 Colloques INSERM/John Libbey Eurotext Ltd, All rights reserved
Unauthorized publication contravenes applicable laws

This book contains the 17 lectures given at the International Symposium on « Liver cells and drugs » held in Rennes on July 7-10, 1987 as well as 50 communications presented at the poster sessions. Two of them concerning nephrotoxicity, together with three on hepatotoxicity, were presented as the final report for a special program on « Hepato-nephrotoxicity » supported by the French Ministry of Research. Only the lectures have English and French abstracts. A special note of gratitude should be given to Mrs Maryvonne André and Annie Vannier for their invaluable assistance in the preparation of this book.

Ce livre contient 17 conférences et 50 communications par affiche présentées au Colloque International « Cellules hépatiques et médicaments » qui s'est tenu à Rennes du 7 au 10 juillet 1987. Deux communications portent sur la néphrotoxicité. Avec trois communications sur l'hépatotoxicité, elles ont été présentées dans le cadre du bilan de l'action « Hépato-néphrotoxicologie » financée par le Ministère de la Recherche. Seules les conférences ont un résumé en français et en anglais. Nous tenons à remercier particulièrement Mmes Maryvonne André et Annie Vannier pour leur aide très efficace à la préparation de ce livre.

A. Guillouzo

Scientific committee
Comité scientifique

M. Bourel (Rennes)
P. Berthelot (Paris)
R. Deraerdt (Romainville)
J.R. Kiechel (Rueil-Malmaison)
J.P. Leroux (Paris)
D. Mansuy (Paris)
D. Pessayre (Clichy)

Scientific secretary
Secrétaire scientifique

A. Guillouzo

Local organizing committee
Comité d'organisation local

M. Bourel (Chairman)
J.M. Bégué
P. Brissot
B. Clément
C. Guguen-Guillouzo
A. Guillouzo
R. Leverge
D. Ratanasavanh
C. Riché

Secretary
Secrétariat

M. André
L. Hartel
A. Vannier

Preface

At the instigation of the Unité de Recherches Hépatologiques U. 49 an International Symposium entitled « Liver Cells and Drugs » was held in Rennes for three days, on July 7-10 1987, which united 300 participants of 14 nations from the world of Clinical and Biological Research and the Pharmaceutical Industry.

The scope of the conference title was kept as broad as possible so as to encompass the biotransformation and the toxicity of drugs in the liver. It seemed an appropriate time to review these themes :
— from the Public Health point of view account must be taken of the frequency of drug induced hepatitis which, today, can represent nearly 1/2 of the hepatitis suffered by people over 50;
— the fundamental knowledge of the mechanism of hepatic transformation of molecules, since at the time of their introduction into human clinical medicine 10 % of these carry a risk of causing deleterious effects on the organism either via themselves or through a metabolic intermediary.

For the scientific community gathered at Rennes, I would like to thank :
— INSERM for financial support; its General Director Philippe Lazar, who has so efficiently promoted exchange between the Laboratories under his direction and Pharmaceutical Companies;
— The City Chambers of Rennes and particularly to the Major, Mr Edmond Hervé, who by virtue of his position and by personal dedication is brought so close to the problems of Health;
— The Ecole Nationale de la Santé Publique whose existence in Rennes perpetuates the memory of its lounder, Prof. Robert Debré and to its present Director Mr Rollet;
— The Ministère de la Recherche et de l'Enseignement Supérieur, the Conseil Général d'Ille-et-Vilaine, the University of Rennes I, the Crédit Mutuel de Bretagne, all of whom provided material support for the conference;
— The Société de Chimie Biologique and the group GERCHIC both of which provided animated leaders for the debates;
— The Pharmaceutical Laboratories who supported the meeting : Abbott, Beckman, Boehringer Ingelheim, Boehringer Mannheim, Fabre, Fournier, Logeais, Merck Sharp & Dohme, Packard, Pasteur « Vaccins », Roche, Roussel, Sandoz, Servier, Synthex France, Wyeth-Byla, Zyma;
— The authors of lectures who presented their message in such diverse domains as clinical aspects of drug induced hepatic toxicity, enzymes of

biotransformation and their regulation and mechanisms of the toxicity of molecules introduced into the organism. As was stated in the introduction of Professor Dame Sheila Sherlock, drug accidents in man can be understood by induced biological reactions and should, *in fine,* depend upon useful predictions given by *in vitro* liver model systems before the new molecules are put on the market.

— André Guillouzo, Director of the Unité de Recherches Hépatologiques U. 49 who, with Christiane Guguen-Guillouzo and the other members of the Unit, organized this meeting.

It is hoped that by reading the results and communications gathered for this book will make valid comments on a wide range of themes and provide a valuable aide-mémoire to those who took part in the symposium.

Professor Michel Bourel
President

Préface

Pendant trois jours, du 7 au 10 Juillet 1987, plus de trois cents personnalités du monde de la recherche biologique et clinique, de l'Industrie Pharmaceutique, venues de quatorze nations, se sont réunies à Rennes à l'instigation de l'Unité de Recherches Hépatologiques U. 49 pour un Colloque International « Cellules hépatiques et médicaments »; intitulé volontairement équilibré laissant aussi bien la place à l'évocation de la biotransformation des molécules (cellules hépatiques et médicaments) qu'à celle de leur toxicité hépatique (médicaments et cellules hépatiques). Le moment semblait venu de faire le point sur cette thématique au double point de vue :
— de la Santé Publique, compte tenu de la fréquence des hépatites médicamenteuses dont on sait aujourd'hui qu'elles peuvent représenter près de la moitié des hépatites frappant le sujet de plus de 50 ans;
— de la connaissance fondamentale des mécanismes de la biotransformation hépatique des molécules dont près de 10 % risquent, au moment de leur proposition en clinique humaine, d'avoir des effets délétères sur l'organisme directement ou par l'intermédiaire de leurs métabolites.

Au nom de la communauté scientifique réunie à Rennes, je voudrais remercier :
— l'Institut National de la Santé et de la Recherche Médicale (INSERM), co-éditeur de ce livre et contributeur essentiel du support financier de la rencontre; son Directeur Général, Philippe Lazar, dont l'une des actions s'inscrit dans le cadre de la valorisation de la Recherche par le moyen d'échanges entre les Laboratoires de l'organisme qu'il dirige et les grandes maisons de l'industrie pharmaceutique;
— la mairie de Rennes, et particulièrement Monsieur le Député-Maire Edmond Hervé, demeuré par conviction et engagement personnel si proche des problèmes de santé;
— l'Ecole Nationale de Santé Publique qui pérennise à Rennes le souvenir du Professeur Robert Debré et dont la Direction, assumée par Monsieur Rollet, sait toujours équilibrer pour les rencontres scientifiques la sérénité du travail et le charme de la détente;
— le Ministère de la Recherche et de l'Enseignement Supérieur, le Conseil Général d'Ille-et-Vilaine, l'Université de Rennes I, le Crédit Mutuel de Bretagne qui ont contribué à l'organisation matérielle de ces journées;
— la Société de Chimie Biologique et le groupe thématique GERCHIC qui en émane, dont certains des leaders animaient les débats;

— les Laboratoires Pharmaceutiques qui avaient répondu nombreux à l'appel et dont chacun pourra identifier la présence en ce document : Abbott, Beckman, Boehringer Ingelheim, Boehringer Mannheim, Fabre, Fournier, Logeais, Merck Sharp & Dohme, Packard, Pasteur « Vaccins », Roche, Roussel, Sandoz, Servier, Synthex France, Wyeth-Byla, Zyma;
— les auteurs d'exposés dont le message a permis une actualisation des connaissances de chacun dans des domaines aussi divers que les aspects cliniques de la toxicité hépatique des médicaments, l'étude des enzymes de biotransformation et leur régulation, le mécanisme de la toxicité des molécules introduites dans l'organisme. Comme le faisait remarquer dans son introduction le Professeur Dame Sheila Sherlock, la prévention des accidents médicamenteux repérés chez l'homme passe par la compréhension des réactions biologiques induites et devrait reposer *in fine,* grâce à la culture des cellules hépatiques *in vitro,* sur des données prédictives utilisables avant la mise sur le marché de nouvelles molécules;
— Monsieur André Guillouzo, Directeur de l'Unité de Recherches Hépatologiques U. 49 qui, avec Madame Christiane Guguen-Guillouzo et les autres membres de l'Unité, fut largement impliqué dans l'organisation de la rencontre.

Que la lecture des rapports et communications ici rassemblés contribue à faire le point d'une thématique en plein essor et à ranimer le souvenir des participants du colloque.

Professeur Michel Bourel
Président du Colloque

Contents
Sommaire

VII Preface
IX *Préface*

CLINICAL ASPECTS OF DRUG HEPATOTOXICITY/*LES ASPECTS CLINIQUES DE L'HÉPATOTOXICITÉ MÉDICAMENTEUSE*

3 **J.P. Benhamou**
Drug-induced hepatitis : clinical aspects
Les hépatites médicamenteuses : aspects cliniques

13 **O.F.W. James, M.D. Rawlins, H. Wynne, K.W. Woodhouse**
The liver, ageing and drugs
Foie, vieillissement et médicaments

23 **G. Danan**
Diagnosis of drug-induced liver injury
Diagnostic d'une atteinte hépatique médicamenteuse

DRUG METABOLISM AND ITS REGULATION/*LE MÉTABOLISME DES MÉDICAMENTS ET SA RÉGULATION*

31 **F.P. Guengerich, D.R. Umbenhauer, C. Ged, T. Muto, R.W. Bork, N. Shinriki, G.A. Dannan, Ph. Beaune, M.V. Martin, R.S. Lloyd**
Purification and characterization of human liver cytochrome P-450 enzymes
Purification et caractérisation des cytochromes P-450 hépatiques humains

41 **M. Daujat, P. Clair, T. Pineau, L. Pichard, C. Bonfils, C. Dalet, P. Maurel**
Regulation of cytochrome P-450 3c from rabbit liver microsomes
Régulation du cytochrome P-450 3c des microsomes hépatiques de lapin

51 **T. Cresteil, H.J. Eisen**
Regulation of human cytochrome P1-450 gene
Régulation du gène du cytochrome P1-450 humain

59 **P.I. Mackenzie, S.J. Haque**
The structure and regulation of UDP glucuronosyltransferases in the rat
Structure et régulation des UDP glucuronosyltransférases de rat

69   B. Ketterer, D.J. Meyer, B. Coles, J.B. Taylor
Glutathione transferases
Les glutathion-transférases

81   D. Müller-Enoch, J. Santak, T. Nagenrauft
The interaction of sulmazole, isosulmazole and pimobendan, three orally active cardiotonic agents, on the monooxygenase system of animals and man
Interaction du sulmazole, de l'isosulmazole et du pimobendane, trois agents cardiotoniques oraux actifs, avec les monooxygénases de foie animal et humain

85   D. Müller-Enoch, A. Greischel
A direct HPLC-method for measuring cytochrome P-450 activities with scoparone as substrate
Une méthode d'HPLC directe pour la mesure de l'activité du cytochrome P-450. Utilisation du scoparone comme substrat

89   D. Müller-Enoch, F. P. Guengerich
Genetic polymorphism in oxidative quinidine metabolism
Le polymorphisme génétique de l'oxydation de la quinidine

95   S. Claeyssens, A. Lavoinne, J. Peret, A. Chedeville, F. Matray
Rat liver glutathione during growth : study in weanling rats fed normal and low protein diet
Le taux de glutathion hépatique au cours de la croissance : une étude chez des rats sevrés, nourris avec un régime normal ou pauvre en protéines

99   C. Esnault, H. Lafont, F. Chanussot, M. Chautan, J. Hauton, C. Laruelle
Inhibition of hepatic HMG-CoA reductase activity by two new hypocholesterolemic drugs
Inhibition de l'activité de la HMG-CoA réductase par deux nouvelles molécules hypocholestérolémiantes

103   D. Ratanasavanh, J. Pazo-Carrera, Ph. Beaune, Y. Cariou, M. Nicol
Effect of vitamin A depletion on cytochrome P-450 isozymic pattern and glutathione transferase activity in rat liver
Effet d'un déficit en vitamine A sur le profil isozymique du cytochrome P-450 et l'activité des glutathion S-transférases dans le foie de rat

111   P. du Vignaud, P. Gelé, J.M. Delbos, N. Bromet, L. Grislain, E. Mocaer
Comparative metabolic pattern of amineptine in rat, dog and human
Etude comparative du métabolisme de l'amineptine chez le rat, le chien et l'homme

113   M.C. Malet-Martino, R. Martino, J. Bernadou, P. Chevreau
Identification of new metabolites of antineoplastic fluoropyrimidines in human bile using fluorine-19 NMR
Identification de deux nouveaux métabolites de fluoropyrimidines anticancéreuses dans la bile humaine par RMN du fluor-19

117 P.V. Chiapetta, K.W. Renton
The interaction between carbamazepine and erythromycin
Interaction entre la carbamazépine et l'érythromycine

123 K. Groen, G.J.J.M. Trommelen, K.F.A. van Bezooijen
The influence of age on the metabolism of theophylline in uninduced rats
Influence de l'âge sur le métabolisme de la théophylline chez des rats non induits

MECHANISMS OF DRUG HEPATOTOXICITY/*LES MÉCANISMES DE L'HÉPATOTOXICITÉ MÉDICAMENTEUSE*

129 D. Pessayre, D. Larrey
Mechanisms of drug-induced hepatitis
Les mécanismes des hépatites médicamenteuses

143 D. Larrey, D. Pessayre
Genetic factors in hepatotoxicity
Facteurs génétiques de l'hépatotoxicité

153 L.F. Prescott
Paracetamol: a model for toxic injury mediated by the formation of active metabolites
Paracétamol: un modèle de toxicité induite par des métabolites actifs

161 J. Neuberger, J.G. Kenna
Halothane hepatitis: a model of immunoallergic disease
L'hépatite à l'halothane: un modèle d'hépatite immunoallergique

175 Ph. Beaune, P.M. Dansette, D. Mansuy, L. Kiffel, C. Amar, J.P. Leroux, J.C. Homberg
Autoantibodies anticytochrome P-450 during autoimmune hepatitis
Auto-anticorps anti-cytochrome P-450 au cours d'hépatites auto-immunes

181 J.M. Warnet, D. Gouy, N. Agheli, P. Vic, R. Aubert, J.R. Claude
Phospholipid fatty acids in the liver phospholipidosis induced by amiodarone in the rat
Composition en acides gras des phospholipides dans la phospholipidose hépatique induite par l'amiodarone chez le rat

185 M.A. Pellissier, M. Boisset, S. Atteba, R. Albrecht
Influence of dietary vitamin E on liver microsomal lipid peroxidation in rats fed vitamin A and/or ascorbate-free diets
Influence de la vitamine E sur la peroxydation lipidique microsomale hépatique chez le rat nourri avec des régimes dépourvus de vitamine A et/ou d'ascorbate

191 A.K. Connolly, S.C. Price, D. Stevenson, J.C. Connelly, R.H. Hinton
Factors influencing the toxicity of alpha-naphthylisothiocyanate towards bile duct lining cells
Facteurs influençant la toxicité de l'alpha-naphtylisothyocyanate sur les cellules des canaux biliaires

197 J.F. Narbonne, P. Cassand, C. Colin, E. Antignac
In vivo and in vitro effects of some vitamins and glutathione on benzo(a)pyrene activation in rat liver
Effets in vivo et in vitro de quelques vitamines et du glutathion sur l'activation du benzo(a)pyrène dans le foie de rat

203 C. Cosson, I. Myara, P.F. Plouin, N. Moatti
Inhibition of the two isoforms of human hepatic prolidase by the converting enzyme inhibiting antihypertensives
Inhibition de deux isoformes de la prolidase hépatique humaine par des agents hypertenseurs inhibiteurs de l'enzyme de conversion

IN VITRO LIVER MODELS: NEW SYSTEMS FOR THE STUDY OF DRUG METABOLISM AND CYTOTOXICITY/*LES SYSTÈMES IN VITRO: DE NOUVEAUX MODÈLES POUR L'ÉTUDE DU MÉTABOLISME ET DE LA CYTOTOXICITÉ DES XÉNOBIOTIQUES*

211 J.F. Le Bigot, J.R. Kiechel
In vitro models in the study of the fate of drugs in research and development
Utilisation de modèles in vitro pour la recherche et le développement de médicaments

221 K.S. Santone, D. Acosta, S.A. Stavchansky, J.V. Bruckner
The use of primary cultures of postnatal rat hepatocytes to investigate carbon tetrachloride-induced cytotoxicity
L'utilisation de cultures primaires d'hépatocytes de rats nouveau-nés pour l'étude de la cytotoxicité induite par le tétrachlorure de carbone

235 A Guillouzo, J.M. Bégué, D. Ratanasavanh, C. Chesné, B. Meunier, C. Guguen-Guillouzo
Drug metabolism and cytotoxicity in long-term cultured hepatocytes
Métabolisme et cytotoxicité des médicaments dans des cultures prolongées d'hépatocytes

245 P. Kremers
Drug metabolism and cytotoxicity in cultured fetal hepatocytes
Métabolisme et cytotoxicité des médicaments dans des cultures d'hépatocytes fœtaux

253 F. Collignon, P. Gires, Y. Vedrine, V. Piguet, S. Martin, J. Gaillot
In vitro models: liver microsomes and isolated perfused liver; a comparison with in vivo metabolism (i.e. pefloxacin)
Etude comparative du métabolisme des médicaments dans des modèles in vitro (microsomes hépatiques et foie isolé perfusé) et in vivo: l'exemple de la pefloxacine chez le rat

259 M.C. Malet-Martino, S. Cabanac, J.P. Vialaneix, M. Bon, R. Martino
In vivo fluorine-19 NMR study of 5-fluoro-uracil metabolism in isolated perfused mouse liver
Etude du métabolisme du 5-fluoro-uracile dans le foie isolé perfusé de souris par RMN du fluor-19

263 E. Rouer, P. Rouet, J.P. Leroux
Microsomal aldrin epoxidase activity in liver of diabetic (insulin deficient) rats and studies of its regulation by glucagon in isolated hepatocytes
Activité de l'aldrine époxydase microsomale dans le foie de rat diabétique (insulinoprive) et étude de sa régulation par le glucagon dans les hépatocytes isolés

269 B. Ribon, Y. Benchekroun, M. Désage, J.P. Riou, J.L. Brazier
Metabolism of caffeine and three of its tri-deuteromethyl isotopomers
Métabolisme de la caféine et de trois de ses isotopomères tri-deutérométhylés

275 M. Jonsson, M. Martinez, L. Dock, B. Jernström
Isolated hepatocytes as a model to study the disposition of carcinogenic benzo(a)pyrene metabolites
Les hépatocytes isolés : un modèle pour l'étude de la disponibilité des métabolites du benzo(a)pyrène

281 M.K. Bayliss, J.A. Bell, A. Bradbury, K. Wilson
The metabolism of ^{14}C-loxtidine by isolated rat and dog hepatocytes
Métabolisme de la loxtidine par des hépatocytes isolés de rat et de chien

287 F. Berthou, D. Ratanasavanh, C. Riché, A. Guillouzo
Caffeine metabolism by human and rat hepatocytes in primary culture
Métabolisme de la caféine par des hépatocytes humains et de rat en culture primaire

293 D. Ratanasavanh, J.M. Bégué, P. Gelé, L. Grislain, N. Bromet, P. du Vignaud, R. Defrance, E. Mocaer, A. Guillouzo
Cytotoxicity and metabolism study of amineptine (S-1694-1) in cultured adult rat and human hepatocytes
Cytotoxicité et métabolisme de l'amineptine (S-1694-1) dans des cultures d'hépatocytes adultes humains et de rat

301 J.P. Cano, R. Rahmani, G. Fabre, B. Richard, B. Lacarelle, P. Boré, P. Bertault-Peres, G. de Sousa, I. Fabre, M. Placidi, C. Coulange, M. Ducros, M. Rampal
Human hepatocytes as an alternative model to the use of animal in experiments
Les hépatocytes humains : un modèle alternatif à l'expérimentation animale

309 A. Rolland, J.M. Bégué, F. Chevanne, R. Le Verge, A. Guillouzo
Comparative penetration of free and polymethacrylic nanoparticle — bound doxorubicin in cultured rat hepatocytes
Etude comparative de la pénétration de doxorubicine libre et liée à des nanoparticules polyméthacryliques dans des hépatocytes de rat en culture

315 B. Chindavijak, F.M. Belpaire, F. de Smet, N. Fraeyman, M.G. Bogaert
Metabolism of propranolol, lidocaine and antipyrine in hepatocytes isolated from rats with inflammation
Métabolisme du propranolol, de la lidocaïne et de l'antipyrine dans des hépatocytes isolés de rats

321 P. Le Corre, D. Ratanasavanh, D. Gibassier, A.M. Barthel, P. Sado, R. Le Verge, A. Guillouzo
Rat hepatocyte cultures and stereoselective biotransformation of disopyramide enantiomers
Biotransformation stéréosélective des énantiomères du disopyramide dans des cultures d'hépatocytes de rat

325 J.C. Peleran, M. Baradat, J.F. Sutra, G.F. Bories
Metabolic profiling of the mutagenic heterocyclic amine IQ using rat isolated hepatocytes
Obtention de profils métaboliques de l'amine hétérocyclique mutagène IQ au moyen d'hépatocytes isolés de rat

329 V. Rogiers, A. Callaerts, W. Sonck, A. Vercruysse
Biotransformation of sodium valproate in isolated rat hepatocytes
Biotransformation du valproate de sodium dans des hépatocytes isolés de rat

335 U.A. Boelsterli, P. Bouis, P. Donatsch
Effects of ciclosporin A on bile acid uptake, conjugation and release in cultured rat hepatocytes
Effets de la ciclosporine A sur le captage, la conjugaison et l'excrétion des acides biliaires dans des cultures d'hépatocytes de rat

343 C. Chesné, P. Gripon, A. Guillouzo
Primary culture of cryopreserved rat hepatocytes
Culture primaire d'hépatocytes congelés de rat

351 W.C. Mennes, B.J. Blaauboer, C.W.M. van Holsteijn
Biotransformation and cytotoxicity studies in primary hepatocyte cultures derived from different mammalian species
Etudes de biotransformation et de cytotoxicité dans des cultures primaires d'hépatocytes obtenus à partir de différentes espèces animales

357 L. Grislain, D. Ratanasavanh, M.T. Mocquard, L. Raquillet, J.M. Bégué, P. du Vignaud, P. Génissel, A. Guillouzo, N. Bromet
Primary cultures of rat and human hepatocytes as a model system for the evaluation of cytotoxicity and metabolic pathways of a new drug S-3341
Utilisation des cultures primaires d'hépatocytes humains et de rat pour l'évaluation de la cytotoxicité et des voies métaboliques d'un nouveau médicament : le S-3341

365 M.A. Le Bot, J.M. Bégué, D. Kernaleguen, J. Robert,
D. Ratanasavanh, Y. Guédes, C. Riché, A. Guillouzo
Metabolism of doxorubicin, epirubicin and daunorubicin by human and rat hepatocytes in primary culture
Métabolisme de la doxorubicine, de l'épirubicine et de la daunorubicine par les hépatocytes humains et de rat en culture primaire

371 M.J. Gómez-Lechón, A. Larrauri, T. Donato, P. López, A. Montaya, J.V. Castell
Predictive value of the in vitro test for hepatotoxicity of xenobiotics
Valeur prédictive des tests in vitro pour l'hépatotoxicité des xénobiotiques

379 F. Braut-Boucher, S. Achard-Ellouk, H. Hoellinger, D. Pauthe-Daide, M. Henry
Isolated and cultured rat hepatocytes as models for studying the cytotoxicity of two triterpenoid saponins
Hépatocytes isolés et en culture : des modèles pour l'étude de la cytotoxicité de deux saponines triterpénoïdes

385 R. Fellous, M.A. Verjus, D. Coulaud, A. Gouyette
Effects of ditercalinium in cultured rat hepatocyte : cytolocalization and ultrastructural mitochondrial damages
Effets du ditercalinium sur les hépatocytes de rat en culture : localisation cellulaire et lésions ultrastructurales des mitochondries

391 R.G. Ulrich, J.W. Cox
Acute hepatocellular changes elicited by various antibiotics in the perfused liver and cultured hepatocytes from the rat
Altérations hépatocellulaires aiguës induites par divers antibiotiques dans le foie isolé perfusé et des cultures d'hépatocytes de rat

397 B. Clément, J.M. Dumont, D. Ratanasavanh, M.F. Latinier, P. Brissot, A. Guillouzo
Effects of malotilate on human and rat hepatocytes in short-term and long-term primary culture
Effets du malotilate sur des hépatocytes humains et de rat maintenus en culture à court terme et à long terme

405 P. Villa, A. Guaitani
Effect of DMSO on microsomal monooxygenase activities in cultured rat hepatocytes
Effet du DMSO sur les activités mono-oxygénasiques microsomales d'hépatocytes de rat en culture

411 D. Müller-Enoch, G. Vergani, T. Nagenrauft
The influence of polycyclic aromatic hydrocarbons on the morphology and the cytochrome P-450 enzyme expression in cultured hepatocytes
Influence des hydrocarbures polycycliques aromatiques sur la morphologie et l'expression du cytochrome P-450 dans des cultures d'hépatocytes

417 Y. Vandenberghe, V. Seneca, A. Vercruysse, A. Guillouzo, B. Ketterer
Expression of glutathione S-transferase isoenzymes in cultured and co-cultured rat hepatocytes
Expression des isoenzymes de la glutathion S-transférase dans des cultures et des co-cultures d'hépatocytes de rat

423 J. Pazo-Carrera, G. Baffet, M. Rissel, A. Guillouzo
Effect of ethanol on the synthesis and secretion of proteins in cultured adult rat hepatocytes
Effet de l'éthanol sur la synthèse et la sécrétion protéiques dans des cultures d'hépatocytes de rat

431 G. Lescoat, B. Desvergne, N. Pasdeloup, D. Glaise, J.P. Gazeau, R. Molimard, Y. Deugnier, P. Brissot, M. Bourel
Effects of ornithine alpha-ketoglutarate on albumin secretion by adult rat hepatocyte co-cultures
Effets de l'alpha-cétoglutarate d'ornithine sur la sécrétion d'albumine par des hépatocytes de rat en co-culture

437 M. Decastel, G. Haentjens, M. Aubery, Y. Goussault
Studies of the toxic activity of ricin on Zajdela's hepatoma cells
Etude de la toxicité du ricin sur les cellules de l'hépatome Zajdela

445 L. Corcos, J.P. Rousset
Phenobarbital induces cytochrome P-450 mRNAs and enhances aflatoxin B1 toxicity in rat hepatoma cells
Le phénobarbital induit les ARNm de certains cytochromes P-450 et augmente la toxicité de l'aflatoxine B1 dans des cellules d'hépatomes de rat

451 M. Levy, D. Bagrel, N. Sabolovic, M.M. Galteau, M. Wellman, S. Rolin, G. Siest
Effects of ethanol on gamma-glutamyltransferase of a rat hepatoma cell line
Effet de l'éthanol sur la gamma-glutamyltransférase d'une lignée cellulaire d'hépatome de rat

459 P. Martel., C. Chaumontet, V. François, K. Ben Reddad, G. Pascal
An in vivo-in vitro model to study the cellular transformation elicited by liver tumor promoters: application to phenobarbital, butylated hydroxytoluene and butylated hydroxyanisole
Un modèle in vivo/in vitro pour l'étude de la transformation cellulaire induite par des promoteurs tumoraux hépatiques : le phénobarbital, le butyl hydroxytoluène et le butyl hydroxyanisole

465 C. Lafarge-Frayssinet, M. Garcette, R. Emanoil-Ravier, E. Morel-Chany, C. Frayssinet
Expression of Ki-ras, myc and fos protooncogenes during progression of spontaneous malignant transformation of epithelial rat liver cells in culture
Expression des proto-oncogènes Ki-ras, myc et fos au cours de la progression de la transformation spontanée maligne des cellules épithéliales de foie de rat en culture

NEPHROTOXICITY/*NÉPHROTOXICITÉ*

475 **G. Martin, J. Besson, B. Ferrier, C. Michoudet, M. Martin, D. Durozard, G. Baverel**
Stimulation of renal ammoniagenesis by the antiepileptic drug: sodium valproate. In vivo and in vitro studies
Stimulation de la synthèse rénale d'ammoniaque par un antiépileptique: le valproate de sodium. Etude in vivo et in vitro

481 **J.C. Cal, F. Larue, C. Dorian, J. Guillemain, P. Dorfman, J. Cambar**
Chronobiological approach of mercury-induced toxicity and of the protective effect of high dilutions of mercury against mercury-induced nephrotoxicity
Chrononéphrotoxicité du mercure et effet protecteur de dilutions élevées de ce métal

487 Author Index
Index des auteurs

490 Subject Index
Index des mots-clés

Clinical aspects of drug hepatotoxicity
Les aspects cliniques de l'hépatotoxicité médicamenteuse

Drug-induced hepatitis : clinical aspects

Jean-Pierre Benhamou

INSERM U. 24, Hôpital Beaujon, 92118 Clichy, France

SUMMARY

Drugs can induce a variety of liver lesions, the commonest of which is hepatitis. There are three main types of drug-induced hepatitis: cytolytic, cholestatic, and mixed; the course of acute hepatitis is usually benign, except for the cytolytic form which exposes the patient to a risk of fulminant liver failure. Drug-induced chronic hepatitis is uncommon and includes three types: chronic active hepatitis, alcoholic-like hepatitis, and chronic cholestatic hepatitis.

keywords

Drug-induced hepatitis

INTRODUCTION

Drugs can induced almost all types of liver injury (Table 1). However, the commonest drug-induced liver lesion is hepatitis: hepatitis is defined as necrosis or dysfunction of hepatocytes, resulting in liver failure and/or cholestasis. Drug-induced hepatitis may be isolated or associated with other types of liver injury (Table 1).

Drug-induced hepatitis is an increasing cause of liver injury in developed countries, obviously as the consequence of the increasing consumption of drugs. In French adults, drug hepatotoxicity is the cause of 10% of cases of acute hepatitis (Table 2). In adults over 50 years, drug hepatotoxicity represents the cause of 45% of cases of acute hepatitis (Table 2): this high percentage is related to the high consumption of drugs in adults over 50 years and, possibly, to the higher risk of drug-induced hepatitis in older than in younger adults.

DIAGNOSIS OF DRUG-INDUCED HEPATITIS

Indirect arguments
(a) Drug hepatotoxicity must be suspected in any case of acute or chronic hepatitis in patients over 50. (b) Drug hepatotoxicity must be envisaged as a cause of hepatitis in individuals with large consumption of drugs. (c) Drug hepatotoxicity must be considered in patients in whom other causes of hepatitis have been excluded, in particular infection with hepatitis A virus and hepatitis B virus.

Table 1. Drug-induced liver lesions

Hepatitis
    acute
            cytolytic
            cholestatic
            mixed
    chronic
            chronic active hepatitis
            alcoholic-like hepatitis
            chronic cholestatis
Granuloma*
Storage liver disease
    triglycerides (steatosis)
        macrovesicular steatosis*
        microvesicular steatosis*
    phospholipids
    vitamin A
    iron (hemosiderosis and hemochromatosis)
Vascular and sinusoidal lesions
    portal vein thrombosis
    hepatic artery thrombosis and hepatic infarction
    sinusoidal dilatation
    peliosis
    veno-oclusive disease
    hepatic vein thrombosis
Tumors
    liver cell adenoma
    hepatocellular carcinoma
    cholangiocellular carcinoma
    angiosarcoma
Sclerosing cholangitis

*These lesions may be associated with hepatitis

Table 2. Causes of acute hepatitis in adults admitted to, or consulting at, Hôpital Beaujon

		Over 50 years
Hepatitis A	420 (36.8%)	0
Hepatitis B	380 (33.3%)	41 (25,2%)
Hepatitis non A non B, B-like*	158 (13.9%)	38 (23.3%)
Hepatitis non A non B, A-like**	10 (0.8%)	0
Hepatitis due to EBV infection	12 (1,1%)	0
Hepatitis due to CMV infection	6 (0.6%)	0
Hepatitis due to poisoning***	32 (2.8%)	12 (7.3%)
Drug-induced hepatitis	122 (10.7%)	72 (44.2%)
	1140	163

*   contracted in France
**   contracted during a visit to Asia or Africa
*** mainly due to Amanita phalloides poisoning

Direct arguments (Danan et al, 1987)
The direct arguments for the diagnosis of drug-induced hepatitis are the following: (a) the drug ingested or injected is known to be toxic to the liver: the book by Zimmerman (1978) and the book by Stricker and Spoelstra (1985), which list all the drugs reputed to be hepatotoxic and give a brief description of the liver injury determined by each drug, are especially useful for the clinicians; (b) the chronology of the drug administration is very important for the diagnosis: the drug must have been taken before the onset of hepatitis usually within one week to six months before the first symptoms; the interruption of the administration of the drug must be followed by complete recovery; (c) the recurrence of hepatitis after readministration of the drug is certainly the strongest argument for the diagnosis; (d) the association of liver injury with hypersensitivity manifestations such as rash, fever, arthralgia, nephritis, and eosinophilia is likewise a good argument for the diagnosis; (e) the histologic examination of a liver specimen may provide some interesting arguments for the diagnosis: centrilobular distribution of hepatocyte necrosis, association of hepatic necrosis with macrovesicular or microvesicular steatosis, presence of giant multinucleated hepatocytes (Pessayre et al, 1981), absent or reduced inflammatory reaction, association of hepatocyte necrosis with veno-occlusive disease.

Diagnostic difficulties
Diagnosis of drug-induced hepatitis may be difficult for several reasons: (a) hepatotoxicity of the drug responsible for hepatitis may have not been hitherto reported: this is often the case for a new drug, but may be the case for drugs put in the market for a long time; (b) the hepatotoxic drug may be forgotten or hidden (for instance: oral contraceptives, antidepressants); (c) the notion of recurrent hepatitis after readministration of the drug may be lacking, because the physician has safely decided not to readminister the drug or because the patient has been affected by fulminant liver failure; (d) the hypersensitivity manifestations may be absent; (e) the histological lesions of drug induced hepatitis are often non specific and are often not associated with other more typical lesions; (f) exclusion of non A non B viral hepatitis may be difficult or impossible, because serological markers for this type of viral hepatitis are not available.

RECOGNITION OF THE MECHANISM OF DRUG-INDUCED HEPATITIS

In most of the cases, hepatic injury affects a very small proportion of the individuals taking the drugs: this situation is described as idiosyncrasy (a drug producing liver damage in a large number of individuals obviously would not be put on the market). The idiosyncratic reactions can be divided into two main types: metabolic idiosyncrasy and immunoallergic (or hypersensitivity) idiosyncrasy.

Metabolic idiosyncrasy is related to the conversion of the drug into a reactive metabolite, produced in the hepatocytes, mainly or exclusively by the microsomal enzymes cytochromes P450, and directly toxic to the liver cells. There are two broad categories of metabolic idiosyncratic reactions. In one category, there is destruction of hepatocyte membranes by peroxidation and associated changes: peroxidation is produced by free radicals or by activated oxygen. In the other category, there is production of electrophilic metabolites of the drug, in particular epoxides, which covalently bind to hepatocellular molecules, thus inducing dysfunction and death of the liver cells. Protection against the toxic effect of the reactive metabolites is provided by the microsomal enzymes epoxide hydrolase (which transforms epoxides into non toxic diols) and by intracellular glutathione (which transforms reactive metabolites into non toxic, water soluble, products that are then excreted in urines) and which reduces peroxides (and so provides a protection against peroxidation by activated oxygen).

In metabolic idiosyncrasy, hepatic injury can take place in an individual because the intracellular concentration of the reactive metabolites is abnormally high. This high concentration may be due to several factors. (a) there are several isoenzymes of cytochrome P450 which are determined by genetic factors: conceivably, some individuals having a certain type of cytochrome P450 might produce an abnormally high amount of a reactive metabolite (Larrey et al, 1985). (b) Some individuals might be genetically deficient in one or several enzymes converting reactive metabolites. (c) Hepatocyte glutathione may be depleted, for instance, by fasting or by alcoholism (depletion in hepatocyte glutathione is responsible for liver injury due to therapeutic doses of paracetamol in alcoholic patients (Seef et al, 1986)). (d) Augmentation in hepatocyte cytochrome P450 determined by enzyme-inducers results in elevated production of reactive metabolites and increased risk of hepatotoxicity (an example of this mechanism is provided by increased hepatotoxicity of isoniazid in patients receiving rifampicin, a potent inducer of cytochrome P450 in man (Pessayre et al, 1977)).

The clinical features suggesting metabolic idiosyncrasy are indicated in Table 3. The main clinical argument for this mechanism of hepatotoxicity are the administration of a drug known to be an enzyme inducer (e.g., barbiturates, benzodiazepines, rifampicin) simultaneously with the hepatotoxic agent and the absence of hypersensitivity manifestations.

Immunoallergic idiosyncrasy is supposed to determine liver cell necrosis according to the following steps. (a) A reactive metabolite of the drug would act as a hapten and would bind to an hepatocyte macromolecule, thus forming a complex having immunogenic properties. (b) This immunogen would migrate to the surface of the hepatocytes. (c) The hepatocytes expressing this foreign immunogen would induce an immune reaction, which in turn would destroy the liver cells having the immunogen. The detailed mechanim of immunoallergic idiosyncrasy is less well known than that of metabolic idiosyncrasy; in particular, the respective role of humoral and cell-mediated immunity has not been well established.

The reason or reasons for the development of immunoallergic idiosyncrasy to a drug are not well known. Recent observations suggest the role of genetic factors: patients with hepatic injury due to an immunoallergic reaction to phenytoin had been shown to have a genetically transmitted defect in converting the reactive metabolites, are n oxides, into the inactive dihydrodiol derivatives; the reactive metabolites presumably could serve as a hapten (Spielberg et al, 1980).

Immunoallergic idiosyncrasy is much commoner than metabolic idiosyncrasy. The features suggesting metabolic idiosyncrasy are set out in Table 3. The main clinical arguments for immunoallergic idiosyncrasy are: (a) the association of hepatic injury with extrahepatic hypersensitivity manifestations such as rash, fever, arthralgias, nephritis, and eosinophilia; and (b) the notion of a reduced delay for recurrent hepatic injury after readministration of the drug responsible for liver damage.

Metabolic and immunoallergic idiosyncrasies can be intricated. Mild hepatic dysfunction, which has been noted in a relative large number of patients receiving halothane anesthesia, would be due to metabolic hepatotoxicity, whereas severe hepatitis affecting a small number of patients would be due to immunoallergic idiosyncrasy (Neuberger and Williams, 1984). Likewise, chlorpromazine induces mild hepatic dysfunction in 35 to 50% of the patients receiving the drug, probably through metabolic idiosyncrasy, whereas this compound causes overt liver disease in 1% of the recipients, probably through an immunoallergic idiosyncrasy (Zimmerman, 1963).

Table 3. Features of metabolic idiosyncrasy and immunoallergic idiosyncrasy

	Metabolic idiosyncrasy	Immunoallergic idiosyncrasy
Effect of enzyme inducers	increase hepatotoxicity	no effect
Duration of exposure	1 week-12 months or more	1-5 weeks
Extrahepatic hypersensitivy manifestations	absent	present
Delay after readministration	unchanged	reduced

CLINICOPATHOLOGIC FORMS OF DRUG-INDUCED HEPATITIS

Acute injury
Severity of acute drug-induced hepatitis markedly varies from patient to patient. In most cases, drug-induced hepatitis is asymptomatic and therefore may remain unrecognized. In a number of patients, acute drug-induced hepatitis determines unspecific symptoms, such as fatigue, nausea, or abdominal pain; in patients taking a drug and complaining of these unspecific manifestations, especially when the drug has been well tolerated for the first weeks of its administration, the diagnosis of acute drug-induced hepatitis should be considered and liver tests, at least serum amininotransferases, should be performed. Icteric drug-induced hepatitis is only the tip of the iceberg.

Cytolytic hepatitis. This type of hepatitis is characterized by more or less extended necrosis of the liver cells. Prenecrotic changes, such as ballooning and eosinophilic degenerations, are associated to liver cell necrosis and may be the chief lesion. Liver cell damage usually predominates in the centrilobular areas: this distribution is very suggestive of drug-induced hepatitis. Inflammatory infiltration consisting of lymphocytes and plasmocytes, which is marked in most cases of viral hepatitis, is moderate in most cases of drug-induced hepatitis; in some cases, mononuclear cell infiltration is intricated with neutrophil infiltration, a histological feature suggestive of drug-induced hepatitis. In a few cases, inflammatory infiltration includes a certain proportion of eosinophils. Inflammatory infiltration, when present, may be diffuse, or aggregated around necrotic hepatocytes, or predominant in portal areas. In some cases, macrovesicular or microvesicular steatosis is present. In some cases, granulomas are seen. Drug-induced cytolytic hepatitis can be associated with veno-occlusive disease.

The main manifestations of cytolytic hepatitis are fatigue, nausea, and jaundice. Serum aminotransferases are increased often markedly; the increase is more marked for alanine aminotransferase than for aspartate aminotransferase. Serum gammaglutamyltranspeptidase is almost constantly, but moderately increased. Serum alkaline phosphatase is normal or moderately increased, less than 2 times the upper limit of the normal range. After cessation of drug administration, the patient recovers completely within one or two months.

In cytolytic hepatitis with jaundice, particularly when drug administration has been maintained after the clinical onset, there is a risk of fulminant liver failure. This risk is not well established, but might range from 5 to 20%, a figure which is markedly higher than in acute icteric viral hepatitis B or A. The delay from the onset of jaundice to the onset of encephalopathy is greater in drug-induced than in viral acute hepatitis, usually more than 15 days in the former and less than 15 days in the latter (Bernuau et al, 1986). Because of the low survival rate of drug-induced fulminant hepatitis, emergency liver transplantation has been proposed and performed successfully in a small number of patients (Bismuth et al, 1987).

Numerous drugs have been implicated in the etiology of acute cytolytic hepatitis. In France, the commonest drugs responsible for this type of hepatitis are the following: halothane (particularly when readministered) (Neuberger and Williams, 1984), isoniazid (particularly when associated with rifampicin (Pessayre et al, 1977)), non steroidal anti-inflammatory drugs (Danan et al, 1985), monoamine oxidase inhibitors (particularly when associated with enzyme inducers (Pessayre et al, 1978)), tienilic acid (Zimmerman et al, 1984) (tienilic acid induced hepatitis is often associated with an antibody to a cytochrome P450 isoenzyme metabolizing the drug (Beaune et al, 1987)), valproic acid (often associated with microvesicular steatosis (Zimmerman and Ishak, 1982)), dihydralazine (Pariente et al, 1983), ketoconazole (Bercoff et al, 1985), isaxonine (Baud et al, 1983) (which has been withdrawn), amodiaquine (Larrey et al, 1986), papaverine, clometacine (Goldfarb et al, 1979).

Cholestatic hepatitis. The lesion consists in cholestasis, usually predominating in the centrilobular areas, with no or limited liver cell necrosis. Two main types of drug-induced cholestasis have been recognized. In one type, exemplified by cholestasis induced by oral contraceptives, there is no lesion other than cholestasis; in particular, portal inflammation is absent or very slight; cholestasis is presumed to be due to canalicular lesions (canalicular type). In the other type, exemplified by carbamazepine induced cholestasis (Larrey et al, 1987), portal inflammation, either with mononuclear cells or, more characteristically, with mononuclear and polymorphonuclear cells, is present and, changes affecting cholangioles can be seen (cholangiolar type); this type of cholestasis is invariably related to an immunoallergic mechanism.

The main manifestations of cholestatic hepatitis are asthenia, nausea, pruritus, and jaundice. In the cholangiolar type of drug-induced cholestasis, the patients may complained of fever and abdominal pain; thus, the clinical presentation can resemble that of cholangitis. Serum bilirubin is more or less increased, reflecting the degree of cholestasis. In a few patients, serum cholesterol may be very high. Serum alkaline phosphatase is more than 2 times the upper limit of the normal range. Serum aminotransferases are normal or, more often, mildly increased.

After cessation of drug administration, recovery is usually complete. However, in few patients, anicteric or, more rarely icteric cholestasis, may persist for one year or more (Larrey et al, 1986). The development of chronic cholestasis resembling primary biliary cirrhosis has been described, but is very rare. In drug-induced cholestasis, there is no risk of fulminant liver failure.

In France, the commonest drugs responsible for drug-induced cholestasis are the following: chlorpromazine and other phenothiazines, anabolic and androgenic steroids, estrogens and estrogen containing oral contraceptives (the risk of cholestasis is markedly increased when triacetyloleandomycin is administered simultaneously with estrogens and estrogen containing oral contraceptives), macrolides (Funck-Brentano et al, 1983; Pessayre et al, 1985; Zafrani et al, 1979), tricyclic antidepressants, ajmaline (Pariente et al, 1980). The cholangilitis-like presentation is particularly common in patients with cholestasis induced by macrolides, tricyclic antidepressants, carbamazepine (Larrey et al, 1987), gold-salt (Pessayre et al, 1979), and ajmaline (Pariente et al, 1980).

Mixed hepatitis. In this type of drug-induced hepatitis, the histological lesions, the clinical manifestations, and the biochemical disorders are those of both the cytolytic and the cholestatic forms. However, the cholestatic features are usually predominant.

In France, the commonest drugs responsible for this type of hepatitis are phenylindanedione, ticlopidine, suloctidil (which has been recently withdrawn), and the above mentioned compounds determining drug-induced cholestasis, except for anabolic, androgenic, and estrogenic steroids.

Chronic injury
Prolonged administration of some hepatotoxic drugs can determine 3 types of chronic hepatitis: chronic active hepatitis, alcoholic-like hepatitis, chronic cholestasis.

Chronic active hepatitis. Drug-induced chronic active hepatitis must be systematically suspected in any patient with chronic active hepatitis. The main arguments for this diagnosis are the following: (1) absence of hepatitis B surface antigen in serum; (2) no epidemiological argument for non A non B hepatitis; (3) age more than 50 years (autoimmune chronic active hepatitis mainly affects women less than 40 years); (4) exacerbations with jaundice and serum aminotransferases more than 10 times the upper limit of the normal range (such exacerbations with jaundice and marked increase in serum aminotransferases are unusual in the other types of chronic active hepatitis); (5) histological examination may show liver cell necrosis predominating in the centrilobular areas, multinucleated giant hepatocytes, inflammatory infiltration including not only mononuclear cells but also neutrophils; all these features are unusual in the other types of chronic active hepatitis; (6) prolonged ingestion of a drug known to be hepatotoxic; (7) improvement after withdrawal of the drug; (7) exacerbation after readministration of the drug. In a few patients with drug-induced chronic active hepatitis, antibodies to nuclei, and/or smooth muscle, and/or mitochondria, and/or microsomes can be demonstrated: therefore, the presence of these tissular antibodies is not a definitive argument for autoimmune and against drug-induced chronic active hepatitis. The evolution of drug-induced chronic active hepatitis to cirrhosis has been described, but is very uncommon.

After cessation of administration of the causal drug, chronic active hepatitis improves within the following weeks or months; complete recovery is usual. In a few patients, the improvement is delayed, requiring 1 or 2 years. In a small number of patients, despite cessation of administration of the drug, no improvement and even progressive aggravation can be observed; in such cases, the causal role of the drug in the etiology of chronic active hepatitis cannot be established.

In France, the commonest drugs responsible for chronic active hepatitis are the following: oxiphenisatin (which has been withdrawn), tienilic acid (Zimmerman et al, 1984), clometacin, alpha-methyldopa, methotrexate, papaverine, suloctidil (which has been withdrawn).

Alcoholic-like hepatitis. Prolonged administration of perhexiline maleate and amiodarone can determine hepatic lesions resembling alcoholic hepatitis, consisting of steatosis (usually mild), hepatocyte necrosis, Mallory's bodies, and fibrosis (Pessayre et al, 1979; Poucell et al, 1984). Abnormal lysosomes reflecting phospholipid accumulation, well demonstrated by electron microscopy, are invariably associated with the alcoholic-like hepatitis lesions (Pessayre et al, 1979; Poucell et al, 1984); abnormal lysosomes may be present in the absence of alcoholic-like hepatitis.

The main clinical manifestation is liver enlargement. Serum aminotransferases are normal or mildly increased. In amiodarone-induced liver injury, hepatic density is increased at computed tomography (Goldman et al, 1985). Despite cessation of administration of the drug, chronic hepatitis induced by perhexiline maleate or amiodarone can transform into cirrhosis and cause the patient's death (Pessayre et al, 1979).

The mechanim of injury determined by perhexiline and amiodarone is not well established. However, it has been shown that these drugs are metabolized by hepatic oxidation. Impaired oxidative capacity assessed by using debrisoquine as a test substance has been shown to be severely impaired in patients with perhexiline-induced liver injury (Morgan et al, 1984).

Chronic cholestasis. Drug-induced chronic cholestasis seems to be uncommon. In most of the cases, cholestasis remains anicteric, only reflected by asthenia and increased serum alkaline phosphatase, and improves progressively with complete recovery within a year after the withdrawal of the drug. In a small number of cases, cholestasis is severe, with marked jaundice, and/or lasts for more than 1 year: the presentation then resembles that of primary biliary cirrhosis. In my experience, drug-induced chronic cholestasis affects only patients having suffered from acute icteric drug-induced hepatitis; in other words, chronic cholestasis is always preceded by an acute episode of icteric cholestasis.

In most of the cases, the lesion of drug-induced chronic cholestasis consists of changes in the interlobular bile ducts, associated with mild inflammatory infiltration. In some cases, the affected bile ducts vanish with, as a consequence, paucity of the intrahepatic bile ducts.

In France, the commonest drugs inducing chronic cholestasis are chlorpromazine and other phenothiazines, ajmaline (Larrey et al, 1986), cyproheptadine (Larrey et al, 1987), troleandomycin (Larrey et al, 1987) and tricyclic antidepressants.

REFERENCES

Baud F, Bernuau J, Benmami N, Pariente EA, Bouygues M, Guillan J, Roche-Sicot J, Degott C, Rueff B, Pessayre D, Benhamou JP: Hépatite aiguë due au phosphate d'isaxonine (Nerfactor). Gastroenterol Clin Biol 1983; 7:352-354

Beaune P, Dansette PM, Mansuy D, Kiffel L, Finck M, Amar C, Leroux JP, Homberg JC: Human anti-endoplasmic reticulum autoantibodies appearing in a drug-induced hepatitis are directed against a human liver cytochrome P450 that hydroxylates the drug. Proc Natl Acad Sci 1987; 84:551-555

Bercoff E, Bernuau J, Degott C, Kalis B, Lemaire A, Tilly H, Rueff B, Benhamou JP: Ketoconazole-induced fulminant hepatitis. Gut 1985; 26:636-638

Bernuau J, Rueff B, Benhamou JP: Fulminant and subfulminant liver failure: definitions and causes. Semin Liv Dis 1986; 6:97-102

Bismuth H, Samuel D, Gugenheim J, Castaing D, Bernuau J, Rueff B, Benhamou JP. Emergency liver transplantation for fulminant hepatitis. Ann Intern Med 1987; 107:337-341

Danan G, Benichou C, Begaud B, Biour M, Couzigou P, Evreux JC, Lagier G, Berthelot P, Benhamou JP: Critères d'imputation d'une hépatite aiguë à un médicament. Résultats de réunions de consensus. Gastroenterol Clin Biol 1987; 11:581-585

Danan G, Prunet P, Bernuau J, Degott C, Babany G, Pessayre D, Rueff B, Benhamou JP: Pirprophen-induced fulminant hepatitis. Gastroenterology 1985, 89:210-215

Funck-Brentano C, Pessayre D, Benhamou JP: Hepatites dues à divers dérivés de l'érythromycine. Gastroenterol Clin Biol 1983; 7:362-369

Goldfarb G, Pessayre D, Boisseau C, Degott C, Béraud C, Benhamou JP: Hépatite à la clométacine. Gastroenterol Clin Biol 1979; 3:537-540

Goldman IS, Winkler ML, Raper SE, Barker ME, Keung E, Goldberg HI, Boyer TD: Increased hepatic density and phospholipidosis due to amiodarone. Am J Roentgenol 1985; 144:541-546

Larrey D, Amouyal G, Danan G, Degott C, Pessayre D, Benhamou JP: Prolonged cholestasis after troleandomycin-induced acute hepatitis. J Hepatol 1987; 4:327-329

Larrey D, Castot A, Pessayre D, Merigot P, Machayekhy JP, Feldmann G, Lenoir A, Rueff B, Benhamou JP: Amodiaquine-induced hepatitis. A report of seven cases. Ann Intern Med 1986; 104:810-813

Larrey D, Genève J, Pessayre D, Machayekhy JP, Degott C, Benhamou JP: Prolonged cholestasis after cyproheptadine-induced acute hepatitis. J Clin Gastroenterol 1987; 9:102-104

Larrey D, Hadengue A, Pessayre D, Choudat L, Degott C, Benhamou JP: Carbamazepine-induced acute cholangitis. Dig Dis Sci 1987; 32:554-557

Larrey D, Pessayre D, Benhamou JP: Polymorphisme génétique du métabolisme hépatique des médicaments. Gastroenterol Clin Biol 1985; 9:522-531

Larrey D, Pessayre D, Duhamel G, Casier A, Degott C, Feldmann G, Erlinger S, Benhamou JP: Prolonged cholestasis after ajmaline-induced acute hepatitis. J Hepatol 1986; 2:81-84

Larrey D, Rueff B, Pessayre D, Danan G, Algard M, Genève J, Benhamou JP: Cross hepatotoxicity between tricyclic antidepressants. Gut 1986; 27:726-727

Neuberger J, Williams R: Halothane anaesthesia and the liver. Br Med J 1984; 289:1136-1139

Morgan MY, Reshef R, Shah RR, Oates NS, Smith RL, Sherlock S: Impaired oxidation of debrisoquine in patients with perhexiline liver injury. Gut 1984; 25:1057-1064

Pariente EA, Pessayre D, Bentata-Pessayre M, Capron JP, Marti R, Delcenserie R, Callard P, Benhamou JP: Hépatite à l'ajmaline. Description de 4 observations et revue de la littérature. Gastroenterol Clin Biol 1980; 4:240-246

Pariente EA, Pessayre D, Bernuau J, Degott C, Benhamou JP: Dihydralazine hepatitis: report of a case and review of the literature. Digestion 1983; 27:47-52

Pessayre D, Bentata M, Degott C, Nouel O, Miguet JP, Rueff B, Benhamou JP: Isoniazid-rifampin fulminant hepatitis. A possible consequence of the enhancement of isoniazid hepatotoxicity by enzyme induction. Gastroenterology 1977; 72:284-289

Pessayre D, Bichara M, Feldmann G, Degott C, Potet F, Benhamou JP: Perhexiline maleate-induced hepatotoxicity. Gastroenterology 1979; 76:170-177

Pessayre D, Degos F, Feldmann G, Degott C, Bernuau J, Benhamou JP: Chronic active hepatitis and giant multinucleated hepatocytes in adults treated with clometacin. Digestion 1981; 22:66-70

Pessayre D, de Saint Louvent P, Degott C, Bernuau J, Rueff B, Benhamou JP: Iproclozide fulminant hepatitis. Possible role of enzyme induction. Gastroenterology 1978; 75:492-496

Pessayre D, Feldmann G, Degott C, Ulmann A, Erlinger S, Benhamou JP: Gold-salt induced cholestasis. Digestion 1979; 19:56-60

Pessayre D, Larrey D, Funck-Brentano C, Benhamou JP: Drug interactions and hepatitis produced by some macrolide antibiotics. J Antimicrobiol Chemot 1985; 16:181-189

Poucell S, Ireton J, Valencia-Mayoral P, Downar E, Larratt L, Patterson J, Blendis L, Philips MJ: Amiodarone-associated phospholipidosis and fibrosis of the liver. Light, immunohistochemical, and electron microscopic studies. Gastroenterology 1984; 86:926-936

Seef LB, Brenda A, Cucceherini A, Zimmerman HJ, Adler E, Benjamin B: Acetaminophen hepatotoxicity in alcoholics. A therapeutic misadvanture. Ann Intern Med 1986; 104:399-404

Spielberg SP, Gordon GB, Blake DA, Godstein DA, Herlong HF: Predisposition to phenytoin hepatotoxicity assessed in vitro. N Engl J Med 1981; 305:722-727

Stricker BHCH, Spoelstra P: Drug-induced hepatic injury. Elsevier, Amsterdam, 1985, p.314

Zafrani ES, Ishak KG, Rudzki C: Cholestatic and hepatocellular injury associated with erythromycin esther. Report of nine cases. Am J Dig Dis 1979; 24:385-396

Zimmerman HJ: Clinical and laboratory manifestations of hepatotoxicity. Ann NY Acad Sci 1963; 104:954-969

Zimmerman HJ: Hepatotoxicity. The adverse effect of drugs and other chemicals on the liver. New York. Appleton-Century Crofts, 1978, p.597

Zimmerman HJ, Ishak KG: Valproate-induced hepatic injury. Analysis of 23 fatal cases. Hepatology 1982; 2:591-599

Zimmerman HJ, Lewis JH, Ishak KG, Maddrey WC: Ticrynafen-associated hepatic injury: Analysis of 340 cases. Hepatology 1984; 4:315-323

Résumé

Les médicaments peuvent induire des lésions très diverses, la plus fréquente étant l'hépatite qui peut exister sous trois formes : cytolytique, cholestasique et mixte. L'hépatite aiguë est habituellement bénigne, à l'exception de la forme cytolytique qui expose le patient au risque d'une insuffisance hépatique fulminante. L'hépatite chronique induite par les médicaments est rare et inclut trois types : l'hépatite chronique active, l'hépatite de type alcoolique, et l'hépatite chronique cholestasique.

The liver, ageing and drugs

O.F.W. James, M.D. Rawlins*, H. Wynne, K.W. Woodhouse

Departments of Medicine (Geriatrics) and Clinical Pharmacology*, University of Newcastle Upon Tyne, UK

SUMMARY

The increased variance of pharmacokinetics and pharmacodynamics in old age must partly arise from a lifetime of exposure to genetic and environmental factors. Broadly, however, drugs metabolised via microsomal oxidation show decreased metabolic clearance whereas conjugation appears relatively unaffected by age. We have found no change in specific activity or affinity of 3 "models" of microsomal oxidation in normal human liver over age range 20-74 years. We studied liver size using ultrasound and calculated blood flow (using ICG clearance) in 65 healthy individuals age 24-91 years. Liver volume and estimated liver blood flow and perfusion diminish both absolutely and in proportion to body weight. These changes may explain the alterations in metabolism which accompany ageing.

Because hepatic adverse drug reactions (ADRs) are more frequent in the elderly it has been assumed that they may be more susceptible to ADRs. Evidence is presented from a recent Swedish study of ADRs that when hepatic ADRs were related to the number of prescriptions there was no increased likelihood of ADRs occurring to most drugs in the aged population.

KEY WORDS: Liver volume and blood flow, Ageing, Hepatic Adverse Drug Reactions, Microsomal Oxidation.

Because of the greying of European, American and Japanese populations there has been increasing interest in the effects of age upon hepatic function in general and drug metabolism in particular. There has also been concern about the incidence of hepatic adverse drug reactions (ADR's) since while 12-18% of the population in Westernised countries is now over age 65 this group consumes 30-40% of national drug budgets. This paper will therefore discuss both the effect of age upon liver drug metabolism in man and the incidence and severity of hepatic ADR's with increasing age.

LIVER FUNCTION
There are no major alterations in conventional liver blood tests in relation to advancing age in man (1). Recently Schnegg and Lauterberg have shown decline in such microsomal 'marker' functions as aminopyrine demethylation and caffeine clearance and in non-microsomally mediated galactose elimination capacity (2). Furthermore many studies have shown that the systemic clearance of a variety of drugs, particularly those metabolised by the hepatic microsomal monoxygenase enzyme system, decreases with advancing years in man; in addition drugs with high hepatic clearance and extraction ratio's which undergo extensive first-pass metabolism following oral administration may show substantially increased bioavailability in elderly man (4). By contrast hepatic conjugation reactions - glucuronidation and sulphation for example - appear to be uninfluenced by age in man. Since the classical studies of Kato (5) which showed a decline in the specific activities of a variety of hepatic microsomal monoxygenases with age in rodents it has been assumed that the age related decline in microsomal oxidative metabolism of drugs in man is also due to a decline in specific activities of these enzymes, although it has also been recognised that alterations in body composition (increased body fat, decreased body water) might also play a part in altered clearance (6). Studies subsequent to those of Kato have also shown that some of the age related decline of microsomal function is sex-related - occurring in males rather than females and have confirmed that this is in relation to the content of microsomal protein and liver weight (7,8).

MICROSOMAL MONOXYGENASE FUNCTION IN AGEING MAN
Since virtually no evidence was available concerning the effect of ageing on microsomal monoxygenase enzyme function in man we have undertaken a series of studies to further clarify the reasons for the apparent decline in clearance of at least some drugs metabolised by Phase I reactions in man.

<u>In Vitro Activity</u>
We examined the specific activities of the probe substrates aldrin epoxidation and 7-ethoxycoumarin O-deethylation (high and low affinity forms) in liver tissue obtained either by Menghini needle biopsy during diagnostic work-up in subjects subsequently shown to have normal liver histology, or from histologically normal wedge biopsies obtained at laparotomy (usually for cholecystectomy) after informed consent. Liver from individuals aged 24-78 years was examined. No subject was taking drugs known to influence monooxygenase enzyme activity, alcohol consumption was trivial, smoking history was recorded. We have described the methodology in detail elsewhere (9,10).
There was no correlation between age and either aldrin epoxidase or 7-ethoxycoumarin O-deethylase activity whether smoking was taken into account or not. There was very marked inter individual variation which tended to increase with advancing age. Recovery of microsomal protein also bore no correlation to age.
It is of interest that Sutton et al and Maloney et al have now also shown no age related effect on hepatic microsomal enzyme specific activities in primates (11,12).

For drugs metabolised with first order kinetics not only is the specific activity of the enzyme in question important but also the affinity of the enzyme for substrate. Thus a fall in enzyme affinity (causing a rise in the Michaelis constant (K_m)) would also lead to a reduction in the rate of metabolism. We have therefore examined the enzyme kinetics of 7-ethoxycoumarin O-deethylation at a wide substrate range. The metabolism of this substrate is mediated by atleast two kinetic components (high and low affinity) in human liver microsomes. Using Eadie-Hofstee analysis the K_m values of both components were determined. There was no change in the affinity of either component for the substrate with advancing years.

As a result of this preliminary work we were faced with an apparent paradox - like rodents there is certainly a decline in clearance of some drugs metabolised by Phase I reactions in man, but unlike rodents there is no decline in specific activity or substrate affinity atleast in one 'marker' enzyme substrate system. We therefore hypothesised that this apparent reduction in drug metabolism might be due to a reduction in liver size and blood flow in advancing age.

MEASUREMENTS OF LIVER SIZE AND BLOOD FLOW
Data on liver size in relation to age in man is largely confined to major post mortem series, these are by their very nature 'selective'. There is general agreement however that liver volume does decrease with age, particularly after the middle years. Studies of liver blood flow in relation to age were initiated by Sherlock et al in 1950 (13) and have largely relied upon the measurement of clearance of the anionic dies bromsulphthalein and Indocyanine Green (ICG) (14). However no study has previously examined the effect of age upon both liver volume and liver blood flow in the same subjects. We therefore performed a systematic study to examine the extent of changes both in liver volume and liver blood flow in healthy subjects over a wide age range. By measuring the variables in the same subjects we were able to determine whether any change occurred with ageing in liver blood flow per unit volume of liver (liver perfusion).

Methods
We studied 65 healthy volunteers (33 females) aged 24-91. These were recruited from amongst colleagues and from local social clubs. No subject was suffering from hepatic, renal, respiratory or cardiac disorder as assessed by full clinical history and examination all had normal liver blood tests, blood count and urea creatinine and electrolytes. None were taking medications. Indocyanine Green clearance was calculated following injection of 0.5mg/kl ICG intravenously. ICG concentrations were determined using an absorption spectrophotometer by the method of Ceasar. Plasma clearance of ICG was calculated from dose/area under curve (AUC). Liver blood flow was estimated by dividing the clearance of ICG by one minor haematocrit for each patient. An extraction ratio of one was assumed for all subjects.

Liver volume was determined from serial, parallel, longitudinal beta-scan ultrasound images obtained at 1cm intervals across the liver using a method modified from that of Carr. The volume of liver was calculated from the sum of the area of each of the longitudinal liver images to which was added a computed volume

(v) for the liver lateral to the first longitudinal image. Assuming this to be parabaloid in shape. All scans were performed on fasted subjects in the early afternoon.

Results
Liver volume fell from 21.4±0.8 mls/kg body wt. age < 40 to 19.3±0.7 mls/kg body wt. age 40-65 and 15.5±0.4 mls/kg body wt. age 65+ ($P<0.001$). Using linear regression estimated liver volume was 1470mls age 24, 945mls age 91. Estimated liver blood flow fell from 17.6 mls/min/kg body wt. age < 40 to 15.4 mls/min/kg body wt. age 40-64, 11.4 mls/min/kg body wt. age 65+ ($P<0.001$). Using linear regression estimated liver blood flow was 1260mls/min age 24; 655mls/min age 91. Estimated liver perfusion fell from 0.84mls/min/ml liver age < 40 to 0.81mls/min/ml liver age 40-64; 0.74mls/min/ml liver age 65+ ($P<0.005$). Using linear regression estimated perfusion per ml liver was 0.87 mls/min blood flow age 24, 0.70 mls/min liver blood flow age 91.

Discussion
Because of their nature measurements of liver blood flow and liver volume in fit volunteers must always be carried out indirectly. We have carried out a pilot study of comparison of liver volume using our ultrasound technique compared with that calculated using CT scan in approximately half the subjects studied. The correlation between the estimated liver volume by CT scan and that found using the ultrasound technique was extremely high with a correlation co-efficient of 0.97. Clearly the estimation of liver blood flow by ICG clearance depends on no age related fall in hepatic extraction or transport of ICG. Studies of age related changes in the kinetics of ICG in rats show stability from adulthood to senescence (15).
These significant negative correlations between liver blood per unit volume of liver and age suggest a relative fall in liver perfusion in old age. This finding may contribute in large part to the increased oral bioavailability and decreased systemic clearance demonstrated for such drugs as triazolam, lignocaine and labetolol (3). It may also contribute to the fall in clearance and increased plasma half life such drugs as antipyrine - a drug which is eliminated totally by hepatic oxidation. Indeed the estimated fall of 18.5% in antipyrine clearance in elderly males (mean age 68.7) compared to young males (mean age 32.9) obtained by Vestal et al (16) closely matches our estimation of a 17% fall in liver perfusion between the ages of 24 and 91. In summary this study has shown that not only is there a significant fall in liver volume with age but there is a relative under perfusion of liver tissue in the elderly which may well be the major factor in defects in both microsomal oxidation with increasing age and also first-pass clearance.

DRUG INDUCED LIVER DISEASE
There is an almost universal impression that ADR's in general are much more common in elderly subjects and that hepatic ADR's are no exception to this rule. Furthermore there is also an impression that if hepatic ADR's occur they are more severe in elderly individuals.

Frequency of Hepatic ADR's

In order to critically examine the question of the frequency of hepatic ADR's one of us (KW) in collaboration with Mortimer and Wiholm has recently examined all hepatic ADR's reported to the Swedish Adverse Drug Reactions Advisory Committee in the five years 1980 through 1984 (17). Reporting of ADR's is arguably more thorough in Sweden than in any other major country, in addition prescribing information is monitored by the national corporation of Swedish Pharmacies and from this data the percentage prescriptions for any individual drug given to patients over age 65 may be calculated. The total reported hepatic ADR's was 807 of which 234 (29%) were in individuals over age 65. In Sweden 17% of the population is over 65, superficially therefore there was a marked excess in the proportion of hepatic ADR's occurring in over 65 year olds compared to that expected purely on the basis of the proportion of persons in this age group. From the monitoring of prescribing data however it is possible to show that about 30% prescriptions are given to individuals over age 65. By obtaining prescribing data for the individual drugs most commonly implicated in hepatic ADR's Woodhouse et al were able to derive a ratio: percent reports over 65 years/percent prescriptions over 65 years, in this way a true reflection as to whether elderly individuals were really more susceptible to the development of hepatic ADR's in individual drugs could be obtained. A high ratio indicating increased susceptibility in the elderly, a ratio of 1 being that which would be expected in the population as a whole, a ratio substantially below 1 indicating reduced susceptibility to the particular ADR in the elderly. It will be seen from Table 1 that for the 11 most freqently reported hepatic ADR's there was no marked increase in susceptibility (no ratio > 1.5) for any drug although there was a suggestion that a higher proportion of elderly individuals receiving nitrofurantoin over 65 might be susceptible to an hepatic ADR (ratio 1.43).

TABLE 1

HEPATIC ADR AND THE EFFECT OF AGE, CORRECTED FOR AGE-RELATED PRESCRIBING VARIABLES

Drug	% Reports >65 years	% Prescription >65 years	Ratio: % Reports >65 years / %Prescription >65 years
Zimelidine	24%	24%	1.00
Co-trimoxazole	40%	34%	1.18
Cimetidine	32%	27%	1.18
Sulindac	50%	37%	1.32
Carbamazipine	18%	17%	1.05
Nitrofurantoin	43%	30%	1.43
Chlorpromazine	20%	32%	0.63
Hydrallazine	37%	55%	0.67
Phenytoin	12%	23%	0.52
Naproxen	37%	37%	1.00
Piroxicam	20%	44%	0.45
OVERALL	30%	32%	0.94

It will be seen that the mean ratio percent reports over 65/percent prescriptions over 65 is only 0.94 indicating no

increased susceptibility to the development of hepatic ADR's in this Swedish population. It is suggested that the impression that the elderly are more susceptible to hepatic ADR's has been given because of the substantially greater number of drugs which they receive.
Woodhouse et al also examined the possibility that ADR's were less commonly reported in the elderly thus biasing the sample, from the pattern of ADR's recorded and from other data available in Sweden they concluded that this was most unlikely. In the United Kingdom Weber and Griffin (18) also calculated that for ADR's in general there was no increased incidence in the elderly when frequency of drug prescriptions was taken into accocunt. However Pickles (19) argued that in some instances - not specifically related to the liver - only more severe ADR's were reported in elderly individuals thus introducing a bias into the figures.

Severity of Hepatic ADR's
In relation to the possibility that if hepatic ADR's do occur in elderly individuals they are liable to be more severe there is little data with which to form an opinion. There is some theoretical basis for suggesting that the aged liver might be more susceptible to a specific damaging influence since Platt (20) showed that, atleast in the rat, the aged liver developed far more serious hepatic necrosis after experimental injury with galactosamine than the young liver.
Despite the general lack of data and the findings of Woodhouse et al it seems possible that in one or two instances hepatic ADR's are more severe in aged man as might be predicted from the data of Platt. In the case of halothane Neuberger and Williams reviewed the age distribution of patients admitted to the King's College Hospital, Liver Failure Unit with halothane associated fulminant hepatic failure and compared this to data on the distribution of patients undergoing anaesthesia in general and individuals with viral fulminant hepatic failure. Among 48 patients with halothane associated fulminant hepatic failure the median age was 57 years with a considerable shift towards an older age group among individuals with halothane associated FHF compared to the generality of individuals undergoing anaesthetic (the majority receiving halothane). In a national study of halothane associated hepatic damage Inman and Mushin (22) also found a skew of mortality from FHF towards the older end of the age spectrum. In this as in most hepatic ADR's there appears to be a preponderance of women. The reason for this is unknown but it is of interest that sex related differences in hepatic drug metabolising enzymes are now becoming increasingly recognised (23).
In the case of the NSAID benoxaprofen unpublished data from the UK, DHSS suggests that while the mean age of individuals receiving the drug was about 59 years the mean age of those sustaining ADR's was about 66 and in individuals with severe or fatal ADR's (almost always hepatic) the mean age was 75. Of the 9 patients described by Taggart and Alderdice (24) and Goudie et al (25) with fatal hepatic failure associated with benoxaprofen, six were over age 80, the remainder over age 70. At present one should probably conclude therefore on the still insubstantial evidence that the liver does not grow more likely to develop drug related disease as age progresses, possibly however, if damage does develop it is more likely to be severe in some instances and this is perhaps not surprising.

REFERENCES
1. Popper H. (1986): Ageing and the Liver. In Progress in Liver Diseases. Vol VIII eds. Popper H., Schaffner F. Grune and Stratton, New York, 659-684

2. Schnegg M. and Lauterberg B.H. (1986): Quantitative Liver Function in the Elderly assessed by Galactose Elimination Capacity, Aminopyrine Demethylation and Caffeine Clearance. J. Hepatol., 164-171

3. Greenblatt D.J., Sellers E.M., Shader R.I. (1982): Drug Disposition in Old Age. N. Engl. J. Med., 1081-1088

4. Stevenson I.H. (1983): Drugs for the Elderly. In "Proceedings of the Second World Conference on Clinical Pharmacology & Therapeutics" edited by L. Lemberger & M.M. Reidenberg. American Society for Pharmacology & Experimental Therapeutics: Bethesda, 64-73

5. Kato R. (1978): Hepatic Microsomal Drug Metabolising Enzymes in Rats - History and Future Problems. In: "Liver & Ageing" edited by K. Kitani, Elsvier, Amsterdam, 257-300

6. Koch-Weser K., Greenblatt D.J., Sellers E.M. and Shader R.I. (1982):Drug Disposition in Old Age. N. Engl. J. Med. 306; 222-227

7. Van Bezooijen C.F.A., Sakkee A.N., Boonstra-Nieveld I.H.J., Begue J.M., Guillouzo A. and Knook D.L. (1982): The Effect of Age on Digitoxin Biotransformation by Isolated Hepatocytes. In "Liver & Ageing" edited by K. Kitani, Elsvier, Amsterdam, 167-176

8. Wynne H., Mutch E., James O.F.W., Rawlins M.D. and Woodhouse K.W. (1986): Monoxygenase Enzyme Kinetics in Rat Liver Microsomes: The Effect of Age. In "Modern Trends in Ageing Research" Colloque Inserm-Emage, 147; 153-157

9. Williams F.M., Woodhouse K.W., Middleton D, Wright P., James O.F.W. and Rawlins M.D. (1982): Aldrin Epoxidation in Small Samples of Human Liver. Biochem. Pharmacol., 31; 3701-3703

10. Woodhouse K.W., Williams F.M., Mutch E., Wright P., James O.F.W. and Rawlins M.D. (1984): The Effect of Alcoholic Cirrhosis on the Two Kinetic Components (high and low affinity) of the Microsomal O-Deethylation of 7-Ethoxycoumarin in Human Liver. Eur. J. Clin. Pharmacol., 26; 61-64

11. Sutton M.A., Wood G., Williamson L.S., Strong R., Pickham K. and Richardson A. (1985): Comparison of the Hepatic Mixed Function Oxidase System of Young Adult and Old Non-Human Primates (Macaque Nomestrina). Biochem. Pharmacol., 34; 2983-2987

12. Maloney A.G., Smucker D.L., Vessey D.S., and Wang R.K. (1986): The Effects of Ageing on the Hepatic Microsomal Mixed-Function Oxidation System of Male and Female Monkeys. Hepatology, 6; 282-287

13. Sherlock S., Bearn A.G., Billing B.H. and Patterson J.C.S. (1950): Splanchnic Blood Flow in Man by the Bromsulphthalein Method. J. Lab. Clin. Med., 35; 823-232

14. Mooney H., Roberts R. Cooksley W.G.E., Halliday J.W. and Powell L.W. (1985): Alterations in the Liver with Ageing. Clinics in Gastroenterology, 14; 757-772

15. Kitani K. (1977): Functional Aspects of the Ageing Liver in Liver and Ageing. ed. Platt D, Schattaner Verlag, Stuttgart, 5-17

16. Vestal R.E., Norris A.H., Tobin J.D., Cohen D.H., Shock N.W. and Andres R. (1977): Antipyrine Metabolism in Man: Influence of Age, Alcohol, Caffeine and Smoking. Clin. Pharmacol. and Ther., 18; 425-432

17. Woodhouse K.W., Mortimer O., Wiholm B.E. (1986): Hepatic Adverse Drug Reactions: The Effect of Age in Liver and Ageing, ed. K. Kitani, Elsvier, Amsterdam, 75-80

18. Weber J.C.P., Griffin J.P. (1986): Prescriptions, Adverse Reactions and the Elderly. Lancet, i; 1220

19. Pickles H. (1986): Prescriptions, Adverse Reactions and the Elderly. Lancet, ii; 40-41

20. Platt D. (1977): Age Dependent Morphological and Biochemical Studies of the Normal and Injured Rat Liver. In Liver and Ageing, ed. Platt D., Schattauer Verlag, Stuttgart, 75-83

21. Neuberger J. and Williams R. (1984): Halothane Anaesthesia and Liver Damage. Brit. Med. J. 289; 1136-1139

22. Inman W.H.W. and Mushin W.W. (1978): Jaundice after repeated exposure to halothane. Brit. Med. J. ii; 1455-1456

23. Schmucker D.L., Vessey D.A., Wang R.K. and Maloney A.G. (1986):Ageing, Sex and the Liver Microsomal Drug Metabolising System in Rodents and Primates. In Liver and Ageing, ed. Kitani K., Elsevier, Amsterdam, 3-13

24. Taggart H.Mc.A. and Alderdice J.M. (1982): Fatal Cholestatic Jaundice in Elderly Persons taking Benoxaprofen. Brit. Med. J. 284; 1372

25. Goudie B.M., Birnie G.F., Watkinson G. et al (1982): Jaundice Associated with the use of Benoxaprofen. Lancet i; 959-961

Résumé

Les variations pharmacocinétiques et pharmacodynamiques accrues chez le sujet âgé peuvent provenir au moins en partie de l'exposition, la vie durant, à des facteurs génétiques et environnementaux. Toutefois, d'une façon générale, les médicaments métabolisés par la voie oxydative microsomale montrent une clearance métabolique diminuée tandis que leur conjugaison est peu affectée par l'âge. Nous n'avons observé aucune modification de l'activité spécifique ou de l'affinité de 3 "modèles" d'oxydation microsomale dans le foie humain normal entre 20 et 74 ans. Nous avons apprécié la taille du foie par ultrasons et calculé le flux sanguin (par la clairance du vert d'indocyanine) chez 65 individus sains âgés de 24 à 91 ans. Le volume du foie tout comme le flux sanguin hépatique estimé et perfusé diminuent en valeur absolue et par rapport au poids du corps. Ces changements peuvent expliquer les altérations métaboliques qui accompagnent le vieillissement.

Les lésions hépatiques liées aux médicaments étant plus fréquentes chez le sujet âgé, on peut estimer que celui-ci est plus susceptible à de telles lésions. Une étude suédoise récente montre qu'il n'y a pas augmentation apparente des lésions hépatiques induites par la plupart des médicaments chez le sujet âgé si ces lésions sont rapportées au nombre de prescriptions.

Liver Cells and Drugs. Ed. A. Guillouzo. Colloque INSERM/John Libbey Eurotext Ltd. © 1988. Vol. 164, pp. 23-28.

Diagnosis of drug-induced liver injury (results of consensus meetings)

Gaby Danan

Direction de la Pharmacovigilance, Roussel Uclaf, 35, Boulevard des Invalides, 75007 Paris, France

SUMMARY

The diagnosis of drug-induced liver injury is based on answers to three questions : (a) is the liver involved ? (b) do the chronological and clinical criteria suggest the causal role of the suspected drug(s) ? (c) can other possible causes be excluded ? In order to standardize answers to these three steps, consensus meetings have been organized where hepatologists from University Hospitals, members of the French National Network of Pharmacovigilance and representatives of Roussel Uclaf Drug Monitoring Department were convened. This paper reports an example of results of these meetings concerning (a) the adaptation of chronological and clinical criteria of the current French official drug reaction assessment method and (b) investigations to be performed to eliminate other possible causes, in case of acute cytolytic hepatitis.

KEYWORDS

ADVERSE DRUG REACTIONS - DRUG REACTION ASSESSMENT METHOD - CONSENSUS MEETINGS - DRUG-INDUCED LIVER INJURY - DRUG HEPATOTOXICITY - DRUG MONITORING.

INTRODUCTION

In most cases diagnosis of drug-induced liver injury results from exclusion of other non drug causes. In addition, the recent and large development of drug surveillance and the rapid circulation of drug information require a standardization of recognition and assessment of adverse drug reactions (ADRs).

CAUSALITY ASSESSMENT BY PRACTITIONERS AND EXPERTS

In practice, the diagnosis of drug-induced liver injury is based on three questions : (a) is the liver involved ? (b) do chronological and clinical criteria suggest a drug-induced reaction ? (c) can other causes be excluded ? Answers to these questions are not always similar for the three involved parties : practitioners, regulatory authorities and pharmaceutical industry.

Indeed, for the practitioner, the main issue is to stop or to continue the suspected drug administration since he has in charge the immediate care for his patient. To take the decision, he can ask for all available information, investigate carefully other causes and follow-up the case until the problem is settled. His assessment of the causal relationship is intuitive, based on his experience and also on the current knowledge of the suspected drug hepatotoxicity. In addition, in several countries, he has to report to regulatory authorities all ADRs he faced with.

For experts in drug surveillance, members either of a regulatory agency or of pharmaceutical company, the main objective is to evaluate benefit/risk ratio of the drug on the basis of case-report forms. In general, the information on each case is scarce, selected by the provider and delayed. The experts cannot therefore investigate nor follow-up the case, but they have to assess the causal role of the drug according to a method depending on the country and the firm. Although there is no "gold standard" method for drug assessment (PERE JC et al. 1986), adverse drug reactions are eventually classified according to the level of the causal relationship : unrelated, doubtful, possible, probable or highly probable. Recently, legal requirements forced drug manufacturers to notify ADRs to the regulatory agency not only of the country where the ADR occurred but also of other countries where the same drug is marketed. On their own, regulatory agencies have to transmit ADRs to W.H.O. Operating Center in Uppsala.

Briefly, for the practitioner and for the regulatory agerncy or industry experts, the final assessment is often not reproducible. Therefore, co-operation between the three parties involved is needed. Our goal was to realize this cooperation during consensus meetings.

CONSENSUS MEETINGS

Consensus meetings have been organized by Roussel Uclaf ; the 3 parties involved in drug-induced liver injury were convened : hepatologists from University hospitals ; members of the French network of pharmacovigilance and members of an international drug surveillance department of a pharmaceutical company (Roussel Uclaf). Objectives were to propose guidelines to answer the 3 basic questions including for each ADR : its definition and criteria to assess the causal relationship. The purpose of this communication is to report an example of conclusions of these consensus meetings dealing only with chronological and clinical criteria in order to assess the causal relationship between a drug administration and an acute cytolytic hepatitis.

Method of drug reaction assessment

The French method of drug reaction assessment was taken as a frame. This method, described elsewhere (BEGAUD B et al. 1985), consists of 2 groups of criteria : chronological and clinical (or semiological). Each group is presented in a decision table combining responses to the criteria.

The 3 chronological criteria are : time to onset of the reaction ; the course of the reaction ; the response to the drug readministration (when it is done). The combination of responses to these 3 criteria leads to a chronological score described as : suggestive, possible, dubious or incompatible.

The 3 clinical criteria are : signs and symptoms of the reaction, the result of a specific test which strongly suggests the causal role of the drug ; assessment of other possible non-drug causes. The combination of responses to these 3 criteria leads to a clinical score described as : suggestive, possible or dubious.

Finally, a decision table combines the 2 scores leading to a final assessment of the causal relationship with 5 degrees : unlikely, dubious, possible, likely, very likely.

Assessment of the criteria

Chronological criteria

a) Time to onset of reaction

This criterion is described as : very suggestive (of the causal role of the drug) compatible or incompatible (with the dates of drug administration). The table shows time intervals corresponding to each situation. In addition, intervals are given from the beginning and from the cessation of the drug administration and according to the first or the "nth" treatment with the suspected drug.

Table : Acute cytolytic hepatitis. Time to onset of the reaction.

TIME TO ONSET OF THE REACTION	SUGGESTIVE *	COMPATIBLE		INCOMPATIBLE	
	From beginning of drug administration	From beginning of drug administration	from cessation of drug administration	From beginning of drug administration	from cessation of drug administration
FIRST TREATMENT	8 to 90 days	< 8 days or > 90 days	≤ 15 days	Drug taken after the onset of the reaction	> 15 days **
"Nth" TREATMENT	Immediately to 15 days	> 15 days	≤ 15 days	Drug taken after the onset of the reaction	> 15 days **

* In place of "very suggestive" as proposed by the French method

** except for slowly metabolized drugs (e.g. amiodarone)

b) Course of the reaction

This criterion is described as : suggestive (of the causal role of the drug), non suggestive or non conclusive. Cases after cessation or not of the drug administration are distinguished.
- When the drug is discontinued (dechallenge), the course of the reaction is :

  . very suggestive : when the difference between the peak of aminotransferases and the upper normal value decreases of 50 % or more, within 8 days ;
  . suggestive : when that decrease is ≥ 50 % within 1 month ;

. **non suggestive** : when the decrease is < 50 % within 1 month or when there is persistence or increase of aminotransferases after 1 month ;
. **non conclusive** : when information on liver tests after dechallenge is not available.

- When the drug is not discontinued, the course of the reaction is:
. **suggestive** : when there is a persistence or additional increase of aminotransferases ;
. **non conclusive** : when there is a decrease of aminotransferases.

c) Readministration of the drug (rechallenge)

The readministration of a suspected drug is hazardous, in particular in case of cytolytic hepatitis, and therefore unethical. However, when the readministration is unintentional, responses can be interpretable only if aminotransferases decreased below 5 N (N = upper limit of normal) before the readministration.
The response is **positive** when there is a doubling or more of aminotransferases after the drug has been administered at any dose for any duration, alone or combined with any of the other non-stopped drugs.
The response is **negative** when there is no increase of aminotransferases or an increase below 1 N. The drug should be administered at the same dose, for the same duration, and combined with the same concomitant drugs as during the first course.
The response is **not interpretable** in any other case different from those described above.

Clinical criteria

a) Signs and symptoms suggesting the causal role of the suspected drug.

This criterion cannot be applied to liver injury since there is no specific drug-induced sign. However, concomitant administration of a strong enzyme inducer can be regarded as a "risk factor" and concomitant disorder such as : fever, rash, renal failure or eosinophilia suggest a drug origin.

b) Specific test.

There is no test sufficiently specific to prove the causal role of a drug. However, serum autoantibodies have been shown specific for two drugs : antimitochondrial type M6 (AMA, M6) for iproniazid and anti-liver and kidney microsomes type 2 (LKM_2) for ticrynafen.

c) Assessment of other possible causes.

The following information and investigations are required to assess other possible causes : serological markers for recent viral infection : IgM anti-HAV, IgM anti-HBc ; increase in specific antibodies titres for CMV, EBV and Herpes viruses ; circumstantial arguments for a contamination by a non-A, non-B virus (blood transfusions, intravenous drug addict, recent travel in endemic areas : Africa, Asia) ; hepatobiliary ultrasonography ; alcohol consumption ; heart or vascular disease (ischemic liver necrosis) ; pregnancy ; underlying and previous disease(s).

Current status of Consensus Meetings

The Hepatology Group of these meetings reviewed definitions and assessment criteria for the following liver injuries :

acute cytolytic hepatitis, acute cholestatic hepatitis, acute mixed hepatitis (DANAN G. et al. 1987) have been published ; chronic hepatitis without histological examination of the liver, chronic hepatitis and cirrhosis histologically proven (unpublished) ;
Other liver injuries have not been considered since they require liver biopsy to be diagnosed and should be therefore discussed separately.

CONCLUSION

According to the conclusions of Consensus Meetings, the diagnosis of drug-induced liver injury can be standardized. The French method of drug reaction assessment based on defined criteria is therefore reproducible. In the future, the specificity of that method could be improved by weighting each criterion. Results of these meetings should be considered as the first step of an international agreement for assessing cases of drug-induced liver injury.

REFERENCES

BEGAUD B, EVREUX J.C, JOUGLARD J, LAGIER G. (1985) : Unexpected or toxic drug reaction assessment (imputation). Actualization of the method used in France (English translation). Therapie, 40, 111-8.

DANAN G, BENICHOU C, BEGAUD B, BIOUR M, COUZIGOU P, EVREUX JC, LAGIER G, BERTHELOT P, BENHAMOU JP. (1987) : Critères d'imputation d'une hépatite aiguë à un médicament. Résultats de réunions de Consensus. Gastroenterol. Clin. Biol., 11. 581-585.

PERE J.C, BEGAUD B, HARAMBURU F, ALBIN H. (1986) : Computerized comparison of six adverse drug assessment procedures. Clin. Pharmacol. Ther., 40, 451-461.

Résumé

Le diagnostic d'atteinte hépatique médicamenteuse repose schématiquement sur les réponses aux trois questions suivantes : (a) le foie est-il atteint ? (b) la séquence chronologique des évènements et la sémiologie suggèrent-elles une origine médicamenteuse ? (c) les autres causes possibles peuvent-elles être exclues ? Les réponses des praticiens et des spécialistes en pharmacovigilance sont souvent différentes et difficilement reproductibles : le praticien, à la moindre suspicion, doit immédiatement interrompre l'administration du (des) médicament(s) ; son évaluation de la relation causale est très subjective, fondée sur son expérience de ce type d'effet indésirable ; pour les spécialistes en pharmacovigilance de l'Administration ou de l'Industrie Pharmaceutique, les renseignements fournis sur l'effet indésirable sont souvent incomplets et retardés ; surtout la méthode d'imputation utilisée pour évaluer la relation causale ne peut être validée en l'absence de méthode de référence. Enfin, selon les pays, la loi oblige les prescripteurs et le laboratoire fabricant à signaler tous les effets indésirables qu'ils ont constatés ou qui leur ont été rapportés.

Afin de standardiser les réponses aux trois questions, des réunions de consensus ont été organisées. Elles ont rassemblé des hépatologues hospitalo-universitaires, des représentants du système national français de pharmacovigilance, et des représentants de la Direction de la Pharmacovigilance du groupe Roussel Uclaf. En prenant pour exemple le cas d'une hépatite aiguë cytolytique, cet article rapporte les conclusions ne concernant que l'adaptation des critères chronologiques et sémiologiques de la méthode d'imputation utilisée en France ainsi que la liste des autres causes à rechercher systématiquement.

L'étude des critères chronologiques a permis de préciser (a) le délai de survenue de l'effet indésirable qui peut être **suggestif, compatible ou incompatible** ; les délais ont été fixés à partir du début et de la fin de l'administration du médicament suspecté et en fonction d'un premier ou d'un nième traitement par le même médicament ; (b) l'évolution de l'effet indésirable qui peut être **très suggestive, suggestive, non suggestive ou non concluante** ; les différentes éventualités ont été envisagées selon l'arrêt (dechallenge) ou la poursuite du médicament suspecté ; (c) l'interprétation de la réponse à la réadministration du médicament suspecté qui ne peut être qu'involontaire ; cette réponse **positive, négative ou ininterprétable** dépend des conditions de la réadministration qui ont donc été définies.

L'étude des critères sémiologiques a mis en évidence : (a) l'absence de **signes spécifiques** suggérant le rôle d'un médicament en particulier, mais l'administration concomitante d'un puissant inducteur enzymatique peut être considérée comme un facteur de risque et l'atteinte d'un autre organe suggestive d'une origine médicamenteuse en général ; (b) l'absence de tests spécifiques confirmant le rôle du médicament suspecté ; (c) les autres causes possibles d'hépatite aiguë cytolytique à rechercher.

En conclusion, les réunions de consensus ont permis de mettre au point un langage commun pour l'évaluation de la plupart des atteintes hépatiques médicamenteuses et de rendre reproductible la méthode d'imputation des effets indésirables des médicaments utilisée en France. Dans l'avenir, la pondération de chaque critère permettra d'en améliorer encore la spécificité.

Drug metabolism and its regulation

Le métabolisme des médicaments et sa régulation

Purification and characterization of human liver cytochrome P-450 enzymes

F. Peter Guengerich, Diane R. Umbenhauer, Cecile Ged, Toshiki Muto, Richard W. Bork, Nariko Shinriki, Ghazi A. Dannan, Philippe Beaune, Martha V. Martin, R. Stephen Lloyd

Department of Biochemistry and Center in Molecular Toxicology, Vanderbilt University School of Medicine, Nashville, Tennessee 37232, USA

ABSTRACT

The individual forms of human liver cytochrome P-450 play important roles in the oxidation of drugs and other chemicals. This report discusses the characterization of these enzymes and their genes in this and other laboratories. The liver microsomal P-450s which have been isolated include $P\text{-}450_{MP}$, $P\text{-}450_{NF}$, $P\text{-}450_{DB}$, $P\text{-}450_{PA}$, $P\text{-}450j$, and $P\text{-}450_{0}$. Other preparations described in the literature appear to be closely related to these six enzymes. Evidence for the existence of other cytochrome P-450 proteins has been provided by recombinant DNA and immunochemical methods. The results of recent efforts on the characterization of the $P\text{-}450_{NF}$ and $P\text{-}450_{MP}$ gene families are presented.

KEY WORDS

Cytochrome P-450, mephenytoin hydroxylation, nifedipine oxidation, debrisoquine hydroxylation, phenacetin O-deethylation

INTRODUCTION

Cytochrome P-450 enzymes are important in the oxidation and clearance of drugs and other xenobiotics in the liver, the most important site of processing in the body. The balance between detoxication and bioactivation of these xenobiotics is very important, and the situation is further complicated by the existence of a large number of forms of cytochrome P-450 proteins that have their own catalytic specificities, not only for individual substrates, but also for stereo- and regioselective oxidation of a single compound (Guengerich and Liebler, 1985). Understanding the nature of the cytochrome P-450 enzymes in human liver has been a desired goal for many years. Inter-individual variations in cytochromes P-450 have been suspected for many years--recently considerable evidence for both a genetic basis and for environmental influences has been obtained. It is now possible to apply many biochemical techniques that have been developed in studies with experimental animals to human liver. In this report we review some of the current understanding and present recent work from our own laboratory dealing primarily with genes coding for two of these enzymes, $P\text{-}450_{MP}$ and $P\text{-}450_{NF}$.

METHODS

The methods for isolation of the cytochrome P-450 enzymes have been described for the preparations obtained in this laboratory; combinations of n-octylamino Sepharose, DEAE- and CM-cellulose, and hydroxylapatite chromatography were used (Wang et al., 1980, 1983; Distlerath et al., 1985; Shimada et al., 1986; Guengerich et al., 1986a). Methods for analysis and characterization of these proteins are presented in the same papers. The cloning strategy involved screening a human liver cDNA library (10^7 inserts) with polyclonal and monoclonal antibodies. Selected clones (full-length if possible) were inserted into M13 phage for dideoxy-terminal sequencing (Beaune et al., 1986; Umbenhauer et al., 1987).

RESULTS AND DISCUSSION

The different cytochrome P-450 enzymes are grouped into very closely related families and discussed. Tentative gene classifications, given in Roman numerals in Table 1, use the nomenclature of Nebert et al. (1987).

$P-450_{MP}$

In retrospect this was probably the first P-450 isolated in our own laboratory (Wang et al., 1980), based upon subsequent studies and the chromatographic conditions and immunochemical cross-reactivity. Subsequent preparations designated $P-450_1$ and $P-450_8$ (Wang et al., 1983) were also related to $P-450_{MP}$. Shimada et al. (1986) isolated two proteins differing in molecular weight by 2 kD and designated these as $P-450_{MP-1}$ and $P-450_{MP-2}$. These proteins actively catalyze S-mephenytoin 4-hydroxylation, S-nirvanol 4-hydroxylation, and hexobarbital 3'-hydroxylation. Tolbutamide (methyl) hydroxylation is catalyzed also, although the in vivo relationship with mephenytoin 4-hydroxylation remains unclear (Knodell et al., 1987). Others who have isolated similar proteins now include P. Shaw and M.D. Burke (personal communication), R. Kato and Y. Yamazoe (personal communication), P.S. Guzelian and S.A. Wrighton (personal communication), and Gut et al. (1986b).

We cloned and sequenced a nearly full-length cDNA (MP-8) related to $P-450_{MP}$; the sequence of the clone matched the previously determined N-terminal protein sequence at all residues which could be determined unambiguously (Umbenhauer et al., 1987). The sequence is highly related to those of rabbit P-450 1 (Tukey et al., 1985) and rat P-450 M-1 ($P-450_{UT-A}$) (Yoshioka et al., 1987), two enzymes which have different catalytic activities. Genomic blotting analysis suggests that at least seven related gene sequences are in this subfamily (P450 IIC9, Nebert et al., 1987) (Umbenhauer et al., 1987). We demonstrated that $P-450_{MP-1}$ and $P-450_{MP-2}$ are coded by different mRNAs (Shimada et al., 1986). More recently we have cloned and sequenced two other cDNAs termed MP-4 and MP-12, isolated from the same cDNA library as MP-8 and originating from the mRNA of a single individual. MP-12 is about 75% similar to MP-8; in some regions the correspondence is very high. The MP-4 also shows some similarity but is clearly different. Tukey et al. (1986) have also sequenced a related human clone which differs from MP-8. Most notably R. Kato and Y. Yamazoe (personal communication) have sequenced a cDNA clone which differs from our MP-8 in the coding region by only two residues but has a quite distinct 3' non-coding region. The relationship of none of these cDNA clones to proteins has been clearly established.

The gene family lies on human chromosome 10. The enzyme does not appear to be readily inducible in cultured hepatocytes, although recently in vivo increases in S-mephenytoin clearance have been demonstrated after rifampicin treatment. The basis of the genetic polymorphism has not been identified although several suggestions have been made that structural gene mutations may be involved (Meier et al., 1985; Umbenhauer et al., 1987).

Table 1. Classification of human liver cytochrome P-450 enzymes

Enzyme (class)	Subfamily*	Related preparations from other laboratories	Major catalytic activities
$P-450_{MP-1}$, $P-450_{MP-2}$	IIC8,9	P-450meph--Gut et al., 1986b Wrighton and Guzelian Shaw and Burke Kato and Yamazoe	S-Mephenytoin 4-hydroxylation S-Nirvanol 4-hydroxylation Hexobarbital 3'-hydroxylation
$P-450_{NF}$	IIIA3	$P-450_{HLFa}$--Kitada et al., 1985 $P-450p$--Watkins et al., 1985	Oxidation of nifedipine and other dihydropyridines Testosterone 6β-hydroxylation Estradiol 2- and 4-hydroxylation Cortisol 6β-hydroxylation Erythromycin N-demethylation Dihydroepiandrostene sulfate 16α-hydroxylation Quinidine N- and 3-hydroxylation
$P-450_{DB}$	IID1	$P-450_{BufI}$, $_{II}$--Gut et al., 1986a $P-450_{NT}$--Birgersson et al., 1986	Debrisoquine 4-hydroxylation Bufuralol 1',-hydroxylation Sparteine Δ^2,Δ^3-oxidation Metoprolol hydroxylation Desmethylimipramine 10-hydroxylation Nortryptilline 10-hydroxylation Encainide O-demethylation Propranolol 4-hydroxylation
$P-450_{PA}$	IA2	4--Quattrochi et al., 1986 (?) $P-450_3$--Jaiswal et al., 1986 (?) $P-450d$--Wrighton et al., 1986a (?)	Phenacetin O-deethylation
P-450j	IIE1		N,N-dimethylnitrosamine N-demethylation
$P-450_9$			

* Nebert et al., 1987.

$P-450_{NF}$

In our early attempts to characterize human liver cytochrome P-450 enzymes, a series of proteins denoted $P-450_2$, $P-450_3$, $P-450_4$, $P-450_5$, $P-450_6$, and $P-450_7$ were isolated from various individuals, with more than one preparation derived from the same liver (Wang et al., 1983). These were all found to be immunochemically related to each other and to $P-450_{NF}$, a protein which we subsequently isolated on the basis of its ability to catalyze nifedipine oxidation (Guengerich et al., 1986a). Like $P-450_{MP}$, this protein(s) appears to be relatively abundant in human liver. However, $P-450_{MP}$ has a much more diffuse localization than $P-450_{NF}$, which is primarily centrilobular (Ratanasavanh et al., 1986). Both $P-450_{MP}$- and $P-450_{NF}$-linked catalytic activities appear to depend upon cytochrome b_5 (Shimada et al., 1986). Watkins et al. (1985) also isolated a similar "P-450p" preparation and Kitada et al. (1987) have recently presented strong evidence that $P-450_{HLFa}$, isolated from human fetal liver several years ago (Kitada and Kamataki, 1979; Kitada et al., 1985), is also closely related to $P-450_{NF}$.

It is somewhat difficult to assess the substrate specificity of $P-450_{NF}$, since this protein tends to lose activity upon purification (Guengerich et al., 1986a), like its rat ortholog $P-450_{PCN-E}$ (Guengerich et al., 1982; Shimada and Guengerich, 1985). Inferences about catalytic specificity have been made primarily by the use of immunochemical inhibition of activities in microsomes. Reactions include oxidation of nifedipine and other 1,4-dihydropyridines (Guengerich et al., 1986a; Böcker and Guengerich, 1986), quinidine N- and 3-hydroxylation (Guengerich et al., 1986b), d-benzphetamine N-demethylation (Wang et al., 1983; Guengerich et al., 1986a), aldrin epoxidation (Guengerich et al., 1986a), testosterone 6β-hydroxylation (Guengerich et al., 1986a; Kitada et al., 1987), cortisol 6β-hydroxylation (C. Ged, P. Maurel, I. Dalet-Beluche, and P. Beaune, submitted), 17β-estradiol 2- and 4-hydroxylation (Guengerich et al., 1986a), dihydroepiandrostenedione 17 sulfate 16α-hydroxylation (M. Kitada and T. Kamataki, personal communication), and the N-demethylation of macrolide antibiotics (e.g., erythromycin, triacetyloleandomycin) and their conversion to heme ligands (Watkins et al., 1985).

We cloned and sequenced a full-length cDNA (NF25) related to $P-450_{NF}$ (Beaune et al., 1986). Recently we found another cDNA in the same library which differs only in having an extended 3' non-coding region (with a poly A tail and a second polyadenylation signal) and missing a 3-base region in the coding region which converts a thr-leu to ile. Genomic blotting with overlapping long 3' and 5' probes indicates that at least three genes should be in this family. Molowa et al. (1986) analyzed partial clones obtained from the same library that we did and presented a cDNA sequence based upon these. The 3' clone shows 12 amino acid replacements with our two clones and that sequence may represent a third mRNA. As in the case of $P-450_{MP}$, the extent of expression of these different sequences is unknown, as is the relationship of the different sequences to function in the putative proteins. The genes have been localized to chromosome 7.

6β-Hydroxycortisol excretion, a function related to the presence of $P-450_{NF}$ (C. Ged, P. Maurel, I. Dalet-Beluche, and P. Beaune, submitted), has been known to be elevated after in vivo treatment with several agents and suggests that $P-450_{NF}$ can be induced. Further Watkins et al. (1985) found high levels of the protein(s) in a patient treated with barbituates, steroids, and macrolide antibiotics. Enzyme levels can be elevated by treatment in hepatocyte cultures (Molowa et al., 1986; A. Guillouzo, P.H. Beaune, M.V. Martin, R.W. Bork, and F.P. Guengerich, unpublished results). Both we (Guengerich et al., 1986a, 1986b) and others (Watkins et al., 1985; Kitada et al., 1987) have shown correlations between immunochemically-measured $P-450_{NF}$ and catalytic activity in different livers; however, for unknown reasons the correlations involving mRNA levels exist but are not as strong (Molowa et al., 1986; Beaune et al., 1986). Whether in vivo differences in nifedipine oxidation can be attributed to genetic variation is unclear (Kleinbloessem et al., 1984).

It is of interest to note that $P-450_{NF}$ is a major fetal cytochrome P-450 (Kitada et al., 1985) while $P-450_{MP}$ and related mRNAs are devoid in fetuses (Shimada et al., 1986).

$P-450_{DB}$

Debrisoquine 4-hydroxylation has attracted considerable interest because it was the first cytochrome P-450-related reaction to show monogenic distribution in humans (Mahgoub et al., 1977). $P-450_{DB}$ was isolated using immunochemical reactivity as a guide; the purified enzyme catalyzes oxidations associated with the clinical polymorphism such as debrisoquine 4-hydroxylation, sparteine Δ^5-oxidation, bufuralol 1'-hydroxylation, encainide O-demethylation, and propranolol 4-hydroxylation (Distlerath et al., 1985). Apparently the same enzyme has been isolated by Birgersson et al. (1986) and Gut et al. (1986a)--these preparations also catalyze desmethylimipramine 10-hydroxylation and metoprolol hydroxylation. Gut et al. (1986a) have also presented evidence for the existence of a related form of the protein ($P-450_{Buf\ II}$) which has lower catalytic activity.

Several lines of investigation suggest that debrisoquine 4-hydroxylase activity is refractory to induction. Nebert and Gonzalez (1987) have recently cloned the gene and suggest that several different causes may be responsible for the phenotypic defect, including mRNA splicing problems associated with a DNA polymorphism. The liver data suggest that individuals having the deficient phenotype may contain the same amount of a protein which is defective because of an increased K_m (Osikowska-Evers et al., 1987).

$P-450_{PA}$

This protein was purified on the basis of its low K_m, high affinity activity for phenacetin O-deethylation (Distlerath et al., 1985), an activity previously ascribed to $P-450_{DB}$. Studies with this protein have been limited. Several lines of indirect evidence suggest that this protein may be the one coded for by the P_3-450 gene, although the situation is still not unambiguous (Guengerich et al., 1987). If this is the case, then the protein should be inducible by certain polycyclic aromatic hydrocarbons and other compounds. The human P_3-450 gene has been extensively characterized (Quattrochi et al., 1986; Jaiswal et al., 1986) and an (inactive) protein has been isolated (Wrighton et al., 1986a).

P-450j

Wrighton et al. (1986b) coupled an antibody raised to rat liver P-450j to an immobilized gel and isolated a denatured ortholog from human liver. The N-terminal sequence was similar to the rat liver protein and the amount of immunochemically-detectable protein in different livers could be correlated with the level of N,N-dimethylnitrosamine N-demethylase activity. Song et al. (1986) have recently cloned and sequenced a human cDNA. Several lines of evidence suggest that this enzyme, which appears to be part of only a small gene family, is inducible by ethanol ingestion. Recently we have purified this enzyme to homogeneity from human liver microsomes in our own laboratory, although the catalytic and biochemical properties have not yet been fully investigated.

$P-450_g$

Beaune et al. (1985) isolated a human liver cytochrome P-450 preparation which appears to be distinct from others obtained in our own and other laboratories. $P-450_g$ has, however, not shown striking catalytic properties and its role in the metabolism of drugs and endogenous chemicals is not clear.

Other cytochrome P-450 enzymes

Evidence related to other human cytochrome P-450 enzymes has also been presented although the proteins have not been isolated and characterized.

A number of lines of evidence indicate that P_1-450, which has been cloned and sequenced by Jaiswal et al. (1985), is inducible (by polycyclic hydrocarbons) in extrahepatic tissues. However, there is no direct evidence to date that this protein exists in human liver, although it might be expected to be there after conditions of dramatic induction.

Phillips et al. (1985) isolated and sequenced a partial-length cDNA clone after screening with a strategy based on a phenobarbital-induced rat liver cytochrome P-450. Although the first suggestions were that this sequence was the ortholog of rat P-450$_{PB-D}$, more recent analysis suggests that it is more closely related to rat P-450$_{UT-F}$ (P-450a), a testosterone 7α-hydroxylase in rats (I.R. Phillips, personal communication).

Human microsomal cytochrome P-450 expressed in extrahepatic tissues which have been extensively characterized include aromatase and C-21 hydroxylase (White et al., 1986; Kellis and Vickery, 1987). There is no evidence, however, that these proteins are ever expressed in hepatic tissue.

REFERENCES

Beaune, P., Flinois, J-P., Kiffel, L., Kremers, P., and Leroux, J-P.(1985): Purification of a new cytochrome P-450 from human liver microsomes. Biochim. Biophys. Acta 840, 364-370.

Beaune, P.H., Umbenhauer, D.R., Bork, R.W., Lloyd, R.S., and Guengerich, F.P.(1986): Isolation and sequence determination of a cDNA clone related to human cytochrome P-450 nifedipine oxidase. Proc. Natl. Acad. Sci. U.S.A. 83, 8064-8068.

Birgersson, C., Morgan, E.T., Jörnvall, H., and von Bahr, C.(1986): Purification of a desmethylimipramine and debrisoquine hydroxylating cytochrome P-450 from human liver. Biochem. Pharmacol. 35, 3165-3166.

Böcker, R.H., and Guengerich, F.P.(1986): Oxidation of 4-aryl- and 4-alkyl-substituted 2,6-dimethyl-3,5-bis-(alkoxycarbonyl)-1,4-dihydropyridines by human liver microsomes and immunochemical evidence for the involvement of a form of cytochrome P-450. J. Med. Chem. 29, 1596-1603.

Distlerath, L.M., Reilly, P.E.B., Martin, M.V., Davis, G.G., Wilkinson, G.R., and Guengerich, F.P.(1985): Purification and characterization of the human liver cytochromes P-450 involved in debrisoquine 4-hydroxylation and phenacetin O-deethylation, two prototypes for genetic polymorphism in oxidative drug metabolism. J. Biol. Chem. 260, 9057-9067.

Guengerich, F.P., Dannan, G.A., Wright, S.T., Martin, M.V., and Kaminsky, L.S.(1982): Purification and characterization of liver microsomal cytochromes P-450: electrophoretic, spectral, catalytic, and immunochemical properties and inducibility of eight isozymes isolated from rats treated with phenobarbital or β-naphthoflavone. Biochemistry 21, 6019-6030.

Guengerich, F.P., and Liebler, D.C.(1985): Enzymatic activation of chemicals to toxic metabolites. CRC Crit. Rev Toxicol. 14, 259-307.

Guengerich, F.P., Martin, M.V., Beaune, P.H., Kremers, P., Wolff, T., and Waxman, D.J.(1986a): Characterization of rat and human liver microsomal cytochrome P-450 forms involved in nifedipine oxidation, a prototype for genetic polymorphism in oxidative drug metabolism. J. Biol. Chem. 261, 5051-5060.

Guengerich, F.P., Müller-Enoch, D., and Blair, I.A.(1986b): Oxidation of quinidine by human liver cytochrome P-450. Mol. Pharmacol. 30, 287-295.

Guengerich, F.P., Umbenhauer, D.R., Churchill, P.F., Beaune, P.H., Böcker, R.H., Knodell, R.G., Martin, M.V., and Lloyd, R.S.(1987): Polymorphism of human cytochrome P-450. Xenobiotica 17, 311-316.

Gut, J., Catin, T., Dayer, P., Kronbach, T., Zanger, U., and Meyer, U.A.(1986a): Debrisoquine/sparteine-type polymorphism of drug oxidation: purification and characterization of two functionally different human liver cytochrome P-450 isozymes involved in impaired hydroxylation of the prototype substrate bufuralol. J. Biol. Chem. 261, 11734-11743.

Gut, J., Meier, U.T., Catin, T., and Meyer, U.A.(1986b): Mephenytoin-type polymorphism of drug oxidation: purification and characterization of a human liver cytochrome P-450 isozyme catalyzing microsomal mephenytoin hydroxylation. Biochim. Biophys. Acta 884, 435-447.

Jaiswal, A.K., Gonzalez, F.J., and Nebert, D.W.(1985): Human dioxin-inducible cytochrome P_1-450: complementary DNA and amino acid sequence. Science 228, 80-83.

Jaiswal, A.K., Nebert, D.W., and Gonzalez, F.J.(1986): Human P_3-450: cDNA and complete amino acid sequence. Nucl. Acids Res. 14, 6773-6774.

Kellis, J.T., Jr., and Vickery, L.E.(1987): Purification and characterization of human placental aromatase. J. Biol. Chem. 262, 4413-4420.

Kitada, M., and Kamataki, T.(1979): Partial purification and properties of cytochrome P-450 from homogenates of human fetal livers. Biochem. Pharmacol. 28, 793-797.

Kitada, M., Kamataki, T., Itahashi, K., Rikihisa, T., and Kanakubo, Y.(1987): Significance of cytochrome P-450 (P-450 HFLa) of human fetal liver in the steroid and drug oxidations. Biochem. Pharmacol. 36, 453-456.

Kitada, M., Kamataki, T., Itahashi, K., Rikihisa, T., Kato, R., and Kanakubo, Y.(1985): Purification and properties of cytochrome P-450 from homogenates of human fetal livers. Arch. Biochem. Biophys. 241, 275-280.

Kleinbloessem, C.H., van Brummelen, P., Faber, H., Danhof, M., Vermeulen, N.P.E., and Breimer, D.D.(1984): Variability in nifedipine pharmacokinetics and dynamics: a new oxidation polymorphism in man. Biochem. Pharmacol. 33, 3721-3724.

Knodell, R.G., Hall, S.D., Wilkinson, G.R., and Guengerich, F.P.(1987): Hepatic metabolism of tolbutamide: in vitro characterization of the form of cytochrome P-450 involved in methyl hydroxylation and relationship to in vivo disposition. J. Pharmacol. Exp. Ther., in press.

Mahgoub, A., Dring, L.G., Idle, J.R., Lancaster, R., and Smith, R.L.(1977): Polymorphic hydroxylation of debrisoquine in man. Lancet ii, 584-586.

Meier, U.T., Dayer, P., Malé, P.J., Kronbach, T., and Meyer, U.A.(1985): Mephenytoin hydroxylation polymorphism: characterization of the enzymatic deficiency in liver microsomes of poor metabolizers phenotyped in vivo. Clin. Pharmacol. Ther. 38, 488-494.

Molowa, D.T., Schuetz, E.G., Wrighton, S.A., Watkins, P.B., Kremers, P., Mendez-Picon, G., Parker, G.A., and Guzelian, P.S.(1986): Complete cDNA sequence of a cytochrome P-450 inducible by glucocorticoids in human liver. Proc. Natl. Acad. Sci. U.S.A. 83, 5311-5315.

Nebert, D.W., and Gonzalez, F.J.(1987): P450 genes and evolutionary genetics. Hospital Practice (March 15).

Nebert, D.W., Adesnik, M., Coon, M.J., Estabrook, R.W., Gonzalez, F.J., Guengerich, F.P., Gunsalus, I.C., Johnson, E.F., Kemper, B., Levin, W., Phillips, I.R., Sato, R., and Waterman, M.R.(1987): The P450 gene superfamily: recommended nomenclature. DNA 6, 1-11.

Osikowska-Evers, B., Dayer, P., Meyer, U.A., Robertz, G.M., and Eichelbaum, M.(1987): Evidence for altered catalytic properties of the cytochrome P-450 involved in sparteine oxidation in poor metabolizers. Clin. Pharmacol. Ther. 41, 320-325.

Phillips, I.R., Shephard, E.A., Ashworth, A., and Rabin, B.R.(1985): Isolation and sequence of a human cytochrome P-450 cDNA clone. Proc. Natl. Acad. Sci. U.S.A. 82, 983-987.

Quattrochi, L.C., Pendurthi, U.R., Okino, S.T., Potenza, C., and Tukey, R.H.(1986): Human cytochrome P-450 4 mRNA and gene: part of a multigene family that contains Ala sequences in its mRNA. Proc. Natl. Acad. Sci. U.S.A. 83, 6731-6735.

Ratanasavanh, D., Beaune, P., Baffet, G., Rissel, M., Kremers, P., Guengerich, F.P., and Guillouzo, A.(1986): Immunocytochemical evidence for the maintenance of cytochrome P-450 isozymes, NADPH-cytochrome c reductase, and epoxide hydrolase in pure and mixed cultures of adult human hepatocytes. J. Histochem. Cytochem. 34, 527-533.

Shimada, T., and Guengerich, F.P.(1985): Participation of a rat liver cytochrome P-450 induced by pregnenolone 16α-carbonitrile and other compoounds in the 4-hydroxylation of mephenytoin. Mol. Pharmacol. 28, 215-219.

Shimada, T., Misono, K.S., and Guengerich, F.P.(1986): Human liver microsomal cytochrome P-450 mephenytoin 4-hydroxylase, a prototype of genetic polymorphism in oxidative drug metabolism: purification and characterization of two similar forms involved in the reaction. J. Biol. Chem. 261, 909-921.

Song, B-J., Gelboin, H.V., Park, S-S., Yang, C-S., and Gonzalez, F.J.(1986): Complementary DNA and protein sequences of ethanol-inducible rat and human cytochrome P-450s: transcriptional and post-transcriptional regulation of the rat enzyme. J. Biol. Chem. 261, 16689-16697.

Tukey, R.H., Okino, S., Barnes, H., Griffin, K.J., and Johnson, E.F.(1985): Multiple gene-like sequences related to the rabbit hepatic progesterone 21-hydroxylase cytochrome P-450 1. J. Biol. Chem. 260, 13347-13354.

Tukey, R.H., Quattrochi, L.C., Pendurthi, U.R., and Okino, S.T.(1986): Identification of a human cytochrome P-450 highly related to rabbit liver progesterone 21-hydroxylase P-450 1. Fed. Proc., Fed. Amer. Soc. Exp. Biol. 45, 1663.

Umbenhauer, D.R., Martin, M.V., Lloyd, R.S., and Guengerich, F.P.(1987): Cloning and sequence determination of a complementary DNA related to human liver microsomal cytochrome P-450 S-mephenytoin 4-hydroxylase. Biochemistry 26, 1094-1099.

Wang, P.P., Beaune, P., Kaminsky, L.S., Dannan, G.A., Kadlubar, F.F., Larrey, D., and Guengerich, F.P.(1983): Purification and characterization of six cytochrome P-450 isozymes from human liver microsomes. Biochemistry 22, 5375-5383.

Wang, P., Mason, P.S., and Guengerich, F.P.(1980): Purification of human liver cytochrome P-450 and comparistion to the enzyme isolated from rat liver. Arch. Biochem. Biophys. 199, 206-219.

Watkins, P.B., Wrighton, S.A., Maurel, P., Schuetz, E.G., Mendez-Picon, G., Parker, G.A., and Guzelian, P.S.(1985): Identification of an inducible form of cytochrome P-450 in human liver. Proc. Natl. Acad. Sci. U.S.A. 82, 6310-6314.

White, P.C., New, M.I., and DuPont, B.(1986): Structure of human steroid 21-hydroxylase genes. Proc. Natl. Acad. Sci. U.S.A 83, 5111-5115.

Wrighton, S.A., Campanile, C., Thomas, P.E., Maines, S.L., Watkins, P.B., Parker, G., Mendez-Picon, G., Haniu, M., Shively, J.E., Levin, W., and Guzelian, P.S.(1986a): Identification of a human liver cytochrome P-450 homologous to the major isosafrone-inducible cytochrome P-450 in the rat. Mol. Pharmacol. 29, 405-410.

Wrighton, S.A., Thomas, P.E., Molowa, D.T., Haniu, M., Shively, J.E., Maines, S.L., Watkins, P.B., Parker, G., Mendez-Picon, G., Levin, W., and Guzelian, P.S.(1986b): Characterization of ethanol-inducible human liver N-nitrosodimethylamine demethylase. Biochemistry 25, 6731-6735.

Yoshioka, H., Morohashi, K., Sogawa, K., Miyata, T., Kawajiri, K., Hirose, T., Inayama, S., Fujii-Kuriyama, Y., and Omura, T.(1987): Structural analysis and specific expression of microsomal cytochrome P-450 (M-1) mRNA in male rat livers. <u>J. Biol. Chem. 262,</u> 1706-1711.

Résumé

Les cytochromes P-450 jouent un rôle important dans l'oxydation des médicaments et des xénobiotiques tout comme dans celle de nombreux composés endogènes de l'organisme. Le foie est l'organe principal d'expression de ces enzymes et habituellement un lieu très important d'oxydation. Au cours des dernières années, des approches biochimiques ont été utilisées pour l'étude de ces enzymes dans le foie humain. Au moins six enzymes différents ont été isolés et la plupart semblent constituer des produits de familles multigéniques. Ainsi, il est probable que des formes voisines de cytochrome P-450 sont exprimées dans un même foie, et discerner les propriétés catalytiques de chaque protéine est malaisé. Certaines activités dépendentes du cytochrome P-450 sont liées au polymorphisme génétique dans le foie humain. Pour d'autres, des variations de régulation au niveau transcriptionnel expliquent probablement les différences individuelles. Les caractéristiques des protéines des cytochromes P-450 connus sont rappelées ainsi que nos connaissances actuelles sur les gènes et la spécificité catalytique des protéines. Des études sur les protéines correspondantes chez le rat et le lapin sont utiles mais dans certains cas, les comparaisons peuvent conduire à des erreurs sur les propriétés physiques et fonctionnelles.

Regulation of cytochrome P-450 3c from rabbit liver microsomes

Martine Daujat, Philippe Clair, Thierry Pineau, Lydiane Pichard, Claude Bonfils, Christian Dalet, Patrick Maurel

INSERM U.128, CNRS, Route de Mende, BP 5051, 34033 Montpellier Cedex, France

ABSTRACT

Cytochrome P-450 3c from NZW rabbit liver microsomes is a member of the P-450 III A subfamily which contains genes responsive to macrolide antibiotics (troleandomycin and erythromycin), rifampicin and glucocorticoïds (pregnenolone 16αcarbonitrile and dexamethasone). Other forms of this subfamily expressed in the rat and human include P-450p1, P-450p2 and P-450 PCN-E, and P-450 HLp/NF, respectively. Comparative analysis of primary sequence indicate that this gene family has diverged from the other P-450 families at least 600 millions years ago. Two distinct species of mRNA (1700 and 1850 bases) cohybridize with P-450 3c cDNA in the liver of animals of both sexes. Nucleotide sequence data from several cDNA, RNase H analysis and use of a 3' restriciton fragment from P-450 3c cDNA as a probe in northern blots allowed us to demonstrate that these 2mRNA species exhibit 3'untranslated region of different length. Southern blot analysis genomic DNA digested with various restriction enzymes suggests that there could be $\leq$3 members in the rabbit P-450 III A subfamily. The level of both mRNA is increased several folds by the inducers. Nuclear run-on transcription analysis indicate that P-450 3c genes transcription is activated in the liver of induced animals. While P-450 3c is absent from foetus and new born animal, its level sharply rises between 3 and 4 weeks and after passing through a maximum at 8 weeks decreases in the adult. Cytochrome P-450 3c appears to be transcriptionally regulated during the development but not in a sex dependent fashion.

KEY WORDS : Cytochrome P-450, multigenicity, induction, mRNA heterogeneity, developmental regulation.

INTRODUCTION

Cytochromes P-450 from liver microsomes constitute a multigenic superfamily of hemoproteins involved in the oxidation of numerous endogenous and exogeneous compounds like drugs and carcinogens. On the basis of primary sequence data these cytochromes were recently classified into ten distinct families four of which are involved in the hepatic detoxication function (Nebert et al, 1987). Family I comprises forms (IA1 and IA2) inducible by polycyclic aromatic hydrocarbons like methylcholanthrene (MC) and B-naphthoflavone (BNF). Some, but not all, members of family II are inducible by phenobarbital (PB) and ethanol (II B1 and II B2, and II E1, respectively). Members of subfamily III A are inducible by two distinct classes of chemicals, antibiotics like troleandomycin (TAO), erythromycin (ER) and rifampicin (RIF) and glucocorticoïds like pregnenolone 16α carbonitrile (PCN) and dexamethasone (DEX). Subfamily IV A contains form(s) inducible by clofibrate.

Cytochrome P-450 3c is a member of subfamily III A which also comprises forms from rat (P-450p1, P-450p2 and P-450 PCN-E) and human (P-450 HLp/NF). We recently reported (Bertault-Peres et al, 1987) that this cytochrome was responsible for at least 80 % of the hepatic metabolism of cyclosporin A in the rabbit. Recent findings concerning the sequence and regulation of P-450 3c are reviewed in this communication.

MATERIALS AND METHODS

Animals and treatments

Male and female New-Zealand white rabbits were used in this work. In some experiments animals were treated with rifampicin (i.p. injection of 50 mg/kg), troleandomycin (i. p. injection of 850 mg /kg in 2 % tween 20 or per os as a diet consisting of 1 % (w/w) TAO mixed in the rabbit chow) and 3 methylcholanthrene (i.p. injection of 25 mg/kg).

Preparation of microsomes and western blot analysis

Microsomes were prepared from rabbit liver by differential centrifugation as described previously (Haugen and Coon, 1976). Protein concentration was determined by the method of Lowry, BSA being used as the standard. Electrophoresis and western blotting were carried out as described (Dalet et al, 1986 ; Daujat et al, 1987). The blot was first incubated with 0.1 mg/ml goat anti P-450 3c IgG and then with HRP labeled rabbit anti goat IgG ; diaminobenzidine was used as the substrate.

Preparation of RNA and northern blot and dot blot analysis

Total RNA was prepared from rabbit liver as described (Daujat et al, 1987). Poly A RNA was isolated by two cycles of oligo dT-cellulose chromatography. Northern blot analysis was performed as described (Dalet et al, 1986). Hybridization was carried out with 10 ng of pLM3c 4-1 cDNA insert (^{32}P) radiolabeled (1-210^8 dpm/µg) with the Multiprime DNA labeling system from Amersham (Amersham, U.K.). Dot blot analysis was carried out under the same conditions of prehybridization, hybridization and washing.

Nuclear run-on experiments

In vitro transcription experiments were carried out essentially as described (Dalet et al 1986) with the following modifications : liver nuclei were purified as described by Greenberg et al, 1984) and incubated in 100 µl of reaction buffer (10 mM Tris HCl pH8.0, 5mM MgCl2, 300mM KCl, 0,5mM of ATP, CTP,

GTP and with 100 µCi of $[\alpha-^{32}P]$ UTP for 15 min at 28°C. After DNAse-RNAse free treatment, nascent RNA chains were extracted out ; deproteinized by the hot phenol procedure, precipitated 3 times by ethanol in the presence of 3µg glycogene and ammonium acetate 2,5 M. The same number of cpm $[\alpha-^{32}P]$ RNA was hybridized to DNA (5µg each of p4.1, puc N5gapdh, pBr322) immobilized on nitrocellulose filters, for 48 H. The filters were then washed with several changes 2xSSC at 42°C, air dried and exposed to kodak X Ray Film.

Primary sequence of P-450 3c and homology with other forms of P-450

Primary sequence of P-450 3c was derived from the nucleotide sequence of pLM3c 4.1 cDNA insert, determined by the dideoxy termination reaction of Sanger (Dalet et al, submitted for publication). For comparative analysis of P-450 3c and other sequences, global alignment of protein sequences was carried out using computer programs developed by J. F. Avril (Institut de Programmation, Université de Paris VI,1985).

RESULTS AND DISCUSSION

Primary sequence homology between P-450 3c and other P-450 forms

The aminoacid sequence of P-450 3c was derived from the nucleotide sequence of cDNA 4.1 (plasmid pLM3c 4.1) which encodes the full length protein (Dalet et al, 1986) (Fig. 1). P-450 3c is 501 aminoacids long and has a molecular weight of 57290 daltons (Dalet et al submitted for publication). As reported in Table 1, amino acid sequence homology between P450 3c and other rabbit forms including P-450 1, 2, 3b, 4 and 6 (Tukey et al, 1985 ; Heineman and Ozols, 1983 ; Leighton et al, 1984 ; Okino et al, 1985) averages 25 %.

Table 1 : Aminoacid sequence homology between P-450 3c and other forms from rabbit, rat and human liver microsomes

P-450 Forms	Subfamily	Homology with P-450 3c (%)
Rabbit		
P-450 1	II C 5	26
2	II B 1	27
3 b	II C 3	26
4	I A 2	24
6	I A 1	24
Rat		
P-450 pcn 1	III A 1	71
pcn 2	III A 2	68
Human		
P-450 HLp/NF	III A 3	73

This is currently taken as an indication that family III should have diverged from the other P-450 families roughly between 600 to 900 millions years ago. However, some short regions of these proteins exhibit a higher degree of homology i.e. the socalled conserved tridecapeptide (40 %) and the C-terminal cysteinyl peptide centered on the Cys^{440} residue on P-450 3c, most likely

43

involved in the heme binding (45 %). On the other hand homology between P-450 3c and rat P-450 p1 and p2 (Gonzalez et al, 1986) and human P-450 HLP/NF (Malowa et al, 1986 and Beaune et al, 1986) averages 70 %. As expected from this high homology these forms exhibit close similaries in terms of enzymatic and immunologic properties as well as in terms of regulation, (same specific inducers) (Wrighton et al, 1985 a).

m-RNA heterogeneity and multigenecity

It is clear from Fig. 2 that two distinct species of mRNA (of 1700 and 1850 nucleotides) cohybridize with pLM3c 4.1 cDNA ; similar observation (not shown

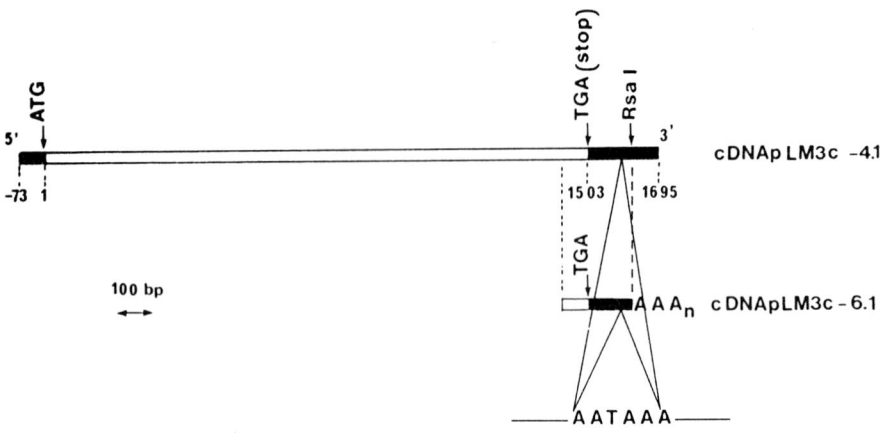

Fig.1. : cDNAs coding for cytochrome P-450 3c.
ATG and TGA : initiation and stop codons. AAAn : poly A tract. AATAAA polyadenylation consensus sequence. RsaI indicates a site which allowed the isolation of the 3' end fragment of cDNA clone 4.1.

here) was made with pLM3c 6.1 cDNA, another cDNA coding for P-450 3c, and isolated from the same rabbit liver cDNA library. It is worth mentioning here that in human liver, two mRNA species (2200 and 2800 nucleotides) were recently reported to hybridize with a cDNA encoding P-450 Hlp the putative ortholog of P-450 3c. Nucleotide sequence data revealed that pLM3c 6.1 cDNA encodes the last 24 amino acids of P-450 3c and further extends 116 nucleotides into the 3' untranslated region ; cDNA 6.1 is 100 % homologous to pLM3c 4.1 cDNA, Fig 1. However, whereas in cDNA 6.1 poly A sequence starts 23 nucleotides down stream from the poly A consensus signal (AATAAA), no poly A tract was found in cDNA 4.1 which exhibits a 3'untranslated region extending 101 nucleotides beyond the polyadenylation signal. These data suggested therefore that both cDNA 4.1 and 6.1 derived from two distinct species of mRNA. Further experiments were carried out to test this hypothesis. First, an RNase H analysis was performed on poly A RNA from RIF induced rabbit liver previously hybridized (or not) with oligo dT. Northern blot (not shown here) revealed that the poly A sequence (100-200 nucleotides in both species), which was digested by RNase H when hybridized with poly T, does not con⁄tribute to the length heterogeneity. On the other hand when the extreme 3'untranslated fragment of cDNA 4.1 downstream from the Rsa I site, (see Fig 1) was used as a probe in northern blot of poly A RNA from RIF induced rabbit liver, only one band at 1850 nucleotides was revealed. In addition to the sequence data these results demonstrate that two distinct species of mRNA cohybridizing with cDNA (P-450 3c) are present in both control and induced rabbit liver and that these species exhibit 3'untranslated region of different length. Southern blots of rabbit genomic DNA digested with various restriction enzymes were carried out. In all cases the probe (pLM3c 4.1 cDNA) hybridized with $\simeq$ 30 kb of DNA ; this suggests therefore but does not definitely prove, that several closely related P-450 3c genes could be present in the rabbit genome, (Dalet et al, 1986). Whether the two mRNA species derive from differential polyadenylation of a single gene, or from two distinct but closely related genes is not yet known and is under current investigation in this laboratory. No evidence has yet been found for the presence of more than one form of P-450 3c in the rabbit liver.

Inducibility

One of the characteristics of the P-450 III A genes subfamily is that their expression is inducible by macrolide antibiotics TAO, ER and RIF and glucocorticoïds PCN and DEX (Bonfils et al, 1985 and Wrighton et al, 1985 b). However, some species and forms specificity have been demonstrated concerning the responsiveness of these genes to these various chemicals. Thus in the rabbit for example, best inducers of P-450 3c are the antibiotics whereas glucocorticoïds are moderate (DEX) or even not inducer (PCN), under standard conditions of treatment, (Wrighton et al, 1985 a).

Table 2 : Nuclear run-on transcription : effect of inducers

Animals and Treatment	Intensity of hybridization relative to untreated animals	
	cDNA probes for	
	P-450 3c	P-450 4
UT	1.0	1.0
RIF (3H)	2.91	-
RIF (24H)	3.01	0.80
TAO (24H) i.p.	2.38	-
TAO (7 days) p.os.	1.16	-
TAO " " "	0.89	-
MC (4H)	0.30	2.12
MC (8H)	0.12	1.80

In the Fig. 2 we report some data concerning the induction of P-450 3c (as revealed by western blot developed with specific anti P-450 3c IgG) and of its specific mRNA (as revealed by northern blot developed with pLM3c 4.1 cDNA) as a function of time after one single injection of RIF (50 mg/kg, i.p.) to adult male rabbits. Same observations were made with females. Cytochrome P-450 3c is expressed at a low level in the untreated animals ($<$ 0.1 nmol/mg). Induction of both mRNA and protein becomes apparent 8 H after the injection of the drug. However, whereas the level of mRNA rapidly reaches a state of equilibrium (between 3 and 8 H) and remains roughly constant between 8 and 48 H, the level of the protein reaches its maximum only between 14 and 24 H. Since translation of mRNA into protein is not a limiting process, the delay we observe between mRNA and protein induction most likely results from the contribution of the protein degradation to the overall equilibrium ; the data presented here

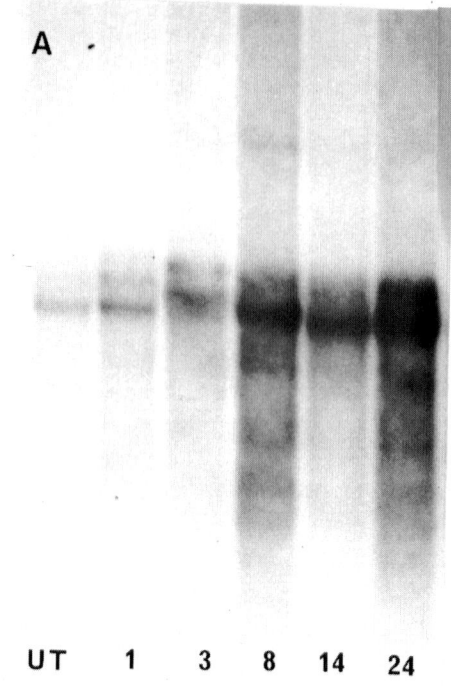
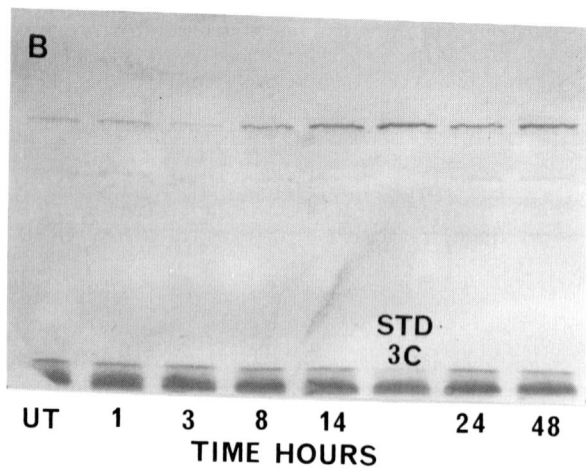

Fig. 2. : Kinetics of induction of P-450 3c (and of its mRNA(s)) after one single injection of RIF (i.p. 50 mg/kg).

(A) Northern blot of total RNA (10µg per lane) probed with (^{32}P) cDNA 4.1.
(B) Western blot of microsomes (2µg per lane) developed with anti P-450 3c IgG.

suggest that the half life of P-450 3c in vivo is of the order of 6 to 10 H. This is comparable to the values of 14 and 10 H determined for P-450 p (the putative rat ortholog of P-450 3c) in vivo and in culture, respectively (Watkins et al, 1986).

In order to evaluate the contribution of gene transcription to the increase in level of P-450 3c mRNA after treatment of the animals with various inducers, newly in vitro transcribed RNA from liver nuclei from untreated (UT) and induced rabbits was quantitated by filter hybridization to two probes (Table 2) coding for P-450 3c and P-450 4, for comparison. Clearly, RIF stimulates P-450 3c gene transcription and this effect becomes apparent 3H after a single injection. Results obtained with TAO are more difficult to interpret. The way of administration seems to affect the influence of this drug at the transcriptional level : 24H after an i.p. injection P-450 3c gene transcription is stimulated whereas it is not, after an overnight fast, with animals maintained 7 days on a diet consisting of 1 % TAO in rabbit chow. However, in both cases, northern blot analysis of liver RNA showed that P-450 3c mRNA level was strongly increased with respect to that determined in untreated animals. These results are not yet clearly understood but they suggest that TAO could increase the accumulation of P-450 3c mRNA by a mixed action at both transcriptional and post-transcriptional (mRNA stabilisation ?) levels. On the other hand, RIF does not affect P-450 4 gene transcription whereas the opposite is observed with 3-methylcholanthrene (MC) a known inducer of P-450 4 and 6 in the rabbit.

Expression of P-450 3c during rabbit development

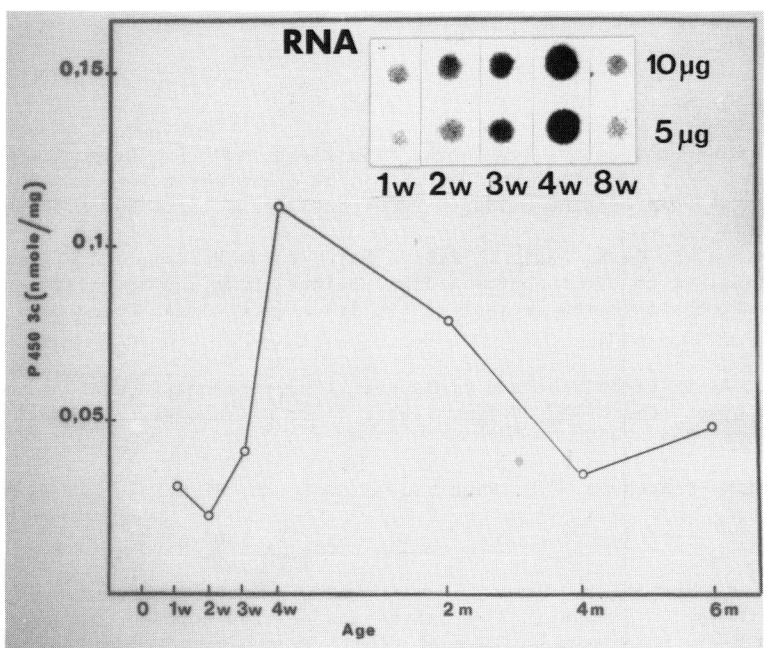

Fig.3. : Developmental expression of P-450 3c and of its mRNA(s) in the rabbit. P-450 3c (nmol/mg) determined from western blots of liver microsomes. Dot blots of total liver RNA (5 and 10µg) hybridized with (^{32}P) cDNA 4.1.

Rabbits of both sexes and of different age, including foetus 1, 2, 3, 4, 8 weeks old animals and adults, were sacrified and liver microsomes and total RNA were prepared. Various P-450 forms were thus tested for their developmental expression by western blot and northern blot developed with specific antibody and probe, respectively. Results concerning P-450 3c are reported in Fig 3. Whereas P-450 3c is undetectable in the foetus, its level sharply rises between 3 and 4 weeks. Other P-450 forms tested including P-450 2, 3b, 4 and 6 exhibited roughly similar behaviour (not shown here). The level of P-450 3c reaches a maximum at 8 weeks and then decreases by at least 50 % in the adults. No influence of sex was evident on this pattern. Fig 3 reveals that same pattern is observed at the level of mRNA which appears to be transcriptionally regulated during development. It should be mentionned here that differential expression of both mRNA (3c) species (1700 and 1850 nucleotides) seems not to be develpmentaly regulated after 3-4 weeks although at 1 week the 1850 nucleotides mRNA is barely detectable in contrast to the 1700 nucleotides species which clearly appears to be expressed. The sharp increase in both mRNA and P-450 3c at 3-4 weeks is probably mediated by a surge in the level of some essential hormone or of endogeneous or exogeneous component. In this respect, it is temptating to correlate the rise in P-450 3c with the onset of the weaning which appears to take place in the rabbit at 3-4 weeks. This, however remains to be definitely established.

ACKNOWLEDGMENTS

This work was supported by grants from INSERM, INRA, DRET and La Fondation pour la Recherche Médicale Française. The cDNA encoding P-450 4, used in the transcription experiments, was isolated and kindly provided by Dr D. Pompon from the Centre de Génétique Moléculaire, Gif sur Yvette. Expert assistance of Mrs. Françoise Couderc in the preparation of the manuscript is gratefully acknowledged.

REFERENCES

Beaune, P, D.R. Umbenhauer, R.W. Bork, R.S. Lloyd and P.F. Guengerich (1986) Isolation and sequence determination of a cDNA clone related to human liver cytochrome P-450 nifedipine oxidase. Proc. Natl. Acad. Sci. 83, 8064-8068.

Bertault-Peres, P, C. Bonfils, G. Fabre, S. Just, J. P. Cano and P. Maurel (1987) Metabolism of cyclosporine A II. Implication of the Macrolide antibiotic inducible cytochrome P-450 3c from rabbit liver microsomes. Drug. Met. and Dispos. (in press).

Bonfils, C, I. Dalet-Beluche and P. Maurel (1985) Triacetyloleandomycin as inducer of cytochrome P-450 3c from rabbit liver microsomes. Biochem. Pharmacol. 34, 2445-2450.

Dalet, C, J.M. Blanchard, P.S. Guzelian, J. Barwich, H. Hartle and P. Maurel (1986) Cloning of a cDNA coding for P-450 3c from rabbit liver microsomes and regulation of its expression. Nucl. Acid. Res. 14, 5999-6015.

Daujat, M., L. Pichard, C. Dalet, C. Larroque, C. Bonfils, D. Pompon, D. Li, P.S. Guzelian and P. Maurel (1987) Expression of five forms of microsomal cytochrome P-450 in primary culture of rabbit hepatocytes treated with various classes of inducers. Biochem. Pharmacol (in press).

Gonzalez, F, B.J. Song and J.P. Hardwick (1986) Pregnenolone 16 -carbonitrile inducible P-450 gene family : Gene conversion and differential regulation. Mol. Cell. Biol. 6, 2969-2979.

Greenberg, M.E. and E.B. Ziff (1984) Stimulation of 3T3 cells induces transcription of c-Fos proto-oncogène. Nature, 311, 433-438.

Haugen, D.A and M.J. Coon (1976) Properties of electrophoretically homogeneous phenobarbital-inducible and B-naphthoflavone-inducible forms of liver microsomal cytochrome P-450. J. Biol. Chem. 251, 7929-7939.

Heinemann, F.S. and Ozols, J. (1983) The complete amino acid sequence of rabbit phenobarbital-induced liver microsomal cytochrome P-450. J. Biol. Chem. 258, 4195-4201.

Leighton, J.K, B.A. Debrunner-Vossbrinck and B. Kemper (1984) Isolation and sequence analysis of three cloned cDNAs for rabbit liver proteins that are related to rabbit cytochrome P-450 (form 2) the major phenobarbital inducible form. Biochemistry. 23, 204-210.

Malowa, D.T, E.G. Schuetz, S.A. Wrighton, P.B. Watkins, P. Kremers, G.A. Parker and P.S. Guzelian (1986) Complete cDNA sequence of a cytochrome P-450 inducible by glucocorticoïds in human liver. Proc. Natl. Acad. Sci., 83, 5311-5315.

Nebert, D.W, M. Adesnik, M.J. Coon, R.W. Estabrook, F.J. Gonzalez, F.P. Guengerich, I.C. Gunsalus, E.F. Johnson, B. Kemper, W. Levin, I.R. Phillips, R. Sato and M.R. Waterman (1987) the P-450 gene superfamily : Recommended Nomenclature. DNA, 6, 1-11.

Okino, S.T, L.C. Quattrochi, H.J. Barnes, S. Osantc, K.J. Griffin, F.F. Johnson and R.H. Tukey (1985) Cloning and characterisation of cDNA encoding 2, 3, 7, 8 tetrachlorodibenzo-p-dioxin-inducible rabbit mRNAs for cytochrome P-450 isozymes 4 and 6. Proc. Natl. Acad. Sci. 82, 5310-5314.

Tukey, R.T, S.T. Okino, H.J. Barnes, K.J. Griffin and E.F. Johnson (1985) Multiple gene-like sequences related to the rabbit hepatic progesterone 21-hydroxylase cytochrome P-450 1. J. Biol. Chem. 260, 13347-13354.

Watkins, P.B, S.A. Wrighton, E.G. Schuetz, P. Maurel and P.S. Guzelian (1986). Macrolide antibiotics inhibit the degradation of the glucocorticoid-responsive cytochrome P-450p in rat hepatocytes in vivo and in monolayer culture. J. Biol. Chem. 261, 6264-6271.

Wrighton, S.A, E.G. Schuetz, P.B. Watkins, P. Maurel, J. Barwick, B.S. Bailey, H. Hartle, B. Young and P.S. Cuzelian (1985, a) Demonstration of multiple species of inducible hepatic cytochromes P-450 and their mRNAs related to the glucocorticoïd-inducible cytochrome P-450 of the rat. Mol. Pharmacol. 28, 312-321.

Wrighton, S.A, P. Maurel, E.G. Schuetz, P.B. Watkins, B. Young and P.S. Guzelian (1985, b) Identification of the cytochrome P-450 induced by macrolide antibiotics in rat liver as the glucocorticoïd responsive cytochrome P-450. Biochemistry, 24, 2171-2178.

Résumé

Le cytochrome P-450 3c des microsomes hépatiques de lapin est un membre de la sous-famille P-450 III A qui regroupe des gènes dont l'expression est inductible par les antibiotiques macrolides (troleandomycine, erythromycine), la rifampicine et certains glucocorticoïdes (pregnenolone 16 carbonitrile et dexamethasone). Les autres formes qui composent cette famille sont chez le rat et l'homme respectivement les P-450p1, P-450p2 et P-450 PCN-E et P-450 HLp/NF. L'analyse comparative des séquences primaires indique que cette famille a divergé des autres il y a au moins 600 millions d'années. Deux espèces de mRNA (1700 et 1850 bases) présentes dans le foie des animaux des deux sexes cohybrident avec les cDNAs codant pour P-450 3c. L'étude des séquences de ces cDNAs, une analyse à la RNase H et l'utilisation d'un fragment 3' d'un cDNA (P-450 3c) comme sonde en northern blots nous ont permis de montrer que ces deux espèces de mRNA (P-450 3c) se distinguent par des longueurs différentes de leur région 3' non codante. L'analyse en Southern blot de l'ADN génomique digéré avec divers enzymes de restriction suggère la présence d'au plus 3 gènes dans la sous-famille P-450 III A chez le lapin. Le niveau des deux mRNA (P-450 3c) est fortement augmenté par les inducteurs. Des expériences de transcription dans des noyaux in vitro indiquent que la transcription du ou des gène(s) P-450 3c est activée dans le foie des animaux induits. Alors que le P-450 3c est absent chez le foetus sa concentration augmente rapidement à partir de 3 à 4 semaines, culmine à 8 semaines puis décroit chez l'adulte. Ce cytochrome est régulé au niveau transcriptionnel, identiquement chez les deux sexes, au cours du développement.

Regulation of human cytochrome P1-450 gene

Thierry Cresteil, Howard J. Eisen

INSERM U.75, CHU Necker, 156 rue de Vaugirard, 75730 Paris Cedex 15, France. Laboratory of Developmental Pharmacology, NIH, Bethesda, USA

This paper is dedicated to the memory of Dr.H.J. EISEN who has initiated this study.

ABSTRACT

The regulation of the human cytochrome P1-450 gene has been investigated in human carcinoma cell lines and tentatively correlated with the presence of regulatory elements. The presence of a TCDD-binding protein has been demonstrated in some lines and corresponds to a highly sensitive induction process. In these lines, the presence of cytochrome P450 MP supporting benzopyrene hydroxylase activity in human liver cannot be detected. Conversely, the P1-450 mRNA concentration is very low in human liver. In fetal liver which is devoid of benzopyrene hydroxylase activity, the expression of P1-450 and P3-450 genes remains unchanged as compared with adult liver. This lack of correlation between P1-450 gene expression and enzymatic activity suggests that cytochrome P1-450 is only a minor component for benzopyrene hydroxylase in human liver.

KEY WORDS
Cytochromes P450, gene expression, human liver.

INTRODUCTION

Since two decades, hepatic monooxygenases have been involved in hydroxylating activities towards hydrophobic molecules like lipids, endogenous steroids and exogenous compounds. Monooxygenase reactions involve an electron transfer chain and an hemoprotein, generally a cytochrome P450 moiety. Different cytochromes P450 have been described and purified: they exhibit an overlapping substrate specificity and can be differently affected by a prior pretreatment of animals with some compounds, resulting in an overexpression of one (or several) isozyme. One of the best well-known reactions is the hydroxylation of polycyclic aromatic hydrocarbons, exemplified with benzopyrene as substrate (aryl hydrocarbon hydroxylase or benzopyrene hydroxylase) leading to the formation of metabolites with mutagenic, teratogenic and/or carcinogenic properties. This activity is

dramatically increased in all tissues by administration of benzopyrene, 3 methylcholanthrene or tetrachlorodibenzo-p-dioxin (TCDD).
In mouse, the raise in benzopyrene hydroxylase activity has been correlated with a marked increase of cytochrome P1-450 isozyme whereas P3-450 is mainly associated with acetanilide hydroxylase activity (Negishi,1979). The mechanism described for induction implies a cytosolic receptor for the inducer, translocated to the nucleus; then, the inducer-receptor complex activates several genes (among them are P1 and P3-450, menadione reductase, UDP-glucuronosyltransferase) leading to an increased mRNA synthesis and finally to an accumulation of each protein (Eisen,1986). In non-responsive mice or in certain tissue culture cell lines, enzymatic activities remained unchanged in response to inducers: the defect can be associated with either the inducer-binding protein (low affinity, absence of nuclear translocation)(Legraverend, 1982) or with the incapacity of the gene to be activated (Cresteil,1987).
Due to its potency to activate procarcinogens into reactive metabolites, P1-450 has been hypothesized to be one element responsive for the initiation/promotion of tumors in humans. Actually, benzopyrene hydroxylase activity is present and can be assayed in human tissues. In liver, benzopyrene hydroxylase activity is positively correlated with the microsomal content in isozyme P450-8 or P450MP, also responsive for 4-nitroanisole demethylase and mephenytoin hydroxylase activities (Cresteil,1985). This correlation is strengthened by the observation that isozyme 8 is absent from human fetal liver which has a very low benzopyrene hydroxylase activity. Only scarce data upon in vivo induction by polycyclic aromatic hydrocarbons are available from the literature. However, a clear relationship between heavy maternal smoking and increased placental benzopyrene hydroxylase activity has been reported (Pelkonen,1972).
Using a human breast carcinoma cell line (MCF 7) it has been possible to markedly stimulate benzopyrene hydroxylase activity by TCDD and benzanthracene A cDNA coding for the P1-450 has been isolated from a cDNA library derived from TCDD treated MCF 7 cells, homologous to the murine P1-450 cDNA cloned previously (Jaiswal,1985).
The aim of the present study was to investigate further the mechanism of induction in a human hepatocarcinoma cell line (Hep G2) in response to polycyclic aromatic hydrocarbons, regarding the presence of a TCDD-binding protein. The second step has been to determine the involvement of the P1-450 gene expression in normal and physiopathological conditions.

MATERIALS and METHODS
Tissue culture solutions and fetal calf serum are from Gibco. $(1,6\ ^3H)$-TCDD (27 Ci/mmol) was a generous gift from Dr.A.POLAND. MonoQ HR5/5 column was purchased from Pharmacia. All other reagents were from the finest grade available. $(\alpha^{32}P)$ dCTP (3000Ci/mmol) and $(\alpha^{32}P)$ UTP (3000Ci/mmol) were from Amersham.
MCF 7 cell line was obtained from Dr.M.LIPPMAN (NIH,Bethesda) and the human hepatoblastoma Hep G2 from Dr.B.KNOWLES (Philadelphia). Cultures were grown as monolayers at 37°C in 95% air and 5% CO_2 in α MEM medium supplemented with 10% fetal calf serum. Adult livers were obtained from donors for kidney transplantation and processed as previously described (Kremers,1981). Fetal livers were those already investigated (Cresteil,1985).
Benzopyrene hydroxylase activity. Tissue culture flasks were washed with Dulbecco's sodium phosphate buffered saline. Cells were scraped, pelleted and homogenized for 5 sec by sonication in 0.25 M Tris buffer, pH 7.6. Activity was determined as previously described (Nebert,1978). In liver, activity was assayed on microsomes according to Van Cantfort et al (1977).
Gel electrophoresis of cellular proteins were performed according to Laemmli (1970) with 50 µg cell homogenate or 10 µg liver microsomes on a 9 percent polyacrylamide gel in presence of SDS. After electrotransfer to nitrocellulose, proteins were visualized by staining with peroxidase-conjugated immunoglobulins and 4-chloronaphtol (Guengerich,1982).

RNA measurement. Total RNA was isolated by the method of Chirgwin et al (1979). 10 to 20 μg of total RNA were applied to nitrocellulose with a Scheicher and Schull Minifold II apparatus and hybridizations conducted as recommended by the manufacturer. Membranes were finally washed with 0.1x SSC, 0.1% SDS at 52°C, then in 0.1x SSC at 45°C. Films were exposed for different times, developed and scanned at 600 nm. A human cardiac genomic DNA (pAc.H8.H) was obtained from Dr.N.BATTULA (NCI,Bethesda). phP1-450 5' was used for kinetic and dose-response investigations. For determinations in human liver, phP1-450 3' (Eco Rl-Eco Rl fragment, 1 kbp in lenght) and phP3-450 3' (Eco Rl-Sall fragment, 1.3 kbp long, devoid of repetitive sequence) were used. Prior to investigations, we have checked that no cross reaction occurred between these fragments. Nick-translations were carried out with the Amersham kit, generating probes with specific radioactivities 10 dpm/μg DNA.

Cytosolic fractions were obtained by homogeneization of cells or tissues in HEDG (25 mM 4-(2-hydroxyethyl)-1-piperazineethansulfonic acid, 1.5 mM EDTA, 1 mM dithiothreitol and 10% glycerol, pH 7.5). The 105,000 g supernatant fraction was stored at -196°C as 2ml aliquots without appreciable loss of binding capacity. Fractions were thawed, incubated for 1 h at 4°C with 5 nM (^{3}H)-TCDD in presence or not of an excess of cold TCDD (500 nM) and then loaded on an anion-exchange column (MonoQ HR5/5) equilibrated with 25 mM Hepes, pH 7.4. A linear gradient up to 0.5 M NaCl in 25 mM Hepes was then developed at a flow rate of 0.5 ml/min. Fractions were collected and counted for radioactivity. In separate experiments, hydroxyapatite adsorption assays were carried out according to Poellinger et al (1985). In another set of experiments, Hep G2 were treated in vivo for 16h with either 6nM (^{3}H)-TCDD or 6nM (^{3}H)-TCDD plus an excess 300 nM cold TCDD. After extensive washes with phosphate buffered saline, the nuclear fraction was prepared as described elsewhere (Legraverend,1982).

RESULTS AND DISCUSSION.

Benzopyrene hydroxylase activity. in MCF 7 and Hep G2 cells, benzopyrene hydroxylase activity (AHH) is very low : about 5 pmoles/min/mg protein. The addition of phenobarbital (1 or 5 mM for 48 h), dexamethasone (10^{-5} or 10^{-7} M for 48 h) or their combination has no effect on AHH activity. On the other hand, the addition of TCDD or benzanthracene to the culture medium for 24 h results in a raise of AHH activity reaching then up to 250-300 pmoles/min/mg protein. If the maximal velocity is about the same in both cell lines, this activity is achieved with different doses of TCDD : thus, the EC50 is around 1 nM in Hep G2 cells and 10 nM in MCF 7. In human liver, basal AHH activity is higher than in cells: 190 pmoles/min/mg microsomal protein corresponding to a 10-20 times higher activity. Of interest, no or very faint activity can be detected in fetal liver (Cresteil,1985).

RNA measurement. In cultured cells, the increased AHH activity has been positively correlated with the accumulation of cellular hP1-450 mRNA (Tukey,1982). Actually, EC50 reported for the accumulation of mRNA in response to TCDD treatment closely correspond to those calculated for AHH activity. In addition, run-off experiments clearly demonstrated that the accumulation of hP1-450mRNA is due to an activation of the gene transcription. In one subclone derived from the original MCF 7 cell line, the activation of transcription is lost and there is no further accumulation of hP1-450mRNA (Cresteil,1987).
Since in human cell lines a positive correlation exists between AHH activity and expression of the hP1-450 gene, the question arises of the expression of hP1-450 gene in the human liver. In previous studies, AHH, mephenytoin hydroxylase and 4-nitroanisole demethylase activities have shown a close relationship with the concentration of one isozyme called P450-8 or P450-MP. Furthermore, fetal livers are deprived of P450-MP and exhibited an extremely low AHH activity. So, two aspects have been examined: - Is P450 MP involved in AHH activity induced in human cell lines by TCDD ? - What is the expression level of P1-450 and P3-450 genes in human liver ?

In "fig 1", a western blot of human cell line proteins immunodetected with anti P450 MP is shown. A positive reaction is observed with 1 pmol P450 MP (homologous antigen) and with 10 μg of human liver microsomes. In both MCF 7

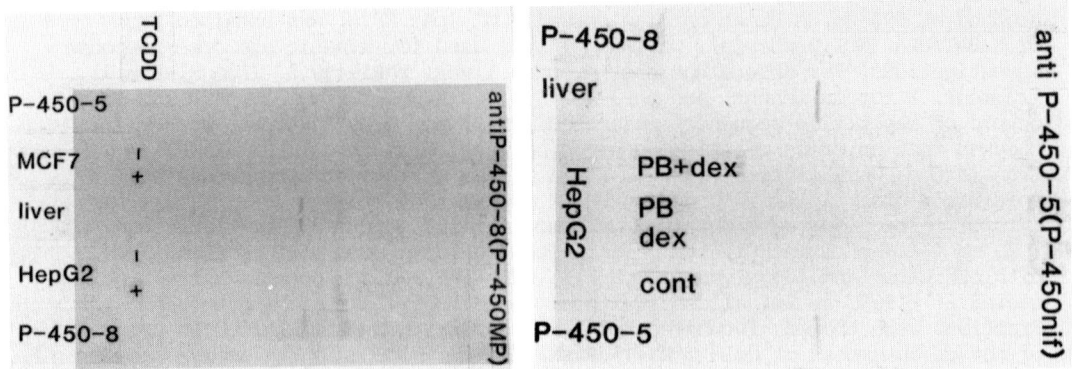

Figure 1: Immunoblot of cellular extracts from MCF 7 and Hep G2 cells treated with TCDD.

Cell homogenates (50μg), pure P450 MP or human liver microsomes (10μg) are detected with anti P450 MP.

Figure 2: Immunoblot of cellular extracts from Hep G2 cells treated with phenobarbital, dexamethasone or their combination.

Proteins are detected with anti P450-5 or nif.

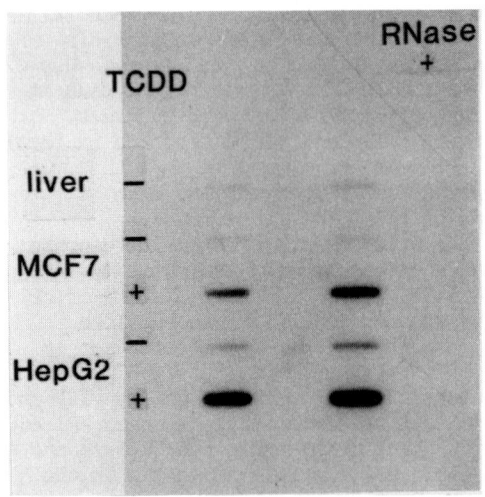

Figure 3: P1-450 mRNA content of MCF 7, Hep G2 and human liver.

10 and 20 μg total RNA were applied to nitrocellulose and hybridized with hP1-450 cDNA. Cells were treated or not with TCDD 16h before RNA isolation. In the lane on the right samples were treated with RNase before loading.

and Hep G2 cells, no cross reaction can be detected, even after an optimal TCDD pretreatment. This clearly demonstrated that the expression of P450 MP, if any, remains extremely low in these cell lines: less than 1 pmole P450 in 50 µg protein. Similarly, Hep G2 cells treated with phenobarbital and/or dexamethasone did not exhibit any cross reactivity with anti P450-5 (or NF), another major P450 isozyme in the human liver (fig 2). So, Hep G2 cell line did not express constitutively or after induction the two major human liver P450 isozymes. In "fig 3", a slot-blot of human mRNAs probed with phP1-450 is shown. RNAs from adult human liver and from untreated MCF 7 or Hep G2 cells give a positive but weak signal. After digestion with RNase no signal are present demonstrating that only RNAs were hybridized. After an optimal TCDD treatment, the signal is dramatically enhanced in both cell lines. To ensure the reliability of this observation, an extended study was carried out on 12 adult and 7 fetal liver RNA preparations. Values are expressed as the ratio hP1-450 mRNA/actin mRNA or hP3-450 mRNA/actin mRNA to eliminate any error due to sample loading. However a large interindividual variation can be reported: for P1-450, values range from 0.4 to 7.1 (mean 3.58 $\pm$ 2.13, n=12) and for P3-450 from 0.2 to 1.4 (mean 0.48 $\pm$ 0.42). In human fetal liver, P1-450 values are from 0.4 to 3.1 (mean 1.22 $\pm$ 0.92, n=7) and P3-450 from 0.15 to 0.96 (mean 0.37 $\pm$ 0.27).

So, the hP3-450mRNA seems less abundant that the hP1-450mRNA in the liver, whatever the age studied. This also demonstrates that the expression of P1 and P3 450 genes remains nearly constant, while AHH exhibits a marked onset of activity. Taken together, these data suggest that P1-450 and P3-450 are not the major isozymes involved in benzopyrene metabolism in the human liver and conversely that TCDD and other polycyclic aromatic hydrocarbons are ineffective to induce P450 MP in cultured human cell lines.

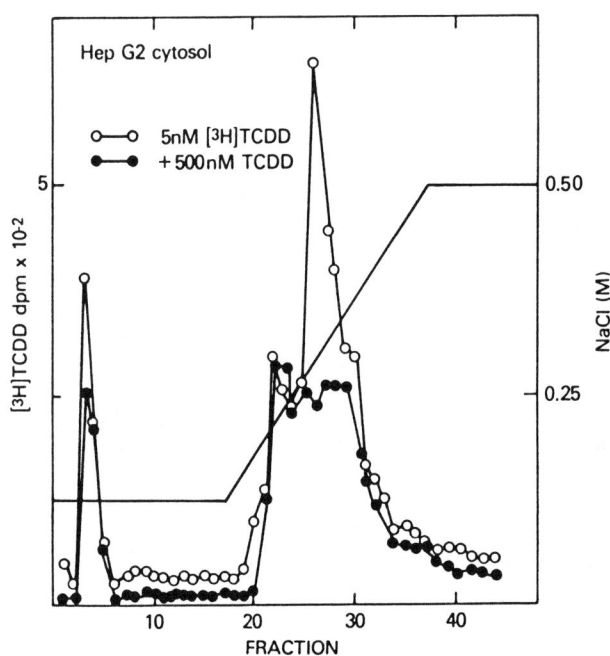

Figure 4: Elution profile of cytosolic TCDD-binding protein from MonoQ column

2.5 mg cytosolic protein were incubated for 1h with 5 nM ^{3}H-TCDD with or without an excess of cold TCDD. Samples were loaded on the column and eluted with a linear gradient of NaCl in 25mM Hepes buffer at a flow rate of 0.5 ml/min.

Another factor implicated in the induction process by TCDD is the cellular TCDD binding protein described in mouse and rat cells. Figure 4 shows a typical elution profile from MonoQ column loaded with Hep G2 cytosol. Two binding proteins were resolved: the first is eluted very soon and may reasonably be hypothesized to correspond to the 4S binding protein described in rat liver (Houser,1985). The second protein is the major ^{3}H-TCDD binding moiety. Its concentration is relatively low: about 8 fmoles/mg protein. In human liver, the binding of ^{3}H-TCDD to cytosolic protein is approximatively 5 fmoles/mg protein. Thus, in Hep G2 cells, the TCDD binding protein remains expressed at the same level as in liver and thus validate this model for induction studies.

When administered ex vivo in the culture medium, ^{3}H-TCDD is translocated to the nuclear compartment. In extracts from isolated nuclei, ^{3}H-TCDD is shown to be specifically associated with a protein retained on MonoQ column, but eluted at a salt concentration (0.23 M NaCl versus 0.30) and with a total binding capacity lower than the cytosolic binding protein (fig 5). In a murine hepatoma cell line (Hepa 1) well characterized for its induction process, the binding capacity is much higher. However, in spite of its low level, the whole pathway implicated in TCDD or other polycyclic aromatic hydrocarbons is present and active in human tissues derived cell lines, suggesting a potential efficency in human beings.

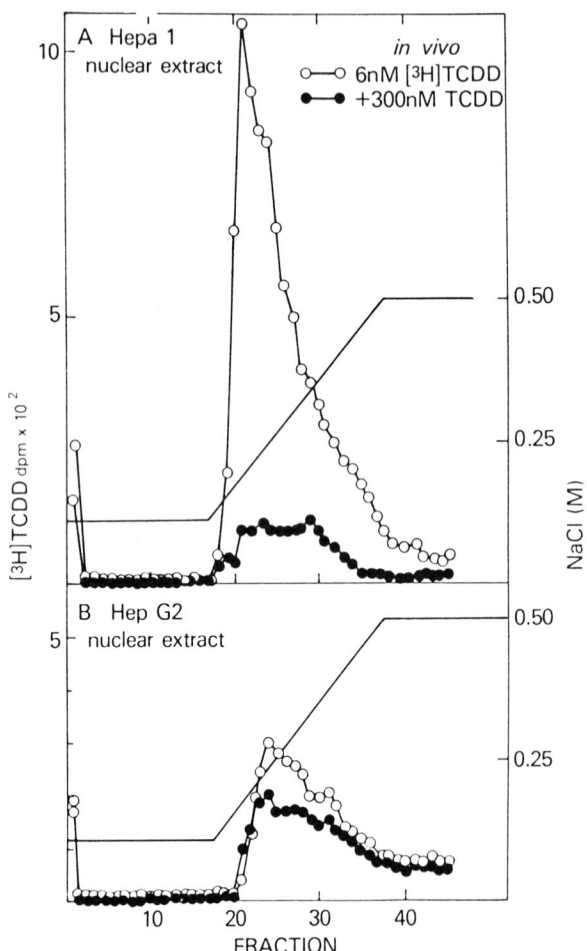

Figure 5: Elution profile of nuclear extracts from Hepa 1 and Hep G2 cells treated with H-TCDD.

Cells were treated for 16h with ^{3}H-TCDD, nuclear extracts prepared and injected on MonoQ column. A linear gradient of NaCl in 25 mM Hepes buffer was developed at 0.5 ml/min.

REFERENCES

Chirgwin,J.M., Przybyla,A.E., MacDonald,R.J., Rutter, W.J. (1979). Isolation of biologically active ribonucleic acid from sources enriched in ribonuclease. Biochemistry, 18, 5294-5299.

Cresteil,T., Beaune,P., Kremers,P., Celier,C., Guengerich,F.P., Leroux,J.P. (1985). Immunoquantification of epoxide hydrolase and cytochrome P450 isozymes in fetal and adult human liver microsomes. Eur.J.Biochem. 151, 345-350.

Cresteil,T., Jaiswal,A.K., Eisen,H.J. (1987). Transcriptional control of human cytochrome P1-450 gene expression by 2,3,7,8 tetrachlorodibenzo-p-dioxin in human tissue culture cell lines. Arch.Biochem.Biophys. 253,233-240.

Eisen,H.J. (1986). Induction of hepatic P450 isozymes. in Cytochrome P450, Ed Ortiz de Montellano, pp 315-344, London, Plenum Press.

Guengerich,F.P., Dannan,G.A., Wright,S.T., Martin,M.V., Kaminsky,L.S. (1982). Purification and characterization of microsomal cytochromes P450: electrophoretic, spectral, catalytic and immunochemical properties and inducibility of eight isoenzymes isolated from rats treated with phenobarbital or naphthoflavone. Biochemistry, 21, 6019-6030.

Houser,W.H., Hines, R.N., Bresnick,E. (1985). Implication of the 4S polycyclic aromatic hydrocarbon binding protein in the transregulation of rat cytochrome P450c expression. Biochemistry, 24, 7839-7845.

Jaiswal,A.K., Gonzalez,F.J., Nebert,D.W. (1985). Human dioxin-inducible cytochrome P1-450: complementary DNA and amino acid sequence. Science, 228, 80-83.

Kremers,P., Beaune,P., Cresteil,T., deGraeve,J., Columelli,S., Leroux,J.P., Gielen,J.E. (1981). Cytochrome P450 monooxygenase activities in human and rat liver microsomes. Eur.J.Biochem. 118,599-606.

Laemmli,U.K. (1970). Cleavage of structural proteins during the assembly of the head of bacteriophage T4. Nature, 227, 680-685.

Legraverend,C., Hannah,R.R., Eisen,H.J., Owens,I.S., Nebert,D.W., Hankinson,O. (1982). Regulatory gene products of the Ah locus. Characterization of receptor mutants among mouse hepatoma clones. J.Biol.Chem. 257, 6402-6407.

Nebert,D.W. (1978). Genetic differences affecting microsomal electron transport: the Ah locus. Methods Enzymol. LII, 226-240.

Negishi,M., Nebert,D.W. (1979). Structural gene products of the Ah locus. Genetic control and immunochemical evidence for two forms of mouse liver cytochrome P450 induced by 3 methylcholanthrene. J.Biol.Chem. 254, 11015-11023.

Poellinger,L., Lund,J., Dahlberg,E., Gustafsson, J.A. (1985). A hydroxyapatite microassay for receptor binding of 2,3,7,8 tetrachlorodibenzo-p-dioxin and 3 methylcholanthrene in various target tissues. Anal.Biochem. 144, 371-384.

Pelkonen,O., Jouppila,P., Karki,N.T. (1972). Effect of maternal cigarette smoking on 3,4 benzopyrene and n-methylaniline metabolism in human fetal liver and placenta. Toxicol.Appl.Pharmacol. 23,399-407.

Tukey,R.H., Hannah,R.R., Negishi,M., Nebert,D.W., Eisen,H.J. (1982). The Ah locus. Correlation of intranuclear appearance of inducer-receptor complex with induction of cytochrome P1-450 mRNA. Cell, 31, 275-284.

Van Cantfort,J., deGreave,J., Gielen,J.E. (1977). Radioactive assay for aryl hydrocarbon hydroxylase. Improved method and biological importance. Biochem. Biophys.Res.Commun. 79, 505-512.

Résumé

La régulation du cytochrome P1-450 humain a été étudié dans des lignées cellulaires d'origine humaine et corrélé avec la présence d'éléments régulateurs. Une protéine liant spécifiquement le TCDD a été mis en évidence dans certaines lignées et permet l'induction par ce composé. Ceci permet de penser que le modèle décrit chez l'animal est également valide dans l'espèce humaine. Dans ces lignées, le cytochrome P450 MP qui catalyse l'hydroxylation du benzopyrène dans le foie humain n'a pu être détecté. Dans le foie foetal, dépourvu d'activité benzopyrene hydroxylase, l'expression des gènes P1-450 et P3-450 n'est pas différente de celles observées dans le foie adulte. L'absence de corrélation entre l'expression du gène P1-450 et l'activité enzymatique suggère que ce cytochrome P1-450 est seulement un constituant mineur de l'activité benzopyrène hydroxylase du foie humain.

The structure and regulation of UDP glucuronosyltransferases in the rat

Peter Ian Mackenzie, Saikh J. Haque

Laboratory of Developmental Pharmacology, National Institute of Child Health and Human Development, National Institutes of Health, Bethesda, Maryland 20892, USA

ABSTRACT

The primary amino acid sequences of several forms of rat liver UDP glucuronosyltransferase (UDPGT) have been established from the cloning and sequencing of their corresponding cDNAs. These enzymes are encoded by a superfamily of genes where the similarities between sequences can vary from 15 to 60 percent. However, despite a sometimes wide divergence in amino acid sequence, each form has similar structural characteristics. These include a signal peptide which is cleaved during insertion of the nascent enzyme into the endoplasmic reticulum and a carboxy-terminal hydrophobic segment preceeding a short basic tail. Based on these structural motifs, a model is proposed in which the enzyme is localized to the luminal surface of the endoplasmic reticulum. The preparation of cDNA probes has also enabled an investigation of the temporal and tissue distribution of UDPGT mRNAs and their regulation by foreign chemicals. The results of these studies demonstrate that the mRNAs of constitutive forms, or that inducible by phenobarbital, are found mainly in the liver and are elevated postnatally, whereas the mRNA of a 3-methylcholanthrene-inducible form is also found in other tissues and is present before birth. These data indicate that the differential glucuronidation of several aglycones during development and in various tissues is a consequence of changes in mRNA levels, rather than membrane-modulated alterations in the enzymes' catalytic properties.

KEYWORDS

UDP glucuronosyltransferases, primary structures, tissue and temporal expression, induction

INTRODUCTION

UDP Glucuronosyltransferase (EC 2.4.1.17) catalyzes the conjugation of the sugar acid moiety of high-energy UDP glucuronic acid to thousands of chemicals to form B-D-glucopyranosiduronic acids (glucuronides). This process increases the polarity of the compound, which is often lipophilic and aids in its solubility in bile or urine and its subsequent excretion from the body (Dutton, 1980). For this reason, glucuronidation often reduces the toxicity of many foreign chemicals, such as polycyclic aromatic hydrocarbons, by decreasing their time of exposure to critical internal targets. Furthermore, reduction of the efficacy of therapeutic drugs may occur by masking their biologically-active moieties with the conjugating molecule. In some cases, however, the glucuronide may be more reactive or toxic. For example, the hepatotoxicity of the hypolipidemic drug, clofibrate, is thought to be a consequence of the reaction of its electrophilic acyl glucuronide with thiol groups on cell proteins (van Breeman and Fenselau, 1985).

Endogenous molecules such as bilirubin, fat-soluble vitamins and steroid hormones are also substrates of UDPGT. The glucuronides are usually excreted although in some cases a glucuronide may be the substrate of another enzyme (e.g. the 3α-glucuronide of 17α-estradiol is a substrate for a phenolic steroid 17α-dehydrogenase; Williamson, 1971), or regulators of physiological processes (e.g. the cholestatic effects of steroid D-ring glucuronides; Meyers et al., 1981).

Several forms of rat liver UDP glucuronosyltransferase have been isolated and purified (Falany and Tephly, 1983; Falany et al., 1983; Burchell and Blanckaert, 1984; Puig and Tephly, 1986; Roy Chowdhury et al., 1986), however, the number of forms which handle this vast array of structurally-diverse chemicals is unknown. The complex induction and developmental profiles and tissue distributions of glucuronidating activities (Dutton, 1980) indicate that each enzyme is regulated differently. The critical nature of this regulation is exemplified well in patients with Crigler Najjar syndrome who lack a fuctional bilirubin UDPGT and accumulate toxic amounts of bilirubin (Billing, 1987), and in infants with grey baby syndrome where a delay in the development of certain forms of UDPGT results in severe chloramphenicol toxicity (Biancaniello et al., 1981).

It is now apparent that recombinant DNA technology offers an excellent tool for investigating the structure of UDPGTs and the molecular mechanisms underlying their regulation. The results of these investigations will be the subject of this report.

STRUCTURE OF UDP GLUCURONOSYLTRANSFERASES

The cDNAs to four forms of transferase have so far been cloned and sequenced (Iyanagi, 1986; Jackson and Burchell, 1986; Mackenzie, 1986a,b, 1987; Harding et al., 1987). Expression of three of these cDNAs in tissue culture demonstrated that one form, $UDPGT_r-2$, encodes a 529 residue polypeptide active in the glucuronidation of the steroids, testosterone and β-estradiol, and foreign chemicals, such as 4-hydroxybiphenyl, 4-methylumbelliferone and chloramphenicol (Mackenzie, 1986a, 1987). A second form, $UDPGT_r-3$, is a 530 residue enzyme which also glucuronidates these steroids, whereas a third form, $UDPGT_r-4$, (530 amino acids) is more active towards androsterone, etiocholanolone and bile acids (Mackenzie, 1986b, 1987). The fourth cDNA encodes a form of transferase (530 residues) which glucuronidates 4-nitrophenol (Iyanagi, 1986) but its capacity to glucuronidate other substrates has not been examined in situ as yet. The percent similarities in protein sequence of the four forms of transferase shown in Table 1, indicate that they are encoded by a superfamily of genes. Despite the wide divergence in protein sequence, however, conserved regions between the proteins can be observed. For example, even though the overall homology between $UDPGT_r-2$ and 4NPGT is 43%, the carboxy-terminal halves of these proteins are more similar ($\approx 60\%$) than the amino-terminal halves ($\approx 30\%$). Furthermore, each form has the following structural characteristics in common: a leader

Table 1. Percent similarity of the deduced amino acid sequence of four UDP glucuronosyltransferase cDNAs*

	$UDPGT_r-2$	$UDPGT_r-3$	$UDPGT_r-4$	4NPGT
$UDPGT_r-2$	100			
$UDPGT_r-3$	68	100		
$UDPGT_r-4$	68	82	100	
4NPGT	43	45	43	100

*Compiled from Iyanagi et al., 1986 and Mackenzie 1986a,b, 1987).

peptide which is cleaved during synthesis of the protein on the endoplasmic reticulum (Mackenzie, 1986a, 1987); a clustering of cysteine residues in the amino half of the protein; and a potential "halt transfer" signal composed of a very hydrophobic segment of 17 residues preceeding a region rich in basic amino acids at the carboxy-terminus (Fig. 1). These common structural motifs suggest that during synthesis, the nascent chain is translocated across the endoplasmic reticulum membrane until this process is halted by the "halt-transfer" signal. Thus, over 95% of the protein would be orientated on the luminal side of the endoplasmic reticulum with the basic carboxy-terminus interacting with phospholipids of the cytoplasic face of the membrane (Iyanagi, 1986; Mackenzie, 1986a). A possible model of this topology is shown in Fig. 2. The more conserved nature of the carboxy-terminal halves of these transferases may indicate the involvement in mutual functions such as the binding of the common cosubstrate, UDP glucuronic acid. This binding site is probably hydrophilic and hence is depicted as being more exposed in the lumen. The amino-terminal half of the protein which shows greater variability may perhaps bind the more varied and hydrophobic aglycone and hence is depicted partly embedded in the membrane. The preponderance of cysteine residues in this area may help to stabilize any tertiary structure via disulfide bonds in a manner analogous to the stabilization of the structure of

```
                    1                     24 Y  Y
UDPGTr-2    MSMKQTSVELLIQLICYFRPGAC G--Y---Y--
                                       ↑
UDPGTr-3    MPGKWISALLLLQISCCFQSGNC G--------
                                       ↑
UDPGTr-4    MPRKWISALFLLQISYCFKSGHC G---Y----
                                       ↑
4NPGT       MACLLPAARLPAGELFLVLWGSVL G--Y_Y_Y--
                                       ↑

            495                                529
UDPGTr-2    VIGFLLLCVVGVVFIIT KFCLFCCRKTANMGKKKKE
                              +       ++  ++++-
UDPGTr-3    VIGFLLTCSAVIAVLTV KCFLFIYRLFVKKEKKMKNE
                              +       + ++-++ + -
UDPGTr-4    VIGFLLTCFAVIAALTV KCLLFMYRFFVKKEKKMKNE
                              +       + ++-++ + -
4NPGT       VIGFLLAIVLTVVFIVY KSCAYGCRKCFGGKGRVFFSHKSHTH
                              +      ++    + +     +
```

Fig. 1. Leader peptides and potential halt-transfer signals in UDP glucuronosyltransferases. The probable cleavage site (Harding et al., 1987) is arrowed, charged residues are denoted, hydrophobic segments are underlined and the number of potential N-linked glycosylation sites are indicated (Y). Sequence data is from Iyanagi, 1986 and Mackenzie, 1986a,b, 1987.

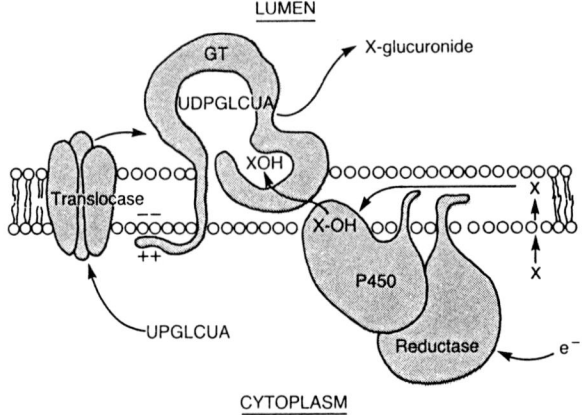

Fig. 2. Model for the orientation of UDP glucuronosyltransferase in the endoplasmic reticulum. A hydrophobic compound (X) is hydroxylated by monooxygenase and binds to the membrane-embedded amino domain of UDP glucuronosyltransferase (GT). UDPglcUA is transported into the lumen by a translocase and binds to the GT carboxy-domain. Conjugation occurs and the glucuronide is released into the lumen of the endoplasmic reticulum. GT remains membrane-bound via its carboxy-terminus and is regulated by the interaction of its aglycone-binding domain with phospholipids.

phospholipase A_2, another membrane-bound enzyme (Maraganore, 1987). This membrane association would also permit the modulation of catalytic activities by phospholipids and other hydrophobic molecules such as detergents (Zakim and Vessey, 1982).

As the endoplasmic reticulum is impermeable to charged sugars, a sugar translocase is needed to transport UDP glucuronic acid, which is made in the cytoplasm, to the lumen. Experimental evidence suggests the plausible existance of such a translocase (Vanstabel and Blanckaert, 1987).

REGULATION OF UDP GLUCURONOSYLTRANSFERASES

Tissue distribution
The transferase cDNAs $UDPGT_r$-2, 3 and 4, belonging to the same family, have mRNA counterparts which are more than 20-fold elevated in liver compared to small intestinal mucosa and which are barely detectable in other organs such as testis, kidney, lung and brain (Fig. 3; Mackenzie, 1987; Roy Chowdhury et al., 1987; unpublished data). In contrast, 4NPGT mRNA levels are high in liver, kidney and small intestinal mucosa (Iyanagi et al., 1986; unpublished data). The tissue specific expression of these genes are in agreement with earlier data demonstrating that the glucuronidation of steroids and foreign compounds such as 4-hydroxybiphenyl, morphine and chloramphenicol which are substrates of $UDPGT_r$-2, 3 and 4, occurs predominantly in the liver whereas activities towards 1-naphthol and 4-nitrophenol are present in several extrahepatic tissues (Lucier et al., 1977; Bock et al., 1980).

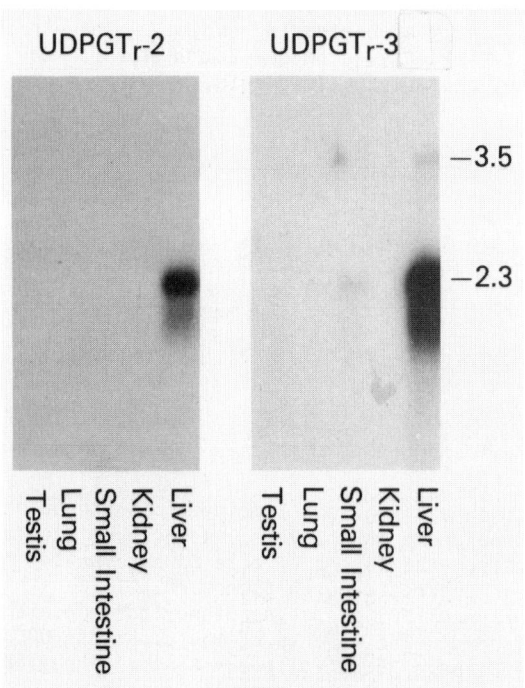

Fig. 3. Levels of UDP glucuronosyltransferase mRNAs in different tissues. Poly(A) RNA was isolated from various tissues, electrophoresed, transferred to nitrocellulose and probed with ^{32}P-labelled UDPGT$_r$-2 and UDPGT$_r$-3 probes.

Induction by foreign chemicals

Phenobarbital elevates the levels of UDPGT$_r$-2 mRNA at least 5-fold in the liver but, under the same experimental conditions, had little effect on the levels of UDPGT$_r$-3, 4 and 4NPGT mRNAs (Fig. 4). This correlates well with the phenobarbital-induced increase in the glucuronidation of the UDPGT$_r$-2 substrates, 4-hydroxybiphenyl and chloramphenicol which has been reported previously (Lilienblum et al., 1982).

3-Methylcholanthrene, which increases the rates of glucuronidation of 4-nitrophenol and 1-naphthol (Lilienblum et al., 1982), also elevates the level of 4NPGT mRNA 15-fold in the liver (Fig. 4). The mRNA levels of 3-methylcholanthrene-inducible P450s which were a positive control in these experiments, were similarly increased. In contrast, the other transferase mRNAs were unaffected.

Pregnenolone-16α-carbonitrile (PCN) has been shown to increase the glucuronidation of digitoxigen monodigitoxide 20-fold, a process believed to be mediated by increased levels of a specific transferase form (Watkins et al., 1982). This chemical had no significant effects on the mRNA counterparts of UDPGT$_r$-2, 3 and 4 (Fig. 4). However, the levels of larger species of mRNA (3.7 and 4.5 kb) were elevated by this compound, suggesting that these RNA's may encode digitoxigenin monodigitoxide-glucuronidating enzymes. The effects of other inducers of drug-metabolizing enzymes on UDPGT mRNA levels were also investigated (Fig. 5). Dexamethasone, rifampicin, imidazole, methylpyrazole and pyrazole

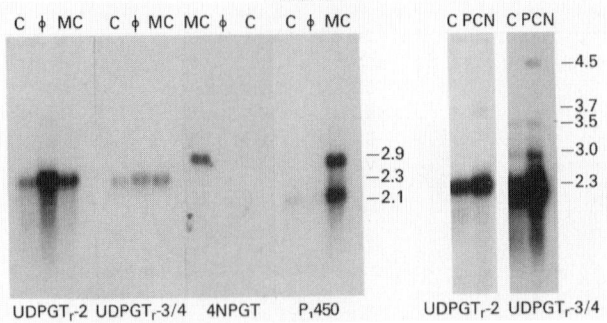

Fig. 4. The effect of phenobarbital and 3-methylcholanthrene on UDP glucuronosyltransferase mRNA levels. A Northern analysis of poly(A) RNA from the livers of male Sprague-Dawley rats untreated (C) or pretreated with phenobarbital (∅) 3-methylcholanthrene (MC) or pregnenolone-16α-carbonitrile (PCN) was performed. The inserts of the plasmids pUDPGT$_r$-2 and 4 and pP$_1$450 and a 36-mer oligomer to the 5'-region of 4NPGT cDNA were radiolabeled and used as probes.

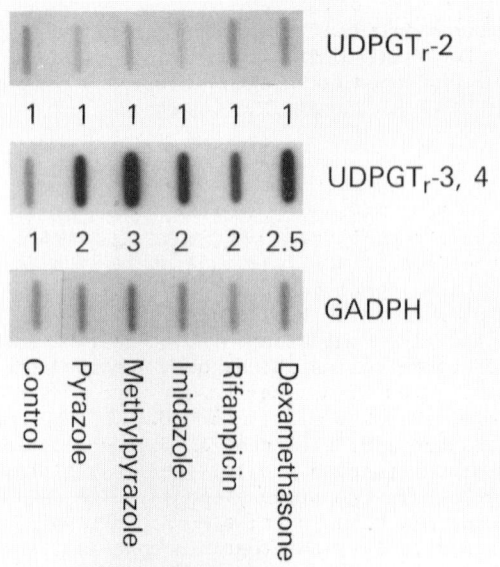

Fig. 5. Effect of xenobiotics on UDPGT mRNA levels. Rats were treated with the indicated compounds and total liver RNA was analyzed on slot-blots using UDPGT$_r$-2, UDPGT$_r$-4 and glyceraldehyde-3-phosphate-dehydrogenase (GADPH) as probes. The fold induction after standardization with the control probe, GADPH, is indicated.

elevated the mRNA levels of members of the subfamily typified by UDPGT$_r$-3 and 4, 2- to 3-fold but had no apparent effect on the more distantly related subfamily represented by UDPGT$_r$-2.

Expression of UDP glucuronosyltransferases during development
Studies in rat liver demonstrate that 4-nitrophenol, 1-naphthol and other substrates of 3-methylcholanthrene-inducible transferases, increase towards adult levels during late gestation whereas activities towards steroids, bilirubin and some substrates of phenobarbital-inducible forms increase after birth (Wishart, 1978). Preliminary data confirm these findings at the mRNA level. Thus, the levels of UDPGT$_r$-2, 3 and 4 mRNAs are elevated after birth whereas the 4NPGT mRNA level is elevated before birth (unpublished data).

CONCLUSION

The use of recombinant DNA techniques has demonstrated that UDPGTs have structural motifs in common and are encoded by a superfamily of genes. These techniques have also provided an alternative approach to analyzing the substrate specificities of each form and have opened the way for investigating the temporal and tissue-specific expression of UDPGT genes and their regulation by xenobiotics and other factors.

REFERENCES

Biancaniello, T., Meyer, R.A. and Kaplan, S.(1981): Chloramphenicol and cardiotoxicity. J. Pediatr. 98, 828-830.
Billing, B.H.(1987): Bilirubin metabolism. In Diseases of the Liver, 6th edn, ed L. Schiff and E.R. Schiff, pp 103-127. Philadelphia: J.B. Lippincott Co.
Bock, K.W., v. Clausbruch, U.C., Kaufmann, R., Lilienblum, W., Oesch, F., Pfeil, H. and Platt, K.L.(1980): Functional heterogeneity of UDP-glucuronyltransferase in rat tissues. Biochem. Pharmacol. 29, 495-500.
Burchell, B. and Blanckaert, N.(1984): Bilirubin mono- and di-glucuronide formation by purified rat liver microsomal bilirubin UDP-glucuronyltransferase. Biochem. J. 223, 461-465.
Dutton, G.J.(1980): Glucuronidation of Drugs and Other Compounds, pp 3-51. Boca Raton, Florida: CRC Press, Inc.
Falany, C.N., Roy Chowdhury, J., Roy Chowdhury, N. and Tephly, T.R.(1983): Steroid 3- and 17-OH UDP-glucuronosyltransferase activities in rat and rabbit liver microsomes. Drug Metab. Disp. 11, 426-432.
Falany, C.N. and Tephly, T.R.(1983): Separation, purification and characterization of three isoenzymes of UDP-glucuronyltransferase from rat liver microsomes. Arch. Biochem. Biophys. 227, 248-258.
Harding, D., Wilson, S.M., Jackson, M.R., Burchell, B., Green, M.D. and Tephly, T.R.(1987): Nucleotide and deduced amino-acid sequence of rat liver 17β-hydroxysteroid UDP-glucuronosyltransferase. Nucl. Acids Res. 15, 3936.
Iyanagi, T., Haniu, M., Sogawa, K., Fujii-Kuriyama, Y., Watanabe, S., Shively, J.E. and Anan, K.F.(1986): Cloning and characterization of cDNA encoding 3-methylcholanthrene inducible rat mRNA from UDP-glucuronosyltransferase. J. Biol. Chem. 261, 15607-15614.
Jackson, M.R. and Burchell, B.(1986): The full length coding sequence of rat liver androsterone UDP-glucuronyltransferase cDNA and comparison with other members of the gene family. Nucl. Acids Res. 14, 779-795.
Lilienblum, W., Walli, A.K. and Bock, K.W.(1982): Differential induction of rat liver microsomal UDP-glucuronosyltransferase activities by various inducing agents. Biochem. Pharmacol. 31, 907-913.

Lucier, G.W. and McDaniel, O.S.(1977): Steroid and non-steroid UDP glucuronyltransferase: Glucuronidation of synthetic estrogens as steroids. J. Steroid Biochem. 8, 867-872.

Mackenzie, P.I.(1986a): Rat liver UDP-glucuronosyltransferase. Sequence and expression of a cDNA encoding a phenobarbital-inducible form. J. Biol. Chem. 261, 6119-6125.

Mackenzie, P.I.(1986b): Rat liver UDP-glucuronosyltransferase. cDNA sequence and expression of a form glucuronidating 3-hydroxyandrogens. J. Biol. Chem. 261, 14112-14117.

Mackenzie, P.I. (1987): Rat liver UDP-glucuronosyltransferase. Identification of cDNAs encoding two enzymes which glucuronidate testosterone, dihydrotestosterone and β-estradiol. J. Biol. Chem., in press.

Maraganore, J.M.(1987): Structural elements for protein--phospholipid interactions may be shared in protein kinase C and phospholipases A_2. Trends Biochem. Sci. 12, 176-177.

Meyers, M., Slikker, W. and Vore, M.(1981): Steroid D-ring glucuronides: Characterization of a new class of cholestatic agents in the rat. J. Pharmacol. Exp. Ther. 218, 63-73.

Puig, J.F. and Tephly, T.R.(1986): Isolation and purification of rat liver morphine UDP-glucuronosyltransferase. Mol. Pharmacol. 30, 558-565.

Roy Chowdhury, J., Roy Chowdhury, N., Falany, C.N., Tephly, T.R. and Arias, I.M.(1986): Isolation and characterization of multiple forms of rat liver UDP-glucuronate glucuronosyltransferase. Biochem. J. 233, 827-837.

Roy-Chowdhury, N., Saber, M., Mackenzie, P. and Roy-Chowdhury, J.(1987): Cloning of multiple UDP-glucuronosyltransferase (UDPGT)-cDNAs: Expression of various isoforms in tissues and in carcinogen-induced liver modules. Gastroenterology 92, 1768.

van Breemen, R.B. and Fenselau, C.(1985): Acylation of albumin by 1-O-acyl glucuronides. Drug Metab. Disp. 13, 318-320.

Vanstapel, F. and Blanckaert, N.(1987): Endogenous esterification of bilirubin by liver microsomes. Evidence for an intramicrosomal pool of UDP-glucose and lumenal orientation of bilirubin UDP-glycosyltransferase. J. Biol. Chem. 262, 4616-4623.

Watkins, J.B., Gregus, Z., Thompson, T.N. and Klaassen, C.D.(1982): Induction studies on the functional heterogeneity of rat liver UDP-glucuronosyltransferases. Toxicol. Appl. Pharmacol. 64, 439-446.

Williamson, D.G.(1972): Evidence for rabbit liver phenolic steroid 17α-dehydrogenase which is more active on estradiol 17α, 3α-glucuronide than on free steroid. Proc. Can. Fed. Biol. Soc. 14, 97.

Wishart, G.J.(1978): Functional heterogeneity of UDP-glucuronosyltransferase as indicated by its differential development and inducibility by glucocorticoids. Demonstration of two groups within the enzyme's activity towards twelve substrates. Biochem. J. 174, 485-489.

Zakim, D. and Vessey, D.A.(1982): The role of the microsomal membrane in modulating the activity of UDP-glucuronosyltransferase. In Membranes and Transport, Vol 1, ed A.N. Martonosi, pp 269-273. New York: Plenum Publishing Corp.

Résumé

Les méthodes d'ADN recombinants ont servi à déduire les séquences primaires d'acides aminés de plusieurs formes d'UDP glucuronyltranférases (UDPGT). Ces études ont démontré que celles-ci sont codées par une superfamille multigénique, les homologies de séquences pouvant varier de 15 à 60 %. Toutefois, même lorsqu'il existe une différence importante dans la séquence d'acides aminés, des motifs structuraux communs sont toujours observés. Ils incluent un peptide "leader" amino-terminal clivable, un ensemble de résidus de cysteine dans la moitié amino la moins conservée du polypeptide et un segment carboxy terminal hydrophobe précédant une courte extrémité basique. A partir de ces motifs, un modèle topographique a été proposé dans lequel l'enzyme est localisé sur la surface luminale du réticulum endoplasmique et est fixé par son groupement carboxy terminal. La modulation de l'activité catalytique par des phospholipides et la fluidité lipidiques sont probablement affectées par l'interaction du domaine amino-terminal avec la membrane. Des clones d'ADNc ont été utilisés pour étudier l'expression temporelle des UDPGT, leur spécificité tissulaire et leur régulation par des composés chimiques exogènes. L'ARNm de l'une des formes, appelée $UDPGT_r$-2 apparaît après la naissance, est augmenté 5 fois par le phénobarbital et est prédominant dans le foie. Les ARNm de deux autres formes, $UDPGT_r$-3 et $UDPGT_r$-4 ont une même expression temporelle et tissulaire mais ne sont pas augmentés par le phénobarbital. En revanche l'ARNm d'une forme plus éloignée, l'UDPGT induite par le méthylcholanthrène est présent dans d'autres tissus et exprimé en fin de gestation. Les différences de glucuroconjugaison de divers aglycones au cours du développement et dans des tissus hépatiques et extrahépatiques peuvent par conséquent provenir de variations dans les taux d'ARNm plutôt que d'altérations des propriétés catalytiques des enzymes modulées par les membranes. Ces résultats illustrent l'utilité des techniques d'ADN recombinant pour caractériser la structure et analyser la régulation de cette superfamille d'enzymes de glucuroconjugaison.

Glutathione transferases

Brian Ketterer, David J. Meyer, Brian Coles, John B. Taylor

Cancer Research Campaign Molecular Toxicology Research Group, Biochemistry Department, University College and Middlesex School of Medicine, Cleveland, London W1P 6DB, UK

SUMMARY

GSH transferases are dimers of subunits of Mr approximately 25,000. In rat and man they are products of at least three multigene families, close homology existing between the two species in corresponding families. GSH transferases catalyse a number of GSH dependent reactions including the GSH conjugation of electrophiles and the reduction of lipid and DNA hydroperoxides. Each subunit has a characteristic substrate specificity and a particular tissue distribution. The latter may 1) vary during development, 2) be under hormonal control, 3) be induced by certain xenobiotics or 4) undergo a change in expression during chemical carcinogenesis or treatment with chemotherapeutic drugs. The role of these enzymes in the direct detoxication of electrophilic metabolites of drugs and carcinogens or the indirect detoxication of redox cycling anticancer drugs is described and discussed. Examples of electrophiles are metabolites of N,N-dimethyl-4-aminoazobenzene, N-acetyl-2-aminofluorene, benzo(a)pyrene, 1-nitropyrene, aflatoxin B1 and paracetamol. The principal redox cycling anti-cancer drug which has been studied is adriamycin. It is suggested that it brings about radical attack on nucleic acids and membranes to produce products which are susceptible to detoxication by GSH transferases.

KEY WORDS

Glutathione transferases, glutathione peroxidases, drugs, carcinogens

INTRODUCTION

The term glutathione (GSH) transferase defines an enzyme which catalyses the reaction of the cellular nucleophile GSH with an electrophile (EC 2.5.1.18) and as a result, these enzymes have been much studied because of their importance for the detoxication of the electrophilic metabolites of a number of drugs and carcinogens (Ketterer et al., 1986). This will be the major concern of this paper, however GSH transferases also have Se-independent GSH peroxidase activity and some of our attention is now being focused on the likely participation of the GSH transferases in systems for the repair of oxygen-centred free radical damage to membrane lipids and DNA (Ketterer et al., 1987). Therefore in this paper some attention will also be given to the possibility that such activity might also contribute to another type of drug detoxication reaction namely the detoxication of those cytotoxic anticancer drugs the activity of which depends on the consequences of oxygen-centred free radical production. The Se-independent GSH peroxidase activity of GSH transferases may be an important determinant of the susceptibility of both normal and tumour cells to these drugs.

STRUCTURES AND GENETIC RELATIONSHIPS OF GSH TRANSFERASES

Soluble GSH transferases are widely distributed throughout the animal and plant worlds where they are seen to consist of dimers of subunits with Mr approximately 25,000. The most detailed studies on the structures and genetic relationships of these enzymes concern rat and man. Of the two species most is known about the rat where at least 12 subunits have been identified. Several nomenclatures exist for the rat, but that devised by Jakoby et al. (1983) is the simplest, each subunit being named numerically in the chronological order of its identification and characterization. So far 3, perhaps 4, multigene families have been identified, namely one containing subunits 1 and 2, a second containing subunits 3, 4 and 6, a third containing subunit 7 and perhaps a fourth containing subunit 5, which is still under study. Full length cDNA clones are available for subunits 1, 2, 3, 4 and 7 (Taylor et al., 1987) and partial sequences for subunits 5 and 6 (D.J. Meyer, C. Southan, K.H. Tan, E. Lalor and B. Ketterer, unpublished information). From this data it is seen that homology is high within a family (at least 70%), but low (about 25%) between families (Taylor et al., 1987). In addition to homodimers, subunits within families can form heterodimers, giving rise to a large number of isoenzymes. Thus in the rat liver the isoenzymes so far identified are 1-1, 1-2, 2-2, 3-3, 3-4, 3-6, 4-4, 4-6 and 5-5. GSH transferase 6-6 is most notable in the spermatogenic tissue of the testis while GSH transferase 7-7 is present in a number of extra-hepatic tissues and is also expressed in hepatocytes during preneoplasia and neoplasia induced by chemical carcinogens (Ketterer et al., 1986).

Similar GSH transferase families occur in man. A number of basic isoenzymes have been separated which are either homodimers or heterodimers of two subunits or subunit classes referred to here (there is no established nomenclature as yet) as α_x and α_y (see Ostlund Farrants et al., 1987). Up to 16 components can be separated and these fall into six classes on chromatofocusing f.p.l.c. Those eluting at the highest extreme of pH are homodimers of α_x and those at the lowest α_y, while the intermediate forms are the heterodimers $\alpha_x\alpha_y$. The basis of the apparent multiplicity of these α-type basic forms remains to be clarified. So far, two cDNA clones for α subunits have been sequenced and shown to be homologous with rat subunits 1 and 2 (Board & Webb, 1987; Rhoads et al., 1987). A neutral human GSH transferase, referred to as µ, has been obtained and its N-terminal sequence shown to have close homology with the N-termini of rat subunits 3, 4 and 6 and an acidic GSH transferase with similar enzymic properties and referred to as ψ also appears to belong to the same class (Hayes et al., 1987). Finally another acidic GSH transferase, first isolated from the placenta and called π, is highly homologous to rat subunit 7 (Cowell et al., 1987). Human GSH transferases ρ and λ from red blood cells and lung respectively are either identical to π or additional homologous forms. Thus, the same three families occur in man as in rat: namely α_x and α_y which are homologous with the rat subunit 1/2 family; µ and ψ which are homologous to the subunit 3/4/6 family; and π, ρ and λ which are homologous to the subunit 7 family. These families in rat and man (and also similar families in mice) are given the designations namely alpha, mu and pi respectively. In general the enzymic activities described below with reference to rat GSH transferase isoenzymes are similar in homologous human GSH transferases (Mannervik et al., 1985). The human equivalent of subunit 5 has yet to be studied.

GSH TRANSFERASES AND THE DETOXICATION OF ELECTROPHILES

General considerations

Lipophilic xenobiotics are often detoxified and excreted in two steps. Phase I involves reaction with mixed function oxygenases such as the cytochrome P-450s: the result is either hydroxylation or the formation of an electrophile. Phase II involves conjugation. Where Phase I results in hydroxylation, sulphation or glucuronidation gives rise to soluble conjugates which are excreted. Where the product of Phase I is an electrophile, reaction with the abundant cellular nucleophile GSH gives a conjugate which is also soluble and readily excreted. In addition to its role in excretion the conjugation of electrophiles with GSH is important because they have the potential to react with other cellular nucleophiles with toxic consequences: for instance, electrophiles which react with DNA may be genotoxic and carcinogenic (Coles, 1984/85). Such is the wide range of chemical structures which is encountered among electrophilic metabolites, that, despite the presence of a number of isoenzymes, success in detoxication varies considerably from one potential substrate to another (See Table 1).

TABLE 1

THE ACTIVITY OF GSH TRANSFERASES TOWARDS SOME ELECTROPHILIC SUBSTRATES

GSH transferases	μmole min^{-1} mg^{-1}					
	HNE	NABQI	BPDE	NPO	BIU	AFO
1-1	2.6	24	0.01	0.01	0.011	0.001
2-2	0.7	48	0.08	0.03	0.114	0.001
3-3	2.7	6	0.03	0.30	0.086	nil
4-4	6.9	3	0.36	0.30	0.063	nil
6-6	nd	nd	nd	nd	nd	nd
7-7	nd	60	0.33	0.02	nd	nil

HNE = 4-hydroxy-non-2-enal; NABQI = N-acetylbenzoquinone imine; BPDE = racemic benzo(a)pyrene-7,8-diol-9,10-oxide; NPO = 1-nitropyrene-4,5-oxide; AFO = aflatoxin B1-8,9-oxide; BIU = racemic α-bromo-isovaleryl urea; nd = not determined

Electrophiles can be put into the following catagories with respect to GSH transferases:-
1. Non-substrates. Examples are electrophilic metabolites of the carcinogen N,N-dimethyl-4-aminoazobenzene and N-acetyl-2-aminofluorene. Because these are not substrates, they are not conjugated catalytically by GSH and consequently an important pathway of detoxication does not reach its full potential; this lack must be presumed to contribute to hepatocarcinogenic properties of these compounds (Ketterer et al, 1986).
2. Poor substrates. An example is the electrophilic metabolite of the hepatocarcinogen and hepatotoxin aflatoxin B1. Aflatoxin-8,9-oxide is a poor substrate for rat subunits 1 and 2 and is not utilized by any of the other subunits. Normal levels of GSH transferases in the rat liver are insufficient to affect significantly the DNA binding and the hepatocarcinogenesis which follows dosage with aflatoxin. If however, compounds which induce these subunits, such

as 1,2-dithiol-3-thiones, are fed, increased detoxication by increased levels of GSH transferases contributes to considerable reduction of DNA binding (Kensler et al., 1987).

3. Good substrates. The term good substrates describes an electrophile the GSH conjugation of which is enzymically catalysed at many times the spontaneous rate, with the result that either its non-enzymic reaction with GSH or its reaction with cellular nucleophiles is very poor. The carcinogenic metabolite of benzo(a)pyrene, i.e. benzo(a)pyrene-7,8-diol-9,10-oxide, is a case in point. This is utilized by all subunits, but particularly well by subunits 4 and 7 (Jernstrom et al., 1985). This may explain the fact that it is not carcinogenic in the liver which is rich in GSH transferases, but is carcinogenic in the skin which is not. Another example is 1-nitropyrene. This gives rise to two epoxides namely 1-nitropyrene-4,5-oxide and 1-nitropyrene-9,10-oxide, both of which are utilized by all the GSH transferases and particularly well by those containing subunits 3 and 4. Kinetic data for the detoxication of 1-nitropyrene-4,5-oxide by GSH and GSH transferases have been obtained which enable catalytic specificity (k_{cat}/K_m) and the rate of the spontaneous reaction (k_2) to be compared. The rate enhancement of the enzymic reaction can be expressed as $k_{cat}/K_m \div k_2$ (see Douglas, 1987) which in the case of 1-nitropyrene-4,5-oxide and GSH transferase 4-4 is 7×10^5. This rate enhancement is responsible for ready detoxication of 1-nitropyrene. On the other hand dinitropyrenes which cannot form these epoxides form very powerful carcinogens, activated at the nitrogen atom (Djuric et al., 1987).

Special cases

1) Alpha-bromoisovaleryl urea. This is an example of a drug which is already an electrophile. It has very low reactivity and is not appreciably toxic. It is also a poor substrate for GSH transferases having a high K_m and a low k_{cat} (J. te Koppele, B. Coles, B. Ketterer & G. Mulder, unpublished information), but because other routes by which it is metabolized are few, GSH conjugation is a major route for its metabolism and excretion.

2) Paracetamol. Paracetamol is metabolized to the highly reactive product N-acetyl-benzoquinone imine (NABQI). It has the highest catalytic specificity (k_{cat}/K_m) for any GSH transferase substrate studied so far. In the case of GSH transferase 2-2 it is greater than $5 \times 10^7 \, M^{-1} s^{-1}$ (B. Coles, I. Wilson, P. Wardman, J. Hinson, S. Nelson & B. Ketterer, unpublished information), which is close to a diffusion controlled rate of association between substrate and enzyme and similar to the catalytic specificity of such very active enzymes as catalase and carbonic anhydrase (Fersht, 1985). This however, does not mean that GSH transferases and NABQI are the best examples of effective GSH transferase-catalysed detoxication. Because the spontaneous rate of reaction of NABQI with GSH is so great, the rate enhancement is only 10^3, i.e. more than two orders of magnitude less than that of the GSH transferase catalyzed conjugation of 1-nitropyrene epoxide. The toxicity of paracetamol in large doses is probably due to the relative inability of the GSH transferases to compete with spontaneous reactions, not only with GSH, but also with critical macromolecular thiols.

GSH TRANSFERASES AND THE DETOXICATION OF HYDROPEROXIDES

GSH transferases catalyse nucleophilic attack of GSH on hydroperoxides, which results in their reduction and the concomitant oxidation of GSH to GSSG. This is Se-independent GSH peroxidase activity (Ketterer et al., 1986). This enzymic reaction is particularly interesting because a number of its known substrates are endogenous e.g. fatty acid hydroperoxides and thymine hydroperoxides (Tan et al., 1986) see Table 2. Fatty acid hydroperoxides can arise from free radical attack on membrane lipids. In vitro GSH and GSH transferases can inhibit microsomal lipid peroxidation and this is now known to be due to the successive actions of membrane bound phospholipase A2 and the soluble GSH transferases. In vivo this sequence, if extended by the action of lysophosphatide fatty acyl transferase, could result in the excision and repair of radical damage to cellular membranes (Ketterer et al., 1987). Se-dependent GSH peroxidase and membrane-bound GSH transferases may also perform the same function, however, not all species are rich in Se-dependent GSH peroxidases (hepatic Se-dependent GSH peroxidases are low in guinea pig and man; see Lawrence and Burk, 1978) and the role of membrane-bound GSH transferases, although they are abundant, is not clear (Ketterer et al., 1986).

TABLE 2

THE ACTIVITY OF GSH TRANSFERASES TOWARDS SOME HYDROPEROXIDE SUBSTRATES

GSH transferases	μmole min^{-1} mg^{-1}				
	CuOOH	LinOOH	AraOOH	HOOMU	DNAOOH
1-1	1.4	2.8	2.8	0.13	nil
2-2	3.0	1.8	1.9	1.01	nil
3-3	0.1	0.2	0.2	0.5	0.018
4-4	0.4	0.2	0.2	0.3	0.032
5-5	12.5	5.3	nd	nd	0.500
6-6	0.04	0.06	nd	1.3	0.010
7-7	0.01	1.5	1.5	1.3	0.005

CuOOH = cumene hydroperoxide; LinOOH = linoleic acid hydroperoxide; AraOOH = arachidonic acid hydroperoxide; HOOMU = 5-hydroperoxymethyl uracil; DNAOOH = peroxidized DNA; nd = not determined

The thymine hydroperoxide, 5-hydroperoxymethyl uracil, is a good substrate for GSH transferases, but is unlikely to exist free in vivo. Most cellular thymine is found as thymine residues in DNA and these are susceptible to peroxidation (Christopherson, 1969). DNA exposed to ionizing radiation in aerated solution contains thymine hydroperoxide residues and is a substrate for GSH transferases (Tan et al., 1987), in particular GSH transferase 5-5, (K.H. Tan, D.J. Meyer, J.B. Taylor, N. Gillies & B. Ketterer, unpublished information) see Table 2. Peroxidized DNA is the first macromolecule to prove to be a substrate for a GSH transferase. It is of considerable interest that it should be such a good substrate. In the cell GSH transferase 5-5 relative to other isoenzymes, is concentrated in the nucleus. Some of it is readily extractable by salt-EDTA, but a similar amount is strongly bound and extractable only with 8.5 M urea (K.H. Tan, D.J. Meyer, J.B. Taylor, N. Gillies & B. Ketterer, unpublished information). GSH transferases may initiate repair of peroxidized thymine residues in DNA. The complete repair sequence would presumably be GSH transferase, DNA glycosylase, endonuclease, DNA polymerase and DNA ligase.

Several lines of information support this hypothesis, for example, hydroxymethyl uracil DNA glycosylase (Hollstein et al., 1984) and thymine glycol DNA glycosylase (Cathcart et al., 1984) have been isolated and the products released, namely hydroxymethyl uracil and thymine glycol, shown to be largely endogenous in origin, are found in urine and (Ames & Saul, 1985).
In vivo, DNA hydroperoxides may have several origins. The stimulation of the cellular immune system causes release of oxygen-centred free radicals with the potential to peroxidize DNA. Polymorphonuclear leukocytes themselves, when stimulated, have been shown to undergo DNA base modification to hydroxymethyl

uracil and thymine glycol (Frenkel & Chrzan, 1987). It may be that this damage arises from the formation of thymine hydroperoxides as a result of the action of active oxygen upon the cells which produce them. The activity of the immune system is unlikely to be the source of all DNA peroxides. Ames and Saul (1985) have suggested that the excretion of thymine glycol and hydroxymethyl uracil is proportional to the rate of oxygen utilization, quantities excreted by mice being greater than those by rats, which are greater than those excreted by man. It is suggested that oxygen metabolism results in the release of oxygen radicals which either directly (or indirectly through the release of lipid radicals) causes DNA damage. Further evidence for the association of oxygen utilization with oxygen radical release is the existence of a low basal level of ethane exhalation (an end product of lipid peroxidation) which is increased substantially under conditions of increased oxygen utilization and impaired antioxidant capacity (Wendel & Feuerstein, 1981) and also the decrease in GSH and increase in GSSG levels in tissues of rats during physical excercise (Pyke et al., 1986).

Certain chemotherapeutic drugs depend for their cytotoxicity on oxygen-centred free radicals formed in the target cell nucleus. Examples are adriamycin and bleomycin. GSH transferases should tend to protect against their cytotoxicity and it is possible that in cases of drug resistance, GSH transferases with GSH peroxidase activity are increased in level, or are expressed de novo. There are a number of examples of adriamycin resistant cells in which GSH transferase activity is elevated but little is known about GSH peroxidase activity (Dahlof et al., 1987). However, there is one case, namely that of an adriamycin-resistant human breast cancer cell line, in which a GSH transferase with high levels of GSH peroxidase activity is expressed de novo (Batist et al., 1986) and it is possible that this new GSH peroxidase is responsible, at least in part, for its adriamycin resistance.

SELECTIVITY OF GSH TRANSFERASE CATALYSED REACTIONS

It is seen in Tables 1 and 2 that there is quite appreciable enzyme specificity for each type of substrate. Where structural isomers are concerned there may also be regioselectivity. For example the Km of GSH transferases with 1-nitropyrene-4,5-oxide is an order of magnitude lower than that with 1-nitropyrene-9,10 oxide: it is probable that the 1-nitro group hinders the adjacent 9,10 oxide. Where optical isomers occur, there may be enantio-selectivity. Thus, GSH transferases, except for 3-3, are highly selective for (+) anti-benzo(a)pyrene-7,8-diol-9,10-oxide, the major enantiomer produced metabolically (Robertson et al., 1987). In the case of racemic α-bromoisovaleryl urea the alpha family of GSH transferases selectively conjugates the (R) form and the mu family the (S) form. In each case described above the reaction has yielded the one product namely the GSH conjugate. NABQI is unusual in that the spontaneous reaction results, not only in conjugation, but also reduction back to paracetamol, via the consumption of a second molecule of GSH. GSH transferases 1-1 and 2-2 catalyse the formation of both products, but GSH transferase 7-7 is selective and catalyses conjugation only.

GSH TRANSFERASES IN DIFFERENTIATION AND DEVELOPMENT

The distribution of GSH transferases varies from tissue to tissue (Ketterer et al., 1985). This is illustrated in Figs 1 and 2 which show the analysis of subunits from liver and kidney in the rat (Ostlund Farrants et al., 1987). The GSH transferase content may change in any particular tissue during development. For instance, the liver of the new born rat contains only small amounts of subunits 2 and "10" (an alpha class enzyme found only in young animals) and the adult pattern develops over the first weeks. At maturity the two sexes differ, the male being richer in the isoenzymes of the mu family and the female in isoenzymes of the alpha family. Tissue distribution is altered by inducers e.g. phenobarbitone and methylcholanthrene induce subunits 1 and 3. Important changes also occur during chemical hepatocarcinogenesis. Preneoplastic nodules have much enhanced levels of subunits 3 and express subunit 7 de novo (Kitahara et al., 1984) and a similar pattern is carried through to the primary hepatoma (Meyer et al., 1985). And as stated above chemotherapeutic agents can produce resistant cell lines which have enhanced GSH transferase gene expression. Most interesting is the observation of Y. Vandenberghe, D. Glaise, D. J. Meyer, A. Guillouzo and B. Ketterer (unpublished information) that when hepatocytes are put into cell culture, striking changes occur in their composition of GSH transferase subunits. Subunits 1 and 2 (the alpha family) are much reduced, while in the case of the mu family levels of subunit 4 are maintained and those of subunit 3 are increased. Also, as in hepatocarcinogenesis, subunit 7 is expressed de novo. It is not yet clear in what way the distribution of these enzymes in a particular tissue is related to its function. The liver is the tissue with the highest concentration of GSH transferases, in keeping with its function as the major organ of detoxication; yet it is surprising that it does not contain subunit 7 which is so effective in the detoxication of hydroxyalkenals, NABQI, BPDE and lipid hydroperoxides. By gaining subunit 7, preneoplastic cells should acquire superior powers of detoxication, compared with surrounding normal liver, which may well assist in tumour promotion and progression.

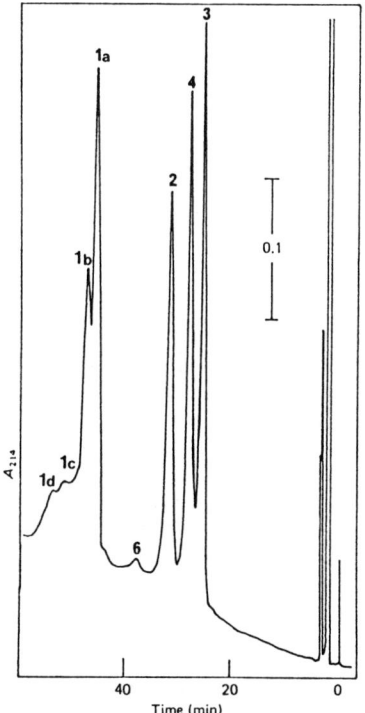

Fig 1 Soluble GSH transferase subunit composition of rat liver determined by reverse phase hplc

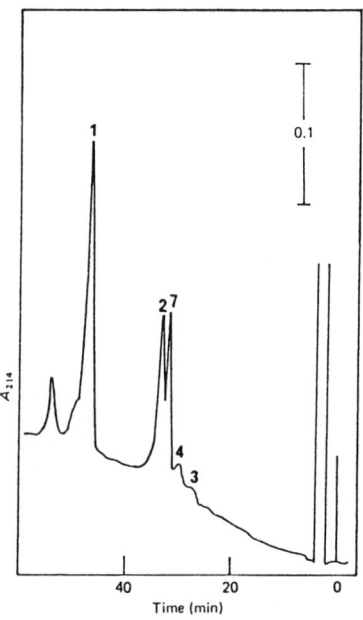

Fig 2 Soluble GSH transferase subunit composition of rat kidney determined by reverse phase hplc

CONCLUSIONS

GSH transferases may first have evolved to deal with endogenous substrates arising from oxygen toxicity such as lipid and nucleic acid hydoperoxides, hydroxy alkenals etc. However, an ability to detoxify electrophilic metabolites of xenobiotics must have been an early force in their evolution, gene multiplication and diversification then being a response to the multiplicity and diversity of xenobiotics. At the moment, the application of recombinant DNA technology is providing much new information concerning the structure, genetics and regulation of these enzymes. One end point of these studies is the elucidation of structure-function relationships which will enable the nature of the active site to be determined in detail. This should make it possible to predict which isoenzyme(s) might detoxify a particular xenobiotic electrophile, and how well. This is not possible at the moment. The problem is simpler where oxygen toxicity is concerned, since a limited number of substrates of endogenous origin are involved. In the long term the identification of regulatory regions in genomic sequences and the mechanism of their regulation should lead to an understanding of the mechanisms of differentiation with respect to GSH transferases. Such information might enable gene expression to be manipulated in order to deal with particular toxicities. The manipulation of GSH transferase gene expression in cultured cells mentioned above (Y. Vandenberghe, D. Glaise, D.J. Meyer, A. Guillouzo & B. Ketterer, unpublished data) may provide a useful starting point for these studies.

New areas are still opening up, the possibility that GSH transferases might be DNA repair enzymes is a case in point. Much has yet to be learnt about mitochondrial GSH transferases and many questions concerning microsomal GSH transferases remained to be answered.

This paper has concentrated upon rat GSH transferases, but similar classes occur in mouse and man. In drug metabolism, the understanding of human detoxication mechanisms is the ultimate goal and progress in this area is rapid. Meanwhile it would seem that the rat has been a good model for man. One important proviso is that the experimental rat is inbred and a relatively uniform population but considerable interindividual variation is present in human populations.

ACKNOWLEDGEMENTS

We would like to thank the Cancer Research Campaign and the Frances and Augustus Newman Trust for generous support throughout this research. We would also like to thank Miss Lucia Christodoulides for assistance in preparing this manuscript.

REFERENCES

Ames, B.N. & Saul, R.L. (1985): Oxidative DNA damage as related to cancer and aging. In Genetic Toxicology of Environmental Chemicals, ed. Alan Liss, pp 1-16, New York.

Batist, G., Tulpule, A., Sinha, B.K., Aspandiar, G.K., Meyers, C.E. & Cowan, K.H. (1986): Overexpression of a novel anionic glutathione transferase in multidrug resistant human breast cancer cells. J. Biol. Chem. 261, 1544-1549.

Board, P.G. & Webb, G.C. (1987): Isolation of a cDNA clone and localization of human glutathione S-transferase 2 genes to chromosome band 6p12. Proc. Natl. Acad. Sci. U.S.A. 84, 2377-2381.

Cathcart, R., Schwiers, E., Saul, R.L. & Ames, B.N. (1984): Thymine glycol and thymidine glycol in human and rat urine: A possible assay for oxidative DNA damage. Proc. Natl. Acad. Sci. U.S.A. 81, 5633-5637.

Christopherson, O. (1969): Reduction of X-ray-induced DNA and thymine hydroperoxides by rat liver glutathione peroxidase. Biochim. Biophys. Acta 186, 387-389.

Coles, B. (1984/85): Effects of modifying structure on electrophilic reactions and biological nucleophiles. Drug Metab. Reviews 15, 1307-1334.

Cowell, I.G., Dixon, K.H., Pemble, S.E., Ketterer, B. & Taylor, J.B. (1987): Characterization of human genomic sequences homologous to rat GSH transferase subunit 7 cDNA. Biochem. Soc. Trans. in press.

Dahlof, B., Martinsson, T., Mannervik, B., Jensson, H. & Levan, G. (1987): Characterisation of multidrug resistance in SEWA mouse tumour cells: increased glutathione transferase activity and reversal of resistance with verapamil. Anticancer Res. 7, 65-70.

Djuric, Z., Coles, B., Fifer, K., Ketterer, B.& Beland, A.F. (1987) In vivo and in vitro formation of glutathione conjugates from the K-region epoxides of 1-nitropyrene. Carcinogenesis in press.

Douglas, K.T. (1987): Mechanism of action of glutathione-dependent enzymes. Adv. Enzymol. Related Areas Mol. Biol. 59, 103-167.

Fersht, A. (1985): Enzyme Structure and Mechanism, 2nd edition, New York: W.H. Freeman and Company.

Frenkel, K. & Chrzan, K. (1987): Hydrogen peroxide formation and DNA base modifications by tumour promotor-activated polymorphonuclear leukocytes. Carcinogenesis 8, 455-460.

Hollstein, M., Brooks, P., Lina, S. & Ames, B.N. (1984): Hydroxymethyl uracil DNA glycosylase in mammalian cells. Proc. Natl. Acad. Sci. U.S.A. 81, 4003-4007.

Jakoby, W.B., Ketterer, B. & Mannervik, B. (1983): Glutathione transferases: nomenclature. Biochem. Pharmacol. 33, 2539-2540.

Jernstrom, B., Martinez, M., Meyer, D.J. & Ketterer, B. (1985): Glutathione conjugation of the carcinogenic and mutagenic electrophile ($\pm$)-7β,8α-dihydroxy-9α,10α-oxy-7,8,9,10-tetrahydro-benzo(a)pyrene catalysed by purified rat liver glutathione transferases. Carcinogenesis 6, 85-89.

Kensler, T.W. Egner, P.A., Dolan, P.M., Groopman, J.D. & Roebuck, B.D. (1987): Mechanism of protection against aflatoxin tumourgenicity in rats fed 5-(2-pyrazinyl)-4-methyl-1,2-dithiol-3-thione and related 1,2-dithiol-3-thiones and 1,2-dithiol-3-ones. Cancer Res. 47, 4271-4277.

Ketterer, B., Meyer, D.J., Coles, B. & Taylor, J.B. (1985): Glutathione transferases: their multiplicity and tissue distribution. In: Microsomes and Drug Oxidation. eds A.R. Boobis, J. Caldwell, DeMatteis, F. & C.R. Elcombe, pp 167-175. London: Taylor and Francis.

Ketterer, B., Meyer, D.J. Coles, B. Taylor, J.B. & Pemble, S. (1986): Glutathione transferases and carcinogenesis. in Antimutagenesis and Anticarcinogenesis Mechanisms, eds D.M. Shankel, P.E. Hartman, T. Kada & A. Hollaender, pp 103-128. New York: Plenum Press.

Ketterer, B., Tan, K.H., Meyer, D.J. & Coles, B. (1987): Glutathione transferases: a possible role in the detoxication of DNA and lipid hydroperoxides. in Glutathione Transferases and Carcinogenesis, eds T. Mantle, C.B. Pickett & J.D. Hayes, pp 149-163. London: Taylor and Francis.

Kitahara, A., Satoh, K., Nishimura, K., Ishikawa, T., Ruiki, K., Sato, K., Tsuda, H. & Ito, N. (1984): Changes in molecular forms of rat hepatic glutathione S-transferases during chemical hepatocarcinogenesis. Cancer Res. 44, 2698-2703.

Lawrence, R.A. & Burk, R.F. (1978): Species, tissue and subcellular distribution of non-Se-dependent GSH peroxidase activity J. Nutrition 108, 211-215.

Mannervik, B., Alin, P., Guthenberg, C., Jensson, H. Tahir, M.K., Warholm, M. & Jornvall, H. (1985): Identification of three classes of cytosolic glutathione transferases common to several mammalian species: correlation between structural data and enzymic properties. Proc. Natl. Acad. Sci. U.S.A. 82, 7202-7206.

Meyer, D.J., Beale, D., Tan, K.H., Coles, B. & Ketterer, B. (1985): Glutathione transferases in primary rat hepatomas: the isolation of a form with GSH peroxidase activity. FEBS Letters 184, 139-143.

Ostlund Farrants, A.-K., Meyer, D.J., Coles, B., Southan, C., Aitken, A., Johnson, P.J. & Ketterer, B. (1987): The separation of glutathione transferase subunits by using reverse-phase high pressure liquid chromatography. Biochem. J. 245, 423-428.

Pyke, S., Lew, H. & Quintanilha, A. (1986): Severe depletion in glutathione during physical exercise. Biochem. Biophys. Res. Commun. 139, 926-931.

Rhoads, D.M., Zarlego, R.P. & Tu, C.-P.D. (1987): The basic glutathione S-transferases from human liver are the products of separate genes. Biochem. Biophys. Res. Commun. 145, 474-481.

Robertson, I.G.C., Jensson, H., Mannervik B. & Jernstrom. B. (1986): Glutathione transferases in rat lung: the presence of transferase 7-7, highly efficient in the conjugation of glutathione with the carcinogenic (+)-7β,8α-dihydroxy-9α.10α-oxy-7,8,9,10-tetrahydrobenzo[a]pyrene. Carcinogenesis 7, 295-299.

Tan, K.H., Meyer, D.J., Coles, B. & Ketterer, B. (1986): Thymine hydroperoxide, a substrate for Se-dependent glutathione peroxidase and glutathione transferase isoenzymes. FEBS Letters. 207, 231-233.

Tan, K.H., Meyer, D.J., Coles, B., Gillies, N. & Ketterer, B. (1987): Detoxication of peroxidized DNA by GSH transferases. Biochem. Soc. Trans. 15, 628-29.

Taylor, J.B. Pemble, S.E., Cowell, I.G., Dixon, K.H. & Ketterer, B. (1987): Molecular biology of glutathione transferases. Biochem. Soc. Trans. 15, 578-581.

Wendel, A. & Feuerstein, S. (1981): Drug-induced lipid peroxidation in mice. Modulation by monooxygenase activity, glutathione and selenium status. Biochem. Pharmacol. 30, 2513-2520.

Illustrations are reprinted by permission from Biochemical Journal, 245, pp.423-428 copywrite (c) 19 The Biochemical Society, London.

Résumé

Les GSH transférases sont des dimères de sous-unités d'environ 25,000 daltons. Chez le rat et l'homme, ils constituent des produits d'au moins trois familles multigéniques. Une étroite homologie existe entre les deux espèces pour chacune des familles. Les GSH transférases catalysent de nombreuses réactions dépendantes du GSH, incluant la conjugaison du GSH avec des électrophiles et la réduction d'hydroperoxydes lipidiques et nucléiques. Chaque sous-unité a une spécificité de substrat caractéristique et une distribution tissulaire particulière. Cette dernière peut 1) varier au cours du développement, 2) être hormono-dépendente ; 3) être induite par certains xénobiotiques ou 4) subir des changements d'expression au cours de l'hépatocarcinogénèse ou du traitement chimiothérapeutique. Le rôle de ces enzymes dans la détoxification directe de certains métabolites électrophiles de médicaments et de cancérogènes ou la détoxification indirecte de drogues anticancéreuses du cycle redox est décrit et discuté. Les exemples d'électrophiles comprennent les métabolites du N,N'-diméthyl-4 aminoazobenzène, du N-acétyl-2-aminofluorène, du benzo(a)pyrène, du 1-nitropyrène, de l'aflatoxine B_1 et du paracétamol. La principale drogue anticancéreuse du cycle redox étudiée est l'adriamycine. On pense qu'elle agit au niveau des acides nucléiques et des membranes en formant des produits qui peuvent être détoxifiés par les GSH transférases.

The interaction of sulmazole isosulmazole and pimobendan, three orally active cardiotonic agents, on the monooxygenase system of animals and man

Dieter Müller-Enoch, Jadranka Santak, Thomas Nagenrauft

Department of Physiol. Chemistry, University of Ulm, FRG

KEYWORDS

Cardiotonic agents, difference spectra, induction of P-450 enzymes, immunochemical quantitation, scoparone O-demethylation.

INTRODUCTION

The interaction of sulmazole, isosulmazole and pimobendan on the cytochrome P-450 dependent monooxygenase system was studied by monitoring difference binding spectra, P-450 enzyme activities, and immunochemical quantitation of different cytochrome P-450 enzymes.

MATERIALS AND METHODS

Chemicals: All reagents were of highest purity available. 2-[2-Methoxy-4-(methylsulfinyl)phenyl]-1H-imidazo[4,5-b]pyridine (Sulmazole) and the isomer 2-[2-Methoxy-4-(methylsulfinyl)phenyl]-1H-imidazo[4,5-c]pyridine (Isosulmazole) and pimobendan were a generous gift from Dr. Karl Thomae GmbH (Biberach an der Riss, FRG). 7-Hydroxy-6-methoxycoumarin (Scopoletin) and 6-hydroxy-7-methoxycoumarin (Isoscopoletin) were purchased from C. Roth (Karlsruhe, FRG). 6,7-Dimethoxycoumarin (Scoparone), [7-O-methyl-^{14}C]6,7-dimethoxycoumarin (spec. act. 51.1 µCi/mmol) and [6-O-methyl-^{14}C]6,7-dimethoxycoumarin (spec. act. 51.1 µCi/mmol) were prepared as described by Müller-Enoch et al. (1979).

Preparation of microsomes: Male Sprague-Dawley rats (260-280 g) were treated p.o. with sulmazole, isosulmazole or pimobendan (15 mg/kg body weight, for 3 days) in 1.0 ml of 0.9 % NaCl or with the same volume of saline. The livers were removed and the microsomal fractions were prepared and washed with potassium pyrophosphate as described by Guengerich (1977). The final microsomal pellets were suspended in 10 mM Tris-acetate buffer (pH 7.4) containing 1 mM EDTA and 20 % (v/v) glycerol and stored at -25°C.

Spectrophotometry: Difference spectra were recorded from 370-500 nm by adding increasing amounts of sulmazole, isosulmazole or pimobendan solutions (10^{-3} M in 0.1 M Tris/HCl buffer pH 7.6) to a final concentration ranging from 10^{-6} to 5×10^{-5} M to microsomes (2 nmol P-450/ml). All difference spectra were performed in a Varian Cary spectrophotometer model 219 (Varian GmbH, Darmstadt, FRG) with fresh microsomal fractions.

Radiochemical determination of the scopoletin/isoscopoletin ratio: The ratios of the radioactive demethylation products scopoletin to isoscopoletin formed by microsomal fractions of sulmazole-, isosulmazole-, and pimobedan-treated rats and from control rats, were determined as described previously by Müller-Enoch et al. (1981) using a 1:1 mixture of the two radioisomers (7-O-methyl-^{14}C)scoparone and (6-O-methyl-^{14}C)scoparone both of which had the same specific radioactivity.

Enzyme assay, P-450 enzymes and antibodies: The scoparone O-demethylation activity was measured by the direct fluorometric assay according to the method of Müller-Enoch et al. (1981), (1985). The four P-450 enzymes used in this study (P-450$_{PB-B}$, P-450$_{\beta NF-B}$, P-450$_{UT-F}$ and P-450$_{\beta NF/ISF-G}$) were isolated from PB- or βNF-treated male Sprague-Dawley rats using techniques described in detail by Guengerich et al. (1980), (1982). Antibodies were raised to the P-450 enzymes in female New Zealand White rabbits using modifications of techniques described by Kaminsky et al. (1981). Antisera were heated at 56°C for 20 min to inactivate complement and stored at -20°C.

Table 1. Difference spectra, λ_{max}-, λ_{min}-, ΔA_{max}- and K_S-values for the interaction of the substrates Sulmazole (AR-L 115 BS), Isosulmazole (AR-L 196 BS) and Pimobendan (UD-CG 115 BS), with liver microsomes of untreated dog, baboon and man.

Liver-microsomal Fractions	Dog		Baboon		Man, Baboon, Dog, Rat and Mouse
Substrate	AR-L 115 BS	AR-L 196 BS	AR-L 115 BS	AR-L 196 BS	UD-CG 115 BS
Diff. Spectrum	Mod. Typ II	Mod. Typ II	Mod. Typ II	Mod. Typ II	–
λ_{max} [nm]	420	424	420	426	–
λ_{min} [nm]	390	390	390	395	–
ΔA_{max} at 20 µM [S]	0.035	0.047	0.008	0.053	–
K_S [µM]	K_S = 10.2	K_S = 8.6	K_S = 4.7	K_S = 6.1	–

RESULTS AND DISCUSSION

The interaction of sulmazole, isosulmazole and pimobendan on the P-450 dependent monooxygenase system was studied by monitoring difference binding spectra with microsomal fractions of rat, mouse, dog, baboon and man (Müller-Enoch et al. 1985, and Table 1). Sulmazole and isosulmazole but not pimobendan show typical modified Type II spectral changes (peak at 420 nm, through at 390 nm) with low apparent spectral dissociation constants (K_S) and spectral responses (ΔA_{max}), see Table 1. These results indicate a strong interaction of the two cardiotonic agents with the heme iron of the P-450 enzymes in microsomal fractions of all species.

Pretreatment of rats with sulmazole and isosulmazole results in a 3-4-fold increase in the scoparone O-demethylation activity (Table 2). The increase of the scoparone O-demethylation activity is accompanied by a significant change of the ratio of the demethylation products scopoletin : isoscopoletin for both drugs (Table 2). A scopoletin/isoscopoletin ratio of 1:2.5 ± 0.1 in microsomal fractions of pretreated rats is referred to as a "3-methylcholanthrene-like"-induction by Müller-Enoch et al. (1985). Therefore the two cardiotonic agents sulmazole and isosulmazole cause a "3-MC-like"-P-450 enzyme induction. Pretreatment of rats with pimobendan shows the same ratio (1: 1.7 ± 0.1) as for controls and has therefore no effect on the product ratio and on the specific demethylation activity (Table 2).

These findings of a "3-MC-like"-P-450 enzyme induction were confirmed by immunochemical quantitation of cytochrome P-450 enzymes. Sulmazole, as well as isosulmazole but not pimobendan are inducers of the P-450βNF-B and the P-450βNF/ISF-G. Table 3 show the results of the immunochemical quantitation of four different P-450 enzymes. In addition the table shows a 8- and 5-fold increase of the "3-MC-inducible"-P-450 enzymes, namely P-450βNF-B and P-450βNF/ISF-G, respectively. The failure to detect a "3-MC-like"-P-450 enzyme induction after pimobendan treatment is important, for this type of induction is notorious for toxic side-effects.

Table 2. Scoparone O-demethylation activities and the ratios of the products Scopoletin : Isoscopoletin obtained with microsomal fractions of rats, pretreated with the cardiotonic benzimidazols Sulmazole (AR-L 115 BS), Isosulmazole (AR-L 196 BS) and Pimobendan (UD-CG 115 BS).

Treatment	spec. Activity [nmol Scoparone demethylated x min^{-1} x nmol P-450^{-1}]	Scopoletin/Isoscopoletin Ratio
Control	0.49	1 : 1.7 ± 0.1
AR-L 115 BS	1.48	1 : 2.4 ± 0.1
AR-L 196 BS	2.35	1 : 2.4 ± 0.1
UD-CG 115 BS	0.60	1 : 1.7 ± 0.1

Table 3. Immunochemical quantitation of individual P-450 enzymes in liver microsomes of controls, Sulmazole- or Isosulmazole- or Pimobendan-treated rats.

Treatment	Immunological form of P-450				Total P-450
	PB-B	βNF-B	UT-F	βNF/ISF-G	
Controls	<0.01	<0.03	0.05	<0.06	1.21
Sulmazole	<0.01	0.21	0.05	0.28	1.30
Isosulmazole	<0.01	0.24	0.05	0.31	1.21
Pimobendan	<0.01	<0.03	0.05	<0.06	1.21

REFERENCES

Guengerich, F.P.(1977): Studies on the activation of a model furan compound-toxicity and covalent binding of 2-(N-Ethylcarbamoylhydroxymethyl)furan. Biochem. Pharmacol. 26, 1909-1915.
Guengerich, F.P. and Martin, M.V.(1980): Purification of cytochrome P-450, NADPH-cytochrome P-450 reductase, and epoxide hydratase from a single preparation of rat liver microsomes. Arch. Biochem. Biophys. 205, 365-379.
Guengerich, F.P., Dannan, G.A., Wright, S.T., Martin, M.V., and Kaminsky, L.S.(1982): Purification and characterisation of rat liver microsomal cytochrome P-450: electrophoretic, spectral, catalytic, and immunochemical properties and inducibility of eight isozymes isolated from rats treated with phenobarbital or β-naphthoflavone. Biochemistry 21, 6019-6030.
Kaminsky, L.S., Fasco, M.J., and Guengerich, F.P., in: Methods in Enzymology, eds. J.J. Laugone, and H. van Vunakis, Vol. 74, pp. 262-272, Academic Press-New York-San Francisco-London (1981).
Müller-Enoch, D., Thomas, H., and Ockenfels, H.(1979): A Fluorometric test for microsomal monooxygenase activity in the rat liver with scoparone as substrate. Z. Naturforsch. 34c, 481-482.
Müller-Enoch, D., Sato, N., and Thomas, H.(1981): O-Demethylation of scoparone and studies on the scoparone-induced spectral change of cytochrome P-450 in rat liver microsomes. Hoppe-Seyler's Z. Physiol. Chem. 362, 1091-1099.
Müller-Enoch, D., Dannan, G.A., Rudolf, B., and Friedl, H.-P.(1985): Induction of cytochrome P-450 isozymes in liver microsomes of rats treated with the cardiotonic agent sulmazole. Arzneim.-Forsch./Drug Res. 35, 698-703.

A direct HPLC-method for measuring cytochrome P-450 activities with scoparone as substrate

Dieter Müller-Enoch, Andreas Greischel*

* Department of Biochemistry (Dr. Karl Thomae, GmbH) Biberach, FRG. Department of Physiol. Chemistry, University of Ulm, FRG

KEYWORDS

Direct HPLC-method, regio selective scoparone O-demethylation, P-450 activities and characterization.

INTRODUCTION

The regio selective metabolism of scoparone (6,7-dimethoxycoumarin) is widely used to characterize microsomal and purified cytochrome P-450 enzymes by fluorimetric and radiochemical methods (Müller-Enoch et al., 1981, and 1985; Legrum et al., 1984). In this study we describe a direct and highly sensitive HPLC-method to measure P-450 activities in microsomal fractions with scoparone as substrate.

MATERIALS AND METHODS

Chemicals

7-Hydroxy-6-methoxycoumarin (scopoletin) and 6-hydroxy-7-methoxycoumarin (isoscopoletin) were purchased from C. Roth (Karlsruhe, FRG). 6,7-Dimethoxycoumarin (scoparone) was prepared by methylation of isoscopoletin with methyl iodide as described by Müller-Enoch et al., (1979).

Preparation of microsomes

Male Sprague-Dawley rats (200-250 g) were treated with phenobarbital (PB) or 3-Methylcholanthrene (3-MC) as described previously (Müller-Enoch et al., 1981). Microsomes were prepared and washed with potassium pyrophosphate as described by Guengerich (1977). The final microsomal pellets were suspended in 10 mM Tris-acetate buffer (pH 7.4) containing 1 mM EDTA and 20 % (v/v) glycerol and stored at -25°C.

High performance liquid chromatography (HPLC)
The separation of the substrate scoparone and the two demethylation products scopoletin and isoscopoletin was carried out on a HPLC-system, consisting on a Model 600/200 HPLC pump (Gynkotek), Autosampler (Perkin-Elmer ISS-100), and a prepacked column, ODS-Hypersil RP 18 (142 mm x 4.6 mm i.d.; 5 µm particle size (Bischoff GmbH).

The compounds were detected with a UV-spectrophotometer (Shimadzu SP-4). Detector outputs were recorded on an integrator (Shimadzu C-R2AX). The spectrophotometer was operated at 345 nm.

The mobile phase consists on 80 % of 0.05 M ammoniumacetate buffer (pH 4.25) and 20 % acetonitrile. Injections of 10-100 µl of the reaction supernatant were performed with an autosampler (Perkin-Elmer ISS-100). The flow rate was 1 ml/min.

Assay for scoparone O-demethylation with microsomes
A standard incubation mixture was incubated under shaking at 30°C for 10 min with scoparone (0.1 mM), liver microsomal fractions (1 nmol P-450/ml), $MgCl_2$ (2 mM), and NADPH (4 mM) in a 0.1 M Tris/HCl buffer (pH 7.6). The reaction was terminated by the addition of 100 µl of TCA (50 %) and centrifuged. The supernatant (10-100 µl) was applied directly on the HPLC-system.

RESULTS AND DISCUSSION

The HPLC chromatogram of a supernatant of a microsomal incubation mixture after TCA-precipitation spiked with scoparone is shown in Fig. 1. It shows, that the substrate is chromatographically pure (t_R = 9.78). Figure 2 shows a HPLC chromatogram of the supernatant of a scoparone O-demethylation assay with a microsomal fraction of control rats. The substrate scoparone (t_R = 9.78), the products isoscopoletin (t_R = 4.38) and scopoletin (t_R = 4.97) are well separated and gave a product ratio of scopoletin to isoscopoletin of 1 : 2.6, with a specific scoparone O-demethylation activity of 0.16 nmol scoparone O-demethylated x min^{-1} x nmol $P-450^{-1}$. Figure 3 and 4 show the results of the HPLC chromatograms of the standard incubation mixtures after TCA-precipitation with microsomal fractions of phenobarbital (PB) pretreated rats and 3-methylcholanthrene (3-MC) pretreated rats, respectively. The ratio of the demethylation products scopoletin to isoscopoletin is 1 : 0.5 ± 0.01 for the phenobarbital induced rats and that of 3-MC induced rats is 1 : 3.4 ± 0.1. The specific activities are 1.07 ± 0.05 or 0.47 ± 0.05 nmol scoparone O-demethylated x min^{-1} x nmol $P-450^{-1}$ with microsomal fractions of PB- or 3-MC-induced rats, respectively (Table 1).

The results of the product ratios and the specific scoparone O-demethylation activities obtained by the direct HPLC-method correlate well with the results received with the direct fluorimetric method and the radiochemical method as described earlier (Müller-Enoch et al., 1981).

Therefore this HPLC-method with scoparone as substrate is a very fast and highly sensitive tool to decide, whether a foreign compound causes an induction of P-450 enzymes, and whether an induction is "3-MC"-like (scopoletin to isoscopoletin ratio 1 : 3.4 ± 0.1) or "phenobarbital"-like (scopoletin to isoscopoletin ratio 1 : 0.5 ± 0.01).

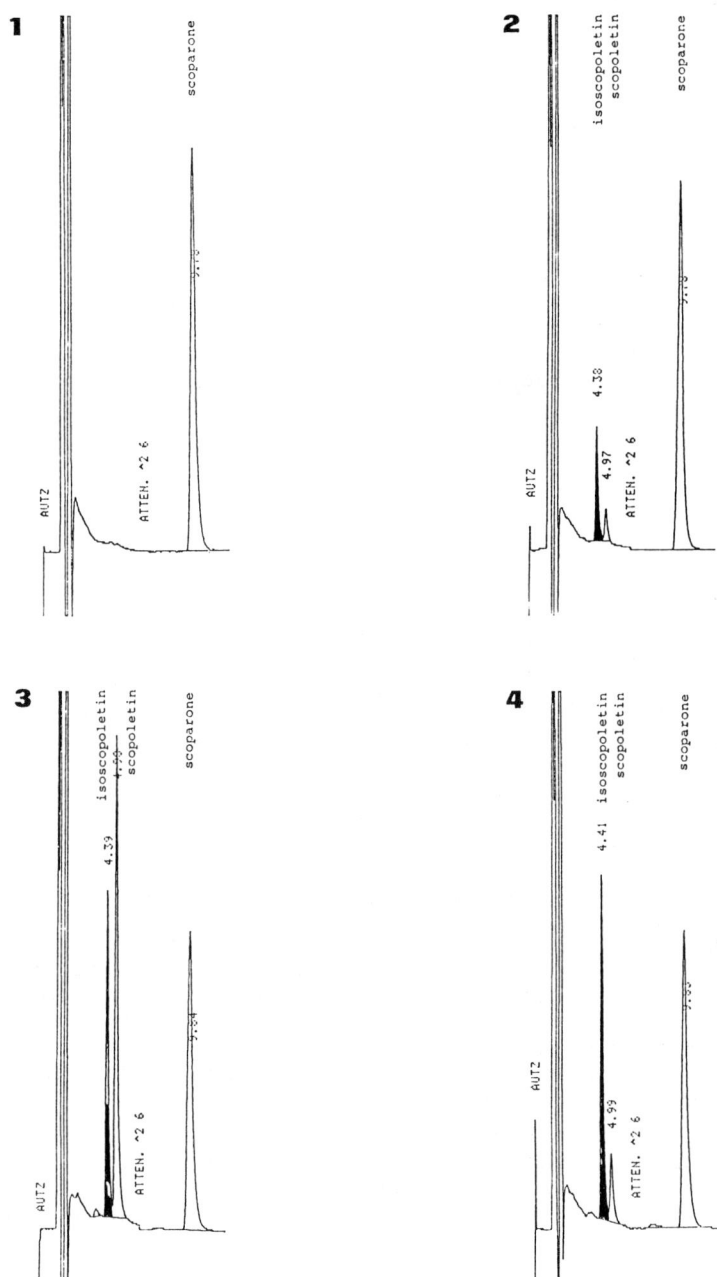

Fig. 1 shows a HPLC-chromatogram of the supernatant of the standard incubation mixture after TCA-precipitation spiked with scoparone. Fig. 2 shows the HPLC-chromatogram of the supernatant of the scoparone O-demethylation assay with a microsomal fraction of control rats, Fig. 3 with microsomes of phenobarbital- and Fig. 4 with 3-methylcholanthrene-treated rats.

Table 1. Scoparone O-demethylation activities and ratios of the two demethylation products scopoletin : isoscopoletin in liver microsomes of untreated, 3-MC- or PB-treated rats.

Microsomal Fractions	Rate			
Treatment	nmol Scopoletin x min^{-1} x nmol P-450^{-1}	nmol Isoscopoletin x min^{-1} x nmol P-450^{-1}	Ratio Scopoletin : Isoscopoletin	nmol Scoparone O-demethylated x min^{-1} x nmol P-450^{-1}
Control	0.04	0.12	1 : 2.6	0.16
3-MC	0.11	0.36	1 : 3.4	0.47
PB	0.73	0.34	1 : 0.5	1.07

REFERENCES

Guengerich, F.P.(1977): Studies on the activation of a model furan compound-toxicity and covalent binding of 2-(N-Ethylcarbamoylhydroxymethyl)furan. Biochem. Pharmacol. 26, 1909-1915.
Legrum, W., Kling, L., and Funke, E.(1983): Radioisomers of Scoparone (6,7-Dimethoxycoumarin) as a Tool for in vivo Differentiation of various hepatic monooxygenase inducers in mice using the breath test technique. J. Pharmacol. Exp. Ther. 228, 769-773.
Müller-Enoch, D., Thomas, H., and Ockenfels, H.(1979): A Fluorometric test for microsomal monooxygenase activity in the rat liver with scoparone as substrate. Z. Naturforsch. 34c, 481-482.
Müller-Enoch, D., Büttgen, E., and Nonnenmacher, A.(1985): Regioselective O-demethylation of Scoparone: Differentation between rat liver Cytochrome P-450 isozymes. Z. Naturforsch. 40c, 682-684.
Müller-Enoch, D., Sato, N., and Thomas, H.(1981): O-Demethylation of scoparone and studies on the scoparone-induced spectral change of cytochrome P-450 in rat liver microsomes. Hoppe-Seyler's Z. Physiol. Chem. 362, 1091-1099.

Genetic polymorphism in oxidative quinidine metabolism

Dieter Müller-Enoch, F. Peter Guengerich

Department of Biochemistry and Center in Mol. Toxicol, Vanderbilt University School of Medicine, Nashville, TN, USA. Department of Physiol. Chemistry, University of Ulm, FRG

KEYWORDS

Quinidine oxidation, human liver $P-450_{NF}$, genetic polymorphism.

INTRODUCTION

While wide inter-individual human responses to drugs have been known to occur for many years, only relatively recently has part of the basis been attributed to polymorphism in P-450 enzymes which catalyze their oxidation.

Probably the most extensively studied oxidative polymorphism involves debrisoquine (DB) 4-hydroxylation, the first for which evidence of monogenic control was presented by Mahgoub et al. (1977). The human P-450 involved in this reaction, $P-450_{DB}$, has been purified and characterized by Distlerath et al. (1985).

With debrisoquine (DB) and mephenytoin (MP), only 2-10 % of Caucasian populations show a poor metabolizer phenotype. In the case of nifedipine (NF) oxidation, the fraction of poor metabolizers was reported by Kleinbloesen et al. (1984) to be as high as 17 % in Dutch Caucasians. A human P-450 with NF-oxidase activity, $P-450_{NF}$, has been purified by Guengerich et al. (1986). The anti-arrhythmic quinidine has been reported to be a competitive inhibitor of the catalytic activities of human liver $P-450_{DB}$, including sparteine Δ^2-oxidation and bufuralol 1'-hydroxylation (Otton et al., (1984; Meyer et al., 1985).

We report here that quinidine is not a substrate of $P-450_{DB}$ or its rat orthology, $P-450_{UT-H}$; instead, using reconstitution and immunoinhibition techniques we find, that $P-450_{NF}$, the human NF-oxidase oxidizes quinidine.

MATERIALS AND METHODS

Chemicals
Quinidine was purchased from Aldrich Chemical Co (Milwaukee, USA). 3S-Hydroxyquinidine was prepared by a modification of the method of Carroll et al., (1976). Quinidine N-oxide was synthesized from quinidine by peracid oxidation. Debrisoquine and 4-hydroxydebrisoquine were provided by Hoffmann-La Roche (Nutley, NJ).

Enzyme preparations and Antibodies
Human liver samples were obtained from organ donors through the Nashville Regional Organ Procurement Agency, Nashville, TN. Rat Liver P-450$_{UT-H}$ was isolated as described by Larrey et al., (1984). Human liver P-450$_{DB}$, P-450$_{MP}$, and P-450$_{NF}$ were isolated as described by Distlerath et al.,(1985), Shimada et al., (1986) and Guengerich et al., (1986), respectively. Polyclonal rabbit and goat antibodies were prepared against rat P-450$_{UT-H}$ (Larrey et al., 1984) and human liver P-450$_{MP}$ (Shimada et al., 1986) and P-450$_{NF}$ (Guengerich et al., 1986); criteria for specificity and other properties are described in these references.

Assays
Quinidine 3-hydroxylase activities and quinidine N-oxidase activities were carried out in amber vials because of the sensitivity of these compounds to light. Microsomal P-450 enzymes or microsomes (generally equivalent to 50 pmol of P-450) were incubated for 10-15 min at 37°C with the substrate and 0.1 M potassium phosphate buffer (pH 7.7) in the presence of an NADPH-generating system in a total volume of 0.50 ml. To separate and quantify the products 3-hydroxyquinidine and the quinidine N-oxide an Altex cyanopropyl column (4.6x250 mm, Beckman Instruments, Palo Alto, CA) and an Altex octadecylsilyl (C_{18}) column were used, respectively. Quantitations were usually done using external standards. Nifedipine oxidation was assayed as described by Guengerich et al., (1986).

RESULTS AND DISCUSSION

Quinidine oxidation by human liver microsomes
Human liver microsomes oxidize quinidine to 3-hydroxyquinidine and quinidine N-oxide which were separate and quantify by two different HPLC systems. The formation of the 3-hydroxyquinidine (K_m = 4 µM) and the quinidine N-oxide (K_m = 33 µM) was absolutely dependent upon the addition of NADPH. No significant amounts of 2-oxoquinidine or O-desmethylquinidine or other fluorescent products were found.

Quinidine oxidation and bufuralol 1'-hydroxylation activities with human and rat liver P-450 forms
Preparations of purified P-450$_{DB}$ and its rat ortholog P-450$_{UT-H}$ catalyzed bufuralol 1'-hydroxylation: 2.7±0.5 and 0.98±0.12 nmol 1'-hydroxybufuralol x min^{-1} x nmol P-450^{-1}, respectively, but, under the same reconstitution conditions, did not catalyze quinidine 3-hydroxylation. Purified P-450$_{MP}$ did not catalyze quinidine 3-hydroxylation either.

Purified P-450$_{NF}$ catalyzed quinidine 3-hydroxylation and N-oxygenation, although the rates were low (0.2 nmol product x min^{-1} x nmol P-450^{-1}) and rather variable.

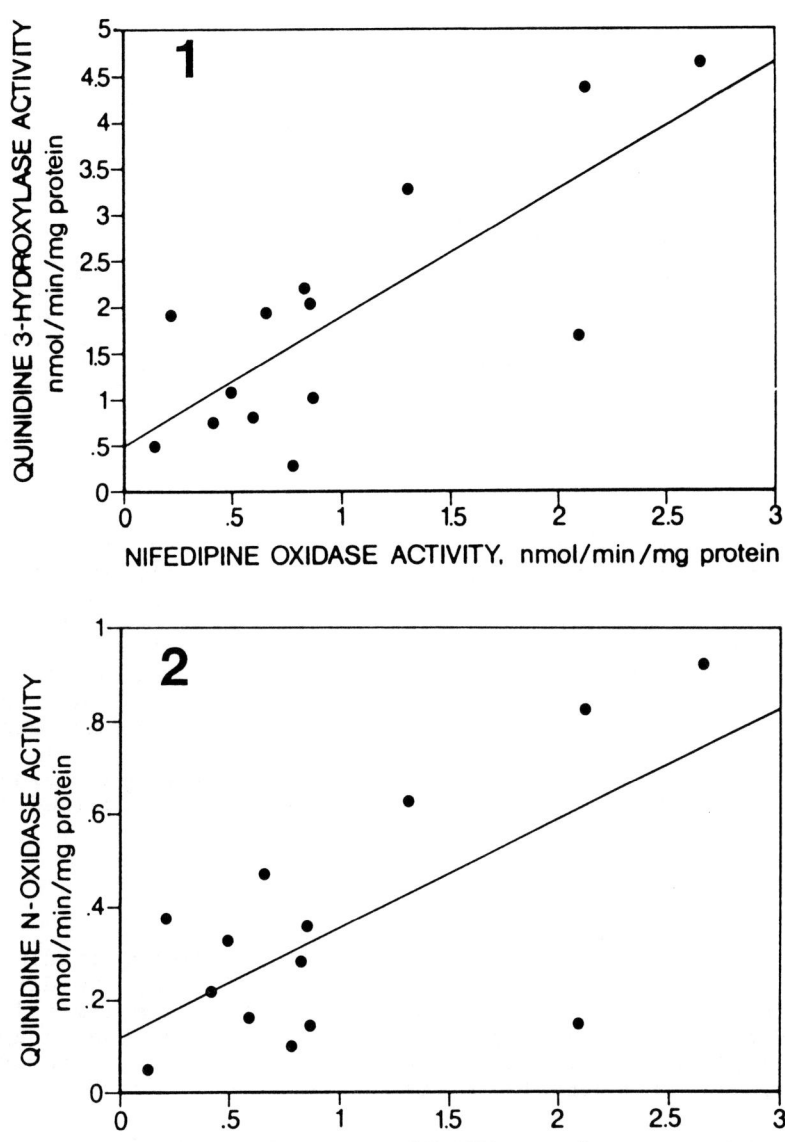

Correlation of nifedipine oxidation with rates of quinidine 3-hydroxylation (1) and quinidine N-oxidation (2) in 14 human liver microsomal preparations. The lines were drawn using linear regression analysis without weighting.

The complexity of reconstitution of P-450$_{NF}$ has been noted by Guengerich et al., (1986) and, in order to circumvent problems in the interpretation of the relative rates of microsomal and purified P-450 forms, we utilized inhibitory antibodies to elucidate the contributions of individual P-450$_S$.

Immunoinhibition studies with antibodies to human and rat liver P-450 forms

Anti-P-450$_{UT-H}$, which extensively inhibits bufuralol 1'-hydroxylation in human liver microsomes, did not affect quinidine 3-hydroxylation or N-oxygenation in human liver microsomes, using goat or rabbit antibody preparations.

Rabbit anti-P-450$_{MP}$ preparations completely inhibits human liver microsomal S-mephenytoin 4-hydroxylation but decreased the quinidine 3-hydroxylation only by < 25 %.

Rabbit anti-P-450$_{NF}$ (10 mg of IgG/nmol of P-450) inhibited > 95 % of the quinidine 3-hydroxylation and > 85 % of the N-oxygenation in several human liver microsomal preparations. Thus, quinidine oxidation appears to be catalyzed primarily by P-450$_{NF}$ and not by P-450$_{DB}$.

Correlation of nifedipine and quinidine oxydation rates

Since the results presented here, indicates that P-450$_{NF}$ is the form of human liver P-450, which is responsible for the oxidation of quinidine, a correlation between rates of nifedipine and quinidine might be expected. Figures 1 and 2 show the correlation of rates of nifedipine oxidation in 14 different human liver microsomal preparations with rates of quinidine 3-hydroxylation ($r = 0.78$) and N-oxygenation ($r = 0.67$). Further analysis of the samples used in this study indicated correlation of both, quinidine 3-hydroxylation and N-oxygenation rates with levels of immunochemically determined P-450$_{NF}$ ($r = 0.82$ in both cases, $p < 0.005$, t test).

It has been shown by Guengerich et al., (1986), who characterize the rat and human microsomal P-450 forms involved in nifedipine oxidation, that the P-450$_{NF}$ levels vary in individuals, and that the NF-oxidase activity is highly correlated with the amount of the protein. Thus, one might expect quinidine oxidation to show a variation in humans similar to that of nifedipine and to possibly show similar induction behaviours.

REFERENCES

Carroll, F.I., Philip, A., and Coleman, M.C.(1976): Synthesis and stereochemistry of a metabolite resulting from the biotransformation of quinidine in man. Tetrahedron Lett., 1757-1760.
Distlerath, L.M., Reilly, P.E.B., Martin, M.V., Davis, G.G., Wilkinson, G.R., and Guengerich, F.P.(1985): Purification and characterization of the human liver cytochromes P-450 involved in debrisoquine 4-hydroxylation and phenacetin O-deethylation, two prototypes for genetic polymorphism in oxidative drug metabolism. J. Biol. Chem. 260, 9057-9067.
Guengerich, F.P., Martin, M.V., Beaune, P.H., Kremers, P., Wolff, T., and Waxman, D.J.(1986): Characterization of the rat and human microsomal cytochrome P-450 forms involved in nifedipine oxidation, a prototype for genetic polymorphism in oxidative drug metabolism. J. Biol. Chem. 261, 5051-5060.
Kleinbloesem, C.H., van Brummelen, P., Faber, H., Danhof, M., Vermeulen, N.P.E., and Breimer, D.D.(1984): Variability in nifedipine phar-

macokinetics and dynamics: a new oxidation polymorphism in man. Biochem. Pharmacol. 33, 3721-3724.

Larrey, D., Distlerath, L.M., Dannan, G.A., Wilkinson, G.R., and Guengerich, F.P.(1984): Purification and characterization of the rat liver microsomal cytochrome P-450 involved in the 4-hydroxylation of debrisoquine, a prototype for genetic variation in oxidative drug metabolism. Biochemistry 23, 2787-2795.

Mahgoub, A., Idle, J.R., Dring, G.L., Lancaster, R., and Smith, R.L. (1977): Polymorphic hydroxylation of debrisoquine in man. Lancet 2, 584-586.

Meyer, U.A., Gut, J., Dayer, P., Kronback, T., Meier, U.T., Skoda, R. (1985): Molecular basis of the oxidation polymorphisms of the "debrisoquine/sparteine-type" and the "mephenytoin-type": clinical and in vitro studies, in Abstracts, Fourth International Symposium on Comparative Biochemistry, Janssen Research Foundation, Beerse, Belgium, 63.

Otton, S.V., Inaba, T., and Kalow, W.(1984): Competitive inhibition of sparteine oxidation in human liver by β-adrenoceptor antagonists and other cardiovascular agents. Life Sci. 34, 73-80.

Shimada, T., Misono, K., and Guengerich, F.P.(1986): Human liver microsomal cytochrome P-450 mephenytoin 4-hydroxylase, a prototype of genetic polymorphism in oxidative drug metabolism: purification and characterization of two similar forms involved in the reaction. J. Biol. Chem. 261, 909-921.

Rat liver glutathione during growth : study in weanling rats fed normal and low protein diet

Sophie Claeyssens, Alain Lavoinne, Jean Peret*, Arlette Chedeville, François Matray

*Groupe de Biochimie et Physiopathologie Digestive et Nutritionnelle, UER Médecine de Rouen. * Centre de Recherches sur la Nutrition, Meudon-Bellevue, France*

KEYWORDS

Glutathione, liver, low protein diet, lactalbumin, weanling rat, growth.

INTRODUCTION

Glutathione plays a key role in the liver detoxication reactions, and in the reduction of peroxides and free radicals. Moreover the ratio of reduced to oxidized glutathione is critical in regulating enzyme functions and protein synthesis, and in the maintenance of the thiol-disulfide status of the cell.

The liver glutathione content is closely related to the nutritional state and previous studies in adult rat and human reported that protein deprivation or starvation induced a fall in the liver glutathione content (Fouin-Fortunet et al., 1986 ; N'djitoyap et al., 1986). However, there is little data concerning the liver glutathione during growth either with a normal or a low dietary regimen, except Golden's studies with protein-malnourished children (Golden, 1984).

The present study was carried out to measure liver glutathione and protein content during the post-weaning growth in rats fed a low but good quality protein diet.

MATERIALS AND METHODS

Animals and diets. Fourty-four weanling male Sprague-Dawley rats, 26 days old (50-60 g), were obtained from Charles River (France). On arrival, the rats were housed in individual cages at 22° C under a 12/12 hour cycle (lights on at 0700 hours). They were fed a 13 % protein diet ad libitum for 7 days before the start of experiment. The 13 % protein diet had the following composition (expressed as g/100 g of diet) : lactalbumin [80 % protein (N x 6.25)] , 16.25 ; peanut oil, 6.0 ; starch, 61.75 ; sucrose, 10.0 ; mineral mixture (Peret et al., 1981), 4.0 ; vitamin mixture (Peret et al., 1981), 1.0 ; powered cellulose, 1.0. The low protein diet contained 6 % protein and starch replaced the protein. The two diets were isocaloric and contained 4.06 kcal per g.

Experimental. Throughout the experiment, food intake and body weight were measured every 2 or 3 days. On day 0, eight rats were killed and others were

divided into two groups and fed either normal (control, n = 26) or low protein
diet (LP, n = 18). Thereafter, on days 7, 14 and 21, six animals of each group
were killed between 09.00 and 10.00 hours. Animals were anaesthetized intraperitoneally with sodium pentobarbital (7 mg per 100 g body weight) and the
liver quickly removed under conditions analogous to freeze-clamping, ground
in fine powder and held in liquid nitrogen (Peret et al., 1981).

Assays. Reduced and oxidized glutathione (GSH and GSSG) were measured in the
neutralized supernatant of perchloric acid extracts as described by Bernt and
Bergmeyer. After homogeneisation of a liver aliquot, protein was assayed by the
method of Lowry. Statistical analysis (analysis of variance and covariance) was
carried out according to Snedecor and Cochran. Results were expressed as mean $\pm$
S.E.M.

RESULTS

Food intake, body and liver weight, liver protein.
Figure 1 presents the food and protein intake, and the body weight gain during
the experiment. The food intake was not different in control and in LP rats.
However, in LP rats, the protein intake and the body weight gain were reduced.

The protein efficiency ratio, which represents the body weight gain per gram of
protein eaten, calculated for the whole period of the study was significantly
higher in LP rats than in control [4.29 $\pm$ 0.12, LP ; 2.96 $\pm$ 0.04, control
(P $<$ 0.05)]. Thus, the low protein diet reduced the growth of rats despite a
greater protein efficiency ratio.

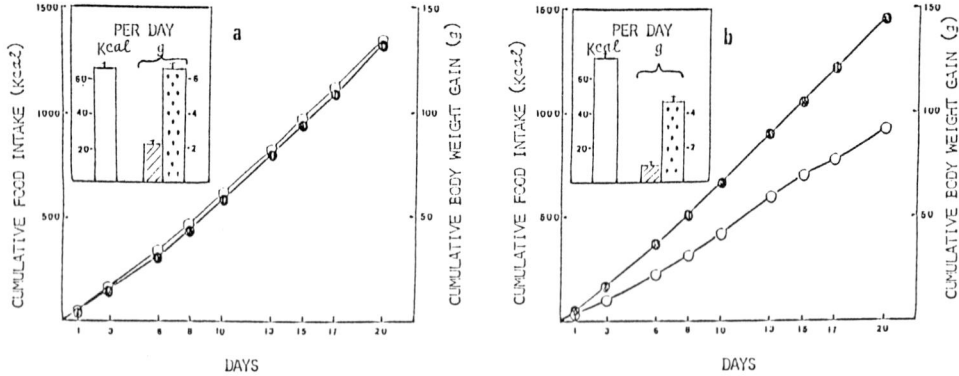

Fig.1 Cumulative food intake (●) and body weight gain (○) for rats fed 13% (a) or 6% (b) protein diets.
Insets represent daily food intake (☐), daily protein intake (▨) and daily body weight gain (▦).

As expected, the liver weight of rats fed normal or low protein diet more
slowly increased than the total body weight (Table 1). In LP rats, the liver
weight expressed as g/100 g body weight was significantly reduced on day 21 as
compared to control.

In control and during growth, the liver protein content increased as described
by Durand et al., 1965 . In LP rats, this increase was immediately curtailed
during the first week on diet and remained significantly reduced from day 7
to day 21 (Table 1).

Liver glutathione. On day 0, the liver GSH content in control was 4.15 $\pm$ 0.20
µmol/g wet weight and the liver GSSG 73.54 $\pm$ 3.76 nmol/g wet weight. The
oxidized liver glutathione content was not different from weanling to adult age

Table 1. Liver weight and protein content in rats
fed 13% or 6% protein diet for 21 days.

The 13% protein diet corresponds to control and the 6% protein
diet to LP. The liver weight was expressed as g per 100 g of body
weight and the liver protein content as mg per g of liver.
Results are given as means ± SEM for 6 rats except on day 0 (n = 8).

DAYS		0	7	14	21
WEIGHT g	CONTROL	4.97 ±0.15	4.65 ±0.05	4.38 ±0.11	4.31 ±0.24
	LP		4.37 ±0.08	4.05 ±0.11	3.61 ±0.26
PROTEIN mg	CONTROL	131.45 ±2.45	134.20 ±2.20	141.73 ±2.73	142.10 ±1.77
	LP		113.96 ±2.90	111.28 ±4.99	120.35 ±2.52

in control but the reduced liver glutathione content was slightly increased
(fig. 2). At the adult age, the average values were similar to those described
by Sies et al. (1983).

In LP rats, on day 7, the liver GSH and GSSG content was significantly decreased
and represented respectively 66.8 and 70.0 per cent of the control value
($P < 0.05$). Then, the liver glutathione content closed to the control values.
The low protein diet did not significantly change the reduced to oxidized
glutathione ratio in LP rats as compared to control (data not shown).

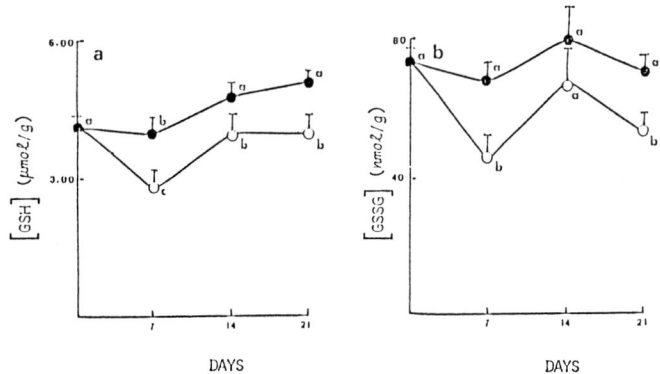

Fig.2 Liver reduced (a) and oxidized (b) glutathione content for rats fed 13% (●) or 6% (○) protein
diets. Each point represents the mean ± S.E.M for 6 rats except on day 0 (n = 8). Means not followed by
the same superscript letter are significantly different ($P < 0.05$).

DISCUSSION

The period in the growth studied in the 26 days old rats corresponds to 2-3
years old humans. In malnourished children, Kwashiorkor appears after weanling

during this period. However, in Kwashiokor, the children are often exposed to both protein and caloric restriction. Thus, it is difficult to estimate the effects of protein restriction and those of caloric restriction. In this work, the rats fed low protein diet were exposed to a pure protein restriction and they were unable to overcome the effects of the protein restriction on both liver and body growth retardation despite an increased protein efficiency ratio (Fig. 1 and Table 1).

This low protein diet induced a fall in the liver glutathione content as was observed on day 7. This emphasizes the importance of the nutritional state to maintain the liver glutathione level in weanling rat without change in GSH/GSSG ratio and confirms the results obtained for the liver glutathione content in adult rat and human (Fouin et al., 1986 ; N'djitoyap et al., 1986). However, in contrast with results obtained in adult rat, the liver glutathione content rapidly closed to the control value within day 7 and 14 (Fig. 2). In these studies, casein was used but not lactalbumin ; so, in weanling rats the quality of the used protein may play a role to explain the adaptative change observed in the liver glutathione content. Indeed, lactalbumin contains sulfur amino-acids which are essential to the glutathione synthesis. However, it should be pointed out that the casein diets were supplemented with a sulfur amino-acid. Lactalbumin also offers the highest nutritive value and the protein efficiency ratio is maximal in the 6 per cent lactalbumin diet (Hegsted and Yet-oy Chang, 1965). In our study the 6 per cent lactalbumin diet may induce a less important protein restriction than that obtained with a 4 per cent casein diet. Thus, it is possible that the observed restoration in liver glutathione may be explained by the difference in the protein supply.

In conclusion, these results suggest that weanling rats, fed a low but good quality protein diet, may rapidly restore their liver glutathione content while they were unable to overcome the effects of the protein restriction on growth retardation.

REFERENCES

Durand, G., Fauconneau, G., Penot, E. (1965) : Etude biochimique de la croissance de l'intestin grêle, du foie et de la carcasse du rat ; rôles respectifs de la multiplication et du grandissement cellulaires. Annal. Biol. Arch. Biophys. 5, 163.

Fouin-Fortunet, H., Lerebours, E., Rose, F., Deschalliers, J.P., Wessely, J.Y., Denis, Ph., Colin, R. (1986) : Cinétique des modifications des enzymes microsomiales et du glutathion hépatique lors d'une carence protidique et lors de la renutrition chez le rat. Gastroenterol. Clin. Biol. 10, 262.

Golden, M.H.N. (1984) : The consequences of protein deficiency in man and its relationship to the features of Kwashiorkor. In Textbook of Nutritional Adaptation in Man, ed. S. Kenneth Blaxter and J.C. Waterlow, pp 169-87. London, Paris : John Libbey.

Hegsted D.M. and Yet-oy Chang (1965) : Protein utilisation in growing rats. 1. Relative growth index as a bioassay procedure. J. Nutr. 85, 159.

N'djitoyap, C., Deschalliers, J.P., Fouin-Fortunet, H., Lerebours, E., Denis, Ph., Colin, R. (1986) : Influence de l'état nutritionnel sur le contenu hépatique en glutathion chez l'homme à foie sain. Gastroenterol. Clin. Biol. 10, 262.

Peret, J., Foustock, S., Chanez, M., Bois-Joyeux, B., Robinson, J.L. (1981) : Hepatic metabolites and amino acids levels during adaptation of rats to a high protein, carbohydrate-free diet. J. Nutr. 111, 1704.

Sies, H., Brigelius, R., Akerboom, T.P.M (1983) : Intrahepatic glutathione status. In Textbook of Functions of Glutathione : Biochemical, Physiological, Toxicological and Clinical Aspects, ed. A. Larsson et al., pp 51-71. New-York : Raven Press.

Inhibition of hepatic HMG-CoA reductase activity by two new hypocholesterolemic drugs

Christine Esnault, Huguette Lafont, Françoise Chanussot, Magali Chautan, Jacques Hauton, Claude Laruelle*

INSERM U.130, 10 avenue Viton, 13009 Marseille. *Laboratoires Pan Medica, 06516 Carros Cedex, France

KEY WORDS

Liver, hypocholesterolemiant drug, HMG CoA reductase activity.

INTRODUCTION

The relationship between hypercholesterolemia and coronary artery disease is well established. In man de novo synthesis of cholesterol plays an important triggering role in the onset of hypercholesterolemia. Thus the availibility of a drug capable of reducing the activity of HMG CoA reductase, the key enzyme in de novo synthesis of cholesterol, has great therapeutic implications.

In this study, we tested the effects of two drugs, PMD 387 and 77 on the HMG CoA reductase activity in the liver. These drugs which are synthesized from pyroglutamic acid are chemically different from fenofibrate (Schlierf et al., 1980) which is a cholesterol lowering agent and mevinoline, a potent new competitive inhibitor of HMG CoA (Albers et al., 1980). It was found that PMD 387 and 77 effectively lowered the cholesterol level in rats rendered hypercholesteremic by treatment with Triton X 100. In view of this finding, we investigated the inhibitory effects of these two drugs and their soluble derivatives on HMG CoA reductase activity. Since the solubility of these drugs in water is low, they were solubilized in mixed micelles thus avoiding the use of solvent (DMSO).

MATERIAL AND METHODS

Microsome Preparation
Microsomes were prepared from the livers of Wistar rats maintained on cholesterol-free rat chow. After homogenization in Tris buffer 0.1 M pH 7.5 sucrose 0.25 M, livers specimens were centrifuged twice at 10.000 g for 15 min and the supernatants submitted to ultracentrifugation at 78.000 for 1 hour (Mac Namara et al., 1972). The resulting pellet containing the microsomes was suspended in a phosphate buffer : KH_2PO_4 50 mM, EDTA 30 mM, KCl 70 mM dithiothreitol 1 mM, pH 7.4 at a volume of 1 ml/g of liver. The purity of microsome preparation was checked by assessing the activity of rotenone unsensitive NADPH cytochrome C reductase.

Micellar Solubilization of the drug
The drug 0.1 mM either PMD 387 or PMD 77 (Pan Medica, Virbac, Nice, France) was solubilized in 10 mg of a benzene solution of phosphatidylcholine purified from egg yolk (Sigma, France). After careful evaporation of the solvent under nitrogen, a solution composed of 82 mg of Na taurocholate (Calbiochem) and 10 ml of phosphate buffer was added to achieve micellar solubilization.

HMG CoA Reductase Assay (Mac Namara et al., 1972)
The isolated microsomes containing 250 ug - 1 mg of protein were added to 100 ul of phosphate buffer 50 mM, EDTA 50 mM, dithiothreitol 1 mM, 5 mM NADP glucose 6P 30 mM, glucose deshydrogenase 2 UI, 5 uM DL ^{14}C HMG CoA (52 MCi/mmoles). After incubation at 37° for 5 to 10 min, the reaction was stopped by adding 20 ul of 2 N HCl. Mevalonate lactone formed overnight was isolated and counted after micro column separation (Albers et al., 1980). To evaluate loss during preparation, a control experiment was performed in which H^3 mevalonate was added to the samples before lactonisation. In this control experiment, 5-10 nm of mevalonate was formed per min per mg protein. Protein levels were measured by the Lowry method.

RESULTS

Solubilization of the Drug
The inhibitory effect of the drug after micellar solubilization achieved in phospholipid bile salt mixed micelles was dose-dependent. In unsolubilized form, no inhibitory effect was observed.

Inhibition of HMG CoA Reductase
"Fig. 1" depicts inhibition of HMG CoA reductase by PMD 77 and PMD 387 in comparison to the effects of fenofibrate and mevinoline solubilized under the same conditions. The concentration required for 50% inhibition was, 2 umoles for PMD 77, 1 umole for PMD 387, 0.2 umole for mevinoline and 3 umoles for fenofibrate. PMD 387 appeared to be more potent than PMD 77. The soluble derivative of PMD 77 appeared to have a lesser effect than native PMD 77. On the other hand, one of the derivatives of PMD 387 appeared to be more potent than native molecule at 2 umoles (76.72% of inhibition).

Fig. 1

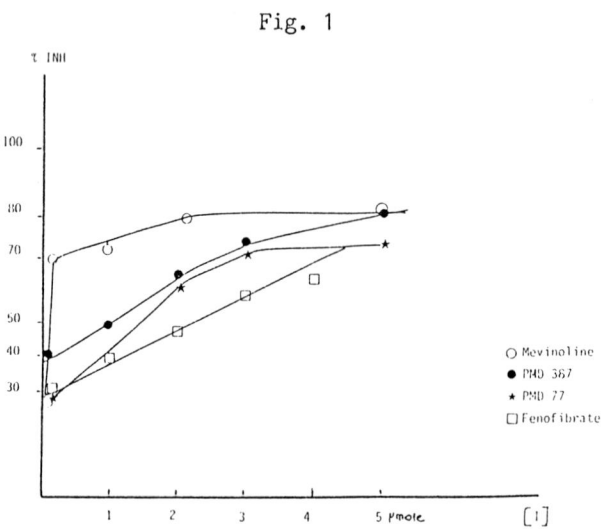

Characterization of the Inhibition of PMD 387 and PMD 77

Under our conditions, these drugs -both in native and derivative form- seemed to act in a non-competitive manner through a complex mechanism involving the Vmax and Km of the enzyme. The inhibitory effect of these drugs seemed to result from changes in the substrates (Fig. 2) and reaction products.

Fig. 2

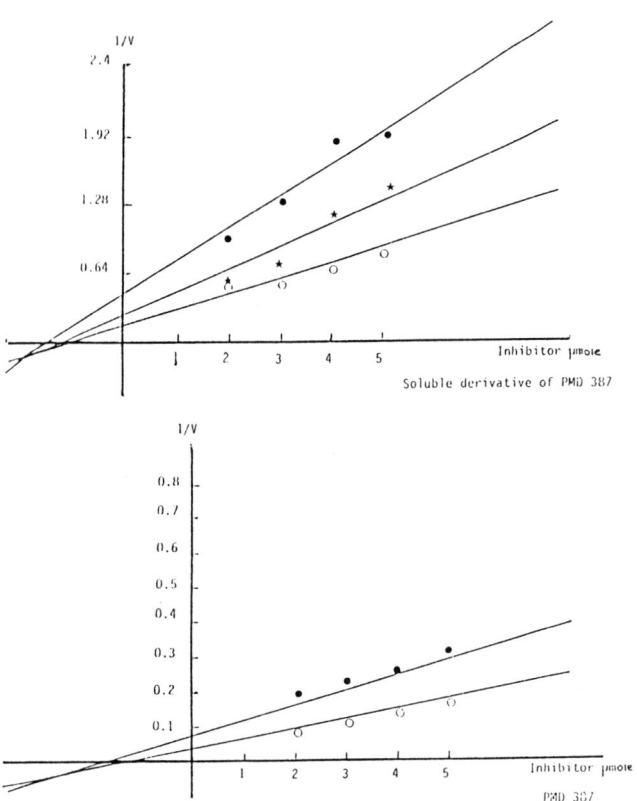

DISCUSSION

The present report describes the inhibitory effects of two new drugs, PMD 387 and PMD 77, on HMG CoA reductase enzyme in the microsomes isolated from rat livers. Because of their highly hydrophobic behavior, the native molecules are inactive if they are not solubilized. Micellar solubilization in mixed micelles seems to have the dual advantage of effectively potentiating inhibition and avoiding the use of a solvent such as DMSO which has a variable, non-reproducible inhibitory effect of its own. Soluble derivatives of the drugs have the same inhibitory effect as the initial molecule after micellar solubilization. PMD 387 which is derived by chemical synthesis from pyroglutamic acid seemed to be the more potent inhibitor.

The kinetic data obtained in this study were compared with similar data for two commercial inhibitors of HMG CoA reductase, namely : mevilonine and fenofibrate. This comparison showed that both PMD 387 and PMD 77 were more potent inhibitors than fenofibrate. Although mevinoline acted faster than with PMD 387, the maximum level of inhibition at the same concentration was identical (80%) (Endo et al., 1976; Alberts et al., 1980). The action of PMD 387 or its soluble derivatives was studied by the method of Dixon. Inhibition was found to result from a non-competitive mechanism involving the substrate and altering the Vmax of the incubation reaction. The present findings together with in vivo inhibitory effect after oral administration in rats strongly suggest that these inhibitors of HMG CoA reductase may be effective in reducing blood cholesterol. Moreover previous results obtained to the fate of cholesterol from the HDL of LDL in the liver showed that the cholesterol-LDL uptake increased markedly under drug injection. Taken as a whole, this evidence indicates that PMD 387 may be a potentially effective therapeutic agent for the treatment of hypercholesterolemia.

REFERENCES

Alberts, A.W., Chen, J., Kuron, G., Hunt, V., Huff, J., Hoffman, C., Rothrock, J., Lopez, M., Joshua, H., Harris, E., Patchett, A., Monaghan, R., Currie, S., Stapley, E., Albers-Schonber, G., Hensens, O, Hirshfield, J., Hoogsteen, K., Liesch, J., Spinger, J. (1980): Mevinolin : a highly potent competitive inhibitor of hydroxymethylglutaryl-coenzyme A reductase and a cholesterol-lowering agent.   Proc. Natl. Acad. Sci. USA, 77, 3957-3961.

Mac Namara, D.J., Quackenbush, F.N., Rodwell, V.W. (1972): Regulation of hepatic 3OH 3CH$_3$ glutacyl CoA reductase, developmental pattern. J. Biol. Chem. 247, 5805-5810.

Endo, A., Kuroda, M., Tanzawa K. (1976): Competitive inhibition of 3OH 3CH$_3$ HMG CoA reductase by ML 236 A and ML 236 B fr metabolites having hypocholes-terolemic activity. Febs Let.,   72, 323-326.

Schlierf, G., Chwat M, Feuerborn, E., Wuelfinghof, E., Heuck, E.E., Kohlmeier M., Oster, P., Stiehl, A. (1980): Biliary and plasma lipids and lipid lowering chemotherapy. Studies with clofibrate-fenefibrate and etofibrate in healthy volunteers. Atherosclerosis 36, 323-329.

Effect of vitamin A depletion on cytochrome P-450 isozymic pattern and glutathione transferase activity in rat liver

Damrong Ratanasavanh[1], Jesus Pazo-Carrera[1,*], Philippe Beaune[2], Yves Cariou[3], Marc Nicol[3]

[1] Unité de Recherches Hépatologiques. INSERM U.49, Hôpital Pontchaillou, Rennes, France.
[2] INSERM U.75, Hôpital Necker, Paris, France. [3] Laboratoire de Biochimie Médicale A, Faculté de Médecine, Hôpital Pontchaillou, Rennes, France. * Present address : Departmento Fisiologia Animal, Faculted de Biologia, Universitad de Santiago de Compostela, Spain.

Key-words : Vitamin A, cytochrome P-450, isozymes, glutathione transferase, rat hepatocytes.

INTRODUCTION

The liver is involved in storage of vitamin A and its transfert via a retinol binding protein to peripheral tissues. Low hepatic vitamin A levels might be responsible for some functional or structural abnormalities in the liver (Leo et al., 1983). Vitamin A deficiency may also enhance susceptibility of a number of organs to carcinogenesis (Goodman, 1984 ; Wilett et al., 1984). The potentiality of xenobiotics to be carcinogenic may depend on the status of drug metabolizing enzyme activities ; this leads us to investigate effect of vitamin A depletion on the levels of these enzymes in liver.
The results reported here show that vitamin A deficiency lowered markedly the cytochrome P-450 isozymic pattern and increased selectively the activity of a glutathione S-transferase isozyme in rat liver.

MATERIAL AND METHODS

Animals

Three groups of 5 weanling male Wistar rats were used. The first group of animals was fed the vitamin A-free diet (Vitamin A-free casein 22 g, salt-mix 4 g, saccharose 5 g, wheat flour 58 g, peanut oil 5 g, barm 6 g, vitamins C, D, E, K physiological dose supplement). The second group was fed the vitamin A-free diet supplemented with 20 µg of retinol per day. The third group was fed the vitamin A-free diet supplemented with 100 µg of retinoic acid per day. After 4 months, the animals were sacrified.

Tissue fixation.

Rat livers were fixed for immunohistochemical analysis according to a procedure previously described (Guillouzo et al., 1982). Briefly, livers were washed with phosphate buffer saline (PBS) pH 7.4 for 5 min, then perfused with a 4 % paraformaldehyde solution buffered with 0.1 M sodium cacodylate pH 7.4. The flow rate was 15 ml/min. After perfusion for 15 min, the samples were cut into fragments and immersed in PBS.

Preparation of antigens and antibodies.
Purified cytochrome P-450-UTA (a constitutive form), P-450-PB-B (an inducible form by phenobarbital) and P-450-BNF-B (an inducible form by B-naphtoflavone) were prepared as described by Guengerich et al. (1982). Corresponding antibodies were obtained in New Zealand female rabbit according to Le Provost et al. (1981).

Immunohistochemical procedure.
Cytochrome P-450 isozymes were localized in cryostat sections. Liver fragments were first soaked in 10 % glycerol in PBS for 1 hour and freezing was performed in liquid nitrogen cooled isopentane. 6 to 8 µm cryostat sections were routinely prepared and incubated in 10 % fetal calf serum in PBS for 1 hour before incubation for 1 additional hour with specific antibodies at the appropriate dilution. After 3 washes (15 min. each), the sections were incubated with peroxidase-labelled immunoglobulins (Institut Pasteur, Paris, France) in PBS. Then, after 3 washes with PBS, staining was performed with 3,3' diaminobenzidine/H_2O_2 for 20 min. (Graham and Karnovsky, 1966). Sera from non immunized rabbits were used as controls.

Glutathione S-transferase assay.
Glutathione S-transferase activities were determined spectrophotometrically in isolated hepatocytes (after sonication) according to the procedures of Habig et al. (1981), with 1-chloro-2,4-dinitrobenzene (CDNB), 1,2-dichloro-4-nitrobenzene (DCNB), paranitrophenyl acetate (PNP) and trans-4-phenyl butene 2-one (tPBO) as substrates. Hepatocytes were obtained by collagenase perfusion according to the method of Guguen-Guillouzo and Guillouzo (1986).

Determination of vitamin A.
Vitamin A content of liver homogenates was determined by the reversed phase HPLC technique. Liver homogenates were mixed in glass-capped tubes with 1 volume of an ethanolic solution of the internal standard (retinol acetate). The samples were extracted with n-hexane, in a vortex mixer. After centrifugation, a part of the upper phase was evaporated under a stream of nitrogen. The residue was dissolved in methanol and injected on top of a RP 18 column. The mobile phase was pure methanol ; flow rate was fixed at 2 ml/min. The detector wavelength was set at 320 nm.

RESULTS

Body weight and hepatic vitamin A content.
As shown in figure 1, the body weight did not differ significantly between the 3 groups at 2 months of regimen. After 3 to 4 months, the body weight of animals fed the vitamin A-free diet was significantly lower than that of the 2 other groups. Hepatic vitamin A content in rats fed vitamin A-free diet was completly abolished whereas in control group retinol and retinol palmitate were characterized (Fig. 2).

Cytochrome P-450 isozymes
As shown in figure 3, immunostaining for P-450 UTA, P-450-PB-B and P-450-BNF-B was easily evidenced in the livers of rats fed the diet supplemented with vitamin A or retinoic acid. These cytochromes P-450 isozymes were found in all cells in the lobules although centrilobular hepatocytes bound slightly more antibodies than did periportal cells. In the liver of rats fed the vitamin A-free diet, immunostaining of these 3 P-450 isozymes was markedly decreased (Figure 3).

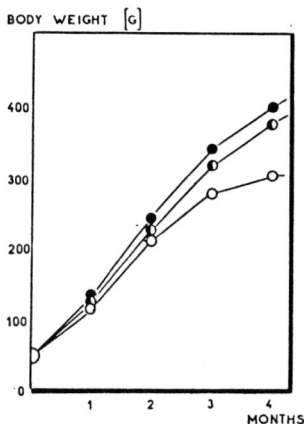

Figure 1 : Effect of vitamin A deficiency on body weight of rats :
+ retinol :●—●; + retinoic acid :◐—◐; retinol deficient :○—○

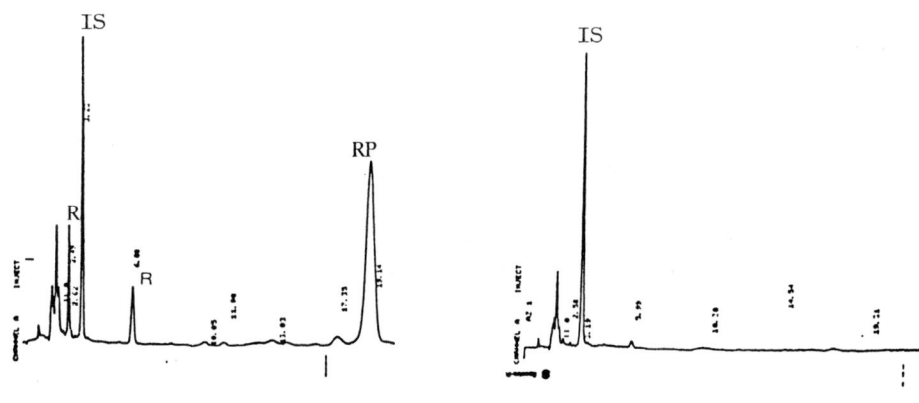

      Vitamin A supplemented diet   Vitamin A deficient diet.

Figure 2 : Chromatograms of hepatic vitamin A content in rat fed vitamin A-free or vitamin A supplemented diet. Retinol acetate was used as internal standard (IS). R : retinol ; RP : retinol palmitate.

Glutathione S-transferase activity.

The values of GST activities with CDNB and DCNB as substrates presented here were slightly lower than those reported by Van den Berghe et al. (1987). The differences could be due to strain and age of animals used. No significant difference in glutathione S-transferase activities was observed between the 3 groups of animals when CDNB, DCNB and PNP were used as substrates. In contrast, when tPBO which is a typical substrate for hepatic transferase isozymes containing subunit 4 (Mannervik, 1985) was used, the enzyme activity was found significantly increased in hepatocytes of rat fed vitamin A-free diet (Figure 4).

Control

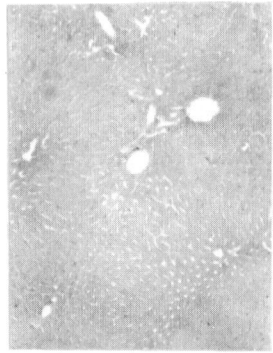

Figure 3 : Immunohistochemical localization of cytochrome P-450 isoenzymes in liver of rats fed retinoic acid or vitamin A supplemented diet and vitamin A-free diet.

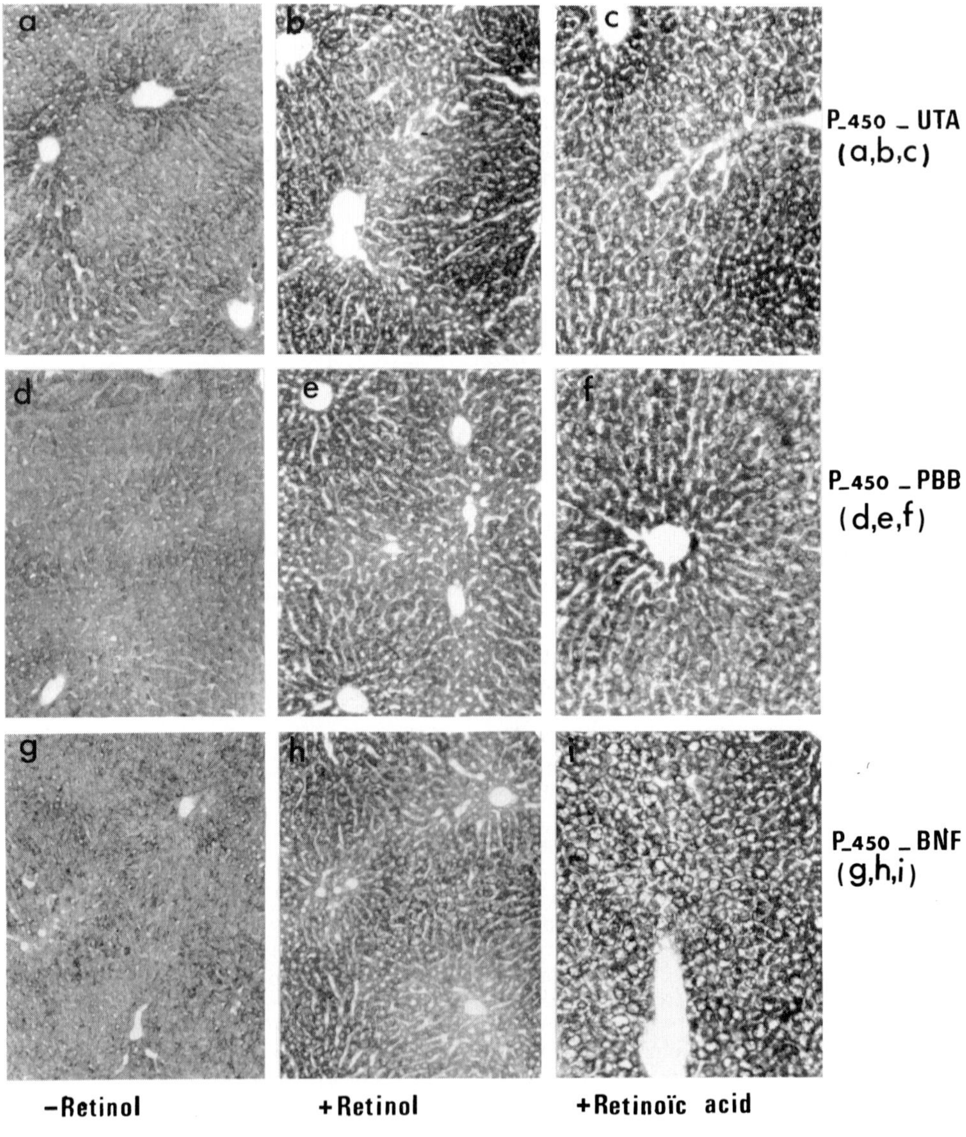

a
b
c
P-450 - UTA
(a,b,c)
d
e
f
P-450 - PBB
(d,e,f)
g
h
i
P-450 - BNF
(g,h,i)
-Retinol
+Retinol
+Retinoïc acid

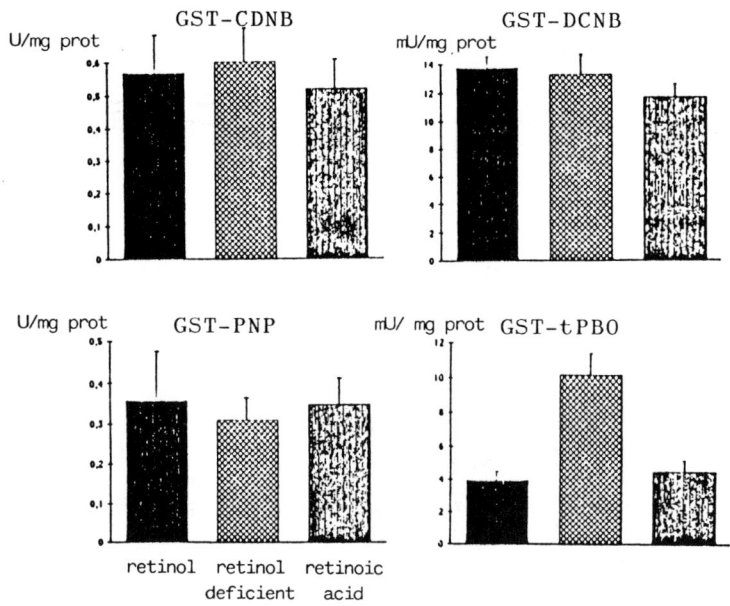

Figure 4 : Effect of vitamin A deficiency on glutathione-S-transferase activities in rat hepatocytes.

DISCUSSION

In control rat liver, the patterns of immunostaining of P-450 isozymes studied are in agreement with those reported in the litterature (see review Baron et al., 1984). Centrilobular hepatocytes are more stained than periportal hepatocytes. The heterogeneous distribution of P-450 isozymes is also described in human liver (Ratanasavanh et al., 1986). The results of the present study provide evidence that levels of P-450 isozymes namely P-450-UTA, P-450-PB-B and P-450-BNF-B are markedly altered in vitamin A deficient rat liver. The decline of the immunostaining of the 3 studied P-450 isozymes could correspond to the decrease in enzymatic activities of P-450. Indeed, it is reported that vitamin A deficiency decreases hepatic P-450 content as well as arylhydrocarbon hydroxylase and aminopyrine N-demethylase (Khanduja et al., 1983 ; Periquet et al., 1986). The vitamin A derivative retinoic acid seems to overcome the effect of vitamin A deficiency on the decrease in P-450 isozymes. The exact mechanism of vitamin A and retinoic acid in the maintenance of P-450 levels in liver remains to be determined but it is noteworthy to notice that microsomal drug metabolizing enzymes can be involved in vitamin A metabolism (Leo and Lieber, 1985) and that retinoic acid has a sparring effect on liver reserves of vitamin A (Periquet et al., 1985) and exerts some retardation in the hepatic vitamin A loss. The glutathione transferases are multifunctional proteins that play also an important role in the detoxification of drugs (Ketterer et al., 1982). As cytochrome P-450 isozymes, these transferases are inducible by a number of drugs (Chasseaud et al., 1979) ; but in contrast to P-450, vitamin A deficiency does not affect GST activities with CDNB, DCNB and PNP as substrates. Even, the deficiency in hepatic vitamin A increases GST activity with tPBO as substrate. The physiological importance in selective increase of GST-tPBO remains to be determined but it is well known that tPBO is specific for GST family containing subunit 4 which has high activity with many epoxides especially with epoxide

leukortriene A4 (Mannervick et al., 1984). In addition, GST has been demonstrated to be involved in the conjugation of activated aflatoxin B_1 during aflatoxin hepatocarcinogenesis in the rat (Neal and Green, 1982).
The results reported here show that vitamin A deficiency affects selectively phase I and phase II drug metabolizing enzymes and suggest that metabolism of various drugs may be altered in rat depleted in vitamin A.

ACKNOWLEDGMENTS

This work was supported in part by the Réseau de Toxicologie Alimentaire (M.R.E.S.).

REFERENCES

Baron, J., Kawabata, T., Knapp, S., Voigt, J.M., Redick, J.A., Jacoby, W.B. and Guengerich, F.P. (1984): Intrahepatic distribution of xenobiotic metabolizing enzymes in foreign compounds metabolism. Eds. J. Caldwell, G.D. Paulson, pp 17-36. London and San Francisco : Taylor and Francis.

Chasseaud, L.F. (1979): The role of glutathione and glutathione S-transferase in the metabolism of chemical carcinogens and other electrophilic agents. Adv. Cancer Res.29, 175-274.

Goodman, D.S. (1984): Vitamin A and retinoids in health and disease. N. Engl. J. Med. 310, 1023-1031.

Graham, R.C. and Karnovsky, M.J. (1966): The early stages of absorption of injected horseradish peroxidase in the proximal tubules of mouse kidney : ultrastrutural cytochemistry by a new technique. J. Histochem. Cytochem. 14, 291-302.

Guengerich, R.P., Dannan, G.A., Wright, S.T., Martin, M.V. and Kaminsky, L.S. (1982): Purification and characterizaiton of liver microsomal cytochromes P-450 : electrophoretic, spectral, catalytic and immunochemical properties and inducibility of eight isozymes isolated from rat treated with phenobarbital or beta-naphtoflavone. Biochemistry, 21, 6019-6030.

Guguen-Guillouzo, C. and Guillouzo, A. (1986): Méthodes de préparation d'hépatocytes adultes et foetaux. In Hépatocytes isolés et en culture, Eds A. Guillouzo, C. Guguen-Guillouzo, pp 1-12, Paris : John Libbey Eurotext.

Guillouzo, A., Beaumont, C., Le Rumeur, E., Rissel, M., Latinier, M.F., Guguen-Guillouzo, C. and Bourel, M. (1982): New findings on immunolocalization of albumin in rat hepatocytes. Biol. Cell. 43, 163-172.

Habig, W.H. and Jakoby, W.B. (1981): Assays for differentiation of glutathione S-transferases. In Methods in enzymology, Ed W.B. Jacoby, pp 396-405. New York : Academic Press.

Ketterer, B., Beale, D. and Meyer, D.J. (1982): The structure and multiple functions of glutathione transferases. Biochem. Soc. Transact. 10, 82.

Khanduja, K.L., Dogra, S.C., Sarita Kaushal and Sharma, R.R. (1984): The effect of anti-cancer drugs on pharmacokinetics of antipyrine in vitamin A deficiency. Biochem. Pharmacol. 33, 449-452.

Le Provost, E., Flinois, J.P., Beaune, P. and Leroux, J.P. (1984): Immunochemical characteriztion of some monooxygenase activities in liver microsomes from untreated and phenobarbital treated rats. Biochem. Biophys. Res. Commun., 101, 545-554.

Leo, M.A., Sato, M. and Lieber, C.S. (1983): Effect of hepatic vitamin A depletion on the liver in humans and rats. Gastroenterology, 84, 562-572.

Leo, M.A. and Lieber, C.S. (1975): New pathway for retinol metabolism in liver microsomes. J. Biol. Chem. 260, 5228-5231.

Mannervik, B., Jensson, H., Alin, P., Orning, L. and Hammarstrom, S. (1984): Transformation of leukortriene A4 methyl ester to leukotriene C4 monomethyl ester by cytosolic rat glutathione transferases. Febs Lett. 175, 289-293.

Mannervik, B. (1985): The isozymes of glutathione transferase. Adv. Enzymol. 57, 357-417.

Neal, G.E. and Green J.A. (1983): The requirement for glutathone S-transferase in the conjugaison of activated aflatoxin B_1 during aflatoxin hepatocarcinogenesis in the rat. Chem. Biol. Inter. 45, 259-275.

Periquet, B., Bailly, A., Periquet, A., Ghisolfi, J. and Thouvenot, J.P. (1985): Evidence fot two subcellular pools and different kinetic behaviour of retinyl palmitate in rat liver. Int. J. Vit. Res. 55, 245-251.

Periquet, B., Periquet, A., Bailly, A., Ghisolfi, J. and Thouvenot J.P. (1986): Effects of retinoic acid on hepatic cytochrome P-450-dependent enzymes in rats under different vitamin A status. Int. J. Vit. Nutr. Res. 56, 223-229.

Ratanasavanh, D., Beaune, P., Baffet, G., Rissel, M., Kremers, P., Guengerich, F.P. and Guillouzo, A. (1986): Immunocytochemical evidence for the maintenance of cytochrome P-450 isozymes, NADPH cytochrome C reductase and epoxyde hydrolase in pure and mixed primary cultures of adult human hepatocytes. J. Histochem. Cytochem. 34, 527-533.

Vandenberghe, Y., Ratanasavanh, D., Glaise, D. and Guillouzo A. (1988): Influence of medium composition and culture conditions on glutathione S-transferase activity in adult rat hepatocytes during culture. In Vitro Cell. Develop. Biol. (in press).

Willet, W.C., Polk, B.F. and Underwood, B.A. (1984): Relation of serum vitamins A and E and carotenoids to the risk of cancer. N. England J. Med. 310, 430-434.

Comparative metabolic pattern of amineptine in rat, dog and human

P. du Vignaud*, P. Gelé*, J.M. Delbos*, N. Bromet*, L. Grislain*, E. Mocaer**

* Technologie Servier, Orléans, France. ** Institut de Recherches Internationales Servier, Neuilly-sur-Seine, France

Keywords : Amineptine, metabolites, rat, dog, human

INTRODUCTION

Amineptine is a compound derived from the tricyclic antidepressants (Ponzio et al., 1986). Its mechanism of action is dopaminergic (Van Amerongen, 1979). The aim of this study was to investigate the metabolism of the amineptine in rat, dog and human after oral administration of ^{14}C-amineptine HCl.

METHODS

Administration and collection of biological samples.

The metabolism of S-1694-1 or amineptine hydrochloride or 7-[(10-11)-dihydro-5H-dibenzo (a, d) cyclohepten-5yl-]amino heptanoic acid was studied in the rat, the dog and in man. ^{14}C-S 1694-1 (amineptine HCl) was administered orally to rats at doses of 2 mg.kg^{-1} and 100 mg.kg^{-1}, to dog at doses of 2 and 50 mg.klg^{-1} and to man at a dose of 100 mg. Blood samples were collected at the following times : rat : 1 h ; dog : 1.4 and 5.5 h ; human 0 , 1 h, 4 h and 12 h. Urine samples were collected at the follwing times : rat and dog : 0-24 h, 24-48 h, human : 0-12 h, 12-24 h, 24-36 h and 38-48 h.

Analytical methods.

The radioactivity in urine and plasma was extracted using a XAD$_2$ column. The different metabolites were separated and purified using TLC and/or HPLC techniques. Quantification was based on the measurement of radioactivity. The identification of the major metabolites was carried out by the combined use of reference compounds and MS/GC-MS.

RESULTS

The results are expressed as percentage of the administered dose. (Fig. 1).

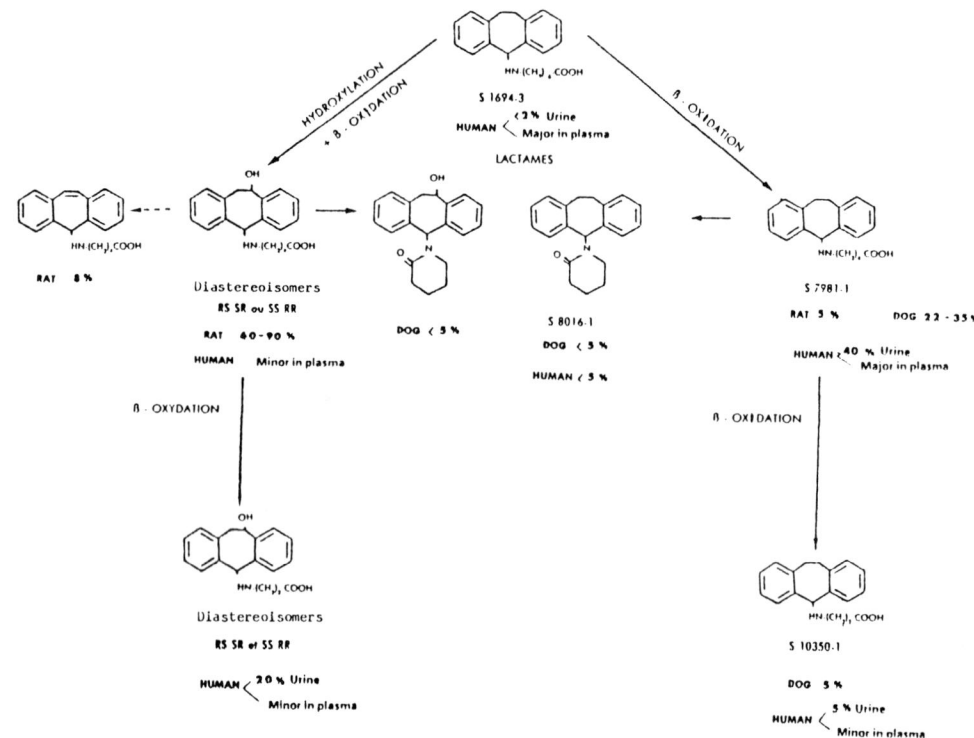

Figure 1 : PROPOSED METABOLIC PATHWAYS

CONCLUSION

The metabolism of amineptine was qualitatively similar in rat, dog and man. The most important phase I reactions for the three species were β-oxidation of the amino heptanoic chain (S 7981-1 metabolite) and hydroxylation of the 10-position of the dibenzocycloheptyl ring which when combined with β-oxidation, resulted in the formation of two diastereoisomers. A minor pathway of biotransformation was the lactamization of these metabolites. In contrast to what observed in dog and man no phase II reactions occurred in the rat. Quantitative differences in metabolic patterns were observed between the three species. Urinary excretion of amineptine and metabolites was higher in man than in rat and dog.

REFERENCES

Ponzio, F., Achilli, G., Garattini, S., Perego, C., Sacchetti, G., Algeri, S. (1986): Amineptine : its effect on the dopaminergic system of rats. J. Pharm. Pharmacol. 38, 301-303.

Van Amerongen, P. (1979): Double-bind clinical trial of the antidepressant action of amineptine. Curr. Med. Res. Opin. 2, 93-100.

Identification of new metabolites of antineoplastic fluoropyrimidines in human bile using fluorine-19 NMR

Marie C. Malet-Martino, Robert Martino, Jean Bernadou, Pascal Chevreau

Laboratoire des IMRCP, Université Paul Sabatier, 118, route de Narbonne, 31062 Toulouse Cedex, France. CHR Purpan, place du Dr. Baylac, 31059 Toulouse Cedex, France

KEY WORDS

Antineoplastic fluoropyrimidines, ^{19}F NMR, biliary metabolites, α-fluoro-β-alanine conjugates with bile acids

INTRODUCTION

5-fluorouracil (5FU) and 5'-deoxy-5-fluorouridine (5'dFUrd), a recent prodrug of 5FU, are used to treat advanced solid tumors. No data exist on the biliary metabolites of 5'dFUrd, and only two studies have examined the human biliary metabolites of 5FU (Douglass, 1974; Heggie, 1986). In bile samples of patients treated with radiolabeled 5FU, Douglass (1974) only found unmetabolized 5FU, and Heggie (1986) reported that the major fraction of radioactivity was a novel metabolite that he did not identify.

Using fluorine-19 nuclear magnetic resonance (^{19}F NMR), a technique requiring no labeled drug and no prior extraction of the biological sample (Malet-Martino, 1986), we demonstrated the presence of novel metabolites of 5'dFUrd or 5FU as human biliary excretion products and identified them as conjugates with bile acids of α-fluoro-β-alanine (FBAL), the main catabolite of fluoropyrimidines.

PATIENTS AND METHODS

The patients
Two patients were evaluated in this study. Patient 1 was a 36-year old male patient being treated for a colon adenocarcinoma. He had a percutaneous transhepatic drainage of the biliary tract. He received 16 g of 5'dFUrd (10 g/m²) by continuous iv infusion over 6 hrs. Patient 2 was a 66-year old male patient with metastatic (rectum adenocarcinoma) liver cancer treated with intraarterial hepatic infusions of 5FU. In the course of an hepatic resection, a bile sample was collected 2 hrs after a bolus injection of 5FU (1 g) via hepatic artery.

^{19}F NMR analysis
The ^{19}F NMR spectra were recorded at 282.4 MHz on a Bruker AM 300 spectrometer, with proton decoupling. The chemical shifts (δ) were reported relative to the chemical shift of trifluoroacetic acid (5 per cent (w/v) aqueous solution).

Reference compounds synthesis

The conjugates of FBAL with bile acids (cholic, deoxycholic and chenodeoxycholic acids) were synthesized using a general method for coupling peptides involving the dicyclohexylcarbodiimide/1-hydroxybenzotriazole combination (Rich, 1979).

RESULTS AND DISCUSSION

A typical ^{19}F NMR spectrum of a bile sample from the patient with an external bile derivation and treated with 5'dFUrd showed the signals of FBAL and fluoride ion that represented ≃ 10% of the excreted fluorinated metabolites. Two other signals were observed, one (X) at -110.68 ppm, the other (Y) at -110.65 ppm (Fig. 1A); X and Y represented ≃ 90% of the biliary metabolites of 5'dFUrd.

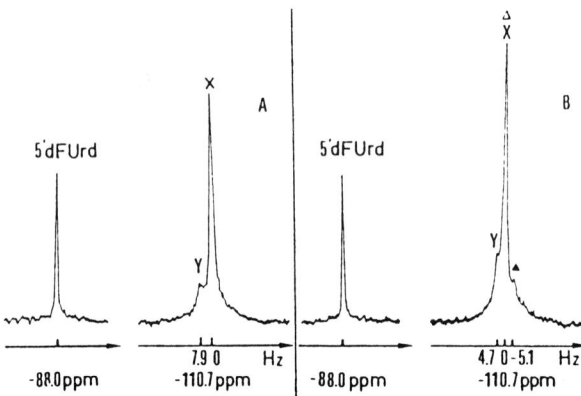

Fig. 1. ^{19}F NMR spectra of bile samples (from patient treated with 5'dFUrd) not spiked (A) and spiked with choloFBAL (B).
X, Y: unknown biliary metabolites; Δ, ▲: choloFBAL. 5'dFUrd is an internal standard. The zero was arbitrarily assigned to the resonance of X.

We verified that X or Y were not already known catabolites of fluoropyrimidines (Fig. 2). 5,6-dihydro-5-fluorouracil (-126.6 ppm), α-fluoro-β-ureidopropionic acid (-111.0 ppm), α-fluoro-β-guanidinopropionic acid (-111.5 ppm) and N-carboxyFBAL (-111.3 ppm) gave rise to 19F NMR signals different from that of X or Y.

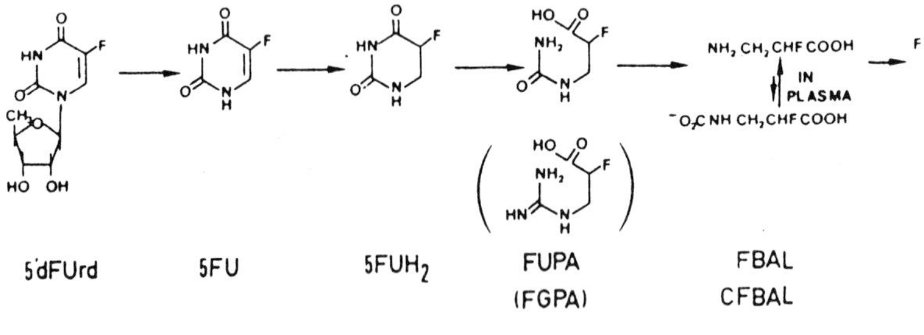

Fig. 2. Catabolic pathway of 5'-deoxy-5-fluorouridine (5'dFUrd) and 5-fluorouracil (5FU).
5FUH2: 5,6-dihydro-5-fluorouracil; FUPA: α-fluoro-β-ureidopropionic acid; FGPA: α-fluoro-β-guanidinopropionic acid; FBAL: α-fluoro-β-alanine; CFBAL, N-carboxy-α-fluoro-β-alanine; F$^-$: fluoride ion.

The ^{19}F NMR characteristics of X and Y and the fact that the acidic hydrolysis of a patient's bile sample gave FBAL led us to assume that these compounds were conjugates of FBAL. A conjugation reaction on the carboxylic acid function of FBAL was discarded since compounds synthesized as models for such a substitution gave 19F NMR signals at much higher field than X or Y. Several hypotheses were considered for a conjugation involving the amine function of FBAL. Glucuronidation and sulfate conjugation were excluded after the unsuccessfull hydrolysis of X or Y by β-D-glucuronidase or sulfatase. N-acetylFBAL (-110.69 ppm) and N-formylFBAL (-110.9 ppm) gave 19F NMR signals that did not correspond to X or Y signals.

Since the structure of FBAL is very close to that of taurine (a β-aminosulfonic acid which conjugates with bile acids) and β-alanine is also a substrate for the bile acid-coA:aminoacid N-acyl transferase (the enzyme that catalyzed the conjugation of glycine or taurine with bile acids (Killenberg, 1980)), we assumed that X and Y could be conjugates of FBAL with bile acids. The conjugates of FBAL with cholic (choloFBAL), deoxycholic and chenodeoxycholic (chenoFBAL) acids were therefore synthesized. The addition of synthetic choloFBAL and chenoFBAL to patient's bile samples led to a sharp increase of the X and Y signals respectively (Fig. 1B and 3B). Since racemic FBAL was used for the synthesis of these compounds, the two diastereoisomers of the bile acid conjugates of FBAL were obtained; the small signals at $\simeq$ 5 Hz (Fig. 1B) or 14 Hz (Fig. 3B) upfield from the main signal of choloFBAL (X) corresponds to the second diastereoisomer of synthetic choloFBAL and chenoFBAL.

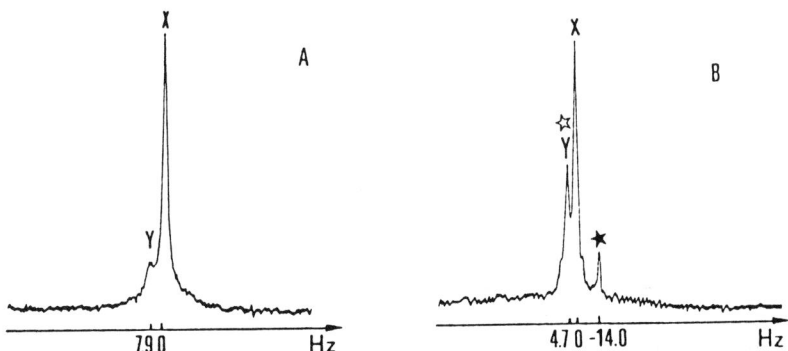

Fig. 3. ^{19}F NMR spectra of bile samples (from the patient treated with 5'dFUrd) not spiked (A) and spiked with chenoFBAL (B).
X, Y: unknown biliary metabolites; ☆, ✶ : chenoFBAL. The zero was arbitrarily assigned to the resonance of X.

Figure 4 shows the ^{19}F NMR spectrum of a bile sample obtained by surgery from the patient treated with intrahepatic 5FU. FBAL represented $\simeq$ 5% and FBAL conjugates $\simeq$ 95% of the biliary metabolites. CholoFBAL (X) and chenoFBAL (Y) were found again but there was also another signal (Z) that corresponds to the conjugate of FBAL with deoxycholic acid.

In conclusion, the biliary excretion of 5FU and 5'dFUrd is mainly constituted by conjugates of FBAL with bile acids. In the patient without external bile drainage, the conjugates of FBAL with "primary" bile acids (cholic and chenodeoxycholic acids)and with the "secondary" bile acid that derives from cholic acid (deoxycholic acid) were observed. In the patient with external bile derivation, only the conjugates of FBAL with "primary" bile acids were formed; this seems not surprising since in cases of bile derivation, the "secondary" bile acids are no longer synthesized due to the suppression of the enterohepatic recirculation. Our study also showed that only one of the two diastereoisomers of each conjugate of FBAL with bile acids was formed in vivo, confirming that metabolic FBAL is optically active.

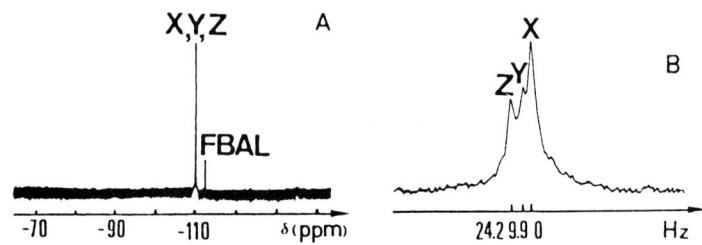

Fig. 4. ^{19}F NMR spectrum of a bile sample from the patient treated with 5FU (A) and expanded area of FBAL conjugates (X, Y, Z) signals (B). The zero was arbitrarily assigned to the resonance of X.

REFERENCES

Douglass, H.O. (1974): Metabolic studies of 5FU. II. Influence of the route of administration on the dynamics of distribution in man. Cancer 34, 1878-1881.

Heggie, G.D. (1986): Catabolism of 5-fluorouracil (FU) in man: evaluation of dihydrofluorouracil (FUH2) formation at different doses of FU with evidence of a novel metabolite in bile. Proc. Amer. Assoc. Cancer Res. 27, 174.

Killenberg, Q.G. (1980): Conjugation by peptide bond formation. In Enzymatic basis of detoxication, vol II, ed W.B. Jacoby, pp 141-67. New York: Academic Press.

Malet-Martino, M.C. (1986): Evidence for the importance of 5'-deoxy-5-fluorouridine catabolism in humans from 19F nuclear magnetic resonance spectrometry. Cancer Res. 46, 2105-2112.

Rich, D.H. (1979): The carbodiimide method. In The peptides. Analysis, synthesis, biology, ed E. Gross and J. Meienhofer, pp 241-61. New York: Academic Press.

The interaction between carbamazepine and erythromycin

Patricia V. Chiappetta, Kenneth W. Renton

Department of Pharmacology, Dalhousie University, Halifax, Nova Scotia, Canada

KEY WORDS
Drug Interaction, Drug Toxicity, Hepatic Drug Metabolism, Erythromycin, Carbamazepine.

INTRODUCTION

In 1977, Dravet and coworkers first described clinical signs of carbamazepine in 8 epileptic patients receiving carbamazepine who had also been given triacetyloleandomycin for mild infections. Since this initial clinical example, Mesdjian et al (1980), Amedee-Manesme et al (1982), Straughan (1982), Hedrick et al (1983), Wong et al (1983), Vajda and Bladin (1984), Carranco et al (1985), Kessler (1985), Wroblewski et al (1986), Jaster et al (1986), Berrettini (1986), and Goulden et al (1986) have all described incidence of carbamazepine intoxication after instituting concurrent erythromycin therapy. In this report we demonstrate that the interaction of carbamazepine and erythromycin results from inhibition at the level of drug biotransformation in the liver.

MATERIALS AND METHODS

Male Sprague-Dawley rats weighing 200 - 250 g were obtained from Canadian Hybrid Farms (Kentville, N.S.) and were housed in wire cages for at least one week prior to use. In the pharmacokinetic studies blood samples (600 µl) were obtained from a cannula inserted into the carotid artery immediately prior to and at 0.25, 0.5, 0.75, 1.0, 1.5, 2.0, 2.5, 3.0, 3.5, 4.0, 5.0 and 5.25 hour intervals following carbamazepine administration. A modification of the HPLC method of Gerson et al (1984) was used to determine serum carbamazepine levels. Microsomes were prepared from rats by the procedure of El Defrawy El Masry et al (1974). Microsomal protein levels were determined by a modification of the method of Lowry et al (1951). Determination of cytochrome P-450 and cytochrome b_5 content followed the procedure of Omura and Sato (1964). Direct measurement of carbamazepine 10,11-epoxide production was used to determine in vitro carbamazepine metabolism by hepatic microsomes using the methods of Grasela and Rocci (1984) and Sladek and Mannering (1968).

RESULTS

The elimination of a single dose of carbamazepine was not affected by erythromycin in normal non-induced rats as illustrated in figure 1A. The elimination half-life ($t_{\frac{1}{2}\beta}$) for the control group was 2.22 ± 0.44 hr and for the

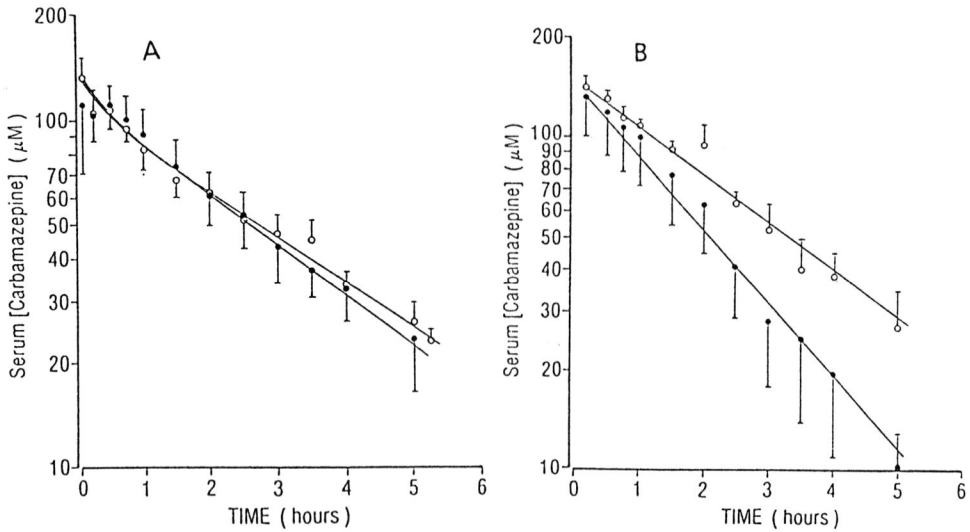

Figure 1: Effect of erythromycin on serum carbamazepine levels in non-induced and carbamazepine induced rats.
Panel A and B illustrates data from normal and carbamazepine induced animals respectively. Closed circles designate saline treated animals and open circles indicate erythromycin treated animals

erythromycin treated rats, it was 2.53 ± 0.08 hr. The clearance rate was 0.145 ± 0.027 1/hr for the controls compared with 0.138 ± 0.020 1/hr for the erythromycin group.

In the multiple dose studies, carbamazepine pretreatment for 4 days was sufficient to induce the in vivo rate of carbamazepine elimination (figure 1B). The elimination rate constants were 0.59 ± 0.06 hr^{-1} (table 1) for the pretreated controls versus 0.35 ± 0.07 hr^{-1} for the untreated controls, indicating that autoinduction of carbamazepine elimination had occurred. In animals induced with carbamazepine for 4 days, erythromycin significantly decreased the rate of carbamazepine elimination compared to the rate observed in saline treated animals (Figure 1B). The clearance rate of carbamazepine was reduced to 0.118 ± 0.016 1/hr compared with 0.233 ± 0.060 1/hr for the controls and the $t_{½\beta}$ after erythromycin treatment was increased to 2.036 ± 0.427 hr from 1.268 ± 0.145 hr

Table 1: Effect of erythromycin on pharmacokinetic parameters of carbamazepine elimination in rats.

	UNINDUCED ANIMALS		CARBAMAZEPINE INDUCED ANIMALS	
	Saline	Erythromycin	Saline	Erythromycin
$t_{½\beta}$ (hr)	2.22 ± 0.44	2.53 ± 0.03	1.27 ± 0.15	2.04 ± 0.43*
Vd_{ss} (1)	0.44 ± 0.09	0.49 ± 0.07	0.43 ± 0.13	0.31 ± 0.01
Cl (1 hr^{-1})	0.15 ± 0.03	0.14 ± 0.02	0.23 ± 0.06	0.12 ± 0.02*
Ke_1 (hr^{-1})	0.35 ± 0.07	0.28 ± 0.01	0.57 ± 0.06	0.39 ± 0.06*

Animals received a single dose of carbamazepine (50 mg/kg) at the beginning of an experiment. Erythromycin (250 mg/kg) treated animals were given the drug at 0 and 5 hours after the start of an experiment. Induced animals received carbamazepine (100 mg/kg) for 4 days prior to pharmacokinetic determinations. Values represent mean ± SEM for 4 rats.
*significantly different from corresponding control, $p<0.05$.

(Table 1). The volume of distribution for carbamazepine remained unchanged in the two treatment groups. From these studies it can be concluded that erythromycin significantly reduced the elimination of carbamazepine in induced but not untreated rats.

Microsomes from the induced rats contained significantly increased cytochrome P-450 levels, 1.086 ± 0.032 nmol/mg protein compared with 0.732 ± 0.026 nmol/mg protein observed for the untreated microsomes, but cytochrome b_5 and protein levels were unaffected.

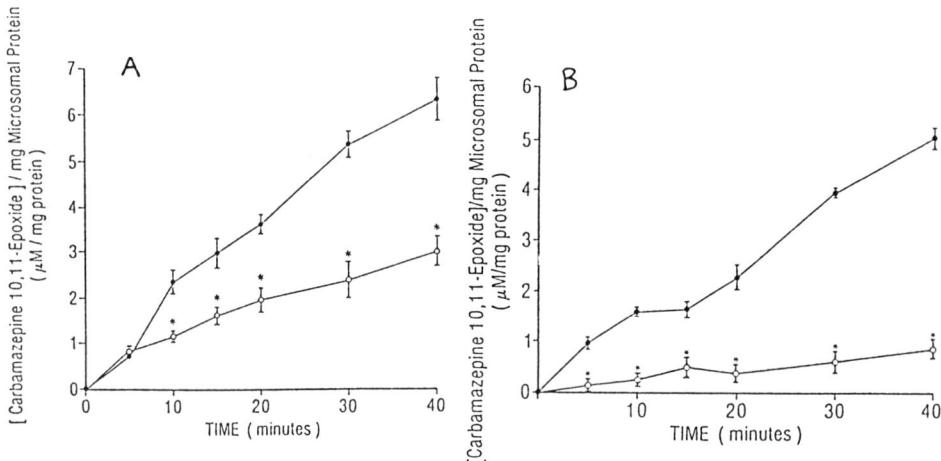

Figure 2: Effect of erythromycin on metabolism of carbamazepine in rat microsomes.
Panel A and B illustrate data form normal and carbamazepine induced animals respectively. Hepatic microsomes were incubated with erythromycin and carbamazepine and the rate of appearance of the major metabolite, carbamazepine 10,11-epoxide was monitored over time (open circles). Control microsomes were incubated with carbamazepine and saline (solid circles). Each point represents mean ± SEM for 4 animals.
* indicates significantly different from controls, $p < .05$

Microsomes were incubated with carbamazepine (7.92 uM) and the rate of formation of the major metabolite, carbamazepine 10,11-epoxide, was monitored in the presence and absence of erythromycin (21.6 uM). Epoxide formation occurred rapidly within 5 minutes of incubation in the untreated control microsomes (figure 2A) and increased to a maximum of 6.35 ± 0.44 uM/mg protein, after 40 minutes of incubation with carbamazepine. In the same experiment, noninduced microsomes incubated with erythromycin were observed to have a significantly decreased rate of production of the metabolite after 10 minutes of incubation; 1.15 ± 0.06 uM/mg protein compared with the controls; 2.36 ± 0.26 uM/mg protein. After 40 minutes of incubation in the presence of erythromycin, the rate of appearance of carbamazepine 10,11-epoxide was found to be over 50% lower than that noted for the control microsomes (3.02 ± 0.34 uM/mg protein), indicating that erythromycin significantly inhibits the in vitro metabolism of carbamazepine.

When carbamazepine-induced microsomes were incubated with carbamazepine, epoxide formation was again found to occur rapidly within 5 minutes (figure 2B). Epoxide production increased throughout the experiment and reached a maximum of

5.04 ± 0.46 uM/mg protein, after 40 minutes. The addition of erythromycin to the pretreated microsomes led to a significant decrease in the rate of metabolite formation (figure 2B). After 5 minutes, the carbamazepine 10,11-epoxide concentration was reduced to 0.15 ± 0.10 uM/mg protein compared with 0.97 ± 0.11 uM/mg protein obtained in the controls. By the end of the experiment, the epoxide concentration in the erythromycin treated microsomes was less than 20% that of the controls; 0.89 ± 0.20 uM/mg protein. It would appear that while both carbamazepine pretreated and untreated microsomes were sensitive to inhibitory effects of erythromycin on carbamazepine metabolism, specifically, the epoxidation route, the induced microsomes were more sensitive to the inhibition, as the concurrent incubation with erythromycin produced a more dramatic reduction in the rate of epoxide formation.

DISCUSSION

The results of this study indicate that carbamazepine elimination is significantly decreased by erythromycin in animals pretreated with carbamazepine but is unaffected in untreated animals. In the carbamazepine-induced rats, the interaction was seen within 24 hours of beginning concomitant erythromycin treatment as is generally the case for reported clinical carbamazepine-erythromycin interactions. Although the dose of carbamazepine used in these studies was at the high end of the therapeutic range for man and the dose of erythromycin was 5 times greater than that recommended for humans, the results suggest that the findings of the current study are relevant to the interaction which has been observed between carbamazepine and erythromycin in humans. In the initial experiments, no significant difference was observed in carbamazepine pharmacokinetics between rats receiving erythromycin and those not receiving it. These observations were perhaps surprising in light of the profound interaction which has been reported to occur between the two drugs in adults and children.

Upon reconsideration of the clinical observations in humans, it was recognized that in all reported incidences of erythromycin or triacetyloleandomycin evoked carbamazepine interactions, patients had been taking carbamazepine for extended periods of time. Therefore, these patients presumably had increased rates of carbamazepine elimination and epoxide formation (Tybring et al, 1981). Thus the use of carbamazepine-induced animals would be a drug interaction model which more closely resembled the clinical situation in humans. Indeed, a 50% reduction in carbamazepine clearance during erythromycin co-administration was observed in induced rats in conjunction with an unmodified volume of distribution, indicating that erythromycin was significantly decreasing the carbamazepine elimination rate (the elimination half-life increased by 60%). It would seem that the findings of the pharmacokinetic studies in induced rats provide a reasonable explanation to account for the high carbamazepine levels which have been reported during the clinical observations of the interaction between erythromycin and carbamazepine in humans. Although no distinguishable effect of erythromycin on epoxide levels was observed in vivo, there were reasonable grounds to believe that this would not be the case in experiments carried out in microsomes. Pachenka et al (1976) and Tybring et al (1981) determined that the epoxide hydrolase activity in rats is much lower in microsomes and the epoxide metabolite is only slowly hydrated to its corresponding diol. This substantial in vitro metabolic difference was observed in microsomes prepared from both induced and uninduced animals. In vitro studies of carbamazepine metabolism can therefore be primarily considered to reflect epoxide formation.

In the current studies, the epoxidation of carbamazepine in untreated rat microsomes was found to decrease by 50% in the presence of erythromycin. In contrast, the rate of epoxide formation in microsomes prepared from carbamazepine-induced rats was inhibited to a greater extent in the presence of the same concentration of erythromycin, indicating that microsomes from carbamazepine-induced animals were more sensitive to the effects of erythromycin. In these microsomes, epoxide formation was decreased by 80% compared to the controls. The greater sensitivity of microsomes from pretreated rats to the effects of erythromycin appears to correlate with the effect of the antibiotic in vivo, where a decrease in carbamazepine elimination by erythromycin was only observed in induced animals. Because a significant reduction in carbamazepine metabolism in the presence of erythromycin was also obtained in untreated microsomes, the potential for an in vivo kinetic interaction also exists in these rats. This likely indicates that the effect of erythromycin in uninduced animals was not of sufficient magnitude to produce a measureable effect (based on serum sampling). These results illustrate that erythromycin is capable of decreasing both the rate of carbamazepine metabolism and subsequent elimination via an inhibition of the epoxide route.

In contrast to the experimental design used in rats in the present study, the only investigation to date which examined the effects of erythromycin on carbamazepine kinetics in healthy human volunteers (Wong et al, 1983) compared the elimination of a single oral dose of carbamazepine with a single oral dose of carbamazepine given after the subjects had been pretreated orally for 5 days with erythromycin. Only the carbamazepine clearance rate was decreased significantly in the study; the elimination rate constant and apparent volume of distribution were unchanged.

In summary this investigation has demonstrated that Erythromycin decreases the elimination of carbamazepine in animals which have been induced by multiple carbamazepine doses. This is caused by a decrease in the metabolism of carbamazepine probably as a result of erythromycin binding to cytochrome P-450 and inhibiting the major route of metabolism to its epoxide. This mechanism likely explains why erythromycin decreases the elimination of carbamazepine and causes a major drug interaction in man.

REFERENCES

Amedee-Menesme, O., Rey, E., Brussieux, J., Goutieres, F., Aicardi, J. (1982): Antibiotiques: à ne jamais associer à la carbamazepine. Arch. Fr. Pediatr., 39, 126.

Berrettini, W.H. (1986): A case of erythromycin-induced carbamazepine toxicity. J. Clin. Psych., 47, 147.

Carranco, E., Kareus, J., Schenley, C.O., Peak, V., Al-Rajeh, S. (1985): Carbamazepine Toxicity Induced by Concurrent Erythromycin Therapy. Arch. Neurol., 42, 187.

Dravet, C., Mesdjian, E., Cenraud, B., Roger, J. (1977): Interaction Between Carbamazepine and Triacetyloleandomycin. Lancet, 1, 810.

El Defrawy El Masry, S., Cohen, G.M., Mannering, G.J. (1974): Sex-Dependent Differences in Drug Metabolism in the Rat. 1. Temporal Changes in the Microsomal Drug-Metabolising System of the Liver During Sexual Maturation. Drug Metab. Disp., 12, 267.

Gerson, B., Bell, F., Chan, S. (1984): Antiepileptic Drugs - Primidone, Phenobarbitol, Phenytoin and Carbamazepine by Reversed-Phase Liquid Chromatography. Clin. Chem., 30, 105.

Goulden, K.J., Camfield, P., Dooley, J.M., Fraser, A., Meek, D.C., Renton, K.W., Tibbles, J.A.R. (1986): Severe Carbamazepine Intoxication After Coadministration of Erythromycin. J. Ped., 109, 135.

Grasela, D.M., Rocci, M.L. (1984): Inhibition of Carbamazepine Metabolism by Cimetidine. Drug Metab. Disp., 12, 204.

Hedrick, R., Williams, F., Morin, R., Lamb, W.A., Cate, J.C. (1983): Carbamazepine - Erythromycin Interaction leading to Carbamazepine Toxicity in Four Epileptic Children. Ther. Drug Monit., 5, 405.

Jaster, P.J., Abbas, D. (1986): Erythromycin - Carbamazepine Interaction. Neurol., 36, 594

Kessler, J.M. (1985): Erythromycin - Carbamazepine Interaction. SA Med. J., 67, 1038.

Lowry, O.H., Rosebrough, N.J., Farr, A.L., Randall, R.J. (1951): Protein Measurement with the Folin Phenol Reagent. J. Biol. Chem., 193, 265.

Mesdjian, E., Dravet, C., Cenraud, B., Roger, J. (1980): Carbamazepine Intoxication Due to Triacetyloleandomycin Administration in Epileptic Patients. Epilepsia, 21, 489.

Omura, T., Sato, R. (1964): The Carbon Monoxide-Binding Pigment of Liver Microsomes. 1. Evidence for its Hemoprotein Nature. J. Biol. Chem., 239, 2370.

Pachenka, J., Salmona, M., Cantoni, L., Mussini, E., Pantarotto, C., Frigerio, A., Belvedere, G. (1976): Activity of liver microsomal mono-oxygenases on some epoxide-forming tricyclic drugs. Xenobiot., 6, 593.

Sladek, N.E., Mannering, G.J. (1969): Induction of Drug Metabolism. 1. Difference in the Mechanisms by Which Polycyclic Hydrocarbons and Phenobarbitol Produce their Inductive Effects on Microsomal N-Demethylating Systems. Mol. Pharmacol., 5, 174.

Straughan, J. (1982): Erythromycin - Carbamazepine Interaction? S.A. Med. J., 61, 420.

Tybring, G., von Bahr, C., Bertilsson, L., Collste, H., Glaumann, H., Solbrand, M. (1981): Metabolism of Carbamazepine and its Epoxide Metabolite in Human and Rat Liver In Vitro. Drug Metab. Disp., 9, 561.

Vajda, F.J.E., Bladin, P.F. (1984): Carbamazepine - erythromycin base interaction. Med. J. Aust., 140, 81.

Wong, Y.Y., Ludden, T.M., Bell, R.D. (1983): Effect of Erythromycin on Carbamazepine Kinetics. Clin. Pharmacol. Ther., 33, 460.

Wroblewski, B.A., Singer, W.D., White, J. (1986): Carbamazepine - Erythromycin interaction : Case Studies and Clinical Significance. JAMA, 255, 1165.

The influence of age on the metabolism of theophylline in uninduced rats

Kees Groen, Gerjan J.J.M. Trommelen, Kees F.A. van Bezooijen

TNO Institute for Experimental Gerontology, PO Box 5815, 2280 HV Rijswijk, The Netherlands

Keywords: aging, cytochrome P-450, theophylline metabolism

INTRODUCTION

It is well known that in the elderly many more adverse drug reactions are observed than in younger people (Seidl et al, 1966; Hurwitz et al, 1969; Smidt et al, 1972).
Since xenobiotics, like drugs, can be eliminated from the body in different ways, there may be different reasons for this increased frequency of adverse drug reactions, of which the possible decreased activity of liver enzymes with age might be an important factor (Van Bezooijen, 1986). The liver cytochrome P-450 complex, which consists of several different isoenzymes, plays an important role in the phase I metabolism of xenobiotics. It is possible that these isoenzymes are differentially influenced by aging.
To characterise the activities of the isoenzymes in vivo, specific model drugs are used (Danhof, 1980; Van der Graaff, 1985; Teunissen, 1984). For this characterisation not only the plasma clearance of the parent drugs are important, but also the formation of the different metabolites (Breimer, 1983; Van der Graaf et al, 1983).
In the present study, the influence of aging on the activity of the isoenzymes involved in the metabolism of theophylline is expected to be mediated by the isoenzymes P-450 c and d (Cyt. P-448) (Teunissen, 1984).

METHODS

Male Brown Norway/BiRij rats of different ages (SPF) from the inbred strain of REP-TNO were used throughout this cross-sectional study. The rats had free access to food and water before and during the study.
Theophylline (dose $\leq$ 13 mg/kg) was injected in a volume of 0.5 ml. intravenously. Serial bloodsamples were taken from the carotid artery via a catheter at regular time-intervals.
During the experiments urine and faeces were collected over a 24 hours period after administration.
Analysis of theophylline in plasma and theophylline and metabolites in urine was performed using the HPLC-method described by Tang-Liu and Riegelman (1982).

RESULTS

The metabolism of theophylline was examined in rats of 3, 12, 24, 30 and 36 months of age. A significant difference ($P \leq 0.05$) was seen between the plasma elimination half-life of theophylline in 3 ($\pm$ 220 min.) and 12 month-old rats ($\pm$320 min.). Only in 36 month-old rats a further increase in the elimination half-life was seen compared to the 12 month-old rats ($\pm$460 min.) (fig. I and fig. II).

The percentage of theophylline excreated in urine as the unchanged drug remained reasonably constant ($\pm$22% of the dose) when the age groups were compared. However, in 2 rats of 24 months an impaired urinairy excretion of the parent compound was found ($\pm$4% of the dose). This phenomenon might be caused by hydronephrosis, a renal disease, which is quite regularly observed in Brown Norway rats.

The intrinsic clearance (CL_i), indicative for the activity of the cytochrome P-450 isoenzymes, was calculated by taking into account the amount of unchanged theophylline excreted in urine.

The protein-binding of theophylline was $\pm$ 12% in the Brown Norway rats and was constant over the age groups.

The intrinse clearance decreased significantly from 1.7 $ml.min.^{-1}kg.^{-1}$ in 3 month-old rats to 1.2 $ml.min.^{-1}kg.^{-1}$ in 12 month-old rats (fig. III). Only in 30 months-old rats a further significant decrease (to $\pm$ 0.90 $ml.min.^{-1}kg^{-1}$) was observed, whereas in the 24-, and 36 month-old rats this phenomenon was masked by a higher standard deviation, though in these groups the mean metabolic clearance was also 0.90 $ml.min.^{-1} kg.^{-1}$.

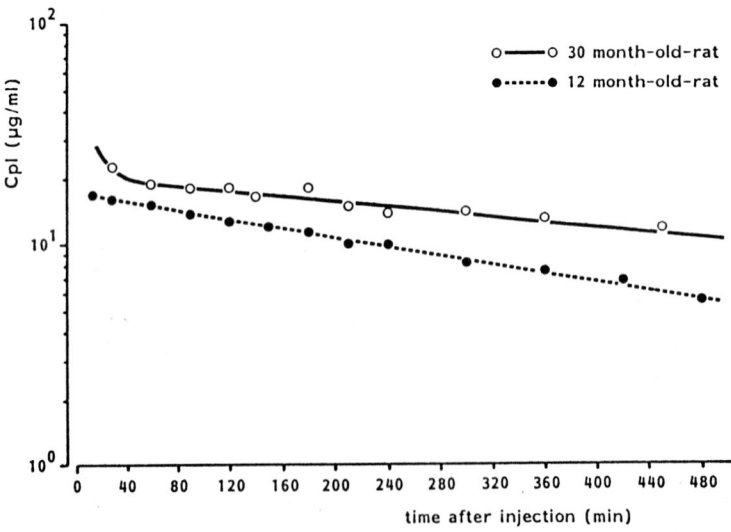

Fig. 1 Plasma disappearance curves of theophylline in male BN/BiRij rats of different age

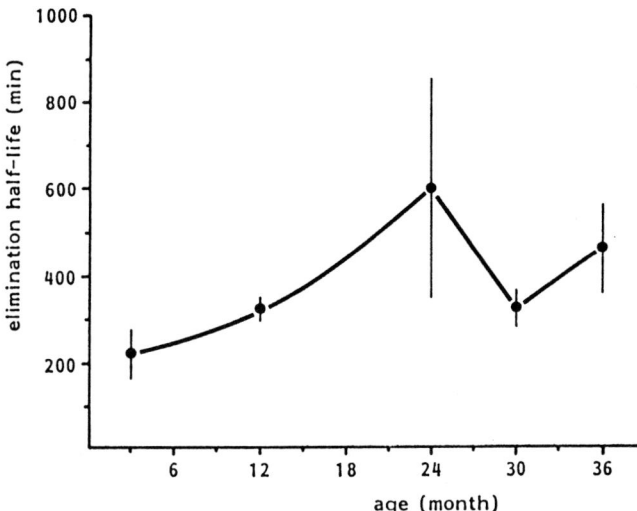

Fig. 2   The influence of age on the plasma elimination half-life of theophylline
means ± S.D. are given for each age group

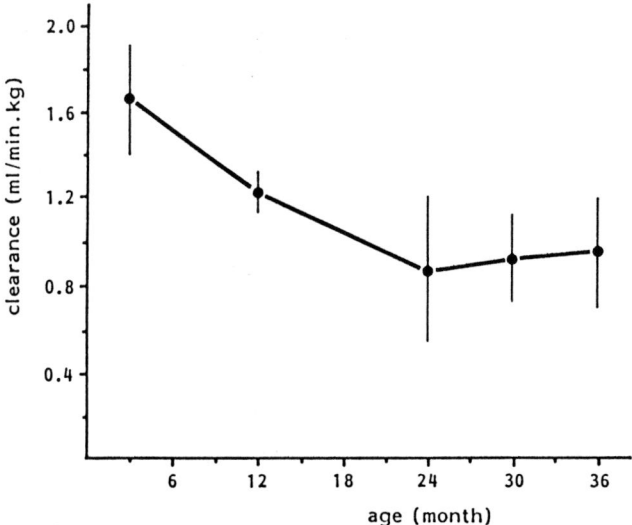

Fig. 3   The effect of age on the hepatic clearance of theophylline
means ± S.D. are given for the age groups

CONCLUSIONS

From the results obtained from the present study it can be concluded that aging decreases the activities of the cytochrome P-450 isoenzymes involved in the metabolism of the theophylline.
It has already been reported (Canada et al, 1986) that in rabbits a comparable decrease in clearance of theophylline from the body was observed, though in their calculation of the clearance the urinary excretion of the parent drug was not taken into account.
Further investigations will be performed to determine to what extend the formation rates of the different metabolites of theophylline are influenced by age.

REFERENCES

Bezooijen, C.F.A. van (1986). Topics in aging research in Europe, In Liver, drugs and aging, ed C.F.A. van Bezooijen, F. Miglio, and D.L. Knook, vol 7, pp 25-32. Rijswijk: EURAGE.

Breimer, D.D. (1983): Interindividual variations in drug disposition: Clinical implications and methods of investigation. Clin. Pharmacokinet., 8, 371-377.

Canada, A., Wilson, J., and Calabrese, E. (1986): Elimination kinetics of theophylline in the rabbit: effect of age and sex. Drug Metab. Disposit. 14, 372-373.

Danhof, M. (1980): Antipyrine metabolite profile as a tool in the assessment of the activity of different drug oxydizing enzymes is man. Thesis, Leiden.

Graaff, M. van der, Vermeulen, N.P.E., Langendijk, M.P.J., and Breimer, D.D. (1983): Pharmacokinetics of simultaneously administered hexo- and heptabarbital in rats. J. Pharmacol. Exp. Ther. 225, 745-751.

Graaff, M. van der (1985) Characterization and prediction of in vivo oxydative drug metabolizing enzyme activity. Thesis, Leiden.

Hurwitz, N. and Wade, D.L. (1969): Intensive hospital monitoring of adverse reactions to drugs. Brit.Med. Journal, 1, 531-536.

Seidl, L.G., Thornton, G.F., Smith, J.W. and Cluff, L.E. (1966): Studies on the epidemiology of adverse drug reactions. Bull. John Hopkins hospital, 199, 299-315.

Smidt, N.A. and McQueen, E.G. (1972): Adverse reactions to drugs: a comprehensive hospital inpatient survey. New Zealand Med. Journal 76, 397-401.

Teunissen, M. (1984): Factors and conditions affecting antipyrine clearance and metabolite formation. Thesis, Leiden.

Mechanisms of drug hepatotoxicity

Les mécanismes de l'hépatotoxicité médicamenteuse

Mechanisms of drug-induced hepatitis

Dominique Pessayre, Dominique Larrey

Unité de Recherches de Physiopathologie Hépatique (INSERM U.24), Hôpital Beaujon, 92118 Clichy, France

KEY-WORDS

Hepatotoxicity, Mechanisms, Reactive metabolites.

SUMMARY

The mechanism for hepatitis remains unknown for most hepatotoxic drugs. A single drug may have several toxic effects on the liver, or may produce either toxic or allergic hepatitis in different patients. Formation of reactive metabolites is relatively frequent. Despite several protective mechanisms, it may lead to the covalent binding of an electrophilic metabolite to proteins, the initiation of lipid peroxidation by a free radical, the depletion and/or oxidation of glutathione. There follows a number of structural and functional lesions, including a sustained increase in cytosolic calcium, eventually leading to cell death.
Formation of reactive metabolites may lead to either toxic or allergic hepatitis in humans. Toxic hepatitis may occur predictably after massive overdoses (see chapter of L.F. Prescott). After therapeutics doses, it occurs in an idiosyncratic fashion, in a few patients only. Both genetic factors (see chapter of D. Larrey) and acquired factors may influence susceptibility. Allergic hepatitis may also occur, as a possible consequence of immunization against metabolite-altered plasma membrane protein epitopes (see chapter of J. Neuberger). In some instances, auto-antibodies (directed against normal protein epitopes) may be detected, as the anti-cytochrome P-450 auto-antibodies found in tienilic acid hepatitis (see chapter of P. Beaune). Determination of the mechanism for hepatitis may lead to therapeutic recommendations, prevention of hepatitis after overdoses, and the rational development of safer analogues.

INTRODUCTION

About 600 drugs are suspected of being possibly hepatotoxic (Stricker and Spoelstra, 1985). The mechanism for hepatitis, however, remains unknown for most compounds. Our present state of ignorance stems from several reasons.

a) For many drugs, including some frequently hepatotoxic, no study has been done to understand the mechanism for hepatitis.

b) The drug itself, a stable metabolite, or a reactive metabolite may be responsible for the toxic effects. Thus, unchanged perhexiline accumulates within lysosomes, where it probably decreases the activity of phospholipases, leading to lysosomal phospholipidosis of the liver (Pessayre et al., 1979b). 5-Fluorouracil is bioconverted to fluorodeoxyuridylic acid which inhibits thymidylate synthetase and DNA synthesis (Albert, 1973). Acetaminophen and several other drugs are transformed into chemically reactive metabolites toxic to the liver (Mitchell and Jollow, 1975).

c) There is not one, but probably many different mechanisms of toxicity. This diversity can be easily apprehended if one thinks of the variety of chemical structures of drugs on the one hand, and the complexity of the liver cell, on the other hand. Clearly, such or such drug may interfere with such or such enzyme, transporter, or regulatory mechanism.

d) A single drug may have several toxic effects on the liver. For example, pirprofen, a non steroidal anti-inflammatory drug, with a 2-arylpropionate structure, is transformed by cytochrome P-450, probably on its pyrroline ring, into reactive metabolites which may be responsible for idiosyncratic hepatocellular jaundice in a few, metabolically susceptible patients (Hayat-Bonan et al., in preparation). At the same time, however, the propionate group of pirprofen may form an acyl-coenzyme A derivative, which inhibits the mitochondrial β-oxidation of fatty acids (Genève et al., 1987b), leading to microvesicular steatosis of the liver in some patients (Danan et al., 1985). Similarly, the antidepressant amineptine is activated by cytochrome P-450, probably on its tricyclic structure, into chemically reactive metabolites that may be responsible for allergic hepatitis in a few patients (Genève et al., 1987a, c,d). In addition, the acyl chain of amineptine inhibits the β-oxidation of fatty acids (Le Din et al., in preparation).

e) In addition to various toxic mechanisms, an allergic phenomenon is frequently responsible for drug-induced hepatitis. Immunoallergic hepatitis is suspected on the following grounds. Hepatitis is uncommon. It is frequently associated with fever and eosinophilia, and may be associated with other allergic manifestations (rash, blood dyscrasia, tubulo-interstitial nephritis...). Even more convincingly, hepatitis quickly recurs after a drug rechallenge, an observation consistent with immune memory.

f) To complicate matters further, it is likely that some drugs may produce toxic hepatitis in some patients and allergic hepatitis in other patients. Thus, while most cases of isoniazid hepatitis are probably toxic in type, a few cases are associated with hypersensitivity manifestations, possibly consistent with an allergic mechanism (Black et al., 1975). Another possible example may be amodiaquine (Larrey et al., 1986a).

Despite these difficulties, much progress has been made in the past decades. One single mechanism has emerged as being particularly frequent, namely the formation of chemically reactive metabolites. This will be the subject of further comments.

FORMATION OF CHEMICALLY REACTIVE METABOLITES

Long before the advent of chemists, pharmacists and doctors, animals and man have been exposed to a variety of foreign compounds (or xenobiotics) which are not part of normal mammalian cell constituents. These xenobiotics had to be eliminated. The kidney may excrete hydrosoluble compounds (which are soluble in urine) but cannot eliminate strictly lipid-soluble xenobiotics. This difficulty is circumvented in the liver, where liposoluble xenobiotics are oxidized by cytochrome P-450 and conjugated with polar compounds, so that the resulting hydrosoluble conjugates can now be excreted in urine.

Cytochrome P-450 is composed of several isoenzymes, with a same oxidizing center (the heme iron) but different apoproteins (Wang et al., 1983). These different apoproteins delineate different hydrophobic pockets, which reversibly bind the substrates. These different pockets have different affinities for such or such substrate. They may also orient differently these substrates towards the heme iron, to that different sites may be oxidized (Kaminsky et al., 1984). Thanks to the multiplicity of these isoenzymes, and the fact that each isoenzyme can metabolize many substrates, cytochrome P-450 represents a versatile system which can metabolize and eliminate an infinity of foreign compounds.

This system is not without drawbacks, however. While some xenobiotics are transformed into stable metabolites, other xenobiotics, including several drugs (Table 1), form reactive, potentially toxic, metabolites.

Table 1. Hepatotoxic drugs known to be transformed into chemically reactive metabolites

Acetaminophen	Estrogens	Nitrofurantoin
Alpha-methyldopa	Ethinyl estradiol	Norethisterone
Benoxaprofen	Fluroxene	Phenacetine
BCNU	Halothane	Phenylbutazone
CCNU	Hycanthone	Phenytoin
Chloramphenicol	Imipramine	Propranolol
Chloroform	Iproniazid	Propylthiouracil
Chlorpromazine	Isaxonine	Tienilic acid
Cyclophosphamide	Isoniazid	Trichloroethylene
Dantrolene	Methimazole	Troleandomycin
Enflurane	Methoxyflurane	Urethane
Erythromycin	Metronidazole	

Such metabolites are usually formed by oxidation mediated by cytochrome P-450 (e.g. the oxidation of acetaminophen into a quinone-imine, or the formation of epoxides from arenes or alkenes). A few reactive metabolites, however, are formed by reduction. In its reduced form, before the binding of molecular oxygen, cytochrome P-450Fe(II) is a good reductant, which can, for example dehalogenate several haloalkanes (e.g. carbon tetrachloride, halothane) to the corresponding free radicals. Microsomal NADPH-cytochrome P-450 reductase may also reduce some drugs into reactive radicals (e.g. formation of semiquinone radicals from quinones; formation of nitro anion radicals from nitroarenes).

It thus appears that the cytochrome P-450 system, albeit highly useful for the elimination of lipid-soluble xenobiotics (and the metabolism of several endogenous compounds) nevertheless represented a serious threat by forming quite a number of potentially toxic metabolites. Obviously, such a system could not have evolved without the preliminary or concomitant development of several protective mechanisms.

PROTECTIVE MECHANISMS

Indeed, several mechanisms concur to limit the toxicity of chemically reactive metabolites.

a) A first mechanism, automatically included in the system, is the auto-inactivation of cytochrome P-450. Indeed, the metabolite which has just been formed inside the hydrophobic pocket of cytochrome P-450 may directly damage cytochrome P-450. It may covalently bind to the apoprotein, or to a nitrogen of heme, may lead to the covalent binding of heme to the apoprotein, or may form a stable complex with the heme iron of cytochrome P-450 (Davies et al., 1986; Franklin, 1977; Halpert et al., 1983; Larrey et al., 1986c; Ortiz de Montellano et al., 1981). In these different ways, the metabolite may inactivate cytochrome P-450, auto-limiting its own formation and toxicity.

b) Epoxide hydrolases convert reactive epoxides into inactive dihydrodiols (Oesh, 1972).

c) Many electrophilic metabolites are conjugated with glutathione and thereby detoxified (Mitchell and Jollow, 1975). This spontaneous reaction is further catalyzed by several glutathione S-transferases.

d) Glutathione, glutathione peroxidase, glutathione S-transferases, glutathione reductase, a glutathione-dependent cytosolic mechanism, vitamin E and vitamin C all concur to limit lipid peroxidation initiated by reactive free radicals.

These various detoxifying mechanisms often act concomitantly, as in the cases of trichloroethylene (Allemand et al., 1978; Pessayre et al., 1979a) and vinyl chloride (Pessayre et al., 1979d). Thanks to these protective mechanisms, natural xenobiotics that we commonly drink, ingest or inhale daily are well tolerated. However, when large amounts of drugs or chemicals are ingested, protective mechanisms may be overwhelmed, leading to molecular and liver lesions.

MOLECULAR LESIONS

Chemically reactive metabolites may lead to three main initial molecular lesions.

Covalent binding to proteins and nucleic acids

Electrophilic metabolites may covalently bind to many different nucleophilic sites of proteins, nucleic acids, or both. Although covalent binding is clearly non specific, there may be at least some degree of selectivity. Both electrophiles and nucleophiles can be classified as being "hard" (with highly polarized charge density) or "soft" (Coles, 1984-85). Soft electrophiles react mainly with soft nucleophiles, while hard electrophiles react mainly with hard nucleophiles (Coles, 1984-85).

Relatively soft electrophilic metabolites react with the relatively soft nucleophilic groups of proteins. The metabolites may react with the -SH group of a cysteine, the sulfur of a methionine, the $-NH_2$ of a lysine, or arginine residue, or the -NH- of an histidine (Coles, 1984-85). Covalent binding of the metabolite may alter protein structure and function, decreasing the activity of enzymes, transporters... and so on.

In contrast, hard electrophilic metabolites covalently bind to the relatively hard nucleophilic sites of nucleic acids, possibly leading to mutagenesis and cancer. This may explain that some reactive metabolites lead mainly to tissue necrosis while other reactive metabolites are mainly mutagenic and carcinogenic. This distinction is not absolute, however. Several compounds are, indeed, both necrogenic and carcinogenic, either because the chemical hardness of the reactive electrophilic metabolite is intermediate, or because they form both hard and soft electrophiles, as in the case of vinyl halides (Coles, 1984-85).

In addition to the chemical hardness or softness of reactive metabolites, other factors may lead to the relative selectivity of covalent binding. A highly unstable intermediate may mainly bind to the apoprotein of cytochrome P-450. Other, still poorly understood, chemical factors may be involved as well (Coles, 1984-85).

Covalent binding to lipids and lipid peroxidation

A second type of molecular lesion is the formation of lipid radicals. Either the additon of a reactive drug radical ($R^{\bullet}$) on a carbon of an unsaturated lipid, or the abstraction by this radical of an hydrogen atom, lead in both cases to a lipid radical (Lipid$^{\bullet}$). This radical quickly adds molecular oxygen to form a peroxy radical (Lipid-OO$^{\bullet}$). This peroxy radical may react with another lipid molecule (Lipid$_2$-H) to form a hydroperoxide and a new lipid radical: lipid$_1$-OO$^{\bullet}$ + lipid$_2$-H $\longrightarrow$ lipid$_1$-OOH + lipid$_2^{\bullet}$. Lipid peroxidation may thus extend from one lipid to the other or along a same lipid chain. Eventually, unsaturated lipids are oxidized and cut into small fragments (alkanes, malondialdehyde, alkenals). These last aldehydes are themselves reactive and can covalently bind to proteins.

Glutatione depletion

Extensive formation of a reactive metabolite, and its conjugation with glutathione may lead to glutathione depletion. Because of the many roles of glutathione in the cell, its depletion has serious toxicological consequences.

a) Once glutathione is depleted, the reactive metabolites which is formed cannot bind to glutathione and massively binds to hepatic proteins (Mitchell and Jollow, 1975).

b) Depletion and/or oxidation of glutathione leads to oxidation of the SH-groups of proteins, which decreases the activity of several enzymes, including that of vital calcium translocases (Bellomo and Orrenius, 1985).

c) Depletion of glutathione permits the onset of lipid peroxidation (Wendel et al., 1979).

STRUCTURAL AND FUNCTIONNAL ALTERATIONS

Subsequent to these initial molecular lesions, there follows a variety of structural and functional alterations. The plasma membrane presents blebs, and it leaks ions. Calcium entry into the cells, together with its reduced captation into microsomes and mitochrondria, and its reduced extrusion out of the cell, lead to sustained increase in cytosolic calcium concentration (Bellomo and Orrenius, 1985). This may in turn activate a non-lysosomal proteolytic system (Nicotera et al, 1986). In addition, there is decreased protein synthesis, reduced formation of ATP, decreased concentration of various cofactors, and inhibition of several enzymes (Thor and Orrenius, 1980).

It is difficult to delineate among these various alterations, which comes first and which is secondary, which is determinant and which is trivial. Considerable evidence, however, has been accumulated in recent years for the role of a sustained increase in cytosolic calcium as an early and determinant step in hepatic injury, at least in several models.

IN SITU LESIONS

While some, slightly reactive metabolites, such as acetaldehyde, may leave their site of formation, most reactive metabolites are so highly unstable and short-lived that they mainly react in situ in the very organ that forms them (Breen et al., 1982). The abundance of cytochrome P-450 in the liver, and the in situ reaction of reactive metabolites explain the unique role of reactive metabolites in drug-induced hepatitis. This in situ binding also contributes to the location of liver cell necrosis. Although different isoenzymes may have different repartition, cytochrome P-450 as a whole predominates in centrilobular hepatocytes. Since such hepatocytes are, in addition, poor in glutathione, covalent binding mainly affects centrilobular areas. This may explain that necrosis usually predominates in centrilobular areas.

CLINICAL ASPECTS

It is increasingly admitted that formation of reactive metabolites may lead to either toxic or allergic hepatitis in humans.

Toxic hepatitis

Drug-induced toxic hepatitis has not the constancy classically expected of a toxic phenomenon. This is because molecules that would produce constant hepatitis at therapeutic doses are not marketed as drugs. This selection imposes that the drug be well tolerated in most subjects. Toxic hepatitis may nevertheless occur in 2 circumtances.

Usual toxicity after overdoses. While therapeutic doses are well tolerated, massive overdoses lead to hepatitis (see the chapter of L.F. Prescott on acetaminophen).

Toxic, idiosyncratic, hepatitis. Although well-tolerated in most patients, therapeutic doses may nevertheless produce toxic hepatitis in a few patients. The reasons explaining the unique susceptibility of these few patients are still poorly understood. There is growing evidence, however, suggesting that individual susceptibility to toxic damage may be either genetic or acquired.

a) Genetic factors may first affect the formation of chemically reactive metabolites. Indeed, levels of a given cytochrome P-450 isoenzyme are quite variable in different subjects (Cresteil et al., 1985). Since a reactive metabolite may be mainly formed by a given isoenzyme, a subject with a high constitutive level of this isoenzyme will form greater amounts of this metabolite and may be uniquely susceptible to its toxicity. Genetic factors may also affect the inactivation of reactive metabolites, as in subjects with a deficiency in glutathione synthetase or in epoxide hydrolase activity (see chapter of D. Larrey).

b) Susceptibililty may also be acquired, as a consequence of physiological, nutritional or therapeutic influences. Pregnancy, for example, decreases the capacity of the liver to resynthetize glutathione, and increases the hepatotoxicity of acetaminophen in mice (Larrey et al., 1986b), and perhaps also in humans (unpublished clinical observations).

Fasting, or protein denutrition, decreases hepatic glutathione content, and dramatically increases the hepatotoxicity of acetaminophen in rats (Pessayre et al., 1979c). Hepatitis has been observed after high therapeutic doses of acetaminophen in a few subjects with malnutrition (Barker et al., 1977; Ware et al., 1978).

Microsomal enzyme induction by concomitantly administered drugs may increase the formation of the reactive metabolite, and the susceptibility to hepatitis. Thus rifampicin, a microsomal enzyme inducer (Pessayre and Mazel, 1976), may increase the formation and toxicity of the reactive metabolites of isoniazid (Pessayre et al., 1977). Microsomal enzyme inducers may have triggered fulminant hepatitis in 3 patients on iproclozide (Pessayre et al., 1978). Chronic ethanol ingestion increases a particular isoenzyme of cytochrome P-450 with a high activity towards acetaminophen, and potentiates the hepatotoxicity of therapeutic doses of acetaminophen in humans (McClain et al., 1980).

Allergic hepatitis

It has been proposed for a decade (Kappus and Remmer, 1976; Pessayre and Benhamou, 1978), and is increasingly admitted, that formation of reactive metabolites may also lead to allergic hepatitis.

Indeed, covalently bound reactive metabolites may not be restricted to the cell inside but may be bound as well to plasma membrane proteins (Satoh et al., 1985a,b). Whether they directly bind there, or whether they first bind to microsomal proteins, which then migrate to the plasma membrane, remains unknown at that time.

Plasma membrane protein epitopes, modified by the covalent binding of a reactive metabolite, may be recognized as foreign and may trigger an allergic response against such modified protein structures. Metabolite-triggered immunologically-mediated hepatitis may be responsible for severe clinical hepatitis due to halothane (see chapter of J. Neuberger), as well as hepatitis due to isaxonine (Fouin-fortunet et al., 1984; Lettéron et al., 1984), α-methyldopa (Neuberger et al., 1985) and amineptine (Genève et al., 1987a,c,d). It may also be responsible for hepatitis due to erythromycin estolate or troleandomycin (Pessayre et al., 1985). Indeed, erythromycin estolate hepatitis is uncommon; it is frequently associated with hypersensivity manifestations (fever, eosinophilia, rash) and recurs within a few days if erythromycin is readministered (Funck-Brentano et al., 1983). Erythromycin and troleandomycin are transformed by glucocorticoid-inducible isoenzyme(s) of cytochrome P-450 into nitroso derivatives in rats (Danan et al., 1981; Pessayre, 1981a), and in humans

(Larrey et al., 1983a; Pessayre et al., 1982). These unstable nitroso derivatives have two adverse effects. a) They form a stable inactive, complex with the iron(II) of cytochrome P-450, decreasing the metabolism of several drugs (Pessayre, 1985) and endogenous substrates (Le Dafniet et al., 1981; Pessayre et al., 1981b). b) The nitroso metabolite (or its nitrone precursor) may react with glutathione or cysteine (Pessayre et al., 1983) and might therefore covalently bind to the SH groups of proteins. Not all macrolides, however, form such nitroso derivatives. Whereas erythromycin and troleandomycin form a nitroso derivative and lead to drug interactions and hepatitis, in contrast, spiramycin and midecamycin do not form nitroso-P-450 metabolite complexes (Delaforge et al., 1983; Larrey et al., 1983b) and do not lead to drug interactions or hepatitis.

Interestingly, whereas halothane, α-methyldopa and isaxonine lead to hepatocellular damage, in constrast, hepatitis due to aminoptine, erythromycin and troleandomycin is mainly cholestatic. Similarly, allergic cholestatic hepatitis due to chlorpromazine or imipramine, might be triggered by the formation of reactive metabolites (De Mol and Busher, 1984; Kappus and Remmer, 1975). It thus appears that metabolite-triggered allergic hepatitis may lead to necrosis, cholestasis, or both (e.g. imipramine).

It is also noteworthy that the same metabolic factors which may predispose some individuals to idiosyncratic, toxic, hepatitis may also predispose them to allergic hepatitis, probably by increasing exposure to allergenic metabolite-altered protein epitopes (see chapter of D. Larrey).

Auto-immunity

In several instances of drug-induced allergic hepatitis, auto-antibodies directed against normal cell constituents can be detected. Thus, iproniazid hepatitis is usually associated with a particular anti-mitochondrial antibody, the "anti-M_6" auto-antibody (Danan et al., 1987). Hepatitis due to tienilic acid is usually associated with an antimicrosomal, anti-cytochrome P-450, auto-antibody (see chapter of P. Beaune).

The mechanism(s) leading to the appearance of such auto-antibodies remain unknown, at present. Perhaps, the immunologic reaction against metabolite-altered plasma membrane protein epitopes may also affect, to some extent (by cross-reactivity), normal protein epitopes.

It is possible that immunization against normal cell constituents may explain the slow aggravation of some cases of iproniazid hepatitis, despite interruption of the drug administration (Pessayre, 1987). Auto-immunity has been considered also as a possible cause of prolonged cholestasis after administration of ajmaline (Larrey et al., 1986d), cyproheptadine (Larrey et al., 1987b) or troleandomycin (Larrey et al., 1987a). In this curious condition, cholestasis may persist several years after withdrawal of the initially offending drug.

THERAPEUTIC CONSEQUENCES

Determination of the mechanism for hepatitis may have useful therapeutic consequences.

Therapeutic recommendations

Understanding the hepatotoxic role of an isoniazid metabolite, and the enhancing effect of enzyme induction, has led to several recommendations: avoid high doses of isoniazid; avoid adding to rifampicin other microsomal enzyme inducers; in case of hepatitis, withdraw isoniazid and not rifampicin ... as was done previously (Pessayre et al., 1977). These recommendations have decreased markedly the incidence of fulminant hepatitis.

Knowing the role of a deficient cytochrome P-450 isoenzyme in perhexiline maleate-induced hepatitis (see chapter of D. Larrey) should allow one to prevent this adverse effect, by determining the drug hydroxylation phenotype, for example, with dextromethorphan.

Prevention of hepatitis after overdoses

Unravelling the protective role of glutathione against the hepatotoxicity of acetaminophen has led to the successful prevention of hepatitis by N-acetylcysteine (see chapter of L.F. Prescott).
Although cytochrome P-450 inhibitors have not been used up to now, they may find use in the future. Methoxsalen, a drug used in the treatment of psoriasis, is a potent, relatively non specific, suicide inhibitor of cytochrome P-450 in rats and in humans (Fouin-Fortunet et al., 1986; Tinel et al., 1987). Methoxsalen administration prevents the hepatotoxicity of acetaminophen and carbon tetrachloride in mice (Lettéron et al., 1986a; Labbe et al., 1987), and decreases the metabolic activation of acetaminophen in humans (Amouyal et al., 1987).

Development of analogues

On two occasions, we have tested a series of already marketed analogues (various macrolides, and various psoralen derivatives). On both accasions, we could find analogues (josamycin, midecamycin and spiramycin in the macrolide groups; trioxsalen in the psoralen group) that did not form (or poorly formed) the reactive metabolites (Larrey et al., 1983b; Lettéron et al., 1986b). This retrospective experience suggests that, in the future, it should be possible to design new analogues that would keep the therapeutic activity, without forming the reactive metabolites.

REFERENCES

Albert, A. (1973): Selective Toxicity. 5th ed, pp 420. London: Chapman and Hall.
Allemand, H., Pessayre, D., Descatoire, V., Degott, C., Feldmann, G. and Benhamou J.P. (1978): Metabolic activation of trichloroethylene into a chemically reactive metabolite toxic to the liver. J. Pharmacol. Exp. Ther. 204, 714-723.
Amouyal, G., Larrey, D., Lettéron, P., Genève, J., Labbe, G., Belghiti, J. and Pessayre, D. (1987). Effects of methoxsalen on the metabolism of acetaminophen in humans. Biochem. Pharmacol (in press).
Barker, J.D., de Carle, D.J. and Anuras, S. (1977): Chronic excessive acetaminophen use and liver damage. Ann. Intern. Med. 87, 299-301.
Bellomo, G. and Orrenius, S. (1985): Hepatology, 5: 876-882.
Black, M., Mitchell, J.R., Zimmerman, H.J., Ishak, K.G. and Eppler, G.R. (1975): Isoniazid-associated hepatitis in 114 patients. Gastroenterology, 69:289-302.

Breen, K., Wandscheer, J.C., Peignoux, M. and Pessayre, D. (1982): In situ formation of the acetaminophen metabolite covalently bound in kidney and lung. Supportive evidence provided by total hepatectomy. Biochem. Pharmacol. 31, 115-116.

Coles, B. (1984-85): Effects of modifying structure on electrophilic reactions with biological nucleophiles. Drug Metab. Rev. 15,1307-1334.

Cresteil, T., Beaune, P., Kremers, P., Celier, C., Guengerich, F.P. and Leroux, J.P. (1985): Immunoquantification of epoxide hydrolase and cytochrome P-450 isoenzymes in fetal and adult human liver microsomes. Eur. J. Biochem. 151, 345-350.

Danan, G., Descatoire, V. and Pessayre, D. (1981). Self-induction by erythromycin of its own transformation into a metabolite forming an inactive complex with reduced cytochrome P-450. J. Pharmacol. Exp. Ther. 218, 509-514.

Danan, G., Homberg, J.C., Bernuau, J., Roche-Sicot, J. and Pessayre, D. (1983). Hépatite à l'iproniazide. Intérêt diagnostique d'un nouvel anticorps anti-mitochondrial, l'anti-M6. Gastroenterol. Clin. Biol. 7,529-532.

Danan, G., Trunet, P., Bernuau, J., Degott, C., Babany, G., Pessayre, D., Rueff, B. and Benhamou, J.P. (1985): Pirprofen-induced fulminant hepatitis. Gastroenterology, 89, 210-213.

Davies, H.W., Britt, S.G., and Pohl, L.R. (1986): Carbon tetrachloride and 2-isopropyl-4-pentenamide-induced inactivation of cytochrome P-450 leads to heme-derived protein adducts. Arch. Biochem. Biophys., 244, 387-392.

Delaforge, M., Jaouen, M. and Mansuy, D. (1983): Dual effects of macrolide antibiotics on rat liver cytochrome P-450. Induction and formation of metabolite-complexes: a structure activity relationship. Biochem. Pharmacol. 32, 2309-2318.

DeMol, M.J. and Busker, R.W. (1984): Irreversible binding of the chlorpromazine radical cation and of photoactivated chlorpromazine to biological macromolecules. Chem. Biol. Interact. 52, 79-92.

Fouin-Fortunet, H., Lettéron, P., Tinel, M., Degott, C., Fléjou, J.F. and Pessayre, D. (1984). Mechanism for isaxonine hepatitis. II. Protective role of glutathione and toxicological studies in mice. J. Pharmacol. Exp. Ther. 229, 851-858.

Fouin-fortunet, H., Tinel, M., Descatoire, V., Lettéron, P., Larrey, D., Genève, J. and Pessayre, D. (1986): Inactivation of cytochrome P-450 by the drug methoxsalen. J. Pharmacol. Exp. Ther. 236, 237-247.

Franklin, M.R. (1977). Inhibition of mixed-function oxidations by substrates forming reduced cytochrome P-450 metabolic-intermediate complexes. Pharmac. Ther. 2, 227-245.

Funck-Brentano, C., Pessayre, D., and Benhamou, J.P. (1983): Hépatites dues à divers dérivés de l'érythromycine. Gastroenterol. Clin. Biol. 7, 362-369.

Genève, J., Degott, C., Lettéron, P., Tinel, M., Descatoire, V., Larrey, D., Amouyal, G., and Pessayre, D. (1987a): Metabolic activation of the tricyclic antidepressant amineptine-II Protective role of glutathione against in vitro and in vivo covalent binding. Biochem. Pharmacol. 36, 331-337.

Genève, J., Labbe, G., Degott, C., Lettéron, P., Freneaux, E., Le Din, T., Larrey, D., Hayat-Bonan, B. and Pessayre, D. (1987b): Inhibition of mitochondrial β-oxidation of fatty acids by pirprofen. Role in microvesicular steatosis due to this non steroidal anti-inflammatory drug. J. Pharmacol. Exp. Ther. (in press).

Genève, J., Larrey, D., Amouyal, G., Belghiti, J. and Pessayre, D. (1987c). Metabolic activation of the tricyclic antidepressant amineptine by human liver cytochrome P-450. Biochem. Pharmacol. (in press).

Genève, J., Larrey, D., Lettéron, P., Descatoire, V., Tinel, M., Amouyal, G. and Pessayre , D. (1987d): Metabolic activation of the tricyclic antidepressant amineptine. I. Cytochrome P-450-mediated in vitro covalent binding. Biochem. Pharmacol., 36, 323-329.

Halpert, J., Näslund, B., and Betner, I. (1983): Suicide inactivation of rat liver cytochrome P-450 by chloramphenicol in vivo and in vitro. Mol. Pharmacol. 23, 445-452.

Kaminsky, L.S., Dunbar, D.A., Wang, P.P., Beaune, P., Larrey, D., Guengerich, F.P., Schnellmann, R.G. and Sipes, I.G. (1984): Human hepatic cytochrome P-450 composition as probed by in vitro microsomal metabolism of warfarin. Drug Metab. Dispos. 12, 470-477.

Kappus, H. and Remmer, H. (1975): Irreversible protein binding of ^{14}C imipramine with rat and human liver microsomes. Biochem. Pharmacol. 24, 1079-1084.

Labbe, G., Descatoire, V., Lettéron, P., Degott, C., Tinel, M., Larrey, D., Carrion-Pavlov, Y., Genève, J., Amouyal, G. and Pessayre, D. (1987): The drug methoxsalen, a suicide substrate for cytochrome P-450, decreases the metabolic activation, and prevents the hepatotoxicity, of carbon tetrachloride in mice. Biochem. Pharmacol. 36, 907-914.

Larrey, D., Amouyal, G., Danan, G., Degott, C., Pesayre, D. and Benhamou J.P. (1987a): Prolonged cholestasis after troleandomycin-induced acute hepatitis. J. Hepatol. (in press).

Larrey, D., Castot, A., Pessayre, D., Merigot, P., Machayekhy, J.P., Feldmann, G., Lenoir, A., Rueff, B. and Benhamou, J.P. (1986a): Amodiaquine-induced hepatitis. A report of seven cases. Ann. Intern. Med. 104, 801-803.

Larrey, D., Funck-Brentano, C., Breil, P., Vitaux, J., Théodore, C., Babany, G. and Pessayre, D. (1983a): Effects of erythromycin on hepatic drug-metabolizing enzymes in humans. Biochem. Pharmacol. 32, 1063-1068.

Larrey, D., Genève, J., Pessayre, D., Machayekhy, J.P., Degott, C. and Benhamou, J.P. (19897b): Prolonged cholestasis after cyproheptadine-induced acute hepatitis. J. Clin. Gastroenterol. 9, 102-104.

Larrey, D., Lettéron, P., Foliot, A., Descatoire, V., Degott, C., Genève, J., Tinel, M. and Pessayre, D. (1986b): Effects of pregnancy on the toxicity and metabolism of acetaminophen in mice. J. Pharmacol. Exp. Ther. 237, 283-291.

Larrey, D., Tinel, M., Lettéron, P., Genève, J. Descatoire, V. and Pessayre, D. (1986c): Formation of an inactive cytochrome P-450 Fe(II)-metabolite complex after administration of amiodarone in rats, mice and hamsters. Biochem. Pharmacol. 35, 2213-2220.

Larrey, D., Tinel, M. and Pessayre, D. (1983b): Formation of inactive cytochrome P-450Fe(II)-metabolite complexes with several erythromycin derivatives but not with josamycin and midecamycin in rats. Biochem. Pharmacol. 32, 1487-1493.

Larrey, D., Pessayre, D., Duhamel, G., Casier, A., Degott, C., Feldmann, G., Erlinger, S. and Benhamou, J.P. (1986d) : Prolonged cholestasis after ajmaline induced hepatitis. J. Hepatol. 2, 81-87.

Le Dafniet, M., Pessayre, D., Le Quernec, L. and Erlinger, S. (1981): Effects of troleandomycin administration on cholesterol 7α-hydroxylase activity and bile secretion in rats. J. Pharmacol. Exp. Ther. 219, 558-562.

Lettéron, P., Descatoire, V., Larrey, D., Degott, C., Tinel, M., Genève, J. and Pessayre, D. (1986a). Pre- or post-treatment with methoxsalen prevents the hepatotoxicity of acetaminophen in mice. J. Pharmacol. Exp. Ther. 239, 559-567.

Lettéron, P., Descatoire, V., Larrey, D., Tinel, M., Genève, J. and Pessayre, D. (1986b) : Inactivation and induction of cytochrome P-450 by various psoralen derivatives in rats. J. Parmacol. Exp. Ther. 238, 685-692.

Lettéron, P., Fouin-Fortunet, H., Tinel, M., Danan, G., Belghiti, J. and Pessayre, D. (1984). Mechanism for isaxonine hepatitis. I. Metabolic activation by mouse and human cytochrome P-450. J. Pharmacol. Exp. Ther. 229, 845-850.

McClain, G.J., Kromhout, J.P., Peterson, F.J. and Holtzman, J.L. (1980): Potentiation of acetaminophene hepatotoxicity by alcohol. JAMA 244, 251-253.

Mitchell, J.R. and Jollow, D.J. (1975): Metabolic activation of drugs to toxic substances. Gastroenterology, 68, 392-410.

Neuberger, J., Kenna, J.G., Nouri Aria, K. and Williams, R. (1985): Antibody mediated hepatocyte injury in methyldopa induced hepatotoxicity. Gut, 26, 1233-1239.

Nicotera, P., Hartzell, P., Baldi, C., Svensson, S.A., Bellomo, G. and Orrenius, S. (1986): Cystamine induces toxicity in hepatocytes through the elevation of cytosolic Ca^{2+} and the stimulation of a nonlysosomal proteolytic system. J. Biol. Chem. 261, 14628-14635.

Oesch, F. (1972): Mammalian epoxides hydrases: Inducible enzymes catalysing the inactivation of carcinogenic and cytotoxic metabolites derived from aromatic and olefinic compounds. Xenobiotica, 3, 305-340.

Ortiz de Montellano, P. R., Beilan, H.S., Kunze, K.L. and Mico, B.A. (1981): Destruction of cytochrome P-450 by ethylene. Structure of the resulting prosthetic heme adduct. J. Biol. Chem. 256, 4395-4399.

Pessayre, D. (1985): Effects of macrolide antibiotics on cytochromes P-450 in rats and in humans. In Drug Metabolism. Molecular Approaches and Pharmacological Implications, ed. Siest, G., pp 51-59, Oxford, Pergamon Press.

Pessayre, D. (1987): Mécanismes des hépatites médicamenteuses. Med. Sci. 2, 373-379.

Pessayre, D., Allemand H, Wandscheer, J.C., Descatoire, V., Artigou J.Y. and Benhamou, J.P. (1979a): Inhibition, activation, destruction and induction of drug-metabolizing enzymes by trichloroethylene. Toxicol. Appl. Pharmacol. 49, 355-363.

Pessayre, D. and Benhamou, J.P. (1978) : Médicaments et foie: Effets toxiques. In Pharmacologie Clinique. Bases de la Thérapeutique, ed. Giroud, J.P., Mathé, G. and Meyniel, G., pp 671-687, Paris, Expansion Scientifique Française.

Pessayre, D., Bentata, M., Degott, C., Nouel, O., Miguet, J.P., Rueff, B. and Benhamou, J.P. (1977): Isoniazid-rifampin fulminant hepatitis. A possible consequence of the enhancement of isoniazid hepatotoxicity by enzyme induction. Gastroenterology, 72, 284-289.

Pessayre, D., Bichara, M., Feldmann, G., Degott, C., Potet, F. and Benhamou, J.P. (1979b): Perhexiline maleate-induced cirrhosis. Gastroenterology, 76, 170-177.

Pessayre, D., de Saint-Louvent, P., Degott, C., Bernuau, J., Rueff, B. and Benhamou, J.P. (1978): Iproclozide fulminant hepatitis. Possible role of enzyme induction. Gastroenterology, 75, 492-496.

Pessayre, D., Descatoire, V., Konstantinova-Mitcheva, M., Wandscheer, J.C., Cobert, B., Level, R., Benhamou, J.P., Jaouen, M. and Mansuy, D. (1981a): Self-induction by triacetyloleandomycin of its own transformation into a metabolite forming a stable 456 nm-absorbing complex with cytochrome P450. Biochem. Pharmacol. 30, 553-558.

Pessayre, D., Dolder, A., Artigou, J.Y., Wandscheer, J.C., Descatoire, V., Degott, C. and Benhamou, J.P. (1979c): Effect of fasting on metabolite-mediated hepatotoxicity in rats. Gastroenterology, 77, 264-271.

Pessayre, D., Konstantinova-Mitcheva, M., Descatoire, V., Cobert, B., Wandscheer, J.C., Level, R., Feldmann, G., Mansuy, D. and Benhamou, J.P. (1981b): Hypoactivity of cytochrome P-450 after triacetyloleandomycin administration. Biochem. Pharmacol. 30, 559-564.

Pessayre, D., Larrey, D., Funck-Bretano, C. and Benhamou, J.P. (1985). Drug interactions and hepatitis produced by some macrolide antibiotics. J. Antimicrob. Chemother. 16, 181-194.

Pessayre, D., Larrey, D., Vitaux, J., Breil, P., Belghiti, J. and Pessayre, D. (1982). Formation of an inactive cytochrome P-450Fe(II)-metabolite complex after administration of troleandomycin in humans. Biochem. Pharmacol. 31, 1699-1704.

Pessayre, D. and Mazel, P. (1976): Induction and inhibition of hepatic drug metabolising enzymes by rifampin. Biochem. Pharmacol. 25, 943-949.

Pessayre, D., Tinel, M., Larrey, D., Cobert, B., Funck-Brentano, C. and Babany, G. (1983): Inactivation of cytochrome P-450 by a troleandomycin metabolite. Protective role of glutathione. J. Pharmacol. Exp. Ther. 224, 685-691.

Pessayre, D., Wandscheer, J.C., Descatoire, V., Artigou, J.Y. and Benhamou, J.P. (1979d): Formation and inactivation of a chemically reactive metabolite of vinyl chloride. Toxicol. Appl. Pharmacol. 49, 505-515.

Pessayre, D., Wandscheer, J.C., Cobert, B., Level, R., Degott, C., Batt, A.M., Martin, N. and Benhamou, J.P. (1980): Additive effects of inducers and fasting on acetaminophen hepatotoxicity. Biochem. Pharmacol. 29, 2219-2223.

Satoh, H., Fukuda, Y., Anderson, D.K., Ferrans, U.J., Gillette, J.R. and Pohl, L.R. (1985a): Immunological studies on the mechanism of halothane-induced hepatotoxicity: immuno-histochemical evidence of trifluoro-acetylated hepatocytes. J. Pharmacol. Exp. Ther. 233, 857-862.

Satoh, H., Gillette, J.R., Davies, H.W., Schulick, R.D. and Pohl, L.R. (1985b): Immuno-chemical evidence of trifluoro-acetylated cytochrome P-450 in the liver of halothane-treated rats. Mol. Pharmacol. 28, 468-474.

Stricker, B.H.Ch. and Spoelstra, P. (1985): Drug-induced Hepatic Injury. Amsterdam: Elsevier.

Thor, H. and Orrenius, S. (1980): The mechanism of bromobenzene-induced cytotoxicity studied with isolated hepatocytes. Arch. Toxicol. 44, 31-43.

Tinel, M., Belghiti, J., Descatoire, V., Amouyal, G., Lettéron, P., Genève, J., Larrey, D. and Pessayre, D. (1987): Inactivation of human liver cytochrome P-450 by the drug methoxsalen and other psoralen derivatives. Biochem. Pharmacol. 36, 951-955.

Wang, P.P., Beaune, P., Kaminsky, L.S., Dannan, G.A., Kadlubar, F.F., Larrey, D. and Guengerich, F.P. (1983): Purification and characterization of six cytochrome P-450 isozymes from human liver microsomes. Biochemistry 22, 5375-5383.

Ware, A.J., Upchurch, K.S., Eigenbrodt, E.H. and Norman, D.A. (1978): Acetaminophen and the liver. Ann. Intern. Med. 88, 267-268.

Wendel, A., Feuerstein, S. and Konz, K.H. (1979): Acute paracetamol intoxication of starved mice leads to lipid peroxidation in vivo. Biochem. Pharmacol. 28, 2051-2055.

Résumé

Le mécanisme de l'hépatite reste inconnu pour la plupart des médicaments. Un même médicament peut avoir plusieurs effets toxiques sur le foie, ou peut produire soit des hépatites toxiques, soit des hépatites allergiques chez différents sujets. La formation de métabolites réactifs est relativement fréquente. Malgré plusieurs mécanismes de protection, elle peut conduire à la fixation covalente d'un métabolite electrophile sur les proteines, le déclenchement d'une péroxydation lipidique par un radical libre, et une diminution ou oxydation du glutathion. Il s'ensuit une série de lésions structurales et fonctionnelles, en particulier une augmentation prolongée du calcium cytosolique, aboutissant finalement à la mort cellulaire.

La formation de métabolites réactifs peut entrainer des hépatites soit toxiques, soit allergiques chez l'homme. L'hépatite toxique peut survenir de façon prévisible après des doses massives (voir chapitre de L.F. Prescott). Après des doses thérapeutiques, elle survient de façon idiosyncrasique, chez quelques sujets seulement. La susceptibilité individuelle est influencée à la fois par des facteurs génétiques (voir chapitre de D. Larrey) et par des facteurs acquis.

Une hépatite allergique peut également survenir, probablement du fait d'une immunisation contre des épitopes protéiques de la membrane plasmique, altérés par la fixation covalente du métabolite. Dans quelques cas, des auto-anticorps (dirigés contre des épitopes protéiques normaux) peuvent être détectés, comme les anticorps anti-cytochrome P-450 présents dans l'hépatite à l'acide tiénilique (voir chapitre de P. Beaune).

La détermination du mécanisme de l'hépatite peut conduire à diverses recommandations d'emploi, à la prévention de l'hépatite après doses massives, ou au développement rationnel d'analogues mieux tolérés.

Genetic factors in hepatotoxicity

Dominique Larrey, Dominique Pessayre

Unité de Recherches de Physiopathologie Hépatique, INSERM U.24, Hôpital Beaujon, 92118 Clichy Cedex, France

ABSTRACT

Drug-induced hepatitis is uncommon and apparently unpredictable. Hepatotoxicity may be related to the drug itself, or to chemically reactive metabolites which can bind covalently to hepatic macromolecules and may lead to either idiosyncratic, toxic hepatitis or to immuno-allergic hepatitis. There is now growing, albeit preliminary, evidence indicating that genetic variations in systems of biotransformation or detoxication may modulate either the toxic or sensitizing effects of some drugs. Thus, the genetic deficiency in a particular hepatic cytochrome P-450 isozyme is involved in perhexiline liver injury. Slow acetylation contributes to sulfonamide hepatitis. The genetic deficiency in glutathione synthetase may increase the susceptibility to several drugs including acetaminophen. A deficiency in epoxide hydrolase activity might be involved in phenytoin hepatotoxicity. A constitutional deficiency in another cell defense mechanism, still not characterized, seems to increase significantly the susceptibility to halothane hepatotoxicity.

KEYWORDS

Pharmacogenetic, hepatotoxicity, drug oxidation, acetylation, glutathione, glutathione synthetase, epoxide hydrolase.

INTRODUCTION

Drug hepatotoxicity is a serious side effect which can lead to death. For some drugs such as paracetamol, hepatotoxicity is dose dependent, results from an overdose and is predictable. In contrast, for many other drugs, hepatotoxicity occurs in a few patients only at therapeutic dose and is apparently unpredictable. The prevalence of such reactions varies widely. It is around 1/100 with isoniazid and iproniazid, 1/10 000 with halothane and ketoconazole, and even below 1/100 000 with cimetidine or penicillin (Zimmermann, 1978; Stricker and Spoelstra, 1985; Pessayre et al., 1985).

In many cases, the mechanism of drug hepatotoxicity remains unknown. Hepatotoxicity may be related to the drug itself or to its transformation into chemically reactive metabolites (Pessayre, 1986). The elimination of liposoluble drugs requires their biotransformation into more hydrosoluble metabolites. These biotransformation reactions are performed mainly in the liver. Two of them are particularly important for the subject of this article: N-acetylation and oxidation by cytochrome P-450 (Park, 1982). The cytochrome P-450 is made up of multiple isozymes having different affinities for different xenobiotics, which enable the oxidation of an infinity of drugs (Guengerich, 1979; Beaune, 1986). The metabolites formed by these biotransformations are generally non toxic. In some cases, however, oxidation by cytochrome P-450 leads to the formation of toxic reactive metabolites (Mitchell and Jollow, 1975; Pessayre, 1986). The potential toxicity of these metabolites is limited by various mechanisms of protection or detoxication: a) suicide inactivation of cytochrome P-450 by reactive metabolites decreasing thereby their formation; b) conjugation of reactive metabolites to glutathione; c) transformation of reactive epoxides into stable dihydrodiols by epoxide hydrolases; d) protection against lipid peroxidation by vitamin E, glutathione peroxidase, and catalase (Pessayre, 1986). These detoxication mechanisms prevent or limit the covalent binding of reactive metabolites to hepatic constituents including proteins, unsaturated lipids and nucleic acids. Formation of reactive metabolites can lead to cell death by interfering with cell homeostasis or by triggering immunologic reactions in which reactive metabolites bound to hepatocyte plasma membrane proteins may act as haptens (Pessayre, 1986).

It has been known for some time that drug hepatotoxicity is influenced by therapeutic, physiologic or nutritional factors interfering with drug elimination, or the formation of reactive metabolites or their detoxication (Pessayre, 1986). Drug accumulation can result from metabolic inhibition caused by another drug. Troleandomycin which forms an inactive complex with glucocorticoid-inducible cytochrome P-450 isozyme(s) involved in estrogen oxidation, increases markedly the risk of cholestasis caused by oral contraceptives (Pessayre et al., 1985). The formation of reactive metabolites can be increased by enzyme induction due to the administration of other drugs (Pessayre, 1986). For instance, isoniazid is transformed by hepatic cytochrome P-450 into a chemically reactive metabolite (Mitchell and Jollow, 1975). Rifampicin which induces hepatic cytochrome P-450, increases the toxicity of isoniazid (Pessayre et al., 1977). On the other hand, several conditions have been shown to decrease the detoxication of reactive metabolites. Denutrition increases the toxicity of acetaminophen, in part by depleting hepatic glutathione (Pessayre et al. 1979). Pregnancy enhances likewise the toxicity of acetaminophen experimentally, probably by decreasing the synthesis of hepatic glutathione (Larrey et al., 1986).

Besides these factors, there is now growing evidence showing that the efficiency of these systems of biotransformation and detoxication is controlled genetically and can modulate the hepatotoxicity of some drugs in humans (Spielberg, 1984; Larrey, 1986).

OXIDATION BY CYTOCHROME P-450

Genetic control of hepatic drug oxidation has been well characterized with the demonstration of a genetic polymorphism in the hydroxylation of debrisoquine into 4-hydroxydebrisoquine (Mahgoub et al., 1977). Two phenotypes have been identified: most subjects with active debrisoquine 4-hydroxylation are named "Extensive Metabolizers" (EM) whereas a minority of subjects with an impaired debrisoquine 4-hydroxylation are named "Poor Metabolizers" (PM) (Mahgoub et al., 1977). The PM phenotype is inherited as an autosomal recessive trait

(Mahgoub et al., 1977; Evans et al., 1980). The impairment of debrisoquine 4-hydroxylation is related to the deficiency of a particular hepatic cytochrome P-450 isozyme, recently identified both in rats (cytochrome P-450 UT-H) (Larrey et al., 1984) and in humans (cytochrome P-450 Db) (Distlerath et al., 1985). The prevalence of PM phenotype for debrisoquine 4-hydroxylation is extremely variable between different populations (0-32%) (Larrey, 1986; Jacqz et al., 1986). In Europe, it ranges from 3 to 10% (Larrey, 1986). More than thirty drugs have been identified as being oxidized by this cytochrome P-450 isozyme including β-blockers, tricyclic antidepressants, chlorpromazine, dextromethorphan and perhexiline maleate (Larrey, 1986; Jacqz et al., 1986). These drugs display an oxidation polymorphism co-segregating with that of debrisoquine. As a result of this polymorphism, serious side-effects can occur, mostly in poor metabolizers who are exposed to excessive drug concentrations after the administration of a standard dose (Larrey, 1986; Jacqz et al., 1986). The relationship between the oxidation polymorphism of debrisoquine and that of perhexiline maleate has been clearly demonstrated (Cooper et al., 1984). Indeed, poor metabolizers of debrisoquine are likewise poor metabolizers of perhexiline maleate and reciprocally (Cooper et al., 1984). Prolonged administration of perhexiline maleate can induce pseudo-alcoholic liver injury associated with phospholipidosis due to the accumulation of phospholipids in lysosomes (Pessayre et al., 1979; Poupon et al., 1980). This phospholipidosis is characterized ultrastructurally by a pattern of pseudo-myeloid figures in enlarged lysosomes (Pessayre et al., 1979). Most patients with perhexiline-induced liver injury were found to be poor metabolizers of debrisoquine (Morgan et al., 1984). Apparently, the observed deficiency in this metabolic pathway did not result from the liver injury due to perhexiline. Indeed, the prevalence of PM phenotype was low (8.6%) (in the range of that found in European control population) in patients with other liver diseases of similar severity (Morgan et al., 1984). This observation strongly suggests that the genetic impairment of perhexiline oxidation is responsible for, or contributes significantly to, the hepatotoxicity of this drug. This view is reinforced by the fact that neuropathy induced by perhexiline occurs mostly in subjects with the PM phenotype (Shah et al., 1982). The following mechanism may be proposed for perhexiline hepatotoxicity. In poor metabolizers, the deficiency of perhexiline oxidation may result in its accumulation in hepatocytes, which would induce phospholipidosis and alcohol-like liver disease (Morgan et al., 1984; Larrey, 1986). It is noteworthy, however, that the case of perhexiline, in which the parent drug itself is hepatotoxic, may be more the exception than the rule. Indeed, we have found that the hepatotoxicity of several other drugs metabolized by hepatic cytochrome P-450 does not appear to be significantly related to the deficiency in debrisoquine oxidation. Indeed, PM phenotype determined by using dextromethorphan as test compound, was found in only one patient out of five with hepatitis due to plethoryl® (an association of cyclovalone, tiratricol and vitamin A), and in none of several patients with hepatitis due to amodiaquine (n = 6) or to tricyclic antidepressants (n = 5).

Genetic polymorphisms of oxidation different from that of debrisoquine, have been demonstrated for mephenytoin, tolbutamide, phenytoin, carboxymethyl-cystein, phenacetin and nifedipine (Jacqz et al., 1986; Larrey, 1986). They are related to the deficiency of other hepatic cytochrome P-450 isozymes. The influence of these genetic oxidation polymorphisms on drug hepatotoxicity is still unknown.

ACETYLATION

The N-acetylation of isoniazid is one of the most remarkable instance of metabolic polymorphism. Indeed, the capacity of acetylation is the prominent factor which determines the plasma concentration of isoniazid after administration

of a standard dose of the drug (Evans et al., 1960). Its evaluation in a
large british population has shown a bimodal distribution corresponding
to two phenotypes, the slow and rapid acetylators (Evans et al., 1960).
The N-acetylation of isoniazid is controlled by two alleles at a single
gene locus and the trait slow acetylator is inherited as an autosomal recessive
trait. The prevalence of the rapid acetylator phenotype varies widely between
different populations (18-100%) (Weber and Hein, 1985). It ranges from 30%
to 60% in Western Europe and in North America (Weber and Hein, 1985). It
was initially reported that rapid acetylators may be predisposed to isonia-
zid-induced hepatitis (Mitchell et al., 1975). In contrast, other studies
suggested that isoniazid hepatotoxicity, may not be significantly influenced
by acetylation phenotype (Weber and Hein, 1985), or may even be slightly
more frequent in slow acetylators (Dickinson et al., 1981). The complexity
of isoniazid metabolism may explain such conflicting results. Isoniazid
is acetylated into acetylisoniazid which is quickly hydrolysed into acetylhydrazine. Acetylhydrazine is then acetylated to diacetylhydrazine or oxidized
by cytochrome P-450 into a reactive metabolite which can bind irreversibly
to hepatic macromolecules and may lead to hepatic necrosis (Mitchell and
Jollow, 1985; Weber and Hein, 1985). Acetylation phenotype is involved both
in the formation and the metabolism of acetylhydrazine. Acetylhydrazine
is formed more rapidly but is likewise eliminated more rapidly in rapid
acetylators than in slow acetylators. Thus, it is conceivable that, in such
a system, the concentration of acetylhydrazine, and subsequently, the formation
rate of reactive metabolites would be finally not significantly different
between both phenotypes (Weber and Hein, 1985). Similarly, the hepatotoxicity
of other hydrazine derivatives such as hydralazine, ecarazine and dihydralazine
does not appear to be significantly influenced by the acetylation phenotype
(Stricker and Spoelstra, 1985).

In contrast, the slow acetylator phenotype may contribute to sulfonamide
hepatotoxicity. Indeed, in a sery of six patients with sulfonamide hepatitis,
all were found to be slow acetylators whereas the prevalence of this phenotype
in a control population was 55% (Shear et al., 1985).

DETOXICATION BY GLUTATHIONE

Glutathione is an essential compound for the detoxication of reactive metabolites
formed from many drugs. Its conjugation to these unstable metabolites transforms
them into non toxic stable metabolites (Pessayre, 1986). Depletion of glutathione
has three adverses consequences. First, it reduces the inactivation of reactive
metabolites and tends to increase their covalent binding to macromolecules
(Pessayre, 1986). Second, it may have several deleterious effects on cell
homeostasis through the oxidation of the SH groups of proteins, which decreases
the activity of several enzymes, including that of vital calcium translocases.
(Bellomo et al., 1982). Third, depletion of glutathione may permit the onset
of lipid peroxidation. Accordingly, depletion of glutathione greatly aggravates
the toxic effects of reactive metabolites. Glutathione is synthetized from
gamma-glutamyl-cysteine and glycine in the presence of glutathione synthetase
(Richman and Meister, 1975). This biosynthesis is performed in many cells
including hepatocytes, renal cells, fibroblasts, erythrocytes, polymorphonuclear
cells, and lymphocytes (Richman and Meister, 1975; Spielberg et al., 1977).
A genetically determined deficiency of glutathione synthesis has been identified
in a few subjects (Spielberg et al., 1977). This deficiency is inherited
as an autosomal recessive trait (Spielberg, 1984). In subjects homozygous
for the deficiency, glutathione synthetase activity is markedly decreased,
and intracellular glutathione levels are very low, being only 15% of normal.
These subjects have a disorder characterized by 5-oxoprolinuria, hemolytic
anemia, polymorphonuclear cell abnormalities, and acidosis (Spielberg, 1984).
In contrast, in heterozygous subjects, glutathione synthetase activity is

moderately decreased (by 50%), glutathione levels are normal in basal conditions, and there is no clinical disorder (Spielberg, 1984). The prevalence of heterozygous subjects for glutathione synthetase deficiency may be 1/10 000, which is similar to the prevalence of idiosyncratic hepatotoxic reaction to many drugs (Spielberg and Gordon, 1981).

The influence of glutathione synthetase deficiency on drug hepatotoxicity has been assessed by an in vitro assay in which lymphocytes are used as target cells for reactive metabolites generated by a hepatic microsomal fraction (Spielberg 1984). Indeed, lymphocytes contain epoxide hydrolase, glutathione and the enzymes necessary to the synthesis and degradation of glutathione (Spielberg, 1984). In constrast, lymphocytes are unable to significantly activate drugs into reactive metabolites. Consequently, lymphocytes can be used to test cell detoxication capacity after exposure to reactive metabolites formed by microsomes. In this assay, lymphocytes from patients with an history of drug hepatotoxicity are incubated for 2 hours with mice hepatic microsomes, a NADPH-generating system, and the test drug at various concentrations (Spielberg, 1984). Cells are then washed to remove microsomes and remaining drug, and resuspended in fresh medium. Sixteen hours later, toxicity is assessed by Trypan blue exclusion and lactate dehydrogenase release into the medium (Spielberg, 1984). Aliquots can be taken at various times during this procedure, to measure lymphocyte glutathione concentration (Spielberg, 1984).

This method has been used to study the effect of glutathione synthetase deficiency on the toxicity of acetaminophen used as test compound. The results showed a higher depletion of glutathione with lymphocytes from subjects homozygous for glutathione synthetase deficiency than with lymphocytes from control subjects (Spielberg and Gordon, 1981). Concomitantly, lymphocyte destruction was higher in the deficient subjects even with low concentrations of acetaminophen (Spielberg and Gordon, 1981). These results tentatively suggested that subjects homozygous for glutathione synthetase deficiency may more susceptible to acetaminophen toxicity, even at low doses of acetaminophen.

The same study has been performed with lymphocytes from subjects heterozygous for glutathione synthetase deficiency. After incubation with acetaminophen, lymphocytes from these subjects exhibited a glutathione depletion and a lymphocyte destruction intermediate between those observed with lymphocytes from control subjects and those observed with lymphocytes from subjects homozygous for glutathione synthetase deficiency (Spielberg, 1984). These results suggest that heterozygous subjects, albeit phenotypically normal in basal conditions, might be more susceptible to the hepatotoxicity of acetaminophen because of their limited ability to resynthetize glutathione in situations of high utilization (Spielberg, 1984). In addition, subjects homozygous for glutathione synthetase deficiency appear to be more susceptible to metronidazole and nitrofurantoin, drugs which are potentially hepatotoxic (Spielberg, 1984).

DETOXICATION BY EPOXIDE HYDROLASE

Epoxide hydrolase is made up of various isozymes. In humans, two epoxide hydrolases have been purified, one present in microsomes, and the other in the cytosol. The physiological activity of epoxide hydrolases is to hydrate various epoxides, several of which are electrophilic and potentially toxic, into non toxic dihydrodiols (Glatt and Oesch, 1984). Epoxide hydrolases are present in many cells, including hepatocytes, lymphocytes, granulocytes and erythrocytes. Large interindividual differences in epoxide hydrolase activities have been found in liver microsomes and in blood cells. For instance,

the activities of microsomal and cytosolic epoxide hydrolases vary by a
factor of 63, and 539, respectively (Glatt and Oesch, 1984). Such interindividual
variations may result from environmental factors but may likewise be compatible
with a genetic polymorphism (Glatt and Oesch, 1984).

Phenytoin is an anticonvulsant drug which can induce hepatocellular or mixed
pattern hepatitis, generally associated with hypersensitivity manifestations
(Stricker and Spoelstra, 1985; Pessayre et al., 1985). Experimentally, phenytoin
is oxidized by cytochrome P-450 into a reactive epoxide, probably an arene
oxide (Spielberg et al., 1981). This metabolite is normally detoxified by
epoxide hydrolase into a non toxic dihydrodiol. The inhibition of epoxide
hydrolase activity by compounds such as trichloropropene oxide (TCPO), results
in an increased covalent binding of phenytoin metabolites to cell macromolecules
(Spielberg et al., 1981). The potential influence of a deficit in epoxide
hydrolase activity in subjects with phenytoin hepatitis, has been studied
by using the same in vitro lymphocyte assay as that described above (Spielberg,
1984). The lymphocytes from 3 patients with previous history of phenytoin-induced
hepatitis were challenged with phenytoin at various concentrations, in presence
of mouse hepatic microsomes and a NADPH-generating system. The results were
compared to those obtained with lymphocytes from 20 control subjects (Spielberg
et al., 1981). After incubation, lymphocyte destruction increased significantly
with the dose of phenytoin in patients with phenytoin hepatitis, but was
absent in control subjects. When epoxide hydrolase activity was inhibited
by adding TCPO in the incubation mixture, cell death was further increased
in patients, and became, now, both apparent and dose-dependent in control
subjects. Lymphocytes from a parent of one patient displayed the same toxicity
patterns as lymphocytes from this patient. These results strongly suggest
that the susceptibility to phenytoin hepatotoxicity may be genetically determined,
and possibly related to a deficiency in epoxide hydrolase activity (Spielberg
et al., 1981). This activity was not measured directly, however.

The hepatotoxicity of phenobarbital, mephenytoin and phenacemide may likewise
be related to epoxide hydrolase deficiency (Spielberg, 1984).

OTHER MECHANISMS OF DETOXICATION

It has also been shown that lymphocytes from subjects with a history of
sulfonamide hepatotoxicity exhibit an enhanced susceptibility to the toxicity
of sulfonamide (Shear et al., 1986). Such a susceptibility to sulfonamide
was also found in some parents of the patients (Shear et al., 1986). The
latter observations suggest that sulfonamide hepatotoxicity may occur in
genetically susceptible subjects with impaired drug detoxication capacity
(Shear et al., 1986). The nature of this presumed deficiency remains unknown,
however.

Halothane anesthesia induces uncommonly cytolytic hepatitis with a high
mortality rate. Obesity, age above 40 years, female sex and previous anesthesia
with this compound, are predisposing factors for halothane hepatotoxicity.
A hereditary susceptibility is suggested by the observation of halothane-induced
hepatitis in several females from the same family (Stricker and Spoelstra,
1985). Halothane hepatotoxicity may be mediated by a reactive metabolite
which would trigger an immune reaction against hepatocytes (Gandolfi et
al., 1980; Neuberger et al., 1981; Stricker and Spoelstra, 1985).

The susceptibility to halothane hepatotoxicity has been recently studied
by using the in vitro lymphocyte destruction test in presence of phenytoin,
rat hepatic microsomes, and TCPO as inhibitor of epoxide hydrolase (Farrell
et al., 1985). After incubation, lymphocyte destruction was markedly higher
in patients with halothane hepatitis than in various groups of control subjects.

Family studies showed an increased lymphocyte cytotoxicity in half of family members of the patients. This argues for a familial, constitutional susceptibility factor predisposing to halothane hepatitis (Farrell et al., 1985). The relationship between epoxide hydrolase deficiency and decreased capacity in detoxication of halothane reactive metabolites is not clear. Indeed, these metabolites are probably not epoxides (Gandolfi et al., 1980). Thus, it is conceivable that TCPO may have interfered with another cell defense mechanism which remains to characterize.

TOXICITY AND IMMUNO-ALLERGY

It is noteworthy that whereas acetaminophen hepatitis is usually toxic in type, in contrast, hepatitis due to phenytoin, sulfonamides and halothane is probably immunologically mediated. This observation suggests that genetic variations in drug metabolism and/or protective mechanisms may influence both toxic and allergic hepatitis. For example, genetic deficiency in epoxide hydrolase might increase the likelihood of an immunologic response to phenytoin by increasing the number of hepatocyte plasma membrane protein molecules altered by the covalent binding of the reactive phenytoin epoxides.

CONCLUSIONS

Albeit often preliminary, these data strongly suggest that susceptibility to drug-induced hepatitis may be explained, at least in some cases, by genetic variations in drug metabolism (oxidation by cytochrome P-450, acetylation) or in the detoxication of reactive metabolites (conjugation to glutathione, epoxide hydrolase). A constitutional deficiency of other mechanisms of detoxication, still not identified, is suggested in the instances of halothane and sulfonamide hepatotoxicity. In the latter case, susceptibility to hepatitis may result from the combination of two different genetic factors. Indeed, sulfonamide hepatitis appeared to occur in subjects who were both slow acetylators, and at the same time, deficient for a specific mechanism of metabolite detoxication. The development of tests for drug oxidation phenotyping and tests of in vitro cytotoxicity should contribute to a better understanding of the influence of genetics on drug hepatotoxicity.

REFERENCES

Beaune, P.H. (1986): Les cytochromes P-450 hepatiques humains. Med. Sci. 2, 358-363.

Bellomo, G., Jewell, S.A., Thor, H. and Orrenius, S. (1982): Regulation of intracellular calcium compartimentation: studies with isolated hepatocytes and t-butyl hydroperoxide. Proc. Natl. Sci. U.S.A. 79, 6842-6846.

Cooper, R.G., Evans, D.A.P. and Whibley, E.J. (1984): Polymorphic hydroxylation of perhexiline maleate in man. J. Med. Genet. 21, 27-33.

Dickinson, D.S., Bailey, W.C., Hirschowitz, B.I., Soong, S.J., Eidus, L. and Hodgkin, M.M. (1981): Risk factors for isoniazid (INH)-induced liver dysfunction. J. Clin. Gastroenterol. 3, 271-279.

Distlerath, L.M., Reilly, P.E.B., Martin, M.V., Davis, G.G., Wilkinson, G.R. and Guengerich, F.P. (1985): Purification and characterization of the human liver cytochromes P-450 involved in debrisoquine 4-hydroxylation and phenacetin O-deethylation. Two prototypes for genetic polymorphism in oxidative drug metabolism. J. Biol. Chem. 260, 9057-9067.

Evans, D.A.P., Mahgoub, A., Sloan, T.P., Idle, J.R. and Smith, R.L. (1980): A family and population study of the genetic polymorphism of debrisoquine oxidation in a white English population. J. Med. Genet. 17, 102-105.

Evans, D.A.P., Manley, K.A. and Mc Kusick, V.A. (1960): Genetic control of isoniazid metabolism in man. Br. Med. J. 2, 485-491.

Farrell, G., Prendergast, D. and Murray, M. (1985): Halothane hepatitis. Detection of a constitutional susceptibility factor. N. Engl. J. Med. 313, 1310-1314.

Gandolfi, A.J., White, R.D., Sipes, I.G. and Pohl, L.R. (1980): Bioactivation and covalent binding of halothane in vitro: studies with |^{3}H| and |^{14}C| halothane. J. Pharmacol. Exp. Ther. 214, 721-725.

Glatt, H. and Oesch, F. (1984): Variations in epoxide hydrolase activities in human liver and blood. In Genetic Variability in Responses to Chemical Exposure, Banbury Report 16, eds G.S. Omenn and H.V. Gelboin, pp 189-203. Cold Spring Harbor Laboratory.

Guengerich, F.P. (1979): Isolation and purification of cytochrome P-450, and the existence of multiple forms. Pharmacol. Ther. 6, 99-121.

Jacqz, E., Hall, S.D. and Branch, R.A. (1986): Genetically determined polymorphisms in drug oxidation. Hepatology 6, 1020-1032.

Larrey, D. (1986): Polymorphisme génétique du métabolisme hépatique des médicaments. Med. Sci. 2, 364-372.

Larrey, D., Distlerath, L.M., Dannan, G.A., Wilkinson, G.R. and Guengerich, F.P. (1984): Purification and characterization of the rat liver microsomal cytochrome P-450 involved in the 4-hydroxylation of debrisoquine, a prototype for genetic variation in oxidative drug metabolism. Biochemistry 23, 2787-2795.

Larrey, D., Lettéron, P., Foliot, A., Descatoire, V., Degott, C., Genève, J., Tinel, M. and Pessayre, D. (1986): Effects of pregnancy on the toxicity and metabolism of acetaminophen in mice. J. Pharmacol. Exp. Ther. 237, 283-291.

Maghoub, A., Idle, J.R., Dring, L.G., Lancaster, R. and Smith, R.L. (1977): Polymorphic hydroxylation of debrisoquine in man. Lancet 2, 584-586.

Mitchell, J.R. and Jollow, D.J. (1975): Metabolic activation of drugs to toxic substances. Gastroenterology 68, 392-410.

Mitchell, J.R., Thorgeirsson, U.P., Black, M., Timbrell, J.A., Snodgrass, W.R., Potter, W.Z., Jollow, D.J. and Keiser, H.R. (1975): Increased incidence of isoniazid hepatitis in rapid acetylators: possible relation to hydrazine metabolites. Clin. Pharmacol. Ther. 18, 70-79.

Morgan, M.Y., Reshef, R., Shah, R.R., Oates, N.S., Smith, R.L. and Sherlock, S. (1984): Impaired oxidation of debrisoquine in patients with perhexiline liver injury. Gut 25, 1057-1064.

Neuberger, J., Mieli-Vergani, G., Tredger, J.M., Davies, M. and Williams, R. (1981): Oxidative metabolism of halothane in the production of altered hepatocyte membrane antigens in acute halothane-induced hepatic necrosis. Gut 22, 669-672.

Park, B.K. (1982): Assessment of the drug metabolism capacity of the liver. Br. J. Clin. Pharmacol. 14, 631-651.

Pessayre, D. (1986): Mecanismes des hépatites médicamenteuses. Med. Sci. 2, 373-379.

Pesssayre, D., Bentata, M., Degott, C., Novel, O., Miguet, J.P., Rueff, B. and Benhamou, J.P. (1977): Isoniazid-rifampin fulminant hepatitis. A possible consequence of the enhancement of isoniazid hepatotoxicity by enzyme induction. Gastroenterology 72, 284-289.

Pessayre, D., Bichara, M., Feldmann, G., Degott, C., Potet, F. and Benhamou, J.P. (1979): Perhexiline maleate-induced cirrhosis. Gastroenterology 76, 170-176.

Pessayre, D., Dolder, A., Artigou, J.Y., Wandscheer, J.C., Descatoire, V., Degott, C. and Benhamou, J.P. (1979): Effect of fasting on metabolite-mediated hepatotoxicity in the rat. Gastroenterology 77, 264-271.

Pessayre, D., Larrey, D. and Benhamou, J.P. (1985): Hepatites médicamenteuses. Sem. Hop. Paris 61, 2049-2071.

Poupon, R., Rosensztajn, L., Prudhomme De Saint-Maur, P., Lageron, A., Gombeau, T. and Darnis, F. (1980): Perhexiline maleate-associated hepatic injury. Prevalence and characteristics. Digestion 20, 145-150.

Richman, P.G. and Meister, A. (1975): Regulation of gamma-glutamyl-cysteine synthetase by nonallosteric feedback inhibition by glutathione. J. Biol. Chem. 250, 1422-1426.

Shah, R.R., Oates, N.S., Idle, J.R., Smith, R.L. and Lockhart, J.D.F. (1982): Impaired oxidation of debrisoquine in patients with perhexiline neuropathy. Br. Med. J. 284, 295-299.

Shear, N.H., Spielberg, S.P., Grant, D.M., Tang, B.K. and Kalow, W. (1986): Differences in metabolism of sulfonamides predisposing to idiosyncratic toxicity. Ann. Int. Med. 105, 179-184.

Spielberg, S.P. (1984): In vitro assessment of pharmacogenetic susceptibility to toxic drug metabolites in humans. Fed. Proc. 43, 2308-2313.

Spielberg, S.P., Garrick, M.D., Corash, L.M., Butler, J.B., Tietze, F., Rogers, L. and Schulman, J.D. (1977): Biochemical heterogeneity in glutathione synthetase deficiency. J. Clin. Invest. 60, 1417-1420.

Spielberg, S.P. and Gordon, G.B. (1981): Glutathione synthetase-deficient lymphocytes and acetaminophen toxicity. Clin. Pharmacol. Ther. 29, 51-55.

Spielberg, S.P., Gordon, G.B., Blake, D.A., Goldstein, D.A. and Herlong, H.F. (1981): Predisposition to phenytoin hepatotoxicity assessed in vitro. N. Engl. J. Med. 305, 722-727.

Stricker, B.H.C. and Spoelstra, P. (1985): Drug-induced hepatic injury. A comprehensive survey of the litterature on adverse drug reactions up to January 1985. Amsterdam: Elsevier.

Weber, W.W., Hein, D.W. (1985): N-acetylation pharmacogenetics. Pharmacol. Rev. 37, 25-79.

Zimmermann, H.J. (1978): Hepatotoxicity. The adverse effects of drugs and other chemicals on the liver. New-York: Appleton-Century-Crofts.

Résumé

Le mécanisme de l'hépatotoxicité des médicaments reste inconnu le plus souvent. Dans certains cas, cependant, l'hépatotoxicité est due au médicament lui-même. Dans d'autres cas, le médicament est transformé par le cytochrome P-450 hépatique en des métabolites réactifs qui se fixent de façon covalente sur des macromolécules hépatiques, et peuvent entrainer, selon les médicaments, soit des hépatites toxiques, soit des hépatites allergiques. Ces métabolites sont normalement détoxiqués par divers mécanismes tels que la conjugaison au glutathion hépatique ou l'hydratation de certains époxydes instables en dihydrodiols non toxiques par l'époxyde hydrolase. Les hépatites médicamenteuses sont rares, n'affectant que quelques sujets seulement. On sait depuis quelques années que des facteurs acquis (induction enzymatique, dénutrition) peuvent modifier la susceptibilité individuelle. Le rôle de facteurs génétiques n'a été démontré que tout récemment. Ces travaux suggèrent que des variations génétiques dans certaines réactions de biotransformation ou de détoxication peuvent expliquer la susceptibilité individuelle non seulement à des hépatites toxiques, mais aussi à des hépatites allergiques. Ainsi, le déficit d'un isoenzyme particulier du cytochrome P-450 hépatique est responsable d'un déficit d'une voie métabolique impliquée dans l'oxydation de la débrisoquine, de la perhéxiline et d'une trentaine d'autres médicaments. Ce déficit d'oxydation, transmis sur le mode autosomal récessif, est présent chez 3 à 10 % des Européens et des Nord-Américains. L'hépatotoxicité de la perhéxiline est observée essentiellement chez les sujets déficitaires. Ceci indique que ce déficit d'oxydation contribue fortement à l'hépatotoxicité de la perhéxiline, en étant responsable de son accumulation dans les hépatocytes. La N-acétylation des médicaments est également contrôlée génétiquement. En Europe et en Amérique du Nord, les phénotypes acétyleurs lents et acétyleurs rapides sont à peu près également répartis. Le caractère acétyleur lent est transmis sur le mode autosomal récessif. L'influence du phénotype d'acétylation sur l'hépatotoxicité de l'isoniazide est très controversée et n'apparaît pas significative. En revanche, le phénotype acétyleur lent semble contribuer à l'hépatotoxicité des sulfamides. Le déficit homozygote en glutathion synthétase, transmis sur le mode autosomal récessif, est caractérisé par une forte diminution du glutathion intra-cellulaire et se manifeste par une maladie, la 5-oxoprolinurie. Ce déficit entraine une susceptibilité accrue à la toxicité de certains médicaments dont le paracétamol. Les sujets hétérozygotes pourraient également avoir une susceptibilité accrue. L'activité de l'époxyde hydrolase est caractérisée par de grandes variations inter-individuelles. L'hépatotoxicité de la phénytoïne est probablement due à son oxydation en un époxyde dont la fixation sur les protéines de la membrane plasmique de l'hépatocyte pourrait entrainer une immunisation contre ces protéines altérées. Il semble exister une susceptibilité génétiquement transmise à ce type d'hépatite dont le mécanisme pourrait être un déficit de l'activité époxyde hydrolase. La survenue d'une hépatite allergique à l'halothane parait être liée en partie à un facteur constitutionnel jouant un rôle dans la défense cellulaire vis-à-vis de métabolites de l'halothane. La nature de ce facteur reste à déterminer. Dans certains cas enfin, l'hépatotoxicité des médicaments fait intervenir plusieurs mécanismes. Ainsi, les hépatites dues aux sulfamides surviennent essentiellement chez des sujets ayant à la fois le phénotype acétyleur lent et un déficit d'un système de défense cellulaire vis-à-vis des métabolites des sulfamides.

Paracetamol: a model for toxic injury mediated by the formation of active metabolites

L.F. Prescott

University Department of Clinical Pharmacology and the Regional Poisoning Treatment Centre, The Royal Infirmary, Edinburgh EH3 9YM, Scotland, UK

ABSTRACT

Paracetamol causes acute hepatic necrosis by conversion to N-acetyl-p-benzoquinoneimine, a minor reactive metabolite. Experimental paracetamol hepatotoxicity depends on microsomal enzyme activity, the capacity of parallel routes of elimination and glutathione status. Species differences in sensitivity seem related to differences in the metabolic activation of paracetamol. In man there is great individual variation both in the oxidative metabolism of paracetamol and in susceptibilty to hepatotoxicity following overdosage. There is extensive metabolic activation in a small minority of individuals. Despite anecdotal reports, microsomal enzyme induction has not been shown to potentiate paracetamol toxicity in man and treatment of overdosage is based on stimulation of glutathione synthesis rather than inhibition of its oxidative metabolism.

KEY WORDS

Paracetamol, overdosage, hepatotoxicity, metabolic activation, microsomal enzyme activity, induction and inhibition, glutathione, individual and species differences.

INTRODUCTION

Over the last thirty years paracetamol (acetaminophen) has become an increasingly popular non-prescription antipyretic analgesic. In comparison with other such drugs it proved remarkably safe when taken in normal doses but in 1966 it was found to cause acute hepatic necrosis when taken in substantial overdosage (Davidson & Eastham, 1966; Thomson & Prescott, 1966). At the same time, hepatic necrosis was observed in rats given paracetamol in the dose range of the LD50 (Boyd & Bereczky, 1966). For the last 20 years, paracetamol overdosage has become an increasing problem in many countries, especially in the United Kingdom.

Mitchell and his colleagues first showed that paracetamol damages the liver by the covalent binding of a minor reactive metabolite generated by cytochrome P-450 dependent mixed function oxidase, and that glutathione plays a vital protective role by preferential conjugation and inactivation of this metabolite (Mitchell et al., 1973a, 1973b; Jollow et al., 1973; Potter et al., 1973). Liver injury does not occur without covalent binding and depletion of hepatic glutathione. The extent of metabolic activation of paracetamol can be assessed by the fractional urinary recovery of the mercapturic acid and cysteine conjugates derived from its glutathione adduct. The toxic metabolite of paracetamol is thought to be N-acetyl-p-benzoquinoneimine formed by N-oxidation (Corcoran et al., 1980), and the critical event leading to cell necrosis is probably arylation of membrane bound ATP-dependent Ca^{2+} translocases (Tsokos-Kuhn et al., 1985; Moore et al., 1985).

FACTORS INFLUENCING EXPERIMENTAL PARACETAMOL HEPATOTOXICITY

Paracetamol hepatotoxicity depends primarily on the balance between the rate of formation of the reactive metabolite and the rate of glutathione synthesis. Both processes can be influenced by physiological, nutritional and pathological factors, and the metabolic activation of paracetamol is further modified by genetic and environmental factors. Microsomal enzyme activity apart, the rate of formation of reactive metabolite also depends on the rate of paracetamol absorption and delivery, and the capacity (and saturability) of the major parallel pathways of elimination by glucuronide and sulphate conjugation. It is therefore not surprising that there are marked species and individual differences in susceptibility to paracetamol hepatotoxicity (Davis et al., 1974; Prescott, 1983; Green et al., 1984). Much of this variation has been attributed to differences in the extent of metabolic activation but this cannot be assumed because of the complex interrelationships between the many factors involved.

Induction and inhibition of liver microsomal enzymes
In their original studies, Mitchell et al. (1973a) showed that paracetamol hepatotoxicity in mice and rats was potentiated by pretreatment with inducing agents such as phenobarbitone and methylcholanthrene, and reduced by treatment with inhibitors such as piperonyl butoxide and cobaltous chloride. Subsequently, other investigators have confirmed that liver damage is enhanced by prior administration of agents which increase microsomal enzyme activity such as phenobarbitone, acetone, chronic ethanol, and ether (McLean & Day, 1975; Moldéus & Gergely, 1980; Sato et al., 1981; To & Wells, 1986). Conversely, protection by a variety of agents has been attributed to their known inhibitory effect on microsomal oxidation. Such compounds include metyrapone, acute ethanol, carbon disulphide, dithiocarb and cimetidine (Goldstein & Nelson, 1979; Sato & Lieber, 1981; Masuda & Nakayama, 1982; Harman & Fischer, 1983; Mitchell et al., 1984). In some studies the expected changes in production of glutathione-derived conjugates have been demonstrated, but other mechanisms have not always been excluded. Anomalous results have been observed with phenobarbitone induction (Poulsen et al., 1985) and cobalt chloride appears to protect not only by inhibiting the metabolic activation of paracetamol, but also by enhancing glucuronide conjugation and increasing the protective capacity of glutathione (Roberts et al., 1986).

Other factors influencing paracetamol metabolism and toxicity
Many factors are known to influence drug metabolising enzyme activity, and corresponding effects on paracetamol toxicity have been demonstrated. However, many of these factors can also modify glutathione status. Thus low protein diets and fasting influence both microsomal enzyme activity and glutathione content of the liver, and the usual effect is potentiation of paracetamol liver injury (McLean & Day, 1975; Miller et al., 1986; Price et al., 1987). Age is another determinant, and as expected, young animals are relatively resistant to paracetamol hepatotoxicity (Hart & Timbrell, 1979; Mancini et al., 1980). Once again however, anomalous results have been reported. Thus in one study isolated hepatocytes from newborn mice were damaged by paracetamol to the same extent as those from adults and covalent binding was actually greater in neonatal liver cells (Harman & McCamish, 1986).

Species differences
There are marked species differences in susceptibility to paracetamol induced liver damage. Hamsters and mice are very sensitive, and doses of 150 - 375 mg/kg produce hepatic necrosis. In contrast, guinea pigs, rabbits and rats are resistant, even with doses in the range of the acute LD50. These species differences are directly related to the degree of

covalent binding of paracetamol and glutathione depletion (Davis et al., 1974). Similar differences have been reported with isolated hepatocytes from these species (Green et al., 1984), and there are also strain differences (Price & Jollow, 1986). Recently, Tee et al., (1987) showed that while isolated hepatocytes from mice and hamsters are much more sensitive to paracetamol injury than those from rats and man, hepatocytes from all four species are equally sensitive to N-acetyl-p-benzoquinoneimine. The species differences in sensitivity seem to be due to differences in the rate of formation of the reactive metabolite rather than to differences in susceptibility to it.

There may be species differences in the effects of microsomal enzyme induction and inhibition on paracetamol toxicity, and also differential effects on its oxidative metabolism and elimination by non-toxic pathways. In addition, there are important species differences in the relative extent of glucuronide and sulphate conjugation of paracetamol. In hamsters, mice and man, glucuronide conjugation is the dominant route of paracetamol elimination, and it may be induced (and inhibited) in parallel with the toxic pathway. The overall effects on the severity of liver injury will then depend on the relative change in capacity of these two routes. In contrast, sulphate conjugation is the major mechanism of paracetamol removal in rats. Sulphate conjugation is not inducible, but it is saturable and dependent on the availability of inorganic sulphate. Sodium sulphate increases the rate of elimination of a large dose of paracetamol in the rat and might be expected to reduce its toxicity (Galinsky et al., 1979) but has no such effect in mice (or presumably man) (Hjelle et al., 1986).

CLINICAL SIGNIFICANCE

On the basis of extensive animal studies, it might be expected that factors which influence drug metabolism in man would be relevant to the incidence and severity of liver damage following overdosage of paracetamol, and perhaps also to its safety in normal therapeutic use. Unfortunately, this animal data cannot be extrapolated directly to man where the effects of microsomal enzyme inducers and inhibitors on paracetamol metabolism seem to be quite different.

The average single acute threshold dose of paracetamol which produces severe liver damage in man is about 250 mg/kg (Prescott, 1983), but in practice there is enormous individual variation. The standard "treatment line" relating plasma paracetamol concentrations to time after ingestion of an overdose can only be used as a guide to prognosis. Some 10% of patients with concentrations of 300 mg/l at four hours may escape liver injury completely, while occasionally others suffer severe liver damage with concentrations of 150 mg/l or less at the same time. Because of this great individual variation and the ethical need for treatment of all patients at risk, it is now virtually impossible to establish whether paracetamol-induced liver damage in man is influenced by factors which change drug metabolising enzyme activity. Nevertheless, such effects have often been assumed and many such claims have been made on the basis of anecdotal case reports.

Age, diet and nutrition
Both increased and decreased sensitivity have been attributed to cachexia and anorexia nervosa respectively but there is no proof either way (Barker et al., 1977; Newman & Bargman, 1979). On the other hand, young children are clearly more resistant to paracetamol toxicity than adults (Rumack, 1986), and they also have a greater capacity for sulphate conjugation than adults (Miller et al., 1976) although it is not known whether this is relevant. The elderly do not appear to be at increased risk (Douglas et al., 1976).

Microsomal enzyme induction
Some time ago we reported that patients who had previously taken drugs likely to cause induction suffered more severe liver damage after taking paracetamol in overdosage than those who had not (Wright & Prescott, 1973). However, the number of patients was small, the differences were not great and there was no independent confirmation of induction.

Nevertheless, it is now widely believed that such individuals are at increased risk and, there have been numerous anecdotal accounts of potentiation of paracetamol hepatotoxicity after overdosage in chronic alcoholics (Emby & Fraser, 1977; Goldfinger et al., 1978; McClain et al., 1980 and others) and in patients previously taking anticonvulsants (Wilson et al., 1978; Smith et al., 1986). It has also been claimed that chronic alcoholics may suffer severe liver damage following the therapeutic use of paracetamol (Leist et al., 1985; Kaysen et al., 1985; Seeff et al., 1986 and others). Chronic alcoholics are notoriously poor historians and analysis of all these reports reveals that most patients had taken overdoses (Prescott, 1986). In none of the reports claiming greater sensitivity on the basis of induction has increased metabolic activation of paracetamol been demonstrated.

Although it is reasonable to expect that inducing agents and chronic consumption of ethanol would enhance the metabolic activation and toxicity of paracetamol in man, this does not appear to be the case. The clinical impression that chronic alcoholics are at increased risk of severe liver damage after overdosage has not been confirmed in a study involving large numbers of poisoned patients (Rumack, 1983). Furthermore, the fractional urinary recovery of glutathione-derived conjugates is not increased in heavy drinkers and induced patients taking rifampicin or anticonvulsants (Prescott & Critchley, 1983). In a more recent report, the excretion of glutathione-derived conjugates in patients receiving diphenylhydantoin was increased by 23% compared with controls, but there was no increase in others taking rifampicin (Bock et al., 1987). On the other hand, induction with agents such as anticonvulsants and sulphinpyrazone (but not ethanol) stimulate glucuronide conjugation and significantly enhance the rate of paracetamol elimination (Prescott et al., 1981; Miners et al., 1984). The latter investigators found no significant increase in the fractional urinary recovery of glutathione-derived conjugates in the induced subjects, and as the metabolic clearances via glucuronide conjugation and oxidative metabolism were increased similarly, little or no potentiation of paracetamol toxicity would be anticipated.

Microsomal enzyme inhibition

Inhibition of the metabolic activation of paracetamol reduces its toxicity in animals and this would seem to be a reasonable approach to the treatment of overdosage in man provided that inhibition was selective. Cimetidine is a general inhibitor of oxidative drug metabolism which reduces the metabolic activation of paracetamol and protects against hepatotoxicity in animals (Mitchell et al., 1984). Cimetidine has been proposed as an antidote for poisoning with paracetamol but it does not inhibit its oxidative metabolism or conjugation as judged by the rate of elimination and the fractional urinary recovery of glutathione-derived conjugates in man (Critchley et al., 1983; Miners et al., 1984). On the other hand, acute ethanol administration dramatically reduces the metabolic activation of paracetamol without inhibiting glucuronide conjugation (Prescott & Critchley, 1983), and it appears to offer some protection against liver damage when taken at the time of overdosage with paracetamol (Rumack, 1986). Many patients take ethanol before an overdose of paracetamol, and in so doing may unwittingly be protecting themselves. Probenecid inhibits the glucuronide conjugation of paracetamol (Abernethy et al., 1985) and might potentiate its toxicity unless oxidative metabolism were correspondingly depressed. At present it seems unlikely that any treatment for paracetamol poisoning based on inhibition of microsomal enzymes will be superior to established therapy with N-acetylcysteine.

Other effects on parallel pathways of elimination

The sulphate conjugation of paracetamol is saturated after overdosage, and the availability of inorganic sulphate is also a limiting factor. N-acetylcysteine is metabolised in part to inorganic sulphate. It produces a modest but delayed increase in the sulphate conjugation of paracetamol but this is unlikely to be relevant to its action in preventing liver damage (Prescott 1980).

It has been claimed that glucuronide conjugation is also saturated after paracetamol overdosage, and that correspondingly enhanced metabolic activation is an important cause of toxicity (Slattery & Levy, 1979). This may be the case in animals, but there is no evidence for saturation of glucuronide conjugation in man except in rare cases of very severe intoxication with plasma paracetamol concentrations of the order of 1000 mg/l and in the newborn (Prescott, 1985).

Individual variation in paracetamol metabolism

There is marked individual variation in the metabolic activation of paracetamol and this undoubtedly contributes to differences in susceptibility to toxicity following overdosage. There are also important ethnic or geographical differences. The fractional urinary recovery of glutathione-derived conjugates following an oral dose in Ghanaians and Kenyans was only about half of that observed in Scots (mean 5.0 compared with 9.3% respectively). Overall, there was a 60-fold range in the extent of the metabolic activation of paracetamol compared with only a 3-fold range in glucuronide and sulphate conjugation (Critchley et al., 1986). It is not known whether this extreme individual variation has a genetic or environmental basis. A finding of particular interest was that a small minority of both the Scots and the Africans converted an abnormally large proportion of the dose of paracetamol (15-25%) to mercapturic acid and cysteine conjugates. There were no obvious environmental causes for this, and such individuals are presumably at increased risk of toxicity from paracetamol and other agents which produce toxicity by the same route of oxidative metabolism. These "extensive metabolic activators" could represent the opposite of the phenotype of "poor hydroxylators" of drugs such as debrisoquine.

SUMMARY

Paracetamol is normally very safe but overdosage can cause acute hepatic necrosis. Liver injury is mediated by its conversion by cytochrome P-450 dependent microsomal oxidase to N-acetyl-p-benzoquinoneimine, a reactive arylating metabolite. Experimental paracetamol hepatotoxicity depends on the rate of absorption, microsomal enzyme activity, the capacity of parallel routes of elimination and glutathione status. Major species differences in sensitivity have been attributed to differences in metabolic activation. In man there are marked individual differences in susceptibility to liver damage after overdosage with paracetamol, and great individual variation (up to 60-fold) in the extent of its metabolic activation. Paracetamol hepatotoxicity would be expected to be modified by factors which influence microsomal enzyme activity in man, and there have been anecdotal case reports to this effect. However, microsomal enzyme induction has not been shown to potentiate paracetamol toxicity and treatment of overdosage is based on stimulation of glutathione synthesis rather than inhibition of its oxidative metabolism. A small minority of individuals are extensive metabolic activators of paracetamol and presumably at increased risk of toxicity after overdosage.

REFERENCES

Abernethy, D.R., Greenblatt, D.J., Ameer, B. & Shader, R.I. (1985): Probenecid inhibition of acetaminophen and lorazepam clearance: direct inhibition of ether glucuronide clearance. J. Pharmacol. Exp. Therap. 234, 345-349.

Barker, J.D., de Carle, D.J. & Anuras, S. (1977): Chronic excessive acetaminophen use and liver damage. Ann. Intern. Med. 87, 299-301.

Bock, K.W., Wiltfang, J., Blume, R., Ullrich, D. & Bircher, J. (1987): Paracetamol as a test drug to determine glucuronide formation in man. Effects of inducers and of smoking. Eur. J. Clin. Pharmacol. 31, 677-683.

Boyd, E.M. & Bereczky G.M. (1966): Liver necrosis from paracetamol. Brit. J. Pharmacol. 26, 606-614.

Corcoran, G.B., Mitchell, J.R., Vaishnav, Y.N. & Horning, E.C. (1980): Evidence that acetaminophen and N-hydroxy-acetaminophen form a common arylating intermediate, N-acetyl-p-benzoquinoneimine. Molec. Pharmacol. 18, 536-542.

Critchley, J.A.J.H., Dyson, E.H., Scott, A.W., Jarvie, D.R. & Prescott, L.F. (1983): Is there a place for cimetidine or ethanol in the treatment of paracetamol poisoning? Lancet i, 1375-1376.

Critchley, J.A.J.H., Nimmo, G.R., Gregson, C.A., Woolhouse, N.M. & Prescott, L.F. (1986): Inter-subject and ethnic differences in paracetamol metabolism. Brit. J. Clin. Pharmacol. 22, 649-657.

Davis, D.C., Potter, W.Z., Jollow, D.J. & Mitchell, J.R. (1974): Species differences in hepatic glutathione depletion, covalent binding and hepatic necrosis after acetaminophen. Life Sciences 14, 2099-2109.

Davidson, D.G.D. & Eastham, W.N. (1966): Acute liver necrosis following overdose of paracetamol. Brit. Med J. 2, 497-499.

Douglas, A.P., Hamlyn, A.N. & James, O. (1976): Controlled trial of cysteamine in treatment of acute paracetamol (acetaminophen) poisoning. Lancet i, 111-115.

Emby, D.J. & Fraser, B.N. (1977): Hepatotoxicity of paracetamol enhanced by ingestion of alcohol. S. Afr. Med. J. 51, 208-209.

Galinsky, R.E., Slattery, J.T. & Levy, G. (1979): Effect of sodium sulfate on acetaminophen elimination by rats. J. Pharm. Sci. 68, 803-805.

Goldfinger, R., Ahmed, K.S., Pitchumoni, C.S. & Weseley S.A. (1978): Concomitant alcohol and drug abuse enhancing acetaminophen toxicity. Amer J. Gastroenterol. 70, 385-388.

Goldstein, M. & Nelson, E.B. (1979): Metyrapone as a treatment for acetaminophen (paracetamol) toxicity in mice. Res. Comm. Chem. Pathol. Pharmacol. 23, 203-206.

Green, C.E., Dabbs, J.E. & Tyson, C.A. (1984): Metabolism and cytotoxicity of acetaminophen in hepatocytes isolated from resistant and susceptible species. Toxicol. Appl. Pharmacol. 76, 139-149.

Harman, A.W. & Fischer, L.J. (1983): Hamster hepatocytes in culture as a model for acetaminophen toxicity: studies with inhibitors of drug metabolism. Toxicol. Appl Pharmacol. 71, 330-341.

Harman, A.W. & McCamish, L.E. (1986): Age-related toxicity of paracetamol in mouse hepatocytes. Biochem. Pharmacol. 35, 1731-1735.

Hart, J.G. & Timbrell, J.A. (1979): The effect of age on paracetamol hepatotoxicity in mice. Biochem. Pharmacol. 28, 3015-3017.

Hjelle, J.J., Brzeznicka, E.A. & Klaassen, C.D. (1986): Comparison of the effects of sodium sulfate and N-acetylcysteine on the hepatotoxicity of acetaminophen in mice. J. Pharmacol. Exp. Therap. 236, 526-534.

Jollow, D.J., Mitchell, J.R., Potter, W.Z., Davis, D.C., Gillette, J.R. & Brodie, B.B. (1973): Acetaminophen-induced hepatic necrosis. II. Role of covalent binding in vivo. J. Pharmacol. Exp. Therap. 187, 195-202.

Kaysen, G.A., Pond, S.M., Roper, M.H., Menke, D.J. & Marrama, M.A. (1985): Combined hepatic and renal injury in alcoholics during therapeutic use of acetaminophen. Arch. Intern. Med. 145, 2019-2023.

Leist, M.H., Gluskin, L.E. & Payne, J.A. (1985): Enhanced toxicity of acetaminophen in alcoholics: report of three cases. J. Clin. Gastroenterol. 7, 55-59.

Mancini, R.E., Sonawane, B.R. & Yaffe, S.J. (1980): Developmental susceptibility to acetaminophen toxicity. Res. Comm. Chem. Pathol. Pharmacol. 27, 603-606.

Masuda, Y. & Nakayama, N. (1982): Protective effect of diethyldithiocarbamate and carbon disulfide against liver injury induced by various hepatotoxic agents. Biochem. Pharmacol. 31, 2713-2725.

McClain, C.J., Kromhout, J.P., Peterson, F.J. & Holtzman, J.L. (1980): Potentiation of acetaminophen hepatotoxicity by alcohol. J. Amer. Med. Ass. 244, 251-253.

McLean, A.E.M. and Day, P.A. (1975): The effect of diet on the toxicity of paracetamol and the safety of paracetamol-methionine mixtures. Biochem. Pharmacol 24, 37-42.

Miller, R.P., Roberts, R.J. & Fischer, L.J. (1976): Acetaminophen elimination kinetics in neonates, children and adults. Clin. Pharmacol. Therap. 19, 284-294.

Miller, M.G., Price, V.F. & Jollow, D.J. (1986): Anomalous susceptibility of the fasted hamster to acetaminophen hepatotoxicity. Biochem. Pharmacol. 35, 817-825.

Miners, J.O., Attwood, J. & Birkett, D.J. (1984): Determinants of acetaminophen metabolism: effect of inducers and inhibitors of drug metabolism on acetaminophen's metabolic pathways. Clin. Pharmacol. Therap. 35, 480-486.

Mitchell, J.R., Jollow, D.J., Potter, W.Z., Davis, D.C., Gillette, J.R. & Brodie, B.B. (1973a): Acetaminophen-induced hepatic necrosis: I. role of drug metabolism. J. Pharmacol. Exp. Therap. 187, 185-194.

Mitchell, J.R., Jollow, D.J., Potter, W.Z., Gillette, J.R. & Brodie, B.B. (1973b): Acetaminophen-induced hepatic necrosis: IV. protective role of glutathione. J. Pharmacol. Exp. Therap. 187, 211-217.

Mitchell, M.C., Schenker, S. & Speeg, K.V. (1984): Selective inhibition of acetaminophen oxidation and toxicity by cimetidine and other histamine H2-receptor antagonists in vivo and in vitro in the rat and in man. J. Clin. Invest. 73, 383-391.

Moldéus, P. & Gergely, V. (1980): Effect of acetone on the activation of acetaminophen. Toxicol. Appl. Pharmacol. 53, 8-13.

Moore, M., Thor, H., Moore, G., Nelson, S., Moldéus, P. & Orrenius, S. (1985): The toxicity of acetaminophen and N-acetyl-p-benzoquinoneimine in isolated hepatocytes is associated with thiol depletion and increased cytosolic Ca^{2+}. J. Biol. Chem. 260, 13035-13040.

Newman, T.J. & Bargman, G.J. (1979): Acetaminophen hepatotoxicity and malnutrition. Amer. J. Gastroenterol. 72, 647-650.

Potter, W.Z., Davis, D.C., Mitchell, J.R., Jollow, D.J., Gillette, J.R. & Brodie, B.B. (1973): Acetaminophen-induced hepatic necrosis. III. cytochrome P-450-mediated covalent binding in vitro. J. Pharmacol. Exp. Therap. 187, 203-210.

Poulsen, H.E., Lerche, A. & Pedersen, N.T. (1985). Phenobarbital induction does not potentiate hepatotoxicity but accelerates liver cell necrosis from acetaminophen overdose in the rat. Pharmacology 30, 100-108.

Prescott, L.F. (1980): Kinetics and metabolism of paracetamol and phenacetin. Brit. J. Clin. Pharmacol. 10 (Suppl. 2), 291-298S.

Prescott, L.F. (1983): Paracetamol overdosage. Pharmacological considerations and clinical management. Drugs 25, 290-314.

Prescott, L.F. (1985): Clinical toxicological aspects of glucuronide conjugation. In Advances in Glucuronide Conjugation, eds S. Matern, K.W. Bock & W. Gerok, pp 329-334. Lancaster: MTP Press.

Prescott, L.F. (1986): Liver damage with non-narcotic analgesics. Med. Toxicol. 1 (Suppl. 1), 44-56.

Prescott, L.F. & Critchley, J.A.J.H. (1983): Drug interactions affecting analgesic toxicity. Amer. J. Med. 75 (Suppl. 5A), 113-116.

Prescott, L.F., Critchley, J.A.J.H., Balali-Mood, M. & Pentland, B. (1981): Effects of microsomal enzyme induction on paracetamol metabolism in man. Brit. J. Cin. Pharmacol. 12, 149-153.

Price, V.F. & Jollow, D.J. (1986): Strain differences in susceptibility of normal and diabetic rats to acetaminophen hepatotoxicity. Biochem. Pharmacol. 35, 687-695.

Price, V.F., Miller, M.G. & Jollow, D.J. (1987): Mechanisms of fasting-induced potentiation of acetaminophen hepatotoxicity in the rat. Biochem. Pharmacol. 36, 427-433.

Roberts, S.A., Price, V.F. & Jollow, D.J. (1986): The mechanisms of cobalt chloride-induced protection against acetaminophen hepatotoxicity. Drug. Metab. Dispos. 14, 25-33.

Rumack, B.H. (1983): Acetaminophen overdose. Amer. J. Med. 75 (Suppl. 5A), 104-112.

Rumack, B.H. (1986): Acetaminophen overdose in children and adolescents. Pediat. Clin. N. Amer. 33, 691-701.

Sato, C., Matsuda, Y. & Lieber, C.S. (1981): Increased hepatotoxicity of acetaminophen after chronic ethanol consumption in the rat. Gastroenterology 80, 140-148.

Sato, C. & Lieber, C.S. (1981): Mechanism of the preventive effect of ethanol on acetaminophen-induced hepatotoxicity. J. Pharmacol. Exp. Therap. 218, 811-815.

Seeff, L.B., Cuccherini, B.A., Zimmerman, H.J., Adler, E. & Benjamin, S.B. (1986): Acetaminophen hepatotoxicity in alcoholics. Ann. Intern. Med. 104, 399-404.

Slattery, J.T. & Levy, G. (1979): Acetaminophen kinetics in acutely poisoned patients. Clin. Pharmacol. Therap. 25, 184-195.

Smith, J.A.E., Hine, I.D., Beck, P. & Routledge, P.A. (1986): Paracetamol toxicity: is enzyme induction important? Human Toxicol. 5, 383-385.

Tee, L.B.G., Davies, D.S., Seddon. C.E. & Boobis, A.R. (1987): Species differences in the hepatotoxicity of paracetamol are due to differences in the rate of conversion to its cytotoxic metabolite. Biochem. Pharmacol. 36, 1041-1052.

Thomson, J.S. & Prescott, L.F. (1966): Liver damage and impaired glucose tolerance after paracetamol overdosage. Brit. Med. J. 2, 506-507.

To, E.C.A. & Wells, P.G. (1986): Biochemical changes associated with the potentiation of acetaminophen hepatotoxicity by brief anesthesia with diethyl ether. Biochem. Pharmacol. 35, 4139-4152.

Tsokos-Kuhn, J.O., Todd, E.L., McMillin-Wood, J.B. & Mitchell, J.R. (1985): ATP-dependent calcium uptake by rat liver plasma membrane vesicles. Effect of alkylating hepatotoxins in vivo. Mol. Pharmacol. 28, 56-61.

Wilson, J.T., Kasantikul, V., Harbison, R. & Martin, D. (1978): Death in an adolescent following an overdose of acetaminophen and phenobarbital. Amer. J. Dis. Child. 132, 466-473.

Wright, N. & Prescott, L.F. (1973): Potentiation by previous drug therapy of hepatotoxicity following paracetamol overdosage. Scott. Med. J. 18, 56-58.

Résumé

Le paracétamol provoque une nécrose hépatique aiguë par biotransformation en un métabolite réactif mineur, le N-acétyl-p-benzoquinonéimine. L'hépatotoxicité expérimentale induite par le paracétamol dépend de l'activité des enzymes microsomaux, de celle des voies d'élimination parallèles et du contenu en glutathion. Il existe des différences interespèces dans la susceptiblité à cette drogue, qui semblent liées à des différences dans l'activation métabolique. Chez l'homme, les variations individuelles sont fortes à la fois dans le métabolisme oxydatif du paracétamol et dans la susceptibilité à l'hépatotoxicité induite par surdosage. Chez une minorité d'individus, l'activation métabolique est très élevée. En dépit de cas anecdotiques, il n'a pas été démontré que l'induction d'enzymes microsomaux potentialise la toxicité du paracétamol chez l'homme et le traitement d'un surdosage est basé sur la stimulation de la synthèse de glutathion plutôt que sur l'inhibition du métabolisme oxydatif.

Halothane hepatitis : a model of immunoallergic disease

James Neuberger, J. Gerald Kenna

The Queen Elizabeth Hospital, Edgbaston, Birmingham B15 2TH, UK. National Institutes of Health, Bethesda, Maryland, 20892, USA

ABSTRACT

Many of the clinical and serological features of this severe form of liver damage that may rarely complicate halothane anaesthesia suggests immune mechanism is involved. Many of these patients have circulating antibodies reacting with both normal liver cell membrane determinants and halothane induced antigens. These latter antigens are generated by oxidative metabolism of the drug. Immunoblotting studies have demonstrated that halothane metabolism results in the generation of at least three different polypeptide antigens recognised by antibodies present in the serum of patients. These antibodies can be detected in the livers of patients anaesthetised with halothane and therefore it would appear that if immune mechanisms are involved in the generation of halothane hepatitis, then the idiosyncracy lies in the nature of the immune response rather than generation of the antigens. Additional studies have suggested that halothane may result in alteration of lymphocyte responsiveness, which may further heighten the immune response. Patients with halothane hepatitis have high titres of antibodies to normal liver cell membranes. Turnover of membrane proteins is fairly rapid and, therefore, if halothane hepatitis is indeed immune mediated, then membrane response may be directed to normal red cell membranes with the halothane antigens merely breaking tolerance.

KEY WORDS

halothane: liver disease: drug related antibodies

INTRODUCTION

Hepatotoxicity, in nearly all instances, is associated with metabolic activation of the drug. In many cases, this hepatotoxicity arises as a direct consequence of the metabolic action and is therefore largely predictable. One of the cardinal features is that the toxicity is dose related, although congenital or acquired factors may modify the likelihood of expression of hepatotoxicity. This type of drug reaction can often readily be studied in vitro using animal models. In contrast are those idiosyncratic drug reactions which are not dose related and where animal models are usually hard to produce. These idiosyncratic drug reactions which, in man at least, have a low incidence, may be due to metabolism of the drug through a usually minor pathway. An example of this includes fluorouracil toxicity which is associated with altered activity of dihydropyrimidine dehydrogenase (Hoft et al 1981). In contrast, other examples of idiosyncratic drug toxicity are thought to be related to the involvement of immune mechanisms. The evidence for immune involvement is largely circumstantial and based on the idiosyncratic nature of the response and the association with features of hypersensitivity, such as rash, fever, arthralgia, circulating immune complexes and the appearance of organ non-specific auto-antibodies. One of the best studied examples of drug reactions in which immune mechanisms are thought to be involved is severe hepatitis that may follow halothane anaesthesia.

FORMS OF HALOTHANE HEPATITIS

Current evidence suggests that halothane associated liver damage may appear in one of two forms. The first occurs relatively commonly and is characterised by minor elevations of serum transaminases and other markers of liver dysfunction (Allen et al 1987, Trowell et al 1975, Wright et al 1975). These may be found in up to 35% of patients exposed to halothane and the changes in liver tests may not be apparent for up to two weeks after halothane exposure. These abnormalities of liver function are rarely associated with any clinical evidence of liver damage, such as jaundice or liver failure. Subsequent re-exposure of such a patient to halothane is not necessarily associated with the reappearance of these abnormalities of liver function. Liver biopsy, in the few cases where it has been performed, shows no more than focal areas of mild hepatitis. This form of liver damage contrasts with the more severe form (halothane hepatitis). This occurs much less commonly, the evidence from the retrospective National Halothane Study (1966) suggests an incidence of otherwise unexplained massive liver cell damage to be about one in 35,000 anaesthetics. Current evidence suggests that not all cases of this severe form of halothane hepatitis are associated with massive liver cell necrosis and therefore the incidence is likely to be greater. Indeed, our own experience suggests that only half of the patients with halothane hepatitis have fulminant hepatic failure (Kenna et al 1987). In those cases where there has been multiple exposure to halothane, the incidence, as assessed by the National Halothane Study, is far greater, approximately one in 3,500 patients. Thus, in contrast to the mild form of liver disease following halothane, the incidence of halothane hepatitis appears far higher in patients who have had more than one exposure to the anaesthetic. There have been reports of patients developing halothane hepatitis after only one exposure and indeed, this has been used to refute the argument that halothane hepatitis is immune mediated (MacKay 1985). This association has to be questioned in view of the recent finding that enough halothane may be absorbed on the rubber of the anaesthetic machine to contaminate any "non-halothane" anaesthetic (Varma et al 1985).

In addition to the strikingly increased frequency of halothane hepatitis after multiple halothane exposures, other features implicating hypersensitivity include a female to male ratio of 1.6:1, the finding of peripheral eosinophilia in 21% and autoantibodies in nearly one third of cases (Neuberger and Kenna 1987). Some authors have drawn attention to the increased incidence of allergy and eczema in such patients, although the incidence does not seem strikingly increased with the normal anaesthetic population. One study from Japan has shown an association with the HLA phenotype DR2, but the validity of this association has to be questioned in view of the statistical analysis

(Otsuka et al 1985). Another feature which suggests a possible genetic association is the occurrence in three pairs of closely related women (Hoft et al 1981).

NATURE OF THE IMMUNE RESPONSE

Early studies to look for evidence of sensitisation to the halothane molecule itself produce conflicting results (Moult et al 1975, Paronetto and Popper 1970, Walton et al 1973, Walton et al 1974). While some of the differences may have been due to different concentrations of halothane used in the leucocyte migration inhibition test or blast cell transformation tests, an alternative explanation was that halothane itself is not the target antigen. Indeed, the molecule is small and therefore unlikely to be a target in the immune response. An alternative explanation was that halothane itself acts merely as a hapten. In order to circumvent the problems of selecting an appropriate antigen for in vitro testing, Vergani and colleagues (1978) used a different technique. Rabbits, which antigenically at least, have some resemblance to man, were given halothane 1% in oxygen and allowed to recover for 18 hours. This interval was to allow time for metabolism of the drug and the appearance of any antigen in the liver. The liver was removed and used as target antigens for in vitro antigen testing. Initial studies using the leucocyte migration test showed sensitisation of lymphocytes in 8 of 12 patients with a presumed diagnosis of halothane hepatitis to an homogenate of liver from these halothane treated rabbits, but not to normal rabbit liver. These studies therefore suggest that patients with halothane hepatitis are sensitised to a liver antigen which is associated with exposure of animals to halothane. Subsequent studies were performed to look for antibodies reacting with these "halothane altered liver cell antigens". The presence of these antibodies were confirmed using both indirect immunoflourescence and antibody dependent cell mediated cytotoxicity (ADCC). In these techniques hepatocytes were isolated by mechanical dissection for indirect immunoflourescence and by collagenase digestion for ADCC (Vergani et al 1980). The studies showed that these "halothane antibodies" were present in the serum of about 70 to 75% of patients with the clinical diagnosis of halothane hepatitis, but not in patients who had been exposed to halothane and had not developed liver damage, or in those patients who, following halothane anaesthesia, had developed liver damage from other causes, such as malignant infiltration of the liver or viral infection (Neuberger et al 1983). Furthermore, the presence of capping in the immunoflourescence experiments indicates that the antigen is present on the liver cell surface.

However, both ADCC and immunoflourescence techniques suffer from limitations in that the techniques are cumbersome and time consuming; neither are quantitative and all, to some extent at least, are dependent on observer assessment. For this reason an enzyme linked immunosorbent assay was developed (Kenna et al 1985). Again, use of this technique showed that the majority of patients with halothane hepatitis have circulating antibodies reacting with halothane altered liver cell determinants and these antibodies are specific to patients with halothane hepatitis. Thus, whether or not these antibodies are involved in the pathogenesis of halothane hepatitis, at least this does provide a rare example in which it is possible to make a positive diagnosis of a drug induced liver disease.

PRIMARY OR SECONDARY RESPONSE?

The presence of halothane antibodies in patients with a clinical diagnosis of halothane hepatitis merely indicates that recognition of halothane altered liver cell determinants has occurred and does not indicate that these antibodies are involved in the pathogenesis of liver disease. Indeed, Smith and colleagues (1980 a, b) have shown clearly that sensitisation to paracetamol damaged liver cells may occur in rats. However, implication of these halothane related antibodies in the pathogenesis of cell damage is suggested by a number of features. Firstly, these antibodies, in vitro, can induce normal lymphocytes to become cytotoxic to the antibody coated target cell and so have the potential to cause liver cell damage. Secondly these antibodies are unlikely to occur as a consequence of a direct halothane toxicity since they cannot be demonstrated in the serum of patients who, following halothane anaesthesia, have developed liver damage from other causes, such as hepatitis A viral infection or malignant infiltration of the liver. In both cases hepatocytes bearing the halothane antigens would be exposed to the general circulation and therefore immune recognition might occur. Finally, IgG class antibodies have been detected even within two weeks of halothane exposure: although switching can occur rapidly, this suggests a secondary response. It is likely that if the appearance of the antibodies were merely secondary to direct damage then IgM class antibodies would be anticipated.

GENERATION OF THE HALOTHANE ALTERED ANTIGENS

It is possible to envisage two mechanisms whereby halothane exposure results in the generation of liver cell antigens. Firstly the halothane molecule itself could directly interact with the liver cell membrane, or alternatively, metabolism of halothane could result in generation of reactive metabolites which bind to and alter liver cell macromolecules which are subsequently expressed on the cell membrane. Halothane itself is metabolised through at least two different pathways, one oxidative and one reductive (Neuberger and Kenna 1987), both are associated with the generation of reactive metabolites which covalently bind to liver cell macromolecules. One pathway is favoured by high oxygen tensions and is stimulated by enzyme inducers such as betanaphthoflavone and is associated with the production of triflouro acetic acid. In contrast to the oxidative pathway, the reductive pathway is preferentially stimulated by lower oxygen tensions and enzyme pretreatment with phenobarbitone. In the reductive metabolism inorganic flouride is released. Experiments involving either enzyme pre-treatment of rabbits with betanaphthaflavone or phenobarbitone or administration of halothane under different oxygen tensions, have shown that the oxidative route of metabolism of halothane is associated with generation of the halothane related antigen (Neuberger et al 1981).

The structure of these halothane associated antigens were investigated using the immunoblotting method. In this technique polypeptides in rabbit liver homogenates are resolved by SDS - polyacrylamide gel electrophoresis and transferred electrophoretically to nitrocellulose. Binding of antibodies in patient's serum to these polypeptides is detected by incubating the serum with nitrocellular strips and the antibody is localised using peroxidase labelled second antibody. Using this technique (Kenna et al 1985), it was possible to show that serum from patients with halothane hepatitis was able to recognise 3 distinct polypeptide antigens of apparent molecular weight 100,000, 76,000 and 57,000 (table I).

Detection in patients' sera of antibodies to halothane induced rabbit liver antigens by immunoblotting

	100 KD	76 KD	100+76 KD	57 KD
Halothane hepatitis (24)	7	3	7	2
Halothane No hepatitis (17)	0	0	0	0
Fulminant hepatic failure (15)	0	0	0	0
Chronic liver disease (10)	0	0	0	0
Normals (24)	0	0	0	0

Use of protease inhibitors showed that the smaller polypeptides were not derived from the larger polypeptides or each other by proteolysis. Furthermore, subcellular fractionation studies showed that the polypeptides antigens were concentrated in the microsomal fraction at 16 hours. This microsomal fraction is composed of membranes from both the endoplasmic reticulum and the plasma membrane and is consistent with the hypothesis that the antigens are generated on the endoplasmic reticulum by the mixed function oxidase system and are transferred by membrane flow to the cell membrane. It was of interest to note that not all sera had antibodies reacting with all three polypeptide antigens and several different patterns of antibody binding were noted. Thus it can be deduced that the patient's antibodies do not recognise a single common epitope consisting of one halothane metabolite bound to different proteins.

WHY IDIOSYNCRATIC?

All the above studies were performed using rabbits and it is clear that all rabbits exposed to halothane under conditions in which the oxidative pathway and metabolism is stimulated produce the halothane associated liver antigen. Studies have shown that in man halothane is also predominantly metabolised through the oxidative pathway. If halothane hepatitis is indeed immune mediated, then does the idiosyncracy lie in idiosyncracy in generation of the antigen or in recognition of the antigen? Initial studies were done using Alexander cells, human derived hepatoma cell lines. Hepatoma cell lines were incubated with extra-cellular NADPH generating system (consisting of human liver microsomes, 1.0 mM NAPDH, 5.0 mM glucose-6-phosphate, 10 mM MgCl2 and G6P dehydrogenase). Those Alexander cells incubated with halothane for one hour were able to generate the halothane associated antigens as shown by indirect immunoflourescence using serum from patients with halothane hepatitis. It was found that both the NAPDH generating system and halothane exposure were necessary for generation of the antigen (table II).

Appearance of immunofluorescence after incubating Alexander cells with serum from either controls or patients with halothane hepatitis or exposed to halothane without hepatitis: cells were exposed to halothane in the presence or absence of NADPH Generating System

Serum (N)	Halothane and NADPH Generating System	NADPH Generating System	Halothane
Control (3)	0	0	0
Halothane hepatitis (4)	3	0	0
Halothane No hepatitis (3)	0	0	0

In the three cases it was possible to obtain liver from patients who had been exposed to halothane, but dying within 24 hours from cardiovascular causes. In both cases, liver was taken immediately post-mortem and used as target antigen in the immunoblotting method. Studies showed that in both cases halothane antigen was detectable in the liver (table III).

Detection by immunoblotting of halothane antigens in human liver

Source of liver	Number	Days after halothane	Antigen detection
Halothane No hepatitis	2	1, 1	2
Halothane hepatitis	3	6, 17, 21	0
Other anaesthetics No hepatitis	3	1, 1, 1	0
Normal liver	1		0

It is of interest that it was not possible to detect halothane antigens in the three livers of patients who had died with halothane hepatitis: clearly, since all three patients had halothane antibodies in the serum, halothane antigens must have been present at some stage in the illness. Thus, based on limited experiments, it would appear that human hepatocytes are capable of generating the liver cell antigen and indeed this seems to be the case in all patients exposed to halothane. Therefore, the susceptibility is likely to lie in the response to the antigen rather than in the generation of that antigen. This hypothesis has an analogy in patients with hepatitis B viral infection. In this instance infection with the virus is associated with the development of antigen (core antigen) on the surface of infected liver cells. It is thought that an impaired immune response, for example in those on renal dialysis or recieving immunosuppression, is associated with chronicity, whereas those with exaggurated immune response have fulminant hepatic failure.

POSSIBLE MECHANISMS OF HALOTHANE HEPATITIS

There are several possible mechanisms whereby halothane exposure may lead to immune mediated liver damage. One possibility is that halothane exposure may lead to a breakdown in tolerance. Current concept suggests that there is a full repetoire of helper-inducer cells that recognise autoantigens and may give help to effector T cells and antibody producing B cells (fig 1).

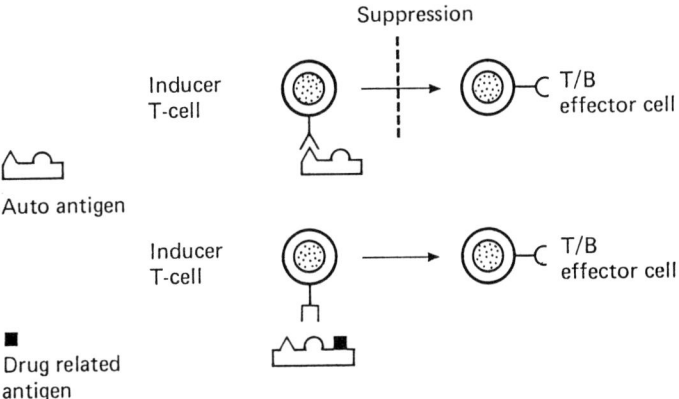

These auto-reactive T cells are normally held in check by antigen specific and non-specific suppressor-cells. If halothane were to inhibit non-specifically T lymphocyte suppressor activity, then an immune mediated response would ensue to auto-antigens. This sort of mechanism has been shown to operate in the case of alpha methyldopa associated liver damage (Kirtland et al 1980). A global reduction in suppressor-cell function would be anticipated to result in the appearance of organ non-specific auto-antibodies and indeed this is found in cases of halothane hepatitis and some other instances of drug associated hepatitis (Homberg et al 1985). Both the stress of surgery and some anaesthetics may be associated with a reduction in suppressor-cell function (Watkins and Salo 1982). Preliminary studies have shown using a concanavallin A induced suppressor cell functional assay of pokeweed mitogen stimulated cells that halothane exposure in vitro will result in a significant decrease in suppressor-cell function in about half the patients examined. Similar results were found with alpha methyldopa which may also cause an immune mediated hepatitis, but not with alcohol (fig 2).

Effect of drugs on Con A induced lymphocyte suppression on PWOM stimulated IgG production. Results are shown as % change in Ts function

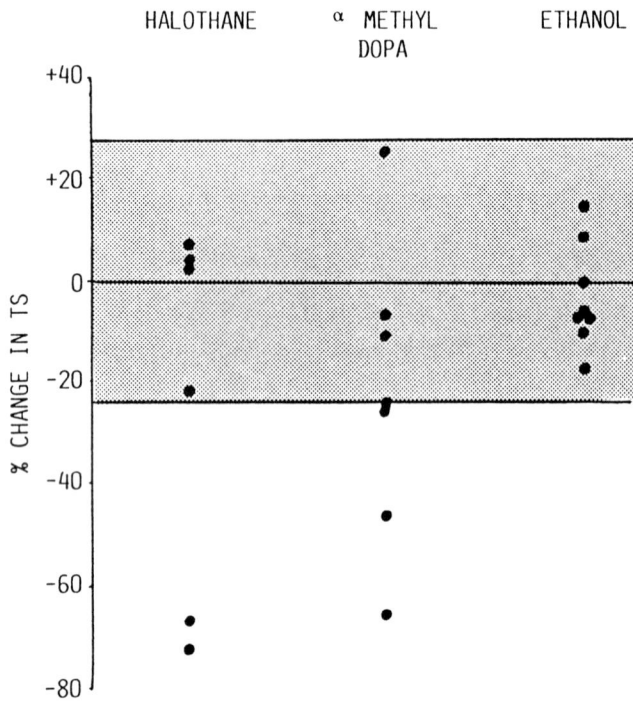

However, if there were a generalised disturbance of immune regulation, then it might be anticipated that halothane exposure would be associated with damage of other organs with the development of haemolytic anaemia or thyroid disturbance.

As indicated above, halothane is predominantly metabolised in the liver and the halothane antigens are directed again to a hapten associated with the metabolism of the drug. However, one major possible criticism to this idea is that the turnover of membrane proteins is usually a matter of hours and evidence of liver dysfunction may not become evident until three or more weeks after halothane exposure. Although the drug itself may be dissolved in adipose tissue, excretion of halothane metabolites is usually over within a few days. Thus an alternative possibility is that the generation of halothane antigens results in the breakdown of tolerance and thus provokes an auto-immune disease. The explantation for this is that inducer and effector lymphocytes recognise different epitopes on the same antigen. While the inducer cells are controlled by the suppressor-cells, introduction of a novel, drug induced epitope will allow different inducer cell population to give help to the effector cell and so lead effectively to T cell bypass. In favour of this hypothesis is the high incidence of antibodies to normal liver cell components found in patients with halothane hepatitis, as shown by the cytotoxicity experiments to normal and halothane treated liver cells (fig 3).

Cytotoxicity to normal and halothane treated rabbit liver cells induced by serum from patients with halothane hepatitis. Dotted line indicates upper limit of normal

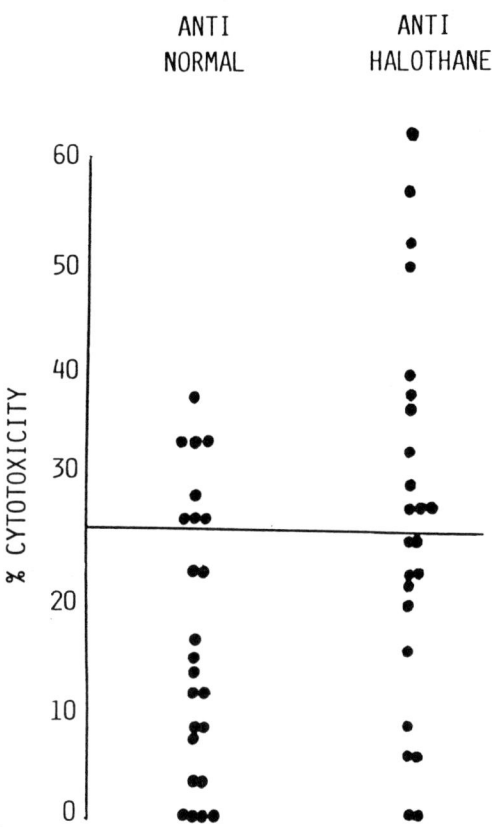

IS HALOTHANE HEPATITIS IMMUNE MEDIATED?

A number of animal models of halothane hepatitis have been reported. In most cases, halothane is given under reductive conditions and there is a rapid onset in susceptible species of animals of liver cell damage within 24 hours (Jee et al 1980, Cousins et al 1979, Sipes and Brown 1976). Death is rarely found. It is thought that these models do not accurately reflect the severe form of halothane hepatitis observed in man; only one exposure of halothane is necessary so the disease is not idiosyncratic and the reaction does not appear to be dose dependant. However, it is not the purpose of this chapter to discuss the possibilities of direct halothane hepatotoxicity.

Based on the above information, it is possible to make a hypothesis of the mechanism of halothane hepatitis. A patient exposed to halothane will metabolise the drug in the liver and halothane antigens will be produced on the surface membrane of the liver cell. Individuals who are susceptible, possibly on the basis of a genetic disposition (Farrell et al 1985), would recognise these antigens as foreign and a primary immune response would be directed to these antigens. Subsequent exposure to halothane in the same individual would lead to a greatly enhanced immune response. The presence of the halothane antigen on the liver cell and its recognition would lead to bypass of the normal mechanisms controlling tolerance and this would lead to a major immune mediated attack on normal liver cells, leading to the appearance of liver cell necrosis and in some cases cell death. Clearly there are many assumptions in this hypothesis and further work is required to refute or deny the involvement of immune mechanisms in a pathogenesis of this drug related hepatotoxicity.

REFERENCES

ALLAN L G, HUSSEY A J & HOWIE J et al. (1987):
Hepatic glutathione-S-transferase release after halothane anaesthesia
Lancet; i: 771-774

COUSINS M J, SHARP J H, GOURLAY G K, ADAMS J F, HAYNES W D & WHITEHEAD R. (1979):
Hepatotoxicity and halothane metabolism in an animal model with application for human toxicity
Anaesthesia and Intensive Care: 7; 9-24

FARRELL G, PRENDERGAST D & MURRAY M. (1985):
Halothane hepatitis: Detection of a constitutional susceptibility factor
New England Journal of Medicine: 313; 1310-1314

HOFT R H, BUNKER J P, GOODMAN H & GREGORY P B. (1981):
Halothane hepatitis in three pairs of closely related women
New England Journal of Medicine: 304; 1023-1024

HOMBERG J C, ABUAF N, HELMY-KHALIL S, BIOUR M, POUPON R, ISLAM S, DARNIS F, LEVY V G, OPOLON P & BEAUGRAND M. (1985):
Drug induced hepatitis associated with anti-cytoplasmic autoantibodies
Hepatology: 5; 722-727

JEE R C, SIPES I G, GANDOLFI A J & BROWN B R. (1980):
Factors influencing hepatotoxicity in the rat hypoxic model
Toxicology and Applied Pharmacology: 52; 267-277

KENNA J G, NEUBERGER J M & WILLIAMS R. (1984):
An enzyme-linked immunosorbent assay for detection of antibodies against halothane altered hepatocyte antigens
Journal of Immunological Methods: 75; 3-14

KENNA J G, NEUBERGER J & WILLIAMS R. (1984):
Characterisation of halothane-induced antigens by immuno-blotting
Biochemical Society Transactions; 13: 910-911

KENNA J G, NEUBERGER J, WILLIAMS R
Specific antibodies to halothane induced liver antigens in halothane hepatitis
Brit Journal of Anaesthesia (in press)

KIRTLAND H, DANIEL M D, MOHLER N & HORWITZ D A. (1980):

Methyl dopa inhibition of suppressor lymphocyte function
New England Journal of Medicine: 302; 825-831

MACKAY I R. (1985):
Induction by drugs of hepatitis and autoantibodies to cell organelles: significance and interpretation
Hepatology: 5; 904-906

MOULT P J A, ADJUKIEWICZ A B, GAYLARDE P M, SARKANY I & SHERLOCK S. (1975):
Lymphocyte transformation in halothane related hepatitis
British Medical Journal: ii; 69-70

NATIONAL HALOTHANE STUDY. (1966):
Summary of the National Halothane Study: possible association between halothane anaesthesia and postoperative hepatic necrosis
Journal of the Americal Medical Association: 197;121-134

NEUBERGER J, MIELI VERGANI G, TREDGER J M, DAVIS M & WILLIAMS R. (1981):
Oxidative metabolism of halothane in the production of altered hepatocyte membrane antigens in acute halothane-induced necrosis
Gut: 22; 669-672

NEUBERGER J M, GIMSON A E S, DAVIS M & WILLIAMS R. (1983):
Specific serological markers in the diagnosis of fulminant hepatic failure following halothane anaesthesia
British Journal of Anaesthesia: 55; 15-19

NEUBERGER J M & WILLIAMS R. (1984):
Halothane anaesthesia and liver damage
British Medical Journal: 289; 1136-1139

NEUBERGER J, KENNA J G. (1987):
Halothane hepatitis
Clin Sci: 72; 263-270

OTSUKA S, YAMAMOTO M, KASUYA S, OHTOMO H, YAMAMOTO Y YOSHIDA T O & ATALA T. (1985):
HLA antigens in patients with unexplained hepatitis following halothane anaesthesia
[Acta Anaesthesiologica Scandinavia: 29; 497-501

PARONETTO F & POPPER H. (1970):
Lymphocyte stimulation induced by halothane in patients with hepatitis following exposure to halothane
New England Journal of Medicine: 283; 277-280

SIPES I G & BROWN B R. (1976):
An animal model of hepatotoxicity associated with halothane anaesthesia
Anaesthesiology: 45; 622-628

SMITH CI, COOKSLEY G E & POWELL L W. (1980a):
Cell-mediated immunity to liver antigens in toxic liver injury - I Occurrence and specificity

Clinical and Experimental Immunology: 39; 607-617

SMITH C I, COOKSLEY G E & POWELL L W. (1980b):
Cell-mediated immunity to liver antigens in toxic liver injury - II Role in pathogenesis of liver damage
Clinical and Experimental Immunology: 39; 618-625

TROWELL J, PETO R & CRAMPTON SMITH A. (1975):
Controlled trial of repeated halothane anaesthetics in patients with carcinoma of the uterine cervix treated with radium
Lancet: i; 821-824

TUCHMAN M, STOECKELER J S, KIANG D T, O'DEA R F, RAMNARAINE M L & MIRKIN B L. (1985):
Familial pyrimidinaemia and pyrimidinuria associated with severe 5-fluorouracil toxicity
New England Journal of Medicine: 313; 245-249

VARMA R R, WHITESELL R C & ISKANDARANI M M. (1985):
Halothane hepatitis without halothane: role of inapparent circuit contamination and its prevention
Hepatology: 5; 1159-1162

VERGANI D, EDDLESTON A, TSANTOULAS D, DAVIS M & WILLIAMS R. (1978):
Sensitisation to halothane altered liver components in severe hepatic necrosis after halothane anaesthesia
Lancet: i; 801-803

VERGANI D, MIELI VERGANI G, ALBERTI A, NEUBERGER J, EDDLESTON A, DAVIS M & WILLIAMS R. (1980):
Antibodies to the surface of halothane altered rabbit hepatocytes in patients with severe halothane associated hepatitis
New England Journal of Medicine: 303; 66-71

WALTON B, DUMONDE D C, WILLIAMS C, JONES D, STRUNIN J M, LAYTON J M, STRUNIN L & SIMPSON R. (1973):
Lymphocyte transformation: absence of increased responses in alleged halothane jaundice
Journal of the American Medical Association: 225; 494-498

WALTON B, HAMBLIN A, DUMONDE D C & SIMPSON R. (1974):
Lymphocyte transformation: absence of cellular hypersensitivity in patients with unexplained jaundice following halothane
Anaesthesiology: 44; 391-397

WATKINS J & SALO M. (1982):
Trauma, stress and immunity in anaesthesia and surgery
Butterworths: London

WRIGHT R, CHISHOLM M, LLOYD B, EDWARDS J C, EADE O E, HAWKSLEY M, MOLES T M & GARDNER M. (1975):
A controlled prospective study of the effect on liver function of multiple exposures to halothane
Lancet: i; 821-823

Résumé

De nombreux signes cliniques et sérologiques de la forme sévère d'hépatotoxicité qui peut exceptionnellement compliquer l'anesthésie à l'halothane suggère un mécanisme immun. Plusieurs de ces patients ont des anticorps circulants qui réagissent avec des déterminants antigéniques normaux membranaires des cellules hépatiques et des antigènes induits par l'halothane. Ces derniers antigènes sont générés par le métabolisme oxydatif de ce composé. Des études d'immunoblotting ont montré que la biotransformation de l'halothane donne naissance à au moins trois polypeptides antigéniques reconnus par des anticorps présents dans le sérum de patients. Ces anticorps peuvent être détectés dans le foie de patients anesthésiés à l'halothane ; par conséquent, si des mécanismes immuns sont impliqués dans la génèse de l'hépatite à l'halothane, l'idiosyncrasie est liée à la nature de la réponse immune plutôt qu'à la formation d'antigènes. Des études complémentaires suggèrent que l'halothane peut entraîner une altération de la réponse lymphocytaire et par la suite aggraver la réponse immune. Des patients ayant développé une hépatite à l'halothane ont des titres élevés d'anticorps dirigés contre les membranes cellulaires hépatiques. Le renouvellement des protéines membranaires est rapide et si l'hépatite à l'halothane est à médiation immune alors la réponse membranaire peut être dirigée contre les membranes des globules rouges normaux et la tolérance est rompue par les antigènes induits par l'halothane.

Autoantibodies anticytochrome P-450 during autoimmune hepatitis

Philippe Beaune[1], Patrick M. Dansette[2], Daniel Mansuy[2], Liliane Kiffel[1], Claudine Amar[2], Jean-Paul Leroux, Jean-Claude Homberg[3]

[1] Laboratoire de Biochimie, INSERM U.75, CHU Necker, 75730 Paris Cedex, France.
[2] Laboratoire de Chimie et Biochimie Pharmacologiques et Toxicologiques, CNRS UA 400, 75270 Paris Cedex 06, France. [3] Laboratoire Central d'Immunologie et hématologie, Hôpital Saint-Antoine, 75571 Paris Cedex 12, France

Abstract

"Anti-Liver/Kidney microsomes" anti-LKM autoantibodies have been found in the serum of patients suffering of different kind of hepatitis : for instance, anti-LKM_1 are associated with cryptogenic hepatitis and cirrhosis and with halothane induced hepatitis; anti LKM_2 were only associated with tienilic acid-induced hepatitis. These autoantibodies were used to study the nature of the macromolecule that they recognized. By using immunoblot and immunoinhibition techniques we have shown that these auto antibodies recognized specifically human cytochrome P-450-8 (=P-450 MP or P-450 II C_9); this cytochrome P-450 is also responsible of the oxidation of tienilic acid and mephenytoin and produced a reactive metabolite covalently bound to proteins. So we can propose a simple scheme describing some of the steps leading to the disease. Finally the study of other auto antibodies seems to show that the scheme we proposed is rather general.

Key words : autoantibodies Cytochrome P-450. Tienilic acid.

Some drugs are able to induce immunoallergic hepatitis in humans. In some case circulating autoantibodies which have been found by immunofluorescence techniques recognized proteins in the endoplasmic reticulum of rat liver and kidney cells (Homberg et al 1984, 1985 Mc Kay 1985). These antibodies have been called anti-LKM (Liver Kidney microsomes) and have been used to study the detailed molecular mechanism of this kind of hepatitis. For instance it has been shown that anti LKM_1 found in halothane-induced hepatitis recognized hepatocytes from halothane-treated rabbits (Neuberger et al 1981).
We used anti-LKM_2 autoantibodies found in tienilic acid induced hepatitis (Homberg et al 1984) in order to identify the protein which is recognized by these autoantibodies and to study their effect on the metabolism of tienilic acid. We have shown here and in a precedent paper (Beaune et al, 1987) that this recognized protein is cytochrome P-450-8 which metabolizes tienilic acid and which is responsible for the production of a reactive metabolite covalently bound to microsomes.

MATERIAL AND METHODS

Chemicals : All chemical reagents were of the highest quality available. Electrophoresis reagents were from Serva (Heidelberg), nitrocellulose was from Biorad and immunochemical reagents from Dako (Copenhagen). ^{14}C tienilic acid (label in the keto group 925 GBQ / mol) was synthetized by CEA Saclay (Herbert and Pichat 1976) and 5-hydroxy-tienilic acid was prepared as described (Mansuy et al 1984).

Human liver : microsomes were prepared from a liver obtain from a renal transplant donor, a woman dead of accidental death : no clinical information was available. The liver was removed as usual and stored at -80°C. Microsomes were prepared as described (Kremers et al 1981).

Animals : rat Sprague-Dawley (180-200g) were used. Phenobarbital (80 mg/kg) was injected intra peritoneally daily for three days. Liver were removed and microsomes prepared as previously described. (Kremers et al 1981)

Human Sera: 19 serum samples containing anti-LKM_2 antibodies (Beaune et al 1987, Homberg et al 1984)) were obtained from patients suffering of hepatitis after tienilic acid treatment. Twenty serum control were from patients that did not contain anti-LKM_2 antibodies. 15 were from individuals who had never taken tienilic acid. Two of them had high serum bilirubin level and one suffered of viral B hepatitis. 5 sera were from patients without hepatitis but taking 250mg of tienilic acid per day for more than one year.

Purified enzymes : cytochromes P-450-5 (= P-450NF or P-450 III A3), 8 (= P-450 MP or II C9) and 9, epoxide hydrolase and the corresponding antibodies were obtained as previously described (Beaune et al 1985, Guengerich et al 1985, Shimada et al 1985, Wang et al 1981)). There was no cross reaction between the cytochromes.

Immunologic analysis : Immunoblot were performed as previously described (Guengerich et al 1985, Towbin et al 1984). For immunoihibitions, microsomes were preincubated with serum 20 min at +4° and then used as described under enzymatic assay section. Preimmune serum was used as control.

Enzymatic assays : tienilic acid hydroxylation was performed as described (Beaune et al 1987). Ethoxycoumarin-O-deethylase was measured as described by Aitio (1978). Inhibition of covalent binding of tienilic acid by various sera : human liver microsomes (0,2 nmol P-450) in 50ul sodium phosphate 0.1 M pH 7.4 were incubated with 50 ul of various dilution of serum in the same buffer for 20 min at 0°C. Then a NADPH generating system (0.15 umol NADP, 1.5 umole glucose-6-phosphate, 0,75 umole $MgCl_2$, 0.2 U glucose-6-phosphate deshydrogenase) and 15 nmol of tienilic acid (^{14}C in keto group, 5 mCi/mmol) in 50 ul total volume was added to start the reaction. After 30min incubation at 37°C a 50ul aliquot was spotted on a whatman GFB glass fiber disc (22 mm) and the disc dipped in 10% trichloroacetic acid. Covalent binding was monitored by a modification of the method of Fenselau (1970) and of Wallin (1981) by successive washes of the glass fiber disc in methanol, then in ethyl acetate and drying. The disc was counted in 2ml of toluene scintillation fluid. Covalent binding was about 1,5 nmol bound in 30 min.

General assays : cytochrome P-450 was spectrally determined as discribed by Omura and Sato (1964). Protein were determined according to Lowry et al (1951).

RESULTS AND DISCUSSION

Immunoblots

Fig 1 shows that sera from patients suffering of tienilic acid induced hepatitis and containing anti-LKM_2 autoantibodies recognized in human liver microsomes a single band by immunoblotting and that this band is very likely cytochrome P-450-8 (Wang et al 1981)) because this purified cytochrome P-450 isozyme is also recognized and because anti cytochrome P-450-8 shows the same pattern of recognition. On the contrary control serum from patients which did not contain anti LKM_2 did not recognize any band in human liver microsomes (Fig.1) and anti cytochrome P-450-5 exibited a different pattern of recognition (Beaune et al 1987). Finally human fetal microsomes which did not contain cytochrome P-450-8 are not recognized by sera of patients containing anti-LKM_2 autoantibodies (Fig 1). It is interesting to note that these sera recognized in liver microsomes from untreated rats only a single band and from phenobarbital-treated rat 2 bands; this is confirmed by results obtained with pure cytochromes P-450 (Fig.2). Cytochrome P-450 UT-A and cytochrome P-450 PB-B are recognized while cytochrome P-450 BNF-B is not. Indeed, UT-A is present in microsomes from both untreated and phenobarbital-treated rats and PB-B is only present in microsomes from phenobarbital-treated rats. These results indicate that sera of these patients contain autoantibodies against human cytochrome P-450-8 which shares epitopes with rat liver cytochrome P-450 UT-A, PB-B but not with cytochrome P-450 BNF-B. Out of 20 sera from patients having anti LKM_2 and suffering from tienilic acid induced hepatitis 12 were able to recognize cytochrome P-450-8 (Beaune et al. 1987). During the electrophoresis preceding immunoblot, proteins are denatured and this could explain why 8 patients sera containing anti-LKM_2 were unable to recognize cytochrome P-450-8. Among all the control sera tested (with hepatitis and no tienilic acid, with tienilic acid but no hepatitis or without both of them) none was able to recognized a band in human liver microsomes.

Covalent binding : Tienilic acid is able to covalently bind to microsomal proteins and this is associated with its metabolisation by cytochrome P-450-8 (Fig 3): this covalent binding is inhibited by anti cytochrome P-450-8, and anti LKM_2. It is not inhibited by control serum a by anti cytochrome P-450-5. (Fig.3). All the anti LKM_2 containing serum were inhibitors (11/11) while control sera were not (the dose inhibiting 50% of the covalent binding was at least one order of magnitude greater for control than for patient sera).

CONCLUSIONS

All together these results with those previously published (Beaune et al. 1987) confirm our hypothesis. Tienilic acid is mostly metabolized by cytochrome P-450-8 in human microsomes to 5-hydroxy tienilic acid but is also covalently bound to microsomal proteins, which could become antigenic proteins. The anti-LKM_2 antibodies recognize not only the native cytochrome P-450-8, but also the covalently modified and the denaturated protein. However the mechanism of formation of these antoantibodies is not known. It is also not clear if they are the cause or the result of the disease. Thus here we have clarified two steps of this mechanism : a) the formation of a neoantigen and b) the specificity of the antibody.
Finally we have found that this mechanism is not unique but might be rather general : Kiffel et al (1986) have recently shown that anti-LKM_1 autoantibodies found in children chronic active hepatitis are directed against P-450 db. Although no drug is known to be implicated in this disease the mechanism of production of anti LKM_1 and anti LKM_2 looks quite similar. Moreover, other anti LM autoantibodies different from anti LKM_1 and anti LKM_2 have recently been found in sera from patients suffering of hepatitis after dihydralazine treatment (Nataf et al 1986). These sera recognize in human liver microsomes only

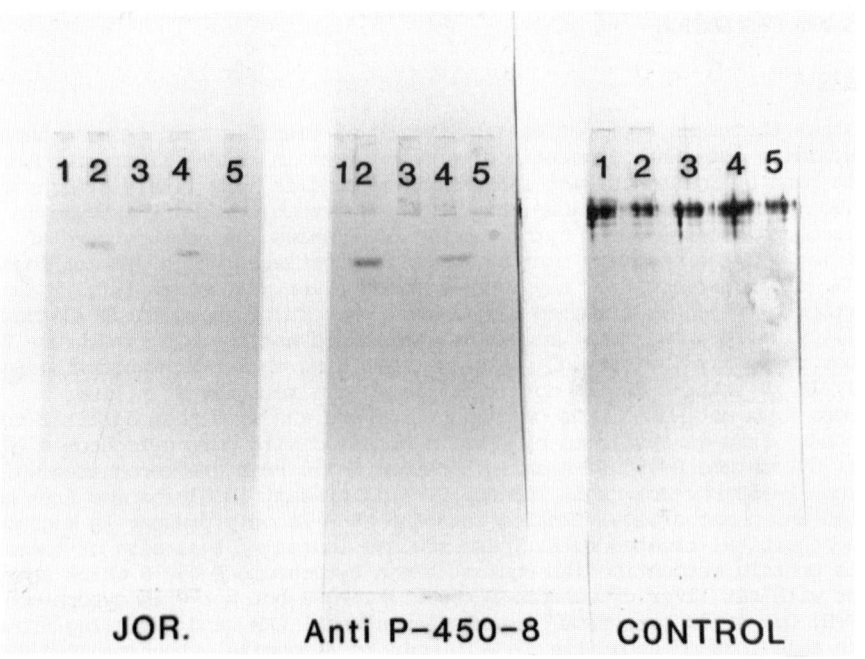

Fig. 1 Immunoblot of human liver microsomes and pure cytochrome P-450
1: cytochrome P-450-5, 2: cytochrome P-450-8, 3: cytochrome P-450-9 (about 1 pmol)
4: adult human liver microsomes, 5: fetal human microsomes (about 2 ug)
JOR, Control, anti-P-450-8 : 1/100 dilution of sera from control, patient JOR
and rabbit immunized with P-450-8 respectively.

Fig. 2 Immunoblot of rat liver microsomes and
pure cytochromes P-450.
1: P-450 UT-A, 2: P-450 PB-B, 3: P-450 BNF-B
(about 1 pmol) 5 and 6 liver microsomes from
untreated (5) and phenobarbital-treated (6)
rats (about 2 ug).

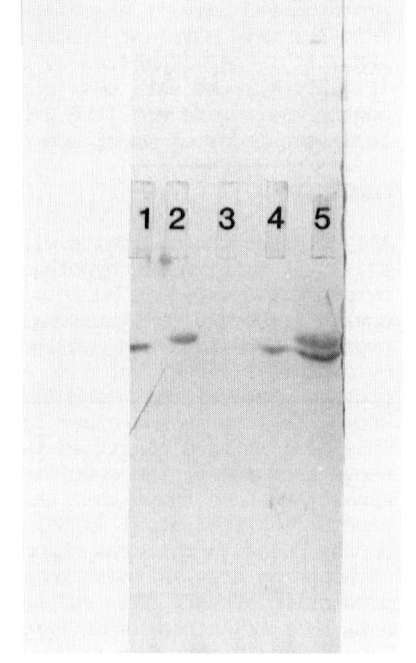

one single band in the 50Kd region, different from P-450-5, P-450-8, P-450-9, P-450 db and P-450 alc. If what is found for tienilic acid holds true, it could be that these antibodies recognize a cytochrome P-450 implicated in the metabolism of the causative drug.

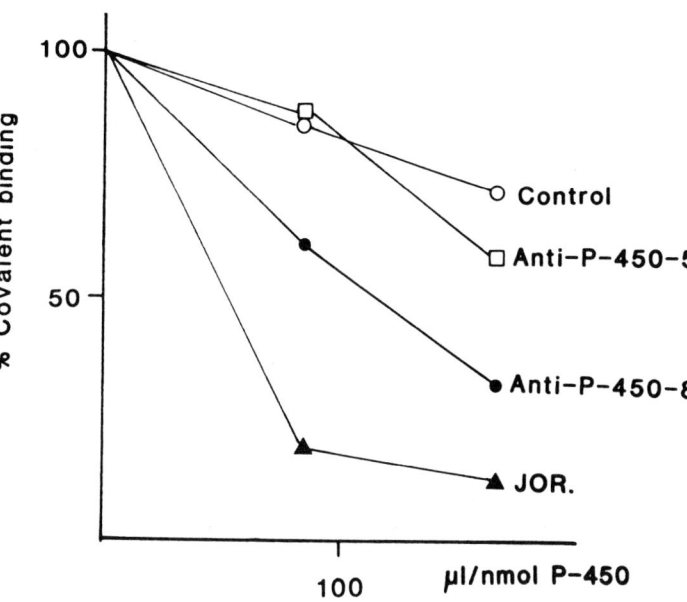

Fig. 3 Immunoinhibition of covalent binding of tienilic acid.
control : control serum
JOR:serum from patient JOR.
anti P-450-5 and 8 : serum from rabbit immunized with P-450-5 and P-450 -8 respectively.
100 percent correspond to no serum added.

AKNOWLEDGEMENTS

The authors thank laboratory ANPHAR-ROLLAND for product supply and Minister for Research and Technology for financial support.

REFERENCES

Aitio, A., (1978):A simple and sensitive assay of 7 ethoxycoumarin-O-deethylation. Anal.Biochem, 85, 488-491.
Beaune, P, Flinois, J.P., Kiffel, L., Kremers, P., and Leroux, J.P.(1985): Purification of a new cytochrome P-450 from human liver microsomes. Biochem. Biophys. Acta, 840, 364-370.
Beaune, Ph., Dansette, P.M., Mansuy, D., Kiffel, L., Finck, M., Amar, C., Leroux, J.P. and Homberg, J.C.(1987): Human anti endoplasmic reticulum autoantobodies appearing in a drug induced hepatitis are directed against a human liver cytochrome P-450 that hyydroxylates the drug. Proc. Natl. Acad. Sci.(U.S.A.) 84, 551-555.
Fenselau, A. (1970): Nicotinamide dinucleotide as an active site director in glyceraldehyde 3-phosphate hydrogenase modification. J. Biol. chem, 245, 1239 1246.
Guengerich, F.P., Wang, P.P., and Davidson, N.K., (1982): Estimation of isozymes of microsomal cytochrome P-450 in rats, rabbits and humans using immunochemical staining coupled with SDS-PAGE. Biochemistry (U.S.A.) 21, 1698-1706.
Guengerich, F.P., Martin, M.W., Beaune, P.H., Kremers, P., Wolf, T., and Waxman D.J. (1985): Characterization of a rat and human liver microsomal cytochrome P 450 forms involved in nifedipin oxidation : a prototype for genetic polymorphism in oxidative drug metabolism. J. Biol. Chem, 261, 5051 -5060.
Herbert, M., and Pichat, L. (1976):.Synthese diocetique marqué au ^{14}C acide dichloro, 2,3 (thenoyl-2 $^{14}C=O$)-4 phenoxy acetique. J. Labelled Compound Radiopharm, 12, 437-453.

Homberg, J.C., Andre, C., and Abuaf, N. (1984): A new anti liver kidney microsome antibody (anti LKM2) in tienilic acid induced hepatitis. Clin. Exp. Immunol, 55, 561-570.

Homberg, J.C., Abuaf, N., Helmy-Khalil, S., Biour, M., Poupon, R., Islam, S., Darnis, F., Levy, V.G., Opolon, P., Beaugrand, M., Toulet, J., Danan, G. and Benhamou, J.P. (1985): Drug induced hepatitis associated with anticytoplasmic organelle autoantibodies Hepatology, NY, 5, 722-727.

Kiffel, L., Loeper, J., Flinois, J.P., Celier, C., Homberg, J.C. and Leroux, J.P. (1986): Does anti liver kidney microsome antibody (anti-LKM$_1$) recognize an isozyme of hepatic cytochrome P-450. 10th European drug metabolism workshop, poster P1/17.

Kremers, P., Beaune, P., Cresteil, T., Degraeve, J., Columelli, S., Leroux, J.P. and Gielen, J.E. (1981): Cytochrome P-450 and monooxygenase activities in human and rat liver microsomes. Eur. J. Biochem, 118, 599-606.

Laemmli, U.K. (1970): Cleavage of structural proteins during to assembly of the head of bacteriophage T4. Nature (London) 227, 580-685.

Lowry, O.H., Rosebrouch, N.J., Farr, A.L. and Randall, R.J. (1951): Protein measurement with the folin phenol reagent. J. Biol. Chem, 193, 265-275.

Mackay, I.R. (1985): Induction of drugs hepatitis and autoantibodies to cell organelles : significance and interpretation. Hepatology (N.Y.), 5, 904-906

Mansuy, D., Dansette, P.M., Foures, C., Jaouen, M., Moinet, C., and Baler, N. (1984): Metabolic hydroxylation of the thiophene ring: isolation of 5 hydroxy tienilic acid as the major urinary metabolite of tienilic acid in man and rat. Biochem. Pharmacol, 33, 1429-1439.

Neuberger, J., Mieli-Vergani, G., Tredge, J.M., Davis, M., and Wiiliams, R. (1981): Oxidative metabolim of halothane in the production of altered hepatocyte membrane antigenes in acute halothane-induced hepatitis. GUT, 22, 669-672.

Omura, T., and Sato, R. (1964): The carbon monoxide binding pigment of liver microsomes. J. Biol. Chem, 237, 1375-1376.

Shimada, T., Misono, K.S. and Guengerich, F.P. (1986): Human liver microsomal cytochrome P-450 mephenytoin 4-hydroxylase, a prototype of genetic polymorphism in oxidative drug metabolism : purification and characterization o two similar forms involved in the reacttion. J. Biol. Chem, 261, 909-921.

Towbin, H.T., Staehlin, T., and Gordon, J., (1979): Electrophoretic transfer of proteins from polyacrylamide gelonto nitrocellulose sheets : procedure and some applications. Proc. Natl. Acad. Sci. USA, 76, 4350-4354.

Wallin, H., Shelin, C., Tunek, A. and Jergil, B. (1981): A rapid and sensitive methode for determination of covalent binding of benzo (a) pyrene to proteins. Chem. Biol. Interaction, 38, 109-118.

Résumé

Le serum de patients atteints de différents types d'hépatites contient dans certains cas des autoanticorps dirigés contre les microsomes de foie et de rein (anti LKM) : par exemple les anti LKM1 sont associés avec une hépatite cryptogénique et avec l'hépatite induite à l'halothane. Les anti LKM2 sont associés uniquement avec l'hépatite induite par l'acide tiénilique. Ces autoanticorps ont été utilisés pour étudier la nature de la macromolécule qu'ils reconnaissent. Grâce à des techniques immunologiques comme l'immunoinhibition et les "Western blots" nous avons montré que ces autoanticorps reconnaissaient spécifiquement les cytochromes P-450 8 humains (=P-450MP ou P-450IIc9); ce cytochrome P-450 est également responsable de l'oxydation de l'acide tiénilique et produit un métabolite réactif lié de façon covalente aux protéines. Ainsi nous avons pu proposer un schéma simple décrivant certaines étapes pouvant conduire à la maladie. Enfin l'étude d'autres autoanticorps semble montrer que le schéma que nous proposons est général.

Phospholipid fatty acids in the liver phospholipidosis induced by amiodarone in the rat

J.-M. Warnet*, D. Gouy**, N. Agheli***, P. Vic**, R. Aubert***, J.R. Claude*

*Laboratoire de Toxicologie, Faculté de Pharmacie, 75270 Paris Cedex 06, France. ** Centre de Recherches Clin-Midy Sanofi, 34082 Montpellier Cedex, France. *** INSERM U.1 (D. Lemonnier), Hôpital Bichat, 75877 Paris Cedex 18, France

KEY WORDS

AMIODARONE - FATTY ACID ANALYSIS - GAS-LIQUID CHROMATOGRAPHY - LIVER - PHOSPHOLIPIDOSIS.

INTRODUCTION

AMIODARONE, an iodine containing benzofuran derivative, was introduced in Europe in 1961 as an antianginal agent ; subsequently it was found to have potent antiarrhythmic properties. However, its chronic use in man is complicated by a wide variety of side effects involving cornea, skin, thyroid, lung, liver, and other tissues. Recently, multilamellar membranous bodies have been demonstrated in the cytoplasm of liver in patients treated with AMIODARONE (POUCELL et al., 1984). Our purpose was to provide an experimental basis of AMIODARONE - Induced lipid disorders since previous data are scanty.

MATERIALS AND METHODS

Groups of 10 male and 10 female 344 Fischer rats weighing about 150 g were used. AMIODARONE was suspended in 10 % aqueous gum-arabic solution and was administered by gastric intubation at doses of 150 mg/kg/ day for 10 days. Controls received gumsolution. Control and dosed rats were killed by exsanguination from the abdominal aorta under pento-barbital sodium anesthesia ; blood was collected and the liver was removed. The total phospholipid (PL), cholesterol (T.C.) and triglyceride (TG) content was determined directly in the serum, and after lipid extraction in the liver (see PIRIOU et al., 1979). Liver lipids were fractionated by thin layer chromatography on 0.2 mm silica gel plates (E MERCK, Darmstadt, Germany) in n-hexane, ethyl ether, and acetic acid (80:20:1.5, vol/

vol). Bands were made visible by spraying the plate with 4'-5'-dibromofluorescein in alcohol (0.10 g/l) and examined under ultraviolet light. The PL fraction was scraped off and treated according to the procedure of TUCKEY and STEVENSON (1979), slightly modified for saponification (20 min at 60° C) and methylation (60 min at 45° C). Methyl esters were extracted by n-hexane and separated with a glass capillary column (52 m x 0.28 mm inside diameter) coated with 20 M Carbowax in a gas chromatograph (GIRDEL model 30) fitted with a hydrogen flame ionosation detector. The temperature was 220° C, and all peaks corresponding to fatty acids from C 12:0 to C 22:6 were measured with a model Icat 50 Delsi integrator. All results are expressed as mean $\pm$ S.D. Statistical differences between control and treated rats were assessed by Student's t test.

RESULTS

Serum lipids (Table I) - In males : AMIODARONE caused an increase in PL and T.C. , and a decrease in TG.
- In females : T.C. is increased, but PL are slightly decreased ; TG are decreased.

Effect of AMIODARONE (150 mg/kg/day for 10 days on serum lipids (g/l) in F 344 rats (+ $p < 0.05$, ++ $p < 0.01$, +++ $p < 0.001$)

Males	PL	T.C.	TG
Controls	0.95 $\pm$ 0.09	0.51 $\pm$ 0.10	0.58 $\pm$ 0.09
Treated	1.37 $\pm$ 0.22	1.18 $\pm$ 0.13	0.42 $\pm$ 0.11
	+++	+++	++
Females			
Controls	1.35 $\pm$ 0.11	0.71 $\pm$ 0.09	0.61 $\pm$ 0.07
Treated	1.21 $\pm$ 0.15	0.99 $\pm$ 0.10	0.45 $\pm$ 0.11
	+	+++	++

Liver Lipids (Table II) - AMIODARONE caused an increase in liver lipid content which was due to an accumulation of PL ; T.C. was increased only in males whereas TG were decreased in both sexes.

Effect of AMIODARONE (150 mg/kg/day for 10 days on liver lipids (mg/g) in F 344 rats. C = Controls T = Treated   T.L. = Total lipids
(+ $p < 0.05$, ++ $p < 0.01$, +++ $p < 0.001$)

Males	T.L.	PL	T.C.	TG
C	44.5 $\pm$ 1.8	34.4 $\pm$ 1.3	1.9 $\pm$ 0.2	6.0 $\pm$ 1.5
T	56.5 $\pm$ 3.2	45.3 $\pm$ 2.2	3.3 $\pm$ 0.6	4.1 $\pm$ 2.0
	+++	+++	+++	+
Females				
C	47.4 $\pm$ 3.1	33.4 $\pm$ 1.4	2.4 $\pm$ 0.3	8.6 $\pm$ 2.4
T	50.5 $\pm$ 1.1	40.2 $\pm$ 1.9	2.6 $\pm$ 0.2	3.7 $\pm$ 1.0
	+	+++		+++

Fatty acid pattern of liver PL (Table III) -

- In males : polyunsaturated fatty acid content (18:2, 20:3, 20:5, and 22:5) markedly decreased and palmitic acid (16:0) slightly decreased, that was balanced by an increase in stearic (18:0) and oleic (18:1) acids.
- In females : 18:0 and polyunsaturated fatty acids decreased (except 22:6), 16:0 and 18:1 increased.

Mean values of relevant fatty acids of liver PL in F 344 rats treated by 150 mg AMIODARONE/kg/day for 10 days. C = Controls   T = Treated
(+ $p < 0.05$, ++ $p < 0.01$, +++ $p < 0.001$)

Males	16:0	18:0	18:1	18:2	20:3	20:5	22:5	22:6
C	21.6	21.8	7.8	16.4	1.2	0.8	1.5	6.0
T	20.1	24.6	11.7	13.2	0.9	0.4	0.7	5.7
	+			+	++	++	++	
Females								
C	15.7	32.1	6.4	12.8	1.5	0.9	1.0	6.2
T	19.2	26.8	8.9	11.4	0.8	0.3	0.7	7.7
	++	++	+++		+++	+++	+	+

DISCUSSION

AMIODARONE-induced liver phospholipidosis may be due to the inhibition of lysosomal PL catabolism since it was shown that AMIODARONE is a potent inhibitor of lysosomal phospholipase A prepared from rat liver (HOSTETLER et al., 1984). Moreover, the changes in fatty acid pattern of liver PL might account for an alteration of hepatocyte PL metabolism that superposes its effect to the inhibition of PL breakdown induced by AMIODARONE.

REFERENCES

HOSTETLER, K.Y., REASOR, M.J., WALKER, E.R., YAZAKI, P.J. and FRAZEE, B.W. (1986) : Role of phospholipase A inhibition in Amiodarone pulmonary toxicity in rats. Biochim. biophys. Acta (Amst.) 875, 400-405.

PIRIOU, A., WARNET J.-M., JACQUESON, A., CLAUDE, J.R., and TRUHAUT, R. (1979): Fatty liver induced by high doses of Rifampicin in the rat : possible relation with an inhibition of RNA polymerases in eukariotic cells. Arch. Toxicol. Suppl. 2, 333-337.

POUCELL, S., IRETON, J., VALENCIA-MAYORAL, P. et al. (1984) : Amiodarone-associated phospholipidosis and fibrosis of the liver : light, immunohisto-chemical, and electron microscopic studies. Gastroenterology 86, 926-936.

TUCKEY, R.C., and STEVENSON, P.M. (1979) : Methanolysis of cholesteryl esters: conditions for quantitative preparation of methyl esters. Anal. Biochem. 94, 402-408.

Influence of dietary vitamin E on liver microsomal lipid peroxidation in rats fed vitamin A and/or ascorbate-free diets

Marie-Agnès Pellissier, Michel Boisset, Sébastien Atteba, Robert Albrecht

Laboratoire de Biologie du CNAM, 292 rue Saint Martin, 75141 Paris Cedex 03, France. Réseau National de Toxicologie Nutritionnelle, France

Key words : Liver microsomes, lipid peroxidation, dietary vitamin E, vitamin A, ascorbate

INTRODUCTION

Oxidative stress in biological cells will depend on many dietary factors (Wills, 1985). The fundamental role of vitamin E is to maintain normal vascular, nervous, muscular and reproductive functions. However, one can also ask about its effect as a lipid-soluble antioxidant such as protecting membrane lipids (Tappel, 1962). Some experimental data suggest that ascorbate acts as an antioxidant in vivo by restoring the propreties of vitamin E (Leung et al., 1981 ; Bendich et al., 1986). On the other hand, Tom et al (1984) found that lipid peroxidation in rat liver microsomes was inversely related to dietary intake of vitamin A.

The present experiment was undertaken to examine the influence of dietary vitamin E on lipid peroxidation and cellular defence systems against oxidative damage in rats fed vitamin A and/or ascorbate-free diets.

MATERIAL AND METHODS

Weanling male Sprague-Dawley rats were maintained on a vitamin E (E)-, vit A (A)-, ascorbate (C)-free semi-synthetic diet (Eo, Ao, Co) for one week and subsequently divided into eight groups fed different diets for 8 weeks ; four groups with normal vit E content   control E+A+C+,   E = 0.17 mg/g, A = 6.0 ug/g, C = 0.80 mg/g ; E+AoC+ ; E+A+Co ; E+ Ao Co ; and four vit E-free groups   EoA+C+ ; EoAoC+ ; EoA+Co ; EoAoCo .

Rats were killed by decapitation. The livers were perfused with ice-cold physiologic saline, rapidly excised, weighed and homogenized in 3 volumes of 10 mM Tris-HCl buffer containing 150 mM KCl and 0.1 mM EDTA (pH = 7.4 at 20°C) and 100,000 xg microsomal and cytosolic fractions were obtained. Microsomes were washed and resuspended with the same buffer without EDTA. Protein (Lowry et al., 1951) and non-protein sulfhydryl groups, mostly reduced glutathione (Sedlak and Lindsay, 1968), were estimated. Total and seleno-dependent glutathione peroxidase activities were assayed spectrophotometrically, using respectively t-butyl-hydroperoxide and hydrogen peroxide as substrates (Burk et al, 1980 ; Günzler et al, 1974). Glutathione reductase was determined according to Calberg and Mannervick (1975). Spontaneous lipid peroxidation (LP) in vitro was assessed by the production of malonic dialdehyde (MDA) (Recknagel et al., 1982). Enzymatic LP was measured in the presence of NADPH and non-enzymatic LP in the presence of L-ascorbic acid ; tetraethoxypropane was used as an external standard.

Statistical evaluation was carried out by the analysis of variance (Lellouch and Lazar, 1974).

RESULTS

Vitamin E deficiency had no effect body weight and relative liver weight at the end of the experiment (see table 1). Daily food intake was not altered by vitamine E deprivation (data not shown).

Table 1
Body and liver weights

Diets* Parameters	Body weight (g)	Liver weight (g/100 g rat)
E+ A+ C+	365 ± 7	3.03 ± 0.09
E+ Ao C+	342 ± 6	2.80 ± 0.07
E+ A+ Co	347 ± 16	2.93 ± 0.08
E+ Ao Co	332 ± 7	2.44 ± 0.06
Eo A+ C+	361 ± 4	3.35 ± 0.10
Eo Ao C+	331 ± 10	2.73 ± 0.12
Eo A+ Co	369 ± 10	3.00 ± 0.06
Eo Ao Co	344 ± 12	2.66 ± 0.06

Results are mean ± S.E.M. of 8 animals

E+ = 0.17 mg vitamin E/g of food   Eo = 0 mg vitamin E/g of food
A+ = 6.0 ug vitamin A/g of food   Ao = 0 ug vitamin A/g of food
C+ = 0.8 mg ascorbate/g of food   Co = 0 mg ascorbate/g of food

No changes in cytosolic reduced glutathione content and glutathione reductase activity were noted (see Table 2).

Table 2
Reduced glutathione content and glutathione-reductase activity

Diets* Parameters	Reduced glutathione (nmoles/mg cyt. prot.)	Glutathione-reductase (nmoles/min/mg cyt.prot.)
E+ A+ C+	37.0 ± 6.4	25.9 ± 2.6
E+ Ao C+	34.1 ± 4.4	24.1 ± 1.6
E+ A+ Co	42.3 ± 4.5	27.1 ± 2.3
E+ Ao Co	25.1 ± 4.6	24.5 ± 2.2
Eo A+ C+	43.4 ± 4.8	25.6 ± 1.7
Eo Ao C+	29.7 ± 4.3	22.8 ± 2.7
Eo A+ Co	32.4 ± 3.9	23.8 ± 1.3
Eo Ao Co	31.4 ± 3.9	24.5 ± 2.2

Results are Mean ± S.E.M. of 8 animals
* See Table 1 for legends

In the case of glutathione-peroxidases, no statistically significant differences were found between the adequate and deficient vitamin E groups (see Table 3).

Table 3
Glutathione-peroxidases activities

Diets* \ Parameters	Total glutathione-peroxidase (nmoles/min/mg cyt. prot.)	Se glutathione-peroxydase (nmoles/min/mg prot.cyt.)
E+ A+ C+	63.4 ± 4.8	45.3 ± 5.8
E+ Ao C+	53.1 ± 8.0	32.4 ± 5.8
E+ A+ Co	64.5 ± 6.6	44.9 ± 5.4
E+ Ao Co	47.4 ± 3.3	32.9 ± 5.2
Eo A+ C+	58.5 ± 6.6	36.2 ± 4.6
Eo Ao C+	53.1 ± 6.0	33.1 ± 5.0
Eo A+ Co	62.0 ± 7.1	34.8 ± 6.0
Eo Ao Co	56.1 ± 7.7	38.2 ± 3.2

Results are Mean ± S.E.M. of 8 animals
* See Table 1 for legends

Vitamin E deprivation increased enzymatic lipid peroxidation in vitamin A-, ascorbate-, and vitamin A plus ascorbate-, deficient rats (x 5.5, x 7.5, x 7.7, respectively). The same effect was observed, although at a lasser extent, in the case of non-enzymatic lipid peroxidation (x 2.6, x 3.3, x 3.8) (see Table 4).

Table 4
Microsomal enzymatic and non-enzymatic lipid peroxidation

Diets* \ Parameters	Enzymatic lipid peroxidation (pmoles MDA/min/mg micr.prot.)	Non-enzymatic lipid peroxidation (pmoles/MDA/min/mg micr.prot.)
E+ A+ C+	21.1 ± 6.1	120 ± 42
E+ Ao C+	19.5 ± 3.7	95 ± 32
E+ A+ Co	15.6 ± 5.8	95 ± 32
E+ Ao Co	14.1 ± 2.1	83 ± 30
Eo A+ C+	9.8 ± 2.9	23 ± 10
Eo Ao C+	108 ± 13	244 ± 29
Eo A+ Co	117 ± 3	309 ± 21
Eo Ao Co	109 ± 17	319 ± 38

Results are Mean ± S.E.M. of 8 animals
* See Table 1 for legends

DISCUSSION

It is generally accepted that peroxidation of polyunsaturated fatty acid is decreased by dietary vitamin E (Wills, 1985). This finding has been overlooked by several investigators who studied lipid peroxidation <u>in vitro</u> by measurement of thiobarbituric acid-reactive substances in liver whole homogenates (Krishnamurthy et al., 1983), microsomes (Rowe et al. 1976 ; Iritami et.al., 1980 ; Hassan et al., 1985) and liposomes (Leung et al., 1981). This phenomenon has been observed in untreated animals or in animals treated with large doses of a pro-oxidant compound such as carbon tetrachloride (Kunert and Tappel, 1983) or a potent inducer of monooxygenases such as 2,3,7,8-tetrachlorodibenzo-p-dioxin (Hassan et al., 1985).

Our data are in accordance with those of other authors only in the case of animals fed either a vitamin A and/or ascorbate-deficient rat. This apparent discrepancy could originate from differences in the experimental procedures : the mode of administration of the vitamin, the duration of the deprivation, the extent of contamination of cell fractions by free iron, the presence of activator (s) during the incubation step of lipid peroxidation study. In our conditions, the level of production of malonic dialdehyde by microsomes is remarkably low because : i) the diet contains 1% (w/w) linoleic acid as the sole source of lipid, ii) the method used to prepare microsomal fraction minimizes contamination by free iron, iii) the measurement of peroxidation is performed without addition of exogenous activator ("spontaneous" lipoperoxidation). Thus it is conceivable that the protection effect of α-tocopherol can only be observed in vitro in systems in which the lipid peroxidation proceeds more actively.

Obviously, peroxidative degradation of fatty acids is a highly deleterious process which can alter the function of cell membranes, disturb intracellular homeostasis and ultimately result in cell death. Under certain condition, protective mechanisms, partly dependent on the balance of dietary components such as vitamin E, can be overwhelmed. Our results suggest that an adequate dietary intake of vitamin E and also vitamin A and ascorbate is required to maintain efficient protection against oxidative damage.

REFERENCES

Bendich, A., Machlin, L.J., Scandurra, O., Burton, G.W. and Wayner, D.D.M. (1986): The antioxidant role of vitamin C. Adv. in Free Radical Biol. Med. 2, 419-444.

Burk, R.F., Lawrence, R.A. and Lane, J.M. (1980): Liver necrosis and lipid peroxidation in the rat as the result of paraquat and diquat administration. Effect of selenium deficiency. J. Clin. Invest. 65, 1024-1031.

Carlberg, I. and Mannervik, B. (1975): Purification and characterization of the flavoenzyme glutathione reductase from rat liver. J. Biol. Chem. 250, 5475-5480.

Günzler, W.A., Kremers, H. and Flohé, L. (1974): An improved, coupled test procedure for glutathione peroxidase in blood. Z. Klin. Chem. Klin. Biochem. 12, 444-448.

Hassan, M.Q., Stohs, S.J. and Murray, W.J. (1985): Effects of vitamin E and A on 2,3,7,8-tetrachlorodibenzo-p-dioxin (TCDD)-induced lipid peroxidation and other biochemical changes in the rat. Arch. Environm Contam. Toxicol. 14, 437-442.

Iritani, N., Fukuda, E. and Kitamura, Y. (1980): Effect of corn oil feeding on lipid peroxidation in rats. J. Nutr. 110, 924-930.

Krishnamurthy, S., George, T. and Jayanthi Bai, N. (1983): Effect of dietary coconut oil and casein and megadoses of vitamin A or C on tissue lipid peroxidation and hemolysis in vitamin E deficiency. Acta Vitaminol. Enzymol. 5, 165-170.

Kunert, K.J. and Tappel, A.L. (1983): The effect of vitamin C on in vivo lipid peroxidation in guinea pigs as measured by pentane and ethane production. Lipids 18, 271-274.

Lellouch, J. and Lazar, P. (1974): Analyse approfondie des expériences biologiques. In Méthodes statistiques en expérimentation biologique, ed. Flammarion, pp. 165-177, Paris.

Leung, H.W., Wang, M.J. and Mavis, R.D. (1981): The cooperative interaction between vitamin E and vitamin C in suppression of peroxidation of membrane phospholipids. Biochim. Biophys. Acta 644, 266-272.

Lowry, O.H., Rosenbrough, N.J., Farr, A.L. and Randall, R.J. (1951): Protein measurement with the folin phenol reagent. J. Biol. Chem. 193, 265-275.

Recknagel, R.O., Glende, E.A., Waller, R.L. and Lowry, K. (1982): Lipid peroxidation. Biochemistry, measurement and significance in liver cell injury. In Toxicology of the liver eds G.L. Plaa and W.R. Hewitt, pp. 213-241. New York : Raven Press.

Rowe, L. and Wills, E.D. (1976): The effect of dietary lipids and vitamin E on lipid peroxide formation, cytochrome P 450 and oxidative demethylation in the endoplasmic reticulum. Biochem. Pharmacol. 25, 175-179.

Sedlak, J. and Lindsay, R.H. (1968): Estimation of total, protein-bound and nonprotein sulfhydryl groups in tissue with Ellman's reagent. Anal. Biochem. 25, 192-201.

Tappel, A.L. (1962): Vitamin E as the biological lipid antioxidant. Vitam. Horm. 20, 493-509.

Tom, W.M., Fong, L.Y.Y., Woo, D.Y.H., Prasongwatana, V. and Boyde, T.R.C. (1984): Microsomal lipid peroxidation and oxidative metabolism in rat liver : influence of vitamin A intake. Chem. Biol. Interact. 50, 361-366.

Wills, E.D. (1985): The role of dietary components in oxidative stress in tissues. In Oxidative stress, ed. H. Sies, pp. 197-218. London : Acad. Press.

This work was supported by grants from PIREN-CNRS : ATP " Alimentation-Santé-Environnement" (n° 955495 et 508005).

Factors influencing the toxicity of alpha-naphthylisothiocyanate towards bile duct lining cells

Ann K. Connolly, Shirley C. Price, Derek Stevenson, John C. Connelly, Richard H. Hinton

Robens Institute of Industrial and Environmental Health and Safety. University of Surrey, Guildford, Surrey, GU2 5XH, UK

KEY WORDS.

ANIT, Cholestasis, bile duct lining cells, intrahepatic jaundice

INTRODUCTION.

Alpha-naphthyl isothiocyanate (ANIT) is a model compound for the induction of intrahepatic cholestasis in experimental animals. A single dose of this compound causes severe damage to the cells lining the intrahepatic bile ducts with little significant damage to the hepatocytes (Eliakim et al. 1959; Goldfarb et al. 1962). The onset of cholestasis occurs 15-20 hours after dosing; however the effects are totally reversible and the liver is completely normal within 4-5 days.

The hepatotoxic effects of ANIT are species specific, cholestasis being observed in rats, mice and guinea pigs but not in hamsters or rabbits (Capizzo and Roberts, 1971), and the role of metabolism in mediating the toxicity of ANIT has also been examined by a number of workers. It has been found that pretreatment of rats with phenobarbitone or chlorpromazine (Roberts and Plaa, 1965), with some steroids or acetohexamide, (Roberts and Plaa, 1966a) potentiates the onset of ANIT induced cholestasis. Conversely treatment with SKF 525A (Roberts and Plaa, 1965) or N-Decylimidazole (Traiger et al 1985) appears to inhibit the toxic effects of ANIT. Thus it is evident that metabolic activation of ANIT plays an important role in mediating its toxicity. This has been supported by the work of Horky, Grasso and Goldberg, (1971) who have demonstated that pretreatment with phenobarbital causes an increase in the toxic effects of ANIT on the intrahepatic biliary system with no apparent increase in parenchymal cell damage, and more recent metabolism studies by Traiger et al (1984; 1985) which indicated that S oxidation is an initial step in the metabolism of ANIT.

This evidence for the requirement of metabolic activation in the hepatotoxicity of ANIT has focussed research upon the role of the hepatocyte, even though pathological evidence has pinpointed the bile duct lining cell as a target for hepatocyte mediated ANIT toxicity.

However, examination of plasma components in ANIT treated rats has shown the presence of 4 major bile components, IgA, FSC, 5'Nucleotidase and conjugated bilirubin at increased concentrations equivalent to their concentrations in bile (Woolley et al. 1979). This suggests that the cholestasis induced by ANIT may be due to mechanical obstruction of the bile duct causing the reflux of biliary constituents into the liver and eventually into plasma, rather than ANIT having any direct toxic effect on bile formation. The mechanisms underlying the toxicity of ANIT have therefore been investigated using a combination of morphological, biochemical and analytical techniques.

MATERIALS AND METHODS.

Male wistar albino rats obtained from the University of Surrey or Charles River and University of Surrey Schneider mice were used in these experiments. ANIT (Sigma Chemical Co. Poole, Dorset) was dissolved in olive oil at a concentration of 60 mg/ml. and sufficient was administered by gavage to give a dose of 300 mg/kg. body weight. Control animals received an approprate dose of olive oil. Animals which were pretreated with phenobarbitone received 80 mg/kg/day by intraperitoneal injection 3 days prior to ANIT treatment.

Animals were killed by cervical dislocation. Tissues for histological examination at light and electron microscope level were prepared as detailed by Connolly et al. (1986).

Bile samples were analysed for the presence of metabolites after extraction with diethyl ether, drying with oxygen free nitrogen, and resuspending in the HPLC eluant: 70% acetonitrile, 30% 0.01M sodium phosphate buffer pH 5. The samples were injected onto a 10 cm. reverse phase HPLC column and metabolite concentrations were calculated by the preparation of standard curves.

RESULTS.

1. Progression of the pathological lesion.

Groups of 4 experimental and control animals were killed at 4, 6, 8, 24 and 48 hours after dosing. Examination of the Haemotoxylin and Eosin stained sections of the liver showed that the damage occured earlier and was more severe in the bile duct lining cells than that observed in the hepatocytes. Ultrastructural studies confirmed this and showed that ANIT induced hepatotoxicity involved a loss of integrity of the tight junction complexes between bile duct lining cells and also between some hepatocytes. (Table 1).

To examine whether ANIT toxicity was mediated via a bile borne toxin the compound was administered to groups of 4 experimental and control mice. The livers and gall bladders of these mice were taken 24 hours after a single dose of ANIT, processed as described earlier and stained with H and E prior to examination. The livers showed very similar damage to that seen in rat liver 24 hours after ANIT administration. The gall bladders were very severely damaged with the whole of the epithelial cell layer which lines the gall bladder being destroyed (Fig.1a), the gall bladders of animals treated only with the vehicle (olive oil) had a normal appearance (fig.1b).

Table 1. Progression of the pathological lesion induced by ANIT.

Time after dosing (Hrs).	Light Microscopy.	Electron Microscopy.
4	NAD*	Bile ducts show loss of microvilli and dilatation of the lumen.
6	Oedema and inflammation visible in some portal areas others show no changes. Loss γ GT activity from bile duct lining cells.	Loss of integrity of TJ complexes between bile duct lining cells and between some hepatocytes.
8	Some bile duct damage with cells exfoliating into duct. Other portal areas still appear normal. Increased loss γ GT from bile duct.	N A** N A
24	Destruction of majority of bile ducts. Focal necrosis in parenchyma. Loss of Alkaline phosphatase from biliary plexus.	N A

* no abnormality detected   ** not available

2. Metabolism investigations.

An attempt was made to extract and identify the components present in the bile of ANIT treated rats which may be responsible for the hepatotoxicity described. Since phenobarbitone pretreatment seemed to enhance the toxic response to ANIT, animals were pretreated with this prior to ANIT dosing in order to increase levels of potential metabolites and thus facilitate extraction and measurement. Animals were anaesthetised with Sagatal (May and Baker) immediately after dosing and bile was collected over 15 minute intervals for upto four hours after dosing.

The bile of the rats induced by treatment with phenobarbitone and then treated with ANIT had four major components which were not observed in control animals (Fig. 2a and b). The first component, ie the least well retained on the column, has been identified as alpha naphthylamine on the basis that the pure standard co-chromatographs with the unknown peak, in a similar way the last of the major components, ie the best retained on the column, co-chromatographs with the parent compound ANIT. The two other major components are as yet unidentified. However their retention time which is between that of alpha-naphthylamine and ANIT indicates that they are at least of intermediate polarity.

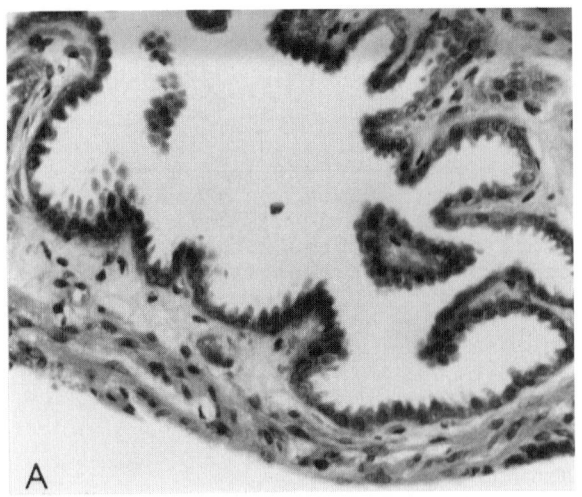
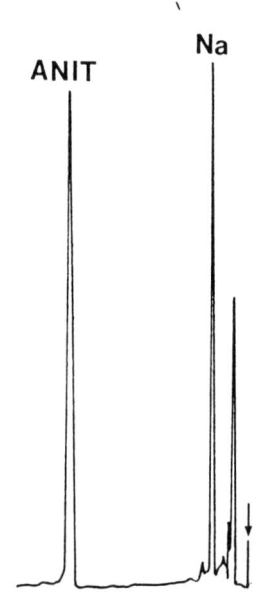

Fig.1a - Section through control gall bladder showing regular arrangement of epithelial layer.
b - Section through gall bladder after ANIT treatment showing total destruction of epithelial layer.

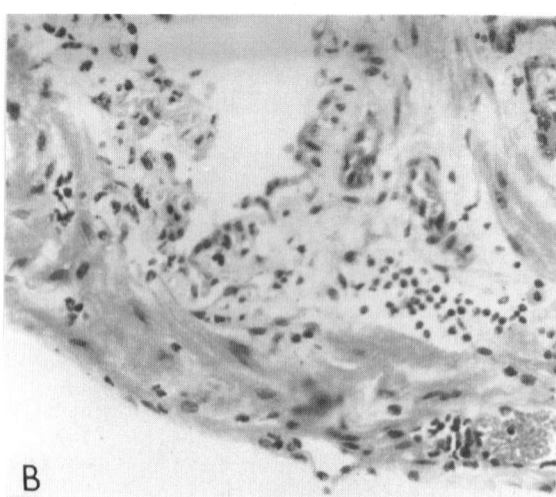
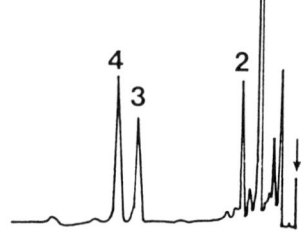

Fig 2. - HPLC trace showing a) retention times of pure standards, b) Retention times of biliary components from rats treated with ANIT.

DISCUSSION.

It is clear that both in control rats and rats pretreated with phenobarbitone the damage caused by ANIT occurs earlier and is more severe in the bile duct lining cells than in hepatocytes. In non-induced animals ultrastructural alterations can be seen within the bile duct at 4 hours after dosing, by 6 hours there is a loss of integrity of the tight junction complexes between bile duct lining cells at 8 hours damage is visible at the light microscope level, and by 24 hours there is almost total necrosis of bile ducts. Pretreatment of the rats with phenobarbitone accelerates these changes so that there is almost total necrosis of bile ducts by 6 hours after a single administration of ANIT. The hepatocytes in non-induced rats show no adverse effects until 8 hours after dosing when there appears to be a loss of integrity of tight junction complexes between some hepatocytes, shown both by electron microscopy and by an increase in biliary albumin. The only significant damage to hepatocytes is seen 24 hours after dosing when focal necrosis is evident in the parenchyma, although no such alteration is found in rats pre-induced with phenobarbitone and examined 6 hours after ANIT treatment. Focal necrosis is however also observed after bile duct ligation and the focal necrosis observed in non-induced rats 24 hours after treatment with ANIT may therefore be attributed to reflux of bile as a consequence of biliary obstruction rather than to any direct effect on hepatocytes.

This evidence indicates that the bile duct lining cell is the primary target for ANIT toxicity. This effect could in theory be attributed to the proximate toxin being carried in bile or to the influence of the periportal hepatocytes. The gall bladder is morphologically similar to the bile duct and is the next organ to receive bile once it has left the liver. Mice, like rats are susceptible to ANIT and both the intrahepatic ducts and the gall bladders of ANIT treated mice showed massive damage 24 hours after dosing. This indicates that ANIT mediated toxicity is effected via a bile borne intermediate which may be a metabolite or the parent compound. The latter is unlikely since it is now almost certain that ANIT toxicity requires metabolic activation and thus the active toxin may be a metabolite of the parent compound produced by the metabolic activity of hepatocytes.

The identity of the toxin was examined by HPLC and the bile of ANIT treated rats showed 4 major components not present in control animals. These have tentatively been identified as alpha naphthylamine, 2 intermediary compounds and ANIT. However it is as yet unknown whether any or all of these components are involved in the toxicity of ANIT towards bile duct lining cells. The mechanism of action of the active metabolite is also unclear, however, one possible mechanism would involve an effect on the integrity of the tight junctional complexes primarily between bile duct lining cells. This would allow the reflux of biliary components into the liver and plasma. It has been shown by Billington et al (1980) that bile is capable of lysing hepatocytes in vitro at bile salt concentrations much less than are present in bile in vivo and this would account for the areas of focal necrosis observed both in bile duct ligation and with ANIT treatment. Thus the mechanism of action of the ANIT metabolites may be the same for bile duct lining cells and hepatocytes, the variation in sensitivity to the toxic effects of ANIT either being due to intrinsic differences in the sensitivities between the cell types or possibly a concentration effect with the toxin being concentrated as it passes down the bile duct. This latter phenomenon has been observed with the chromone FPL52757 (Eason et al 1982). Experiments are currently in progress to identify the metabolites of ANIT and to determine their role in the toxicity of ANIT towards the bile duct lining cell.

REFERENCES.

Billington, D., Evans, C.E., Godfrey, P.P and Coleman, R.(1980): effects of bile salts on the plasma membranes of isolated rat hepatocytes. Biochem. J. 158, 321-327.

Capizzo, F. and Roberts, R.J. (1971). α-Naphthyl isothiocyanate (ANIT) induced hepatotoxicity and disposition in various species. Toxicol. Appl. Pharmacol. 19, 176-187.

Connolly, A.K., Connelly, J.C. and Hinton, R.H.(1986): Early changes in the bile duct lining cells of rats treated with alpha-naphthyl isothiocyanate. Biochem. Soc. Trans. 14, 873.

Eason, C.T., Parke, D.V., Clark, B. and Smith, D.A.(1982): The mechanism of hepatotoxicity of a chromone carboxylic acid FPL52757 in the rat. Xenobiotica, 12, 155-164.

Eliakim, M., Eisner, M. and Ungar, H. (1959). Experimental intrahepatic obstructive jaundice following ingestion of alpha-naphthyl isothiocyanate. Bull. Res. Council. Israel 8E, 7-9.

Goldfarb, S., Singer, E.J. and Popper, H. (1962). Experimental cholangitis due to alpha-naphthyl isothiocyanate (ANIT). Am. J. Pathol. 40, 685-698.

Horky, J., Grasso, P. and Goldberg, L.(1971):Influence of phenobarbital on histological and biochemical changes in experimental intrahepatic cholestasis. Exp. Path. Bd. 5, 200-211.

Roberts, R.J., Plaa, G.L.(1965): Potentiation and inhibition of α-naphthyl isothiocyanate-induced hyperbilirubinaemia and cholestasis. J. Pharmacol. Exp. Ther. 150, 499-506.

Roberts, R.J., Plaa, G.L.(1966a): Effect of norethandrolone, acetohexamide and enovid on ANIT-induced hyperbilirubinaemia and cholestasis. Biochem. Pharmacol, 15 333-341.

Traiger,G.J., Vyas, K.P. and Hanzlik,R.P.(1984): The effect of thiocarbonyl compounds on α-naphthyl isothiocyanate-induced hepatotoxicity and the urinary excretion of [^{35}S]-α-naphthyl isothiocyanate in the rat. Toxicol. Appl. Pharmacol. 72, 504-512.

Traiger, G.J., Vyas, K.P. and Hanzlik, R.P.(1985): Effects of inhibitors of α-naphthyl isothiocyanate-induced hepatotoxicity on the in vivo metabolism of naphthyl isothiocyanate. Chem. Biol. Interactions. 52, 335-345.

Woolley, J., Mullock, B.M. and Hinton, R.H.(1979): Reflux of biliary components into blood in experimental intrahepatic cholestasis induced in rats by treatment with α-naphthyl isothiocyanate. Clin. Chim. Acta. 92, 381-386.

In vivo and *in vitro* effects of some vitamins and glutathione on benzo(a) pyrene activation in rat liver

J.F. Narbonne, P. Cassand, C. Colin, E. Antignac

Laboratoire de Toxicologie Alimentaire, , Université de Bordeaux I, Talence, France. Réseau de toxicologie Nutritionnelle, MRES, France

KEY WORDS

Benzo(a)pyrene, free radical scavengers, mutagenesis, drug metabolizing enzymes.

INTRODUCTION

Benzo(a)pyrene requires metabolic activation to produce biological effects (Conney et al, 1977). Current findings indicate that the mutagenic properties of this compound involve a complex series of metabolic steps to produce the ultimate mutagen. However, when B(a)P is incubated with hepatic S9 from normal rats, the mutagenicity toward Salmonella typhimurium strains is very low (Wood et al, 1976). In order to obtain a significant mutagenicity the rate of B(a)P metabolism is increased by treatment of rats with strong P-450 inducers (like Aroclor 1254). Moreover, many dietary components e.g. proteins, lipids and vitamins have been shown to influence the activities of microsomal enzyme systems wich are involved in the activation and detoxification of xenobiotics (Wade and Norred, 1976; Kalamegham and Krishnaswamy, 1980; Pelissier et al, 1985; Albrecht et al, 1986).

We have previously shown a very high mutagenicity of B(a)P toward Salmonella typhimurium TA 98 when mediated by S9 from rats fed a vitamin A free diet during 8 weeks (Narbonne et al, 1985). In this case the activities of drug metabolizing enzymes (B(a)P-monooxygenase and epoxide hydrolase were decreased while the presence of vitamin A cannot be detected in the liver fractions. Moreover, the liver content in glutathione was decreased (about 30 -50%). Thus in order to elucidate this apparent discrepancy between the activities of B(a)P metabolism and B(a)P mutagenic activity in vitamin A deficient rats, according to a possible intervention of scavengers, we decided to compare both "in vivo" and "in vitro" the role of vitamin A and some free radical scavengers (vitamin E, C and glutathione) on the activation of B(a)P by hepatic S9 fraction.

MATERIAL AND METHODS

Experimental Animals

Weanling male Sprague-Dawley rats were obtained from Charles River (Saint Aubin les Elboeuf- France). They were maintained on a vitamin A free casein based diet (Narbonne, 1979) for 7 weeks. Control animals were fed a diet containing 20 IU of retinyl palmitate per g of food during the same period. Animals had free access to water and food and were kept one per cage. They were injected i.p. 750mg/kg body weight of either liposoluble scavengers (retinyl palmitate or tocopherol acetate) 48 hours before sacrifice or hydrosoluble scavengers (vitamin C or glutathione) 4 hours before sacrifice.

Preparation of cellular fractions
Rats were killed by decapitation. The livers were removed aseptically, minced and homogenized in 3 volumes of 0.15 M KCl. Aliquots of homogenate were stored at -80°C the remaining homogenate was centrifuged for 15 mn at 9 000g.
The supernatants (S9) were pooled, immediately frozen and stored at -80°C until used for mutagenic studies wich were conducted within 1 week from the day of sacrifice. Microsomic and cytosolic fractions were prepared from remaining S9 by centrifugation 1 hr at 105 000g. Final microsomal preparations were suspended in buffer pH =7 (Tris 10mM, KCl 150mM, EDTA 0.1mM) at a protein concentration of 4 mg/ml. The subcellular fractions were stored at -80°C. The protein contents were determined by method of Lowry et al (1951).

Liver parameters
Vitamin A was determined from liver homogenates according to the method of Gyorgy and Pearson (1967). Ascorbic acid was mesured by the method adapted from Roe and Kuether (1943) and described by Pelletier (1985). Liver glutathione burden was determined according with Sedlak and Lindsay (1980).Vitamin E was determined by HPLC analysis (adjusted method by M. Boisset, Laboratory of Biology, CNAM, Paris, unpublished results).

Enzyme assay
Cytochrome P-450 microsomal content was assayed according with Omura and Sato (1964). Benzo(a)pyrene monooxygenase (BaPMO) activity was determined by the radiometric method described by Van Cantfort at al (1977). Microsomal epoxide hydrolase (EH) and cytosolic glutathione S transferase activities were measured with ^{3}H styrene oxide as substrate (Oesh et al, 1971; Marniemi and Parkki, 1975).

Mutagenesis assay
The procedure described by Maron et al (1983) was followed. To 2.5 ml of molten top agar was added in this sequence : 0.1 ml of BaP solution, 0.1 ml of the tested compounds solution, 0.1 ml of the bacterial suspension acid and 0.5 ml of the S9 mix wich contained 20% S9. In order to recover a normal concentration of vitamin A, vitamin C, vitamin E and glutathione in the plates incubated with S9 from deficient rats, the amount of these compounds added were calculated from the levels contained in 100 µl of S9 (30 mg liver) from normal rats : 40 µg retinyl palmitate, 10 µg ascorbic acid, 0.9 µg tocopherol acetate and 30 µg glutathione. The experiments were carried out with 2 concentrations of tested compounds (1 and 10 fold the calculated amounts and 5 concentrations of BaP diluted in DMSO (1, 5, 10, 50 and 100 µg/plate).

RESULTS

In vitamin A deficient rats, hepatic vitamin A was not detectable. The hepatic levels of the others free radical scavengers were also modified. Vitamin E content was significantly increased (45 %). However, it was decreased in both 0 IU and 20 IU vitamin A groups from respectively 10 and 15 % after vitamin A injection. Vitamin C was significantly increased in both 0 and 20 IU vitamin A groups after ip injection (+ 50 and 35 % respectively). It was only increased from 15 % in others deficient vitamin A groups. Glutathione was decreased in vitamin A deficient groups (20 %). However it did not changed with vitamin A injection.

In the microsomal fraction, vitamin A deficiency resulted in a significant decrease in cytochrome P-450 content, BaPMO and EH activities (Fig. 1). The activity of cytosolic GST was enhanced about 20 %. Injection of vitamin C and glutathione did not change the activities of drug metabolizing enzymes while vitamin E treatment increased the BaPMO activity (+ 50 %) in both the 20 IU and 0 IU groups.

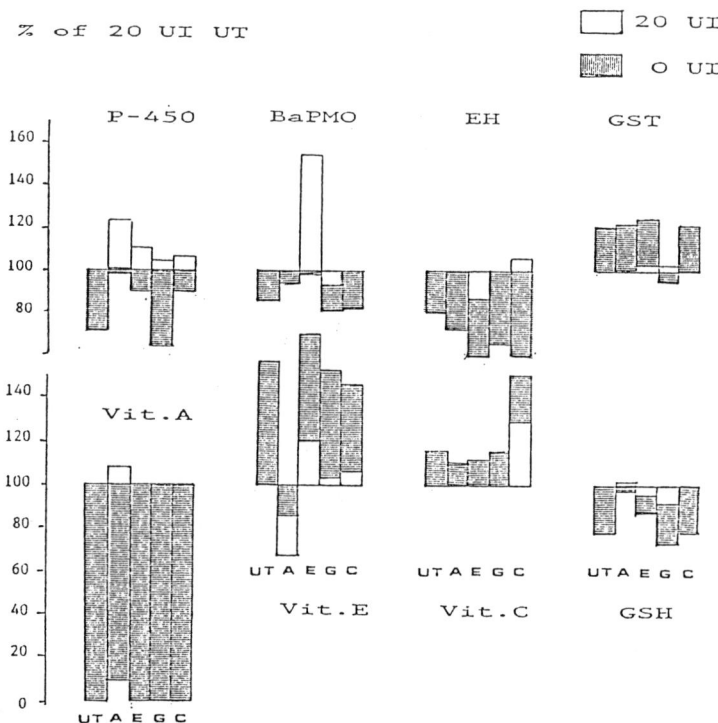

Fig.1 : Benzo(a)pyrene metabolizing enzymes activities and free radical scavengers content in hepatic cellular fractions.

Fig.2 shows that in vivo, vitamins A and E reduced the mutagenicity of BaP in both groups related to vitamin A intake. It is clear that injected in same quantities, vitamin E is more effective than vitamin A. Inversely, the injection of hydrosoluble scavengers increased the BaP mutagenicity. This increase was more pronounced when vitamin C was injected to control rats.

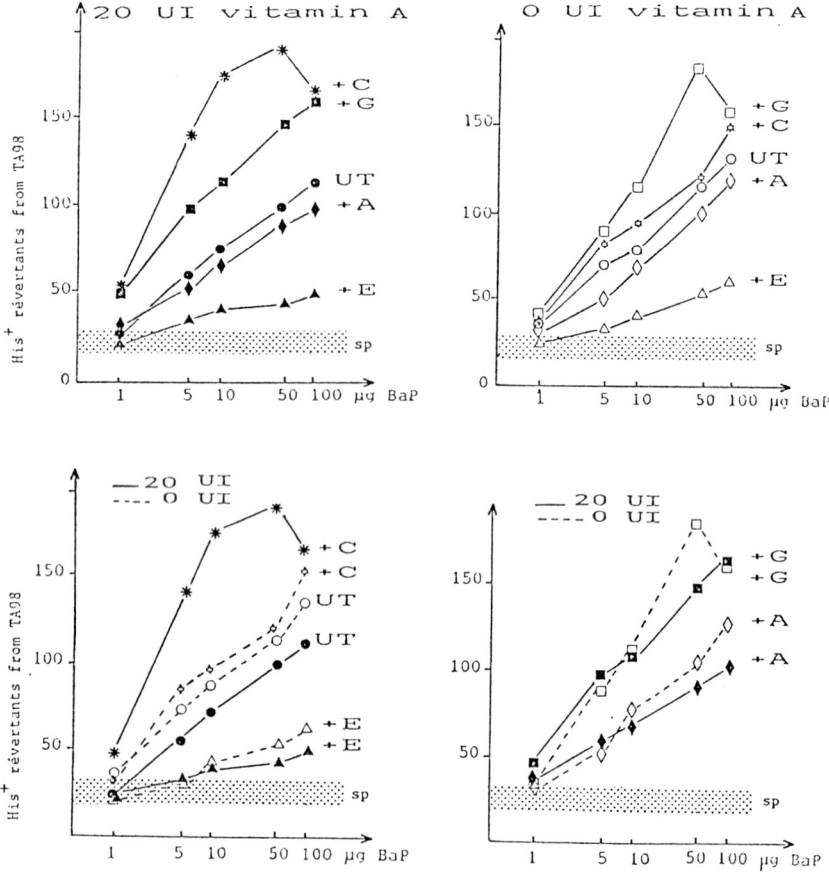

Fig.2 : Mutagenic activity of B(a)P mediated by S9 liver fraction from rats injected i.p. with vitamins A, E, C and glutathione.

In vitro, and at low concentrations (Fig. 3), the addition of vitamins A, E, C and glutathione reduced the genetic toxicity of BaP compared to that obtained with untreated animals. However, at high levels (Fig. 3), the inhibition of mutagenicity by vitamin C and glutathione was lower than that obtained with vitamin A or E. Thus, like in vivo, liposoluble scavengers provide more efficient protection against BaP mutagenicity. Furthermore their action seems dose dependent. The protective effect of hydrosoluble scavengers seems to be related to the cellular content of vitamin A. Nevertheless, in the case of a normal vitamin A intake, they have a little effect or stimulate mutagenesis. This is especially observed with vitamin C.

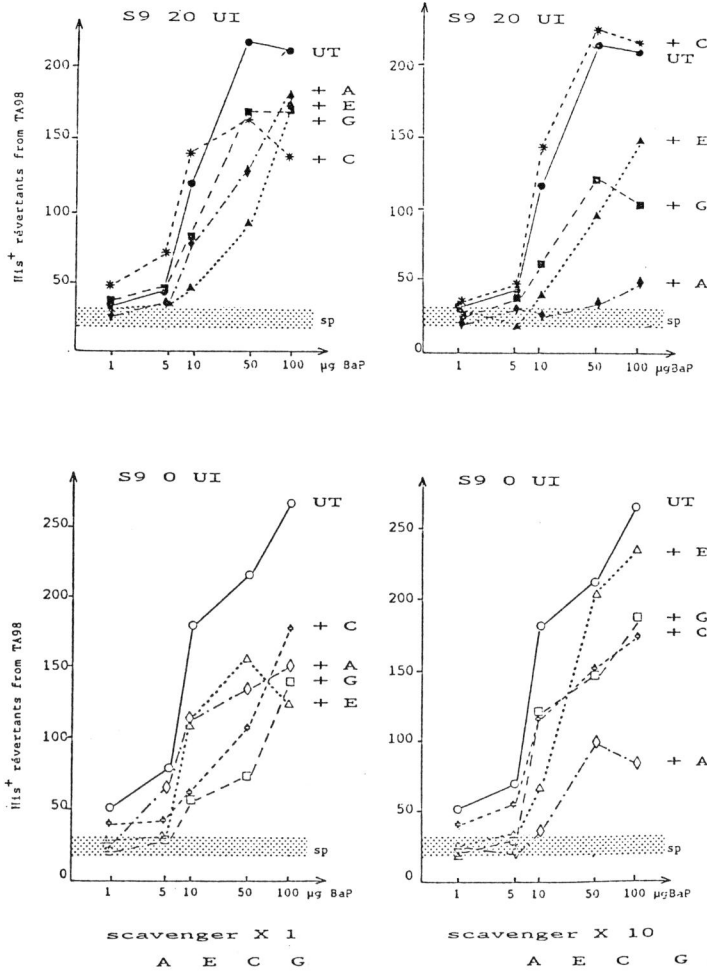

Fig.3 : Mutagenic activity of B(a)P mediated by S9 liver fraction after addition of vitamin A E,C and glutathione into the Ames Plates.

DISCUSSION

We have previously shown that the enhancement of BaP mutagenicity by S9 liver fraction from vitamin A deficient rats cannot be explained as a result of stimulated enzymatic activities of BaP (Narbonne et al, 1985). It seems clearly due to the lack of vitamin A in hepatic S9 fractions. Vitamin E enhanced the BaPMO activity in the control rats. It has been recently shown that it induced BaPMO in human cell line like vitamin K (Chen and Ding (1987). Inversely, it is actually well known that vitamin E inhibits chemically activated cancer in rodents. Our results showed that vitamin E like vitamin A inhibited the mutagenicity of BaP in both the control and vitamin A deficient rats.

In conclusion, the present study demonstrated that the "in vitro" addition of native fat soluble vitamins had the same effects that the "in vivo" treatment in wich the compounds could be metabolized or activated. Our results suggest that a fonctionnal relationship between vitamins A, E and monooxygenase enzymes might exist. Inversely, the addition of soluble scavengers leads to stimulation of BaP toxicity at least in control conditions.

REFERENCES

Albrecht, R., M.A. Pelissier, N. Miladi, S. Atteba, C. Desfontaines and J.F. Narbonne (1986) Restriction protéique et métabolisme des xénobiotiques, Ann. Nutr. Meta., 30, 73-80.
Conney, A.H., E.J. Pantuck, K.C. Hsiano, R. Kuntzman, A.P. Alvares and A. Kappas (1977) Regulation of drug metabolism in man by environmental chemical diet, Fed. Proceedings, 36, 1647-1652.
Gyorgy, P. and W.N. Pearson (1967) The international union of pure and applied chemistry, in : The vitamins Gyorgy, P. and W.N. Pearson (Eds). Acad. Press,VI, 145.
Kalamegham, R. and K. Krishnaswamy (1980) Benzo(a)pyrene metabolism in vitamin A deficient rats, Life Sciences, 27, 33-38.
Lowry, O.H., N.J. Rozenbrough, A.L. Farr and R.J. Randall (1951) Protein measurement with folin phenol reagent, J. Biol. Chem., 193, 265-275.
Marniemi, J. and M.G. Parkki (1975) Radiometric assay of glutathione S epoxide transferase and its enhancement by phenobarbital in rat liver in vitro, Biochem. Pharmacol., 24, 1569-1572.
Maron, D.M. and B.N. Ames (1983) Revised methods for the Salmonella mutagenicity test, Mutation Res., 113, 173-215.
Narbonne, J.F. (1979) Intoxication par les PCB et facteurs nutritionnels : III Influence d'un régime carencé en vitamine A sur l'accumulation des PCB chez le rat, Toxicol. Eur. Res., 1, 41-45.
Narbonne, J.F., P. Cassand, M. Daubèze and P. Alzieu (1985) Carence en vitamine A et activation du benzo(a)pyrène, Sci. Aliments, 5, n° hors série V, 41-46.
Oesch, F., D.H. Jerina and J. Daly (1971) A radiometric assay for epoxide hydrolase activity with (7 ^{3}H) styrene oxide, Biochem. Biophys. Acta, 227, 685-691.
Omura, T. and R. Sato (1971) The carbon monoxide binding pigment of liver microsomes. I : Evidence for its hemoprotein nature, J. Biol. Chem., 239, 2370-2378.
Pelissier, M.A., N. Miladi, S. Atteba, J.F. Narbonne and R. Albrecht (1985) Polychlorobiphényle (Phénoclor DP6) et métabolisme des xénobiotiques : Effets d'un régime hyperlipidique, Fd. Chem. Toxic. 23, 805-808.
Pelletier, O. (1985) Methods of vitamin assay in J. Augustin, P.B. Klein, D. Becker, P.B. Venugopal, J. Wiley and Sons. Ed. NY.
Roe, J.H. and C.A. Kuether (1943) The determination of ascorbic acid in whole blood and urine through the 2-4 dinitrophenylhydrazine derivate of dehydroascorbic acid, J. Biol. Chem., 147, 399-407.
Sedlak, J. and R.H. Lindsay (1968) Estimation of total protein bound and non protein sulfaryl groups in tissue with Ellman's reagent, Anal. Bioch., 25, 195-205.
Van Cantfort, J., J. De Graene and J.E. Gielen (1977) Radioactive assay for aryl hydrocarbon hydroxylase : Improved method and biological importance, Biochem. Res. Comm. 79, 505-512.
Wade, A.E. and W.P. Norred (1976) Effect of dietary lipid on drug metabolizing enzymes, Fed, Proc., 35, 2475-2479.
Wood, A.W., W. Levin, A.Y.H. Lu, H. Yagi, O. Hernandez, M. Jerina and A.H. Conney (1976) Metabolism of benzo(a)pyrene and benzo(a)pyrene derivates to mutagenic products by highly purified hepatic microsomal enzymes, J. Biol. Chem., 251, 4882-4890.
Yuan-Tsong C. and Jia-Huan D. (1987) Vitamins E and K induce Aryl Hydrocarbon Hydroxylase activity in human cell cultures Biochemical and Biophysical Research. Communications, 143, 863-871.

Inhibition of the two isoforms of human hepatic prolidase by the converting enzyme inhibiting antihypertensives

Claudine Cosson[1], Isaac Myara[1], Pierre-François Plouin[2], Nicole Moatti[1]

[1] Laboratoire de Biochimie, and [2] INSERM U.36 et Service de Médecine interne et d'Hypertension artérielle, Hôpital Broussais, 96, rue Didot, 75674 Paris Cedex 14, France

KEY WORDS

Prolidases, isoforms, captopril, converting enzyme inhibitors, liver, collagen.

INTRODUCTION

Prolidase (EC 3.4.13.9) is a dipeptidase that hydrolyzes iminodipeptides of the X-Pro type (X = amino acid; Pro = proline). This enzyme could take part in the metabolism of collagen and, in particular, in the intracellular catabolism of procollagen due to the large amount of imino acids present in this latter molecule. The role of prolidase in pathology is illustrated by the clinical and pathological consequences of its deficiencies (Myara et al., 1984a). Two isoforms of prolidase were recently demonstrated by Butterworth and Priestman (1985) after chromatographic separation on ion exchanger; only the activity of isoform I would be strongly decreased in individuals exhibiting such a deficiency. This isoform I is, however, the most active isoform towards glycyl proline, a dipeptide present in very large amount in the collagen molecule.

During hepatic fibrosis development, characterized by the pathological accumulation of various components of the extracellular matrix, especially collagen, modifications of the prolidase activity were demonstrated both in humans (Myara et al., 1984b) and in carbon tetrachloride intoxicated rats (Myara et al., 1987).

Captopril [N-(3-mercapto-2-methyl-1-oxopropyl)-L-proline] (Fig. 1) is an inhibitor of the converting enzyme used in hypertension treatment. Work by Ganapathy et al. (1985) showed that this antihypertensive has an inhibitory action upon prolidase activity of some tissues, which might cause the cutaneous disorders observed sometimes during treatment.

This study deals with the inhibitory effect of captopril and other antihypertensives belonging to the same class upon the two isoforms of hepatic prolidase.

MATERIALS

The antihypertensives studies were given by the manufacturers: captopril (Squibb), enalapril (Merck, Sharp & Dohme-Chibret), perindopril and its active metabolite perindoprilate (Servier), ramipril and ramiprilate (Hoechst).

CAPTOPRIL

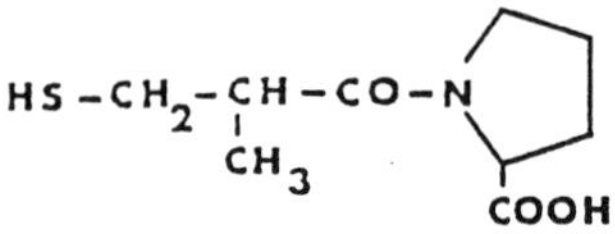

ENALAPRIL

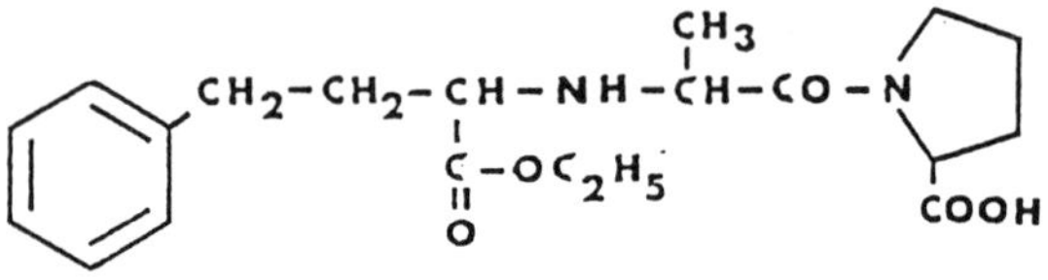

PERINDOPRIL

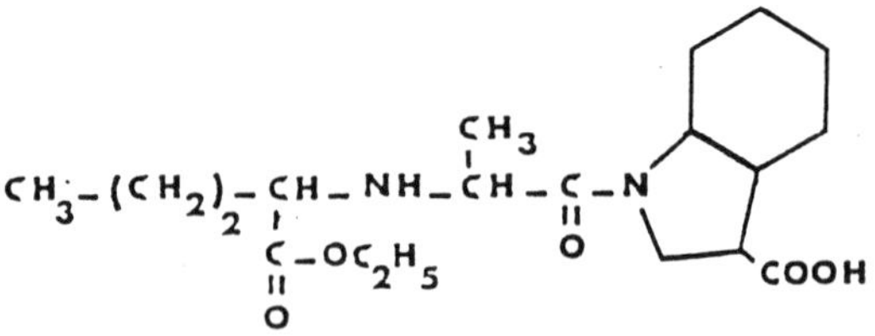

PERINDOPRILATE

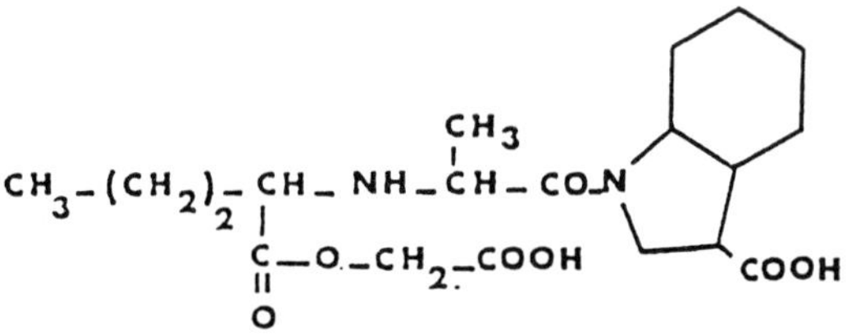

RAMIPRIL

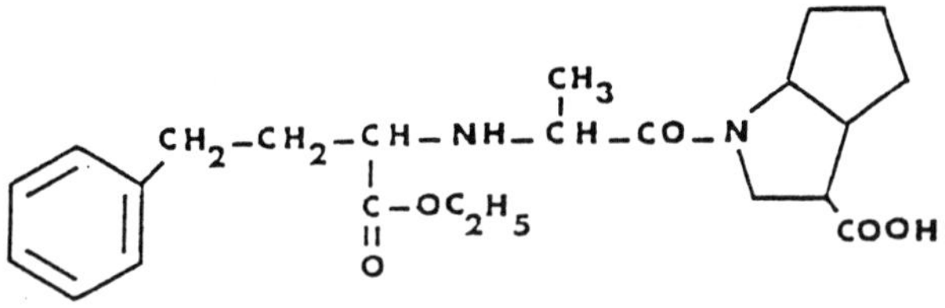

RAMIPRILATE

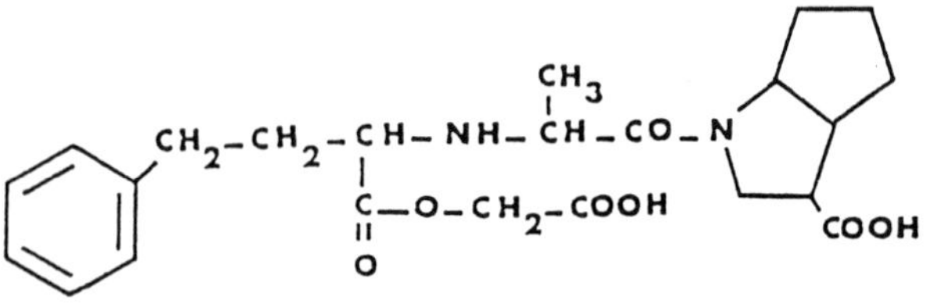

Fig. 1 : Chemical structure of the converting enzyme-inhibiting antihypertensives.

DEAE-Sephadex A-50 was provided by Pharmacia, glycyl-proline and phenylalanyl-proline by Sigma Chemical Co. All other reagents used were of analytical grade.

Human hepatic tissue was collected less than 24 h after death. The integrity of these samples was checked histologically.

METHODS

Separation of the two isoforms of hepatic prolidase

Hundred ml of 1/10 diluted homogenate (w/v) in 0.05 M Tris-HCl buffer pH 7, priorly centrifuged for 60 min at 20,000 g, was introduced at a rate of 30 ml/h into a column (2.6 x 40 cm) containing 10 g DEAE-Sephadex A-50. Elution of prolidase activity was performed by a 0 - 0.5 M gradient of NaCl (total volume: 500 ml) in the 0.05 M Tris-HCl buffer pH 7; 8 ml fractions were collected. Prolidase activity in each chromatographic fraction was determined with phenyl-alanyl-proline as substrate.

Determination of prolidase activity

Prolidase I

The enzyme solution, diluted 1/2 with 0.3 M Tris-HCl buffer pH 7.8 (buffer A) containing 2 mM $MnCl_2$, was preincubated for 24 h at 37 °C. Hundred µl of this mixture was then added to 100 µl of buffer A containing 1 mM $MnCl_2$ (buffer B). The enzymatic reaction was started by the addition of 100 µl of 90 mM glycyl-proline dissolved in buffer B. After 30 min of incubation, the enzymatic reaction was stopped by the addition of 1 ml of 0.45 M trichloroacetic acid. Released proline was determined colorimetrically (Myara et al., 1982).

Prolidase II

The activity of this isoform was determined with phenylalanyl-proline as substrate. With the exception of this modification all operative conditions were identical to those described for prolidase I.

Inhibitory effect

Captopril and the other antihypertensives were dissolved in buffer B at the final concentration of 3 mM.

RESULTS

Chromatographic separation of the two prolidase isoforms (Fig. 2)

Under the conditions described, isoform I was eluted with an NaCl concentration of 175 mM and isoform II with a concentration of 240 mM. Phenylalanyl-proline was chosen as substrate for the enzymatic reaction, because isoform II is very little reactive with glycyl-proline.

Effect of captopril and the other antihypertensives inhibiting the converting enzyme (Table 1)

Captopril inhibits the activity of both isoforms of hepatic prolidase. However, prolidase II is more sensitive to this inhibition than isoform I.

Preincubation for 24 h at 37 °C and pH 7.8 in the presence of 1 mM $MnCl_2$ partially protects both isoforms from this inhibition.

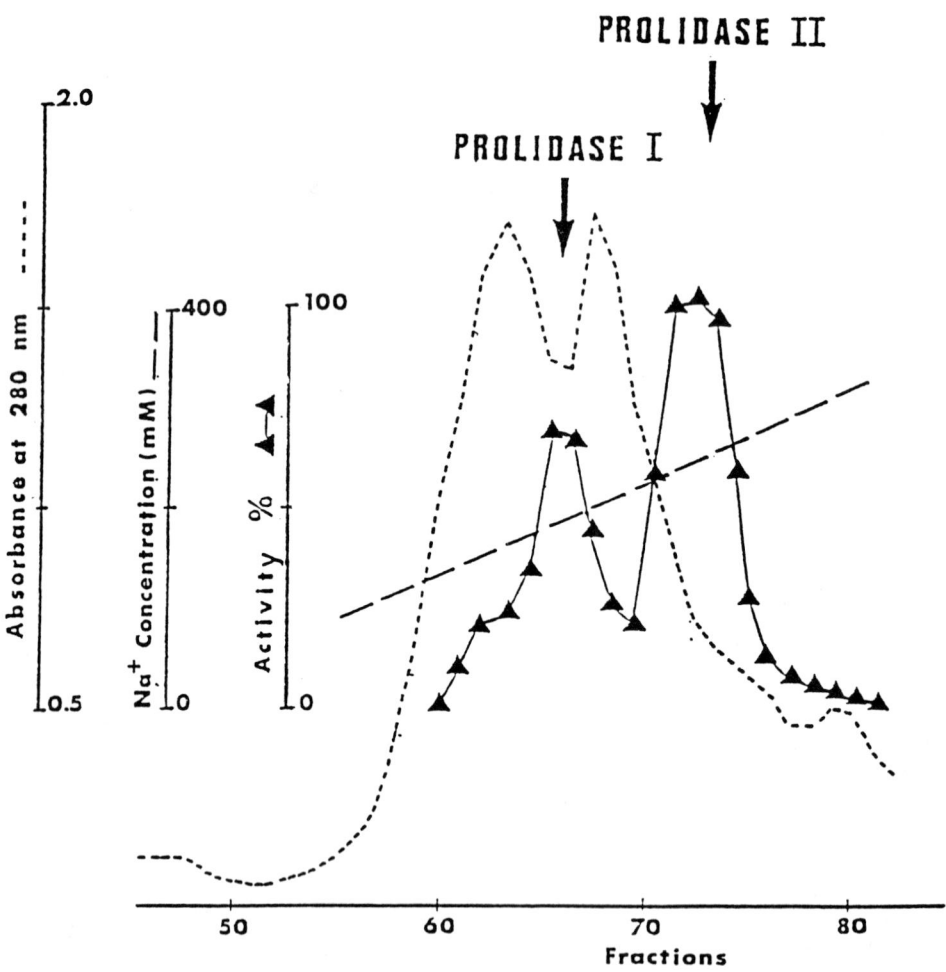

Fig. 2 : Chromatographic separation of the two isoforms of hepatic prolidase.

The inhibitory effect observed in the presence of the other antihypertensives is weaker and mainly apparent for isoform II.

Table 1. Effect of the converting enzyme-inhibiting antihypertensives on the activity (U/l) of the two isoforms of hepatic prolidase.

Inhibitors (3 mM)	PROLIDASE I (gly-pro 30 mM)		PROLIDASE II (phé-pro 30 mM)	
	without preincubation	with preincubation	without preincubation	with preincubation
CONTROL	285 (100)	1 515 (100)	455 (100)	85 (100)
CAPTOPRIL	108 (38)	1 335 (88)	27 (6)	71 (83)
ENALAPRIL	256 (90)	1 425 (94)	195 (43)	26 (31)
PERINDOPRIL	236 (83)	1 425 (94)	340 (75)	74 (87)
PERINDOPRILATE	265 (93)	1 455 (96)	345 (76)	74 (87)
RAMIPRIL	315 (111)	1 290 (85)	175 (38)	24 (28)
RAMIPRILATE	276 (97)	1 395 (92)	28 (6)	14 (17)

Values in brackets are percentages of residual activities. All values are means of triplicate determinations.

DISCUSSION

This work confirms the inhibitory effect of captopril on the activity of human hepatic prolidase. The other antihypertensives that inhibit the converting enzyme also inhibit the prolidase activity. But the two isoforms of prolidase react differently to the action of these antihypertensives. Prolidase isoform I, which is the most active in the intracellular catabolism of procollagen, seems less sensitive to this inhibition than prolidase isoform II.

Among the side effects observed during treatment with that class of drugs, hepatic complications are rare (Vandenburg et al., 1981; Hurault de Ligny et al., 1982; Ryckelynck et al., 1982, Rahmat et al., 1985; Lunel et al., 1987). To the best of our knowledge, no report has ever mentioned the occurrence of liver cirrhosis after taking these drugs.

The inhibitors of the converting enzyme studied in this work have all in common a proline residue. Proline is a competitive inhibitor of pig renal (Manao et al., 1972; Lacoste et al., 1987) and intestinal prolidase (Sjöström et al., 1973). Any modification of the hydrophobic moiety of the pyrrolidine ring partly suppresses the inhibitory effect (Lacoste et al., 1987). The same occurs after desaturation of the ring to 3,4-dehydro-L-proline, hydroxylation at position 4 (4-hydroxyproline) or replacement of the methylene group with an acidic function (pyroglutamic acid). In this study the antihypertensives whose proline residue is substituted still possess all the hydrophobicity properties of the pyrrolidine ring. On the other hand, the nature of the substituted carbon chain on the nitrogen atom also allows the modulation of the inhibitory effect. Thus, N-benzyloxy-carbonyl-L-proline displays a greater inhibitory effect than captopril (King et al., 1987). The presence of a phenyl residue at the chain end in enalapril and ramipril confers to these two antihypertensives a higher inhibitory action than that of perindopril. Finally, substitution of the carboxyl group of proline by phosphoric acid (pyrrolidine-2-phosphonic acid) considerably increases the inhibitory effect (Lacoste et al., 1987). The association within the same molecule of several of these substitutions would allow to envisage the synthesis of a sufficiently inhibitory compound that could be used to conceive an animal or cellular model deficient in prolidase activity.

REFERENCES

Butterworth, J. and Priestman, D.A. (1985): Presence in human cells and tissues of two prolidases and their alteration in prolidase deficiency. J. Inher. Metab. Dis. 8, 193-197.
Ganapathy, V., Paschley, S.J., Roesel, R.A., Pashley, D.H. and Leibach, F.H. (1985): Inhibition of rat and human prolidases by captopril. Biochem. Pharmacol. 34, 1287-1291.
Hurault de Ligny, B., Mariot, A., Keesler, M., Caraman, P. and Netter, P. (1982): Hépatites au cours d'une polythérapie associant le captopril. Thérapie 37, 698-700.
King, G.F., Crossley, M.J. and Kuchel, P.W. (1987): Proton NMR studies of human erythrocyte prolidase. Biomed. Biochim. Acta 46, 302-303.
Lacoste, A.M., Neuzil, E. and Mastalerz, P. (1987): Pyrrolidine-2-phosphonic acid: a new inhibitor of kidney prolidase. Biochem. Soc. Trans. 15, 140-142.
Lunel, F., Grippon, P., Cadranel, J.F., Victor, N. and Opolon, P. (1987): Hépatite aiguë après la prise de maléate d'énalapril (Rénitec). Gastroenterol. clin. Biol. 11, 174-175.
Manao, G., Nassi, P., Cappugi, G., Camici, G. and Ramponi, G. (1972): Swine kidney prolidase: assay, isolation procedure and molecular properties. Physiol. Chem. Physics 4, 75-87.
Myara, I., Charpentier, C. and Lemonnier, A. (1982): Optimal conditions for prolidase assay by proline colorimetric determination: application to iminodipeptiduria. Clin. Chim. Acta 125, 193-205.
Myara, I., Charpentier, C. and Lemonnier, A. (1984a): Prolidase and prolidase deficiency. Life Sci. 34, 1985-1998.
Myara, I., Myara, A., Mangeot, M., Fabre, M., Charpentier, C. and Lemonnier, A. (1984b): Plasma prolidase activity: a possible index of collagen catabolism in chronic liver disease. Clin. Chem. 30, 211-215.
Myara, I., Miech G., Fabre, M., Mangeot, M. and Lemonnier, A. (1987): Changes in prolinase and prolidase activity during CCl_4 administration inducing liver cytolysis and fibrosis in rat. Br. J. exp. Path. 68, 7-13.
Rahmat, J., Gelfand, R.L., Gelfand, M.C., Winchester, J.F., Schreiner, G.E. and Zimmerman, H.J. (1985): Captopril-associated cholestatic jaundice. Ann. Intern. Med. 102, 56-58.
Ryckelynck, J.P., Batho, J.M., Peny, J. and Beuve Mery, J. (1982): Hépatite au captopril. Presse médicale 11, 1950-1951.
Sjöström, H., Noren, O. and Josefsson, L. (1973): Purification and specificity of pig intestinal prolidase. Biochim. Biophys. Acta 327, 457-470.
Taillan, B., Pedinielli, F.T., Blanc, A.P. and Jauffret, P. (1985): Hépatite toxique au captopril. Thérapie 40, 263-267.
Vandenburg, M., Parfrey, P., Wright, P. and Lazda, E. (1981): Hepatitis associated with captopril treatment. Br. J. clin. Pharmacol. 11, 105-106.

In vitro liver models: new systems for the study of drug metabolism and cytotoxicity

Les systèmes in vitro : de nouveaux modèles pour l'étude du métabolisme et de la cytotoxicité des xénobiotiques

Liver Cells and Drugs. Ed. A. Guillouzo. Colloque INSERM/John Libbey Eurotext Ltd. © 1988. Vol. 164, pp. 211-220.

In vitro models in the study of the fate of drugs in research and development

J.F. Le Bigot[1]*, J.R. Kiechel[2]

[1] *Centre de Recherche Pharmaceutique, Laboratoires Sandoz 14, Boulevard Richelieu 92506 Rueil-Malmaison, France.* [2] *Centre de Recherche Bristol-Myers, rue de la Maison Rouge, 77200 Lognes, France*

SUMMARY

The pharmaceutical research and development is a long, complicated and costly process, and failures have often a "biological" origin. With this in mind, the potentialities of several alternatives in vitro experimental models have been investigated.
Using cultured rat, rabbit and human adult hepatocytes an excellent in vitro v.s. in vivo correlation of metabolic pathways and of rates of metabolization has been shown with several drugs. By giving early information, useful in medicinal chemistry (prodrug), in pharmacology (drug interactions) and in toxicology (inter-species comparisons, hepatotoxicity, mutagenicity), cultured hepatocytes are an attractive tool in pharmaceutical research and development.

KEYWORDS : cultured hepatocytes, drug metabolism, in vitro toxicology, ketotifen.

INTRODUCTION

Why to search for in vitro models in research and development ?

Several major pharmaceutical companies are prospecting and searching for in vitro models to improve their research and development. This concern comes from some characteristics of a modern development of a new drug we will briefly discuss. It comes also from the reasons of frequent failures in drug development.

The pharmaceutical research and development : a long, complicated and costly process :

The constant increase in the cost of research and development charaterizes the pharmaceutical industry since more than 12 years. The outlay for developing a new biologically active compound to the stage when it can be released for clinical trials in man is about 40 million french francs, and the human effort put into the product is about 150 man-years. By the time a compound has been developed to the point where it can be launched onto the market as a new drug, approximately 350 million french francs and some 1500 man-years will have been invested (Fig.1 and ref.1).

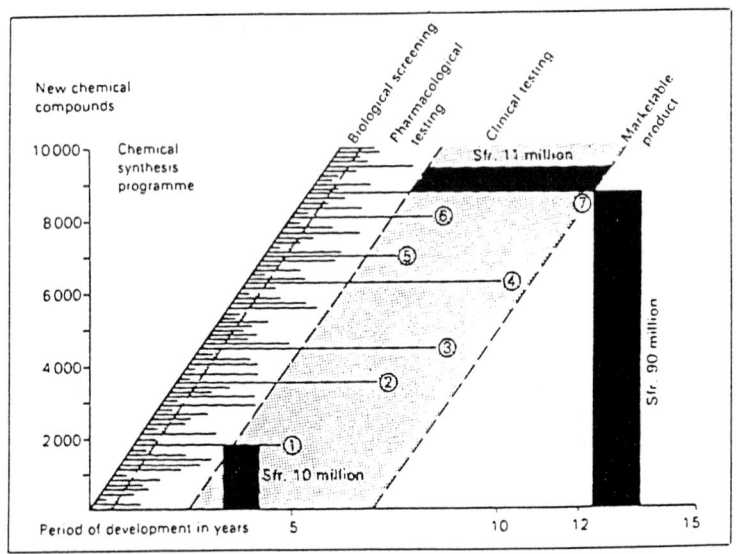

Figure 1 : Diagram showing the development and cost of a new drug (from Berde, 1981)

The second characteristics is the time taken to develop a new medicine which may be expected to run to 7 to 12 years. An highly innovative new drug as cyclosporin (SANDIMMUN®), a new immunosuppresant agent which has greatly improved the organ transplantation in man, gives an example of the time and steps needed for such a development (Fig. 2).

1970	Thiele: discovery of two new strains of fungi imperfecti producing antifungal metabolites.
	Kis: isolation and characterisation of the metabolites as novel neutral polypeptides.
1972	**Borel: discovery of immunosuppressive properties of metabolite 24-556 in rodents.**
1973	Ruegger: purification of cyclosporin A (27-400).
1974	Borel et al.: animal studies of the immunosuppressant activity of cyclosporin A, in vivo and in vitro.
1975	Petcher et al.: Elucidation of the structure of cyclosporin A (x-ray studies).
1976	Toxicity studies (rats, monkeys) demonstrate selectivity of cyclosporin A for lymphocytes and lack of effect on haemopoiesis. World-wide confirmation of specific immunosuppressive effect of cyclosporin A in experimental transplantations and other models.
1978	Calne et al., Powles et al.: first clinical results (renal transplantation, graft-versus-host disease).
1983	Launching in USA, F, GB, RFA, CH, S, N, ...

Figure 2 : Steps of development of cyclosporin (SANDIMMUN®)

Finally, the third charateristics of pharmaceutical R and D is its exceedingly complexity and multidisciplinarity. The activities of the various disciplines are closely interrelated ; some follow consecutively, but most of them are carried out in parallel, and have to be carefully co-ordinated. As simplified network chart of the various activities gives an idea of this complexity (Fig.3).

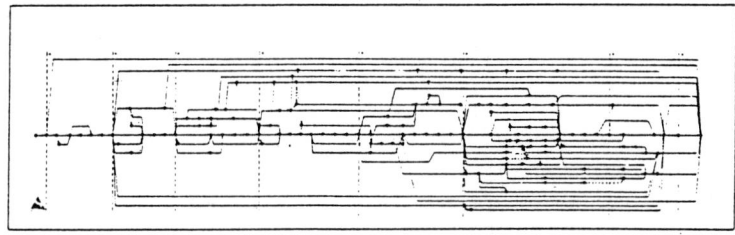

Figure 3 : Simplified network chart of a drug development project

Beside the characteristics of pharmaceutical R and D, it is also interesting to look at the causes of failures in this process. A recent analysis (23) shows that the most frequent causes of failures which lead to stop development of a new drug have a "biological" origin, i.e. toxicological findings or lack of efficacy (Fig.4).

Number of discontinued compounds (Hoechst 1972-1978)			
Reason	Preclinical	Clinical	Total
Synthesis problem	4		4
Patent problem	1	1	2
Instability	4		4
Toxicological finding	12	2	14
Efficacy less than expected	16	16	32
Side effects	5	3	8
Price problems	1		1
Better competitors	3	1	4
Total	46	23	69

Figure 4 : Causes of failure of compounds launched in preclinical and clinical studies (From G. Seidl, 1983)

These economic and strategic constraints explain why the managements and researchers try to improve the R and D process by defining and use of experimental models as simple and rapid as possible and mainly with an high predictive value. That implies all experimental models used in routine have to be previously validated.

With this in mind, since about 8 years, we have study the potentialities of various in vitro models at several stages of the pharmaceutical R and D, and particularly the use of cultures of hepatocytes.

THE USE OF CULTURED HEPATOCYTES IN DRUG METABOLISM STUDIES

Since the liver is the principal organ involved in the biotransformation of xenobiotics and also the first organ met after the gastrointestinal tract by a drug administered by oral route, determination of hepatic metabolic pathways of a new drug is of major importance. For this purpose, various in vitro experimental models have been proposed and used including the isolated perfused liver, liver slices, freshly isolated or cultured hepatocytes and subcellular fractions.

One major problem in such investigations is the species differences in metabolic pathways and rates. Most studies during the last few years have been performed using animal hepatocytes, mainly from rat, and therefore, the extrapolation of results to humans is hazardous. Recently, several groups have developed techniques which allows to isolate viable human adult hepatocytes by perfusing either the whole liver (2,3) or a portion of the liver (7, 8) with collagenase, or by enzymatic treatment of biopsies (14,18,21,24,26).

In order to validate the cultures of animal and human hepatocytes as a model system for drug metabolism studies, including investigation of species polymorphism, we have studied the biotransformation of several drugs in vitro by cultured rat, rabbit and human adult hepatocytes as compared to the biotransformation found in vivo, in collaboration with the group of A. Guillouzo. The first molecule selected for this validation of the hepatocytes model was ketotifen (ZADITEN®) because its metabolic pathways in vivo were well known and were different in man and several animal species (6,10).

Hepatocytes cultured in 25 cm^2 or 80 cm^2 flash at a density of 10^5 hepatocytes/cm^2 were incubated with 50 nmoles of radiolabelled ketotifen per ml. 50 nmoles/ml of medium was selected after a preliminary experiment showing this concentration did not induce any morphological alteration or LDH leakage. After 1, 2, 4, 8, 12 and 24 hours, aliquots of medium were collected. Parent drug and metabolites were analysed by reversed phase high performance liquid chromatography, using an on line continuous radioactivity detector. Structures of metabolites were determined by mass spectrometry.

The metabolism exhibited in vitro in hepatocytes cultures was compared to the in vivo metabolism previously determined in the same species (Fig. 5 and ref.11).

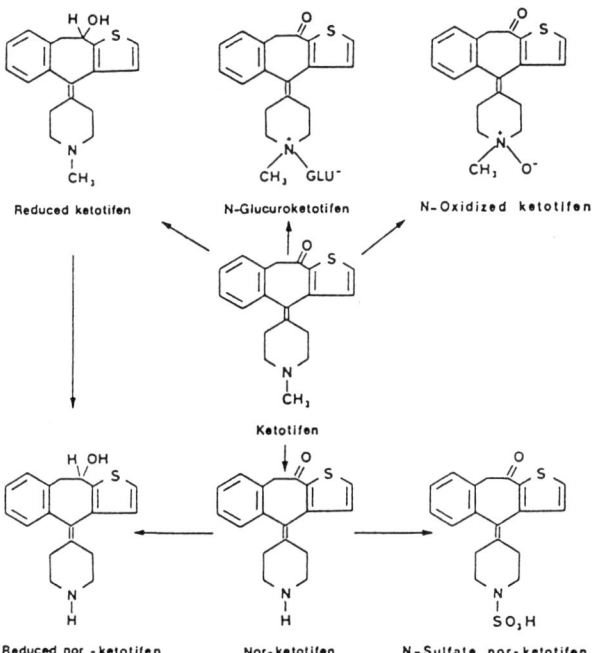

Figure 5 : Metabolic pathways exhibited by cultured rat, rabbit and human adult hepatocytes

(from Le Bigot et al., 1987)

Rat hepatocytes metabolized ketotifen forming two metabolites. The major metabolite was the nor-ketotifen produced by oxidative N-demethylation of ketotifen. The minor metabolite was N-oxidized ketotifen. Nor-ketotifen and N-oxidized ketotifen were also the two metabolites produced in vivo in the rat.

Rabbit hepatocytes metabolized ketotifen forming a major metabolite, the N-sulfate of nor-ketotifen. This metabolite was also the major one found in vivo in urine of treated rabbits. Another metabolite found in vivo was produced also in vitro, i.e. N-glucuroketotifen, which gave unchanged ketotifen after incubation with ß-glucuronidase.

Adult human hepatocytes metabolized ketotifen by two main routes. One is the ketoreduction, giving the 10-hydroxyketotifen, identical to that of the synthetic reference compound, obtained by reduction of ketotifen by sodium borohydride. The other route involves the N-glucuronidation of both unchanged and reduced ketotifen giving conjugates and which formed ketotifen and the free reduced derivative after incubation with ß-glucuronidase. Traces of nor-ketotifen and N-oxidized ketotifen were also found in the medium from human hepatocyte cultures. These metabolites corresponded to the four metabolic pathways found in vivo in man.

This first work of validation clearly demontrates that cultures of rat, rabbit and human adult hepatocytes retain their in vivo specific drug metabolizing activities, and thus can be use to investigate the metabolism of a new drug (11).

More recently, two other compounds, namely pindolol (VISKEN®) and fluperlapine, were also found to be metabolized in human hepatocyte cultures according to the same major pathways found in vivo (16).

Interesting was the result showing not only a qualitative comparison in vitro v.s. in vivo, i.e. same metabolic pathways, but also a qualitative comparison, i.e. intensity of the biotransformation. For pindolol, the studies performed in six animal species permitted to define a full metabolic pathway (9) and showed pindolol is extensively metabolized in animal. In vitro, using cultured human hepatocytes, pindolol was less metabolized than a drug with an higher first pass, like fluperlapine. This result was in agreement with the observation of clinical pharmacology showing an elimination of pindolol in the same order by hepatic and renal clearance.

These results confirmed the excellent in vitro v.s. in vivo correlation of the rates of metabolization and of the metabolic pathways. So, cultured hepatocytes are now routinely used at an early stage of the development of a new drug, before the first clinical trials, and up today, ten new molecules has thus been tested with cultures of hepatocytes.

Cultured hepatocytes can also be used for the preparative biosynthesis of metabolites of reference. This approach makes possible to obtain all metabolites formed in vivo, which is not always possible by chemistry (ex. quaternary ammonium glucuronide of ketotifen) and at a time when the chemist is often working on another serie.

By giving early information on metabolism, the use of such validated in vitro models brings support at several stages of R and D of potential new drugs :

- in medicinal chemistry, the testing of a prodrug-hypothesis or the protection of a metabolic labile site can help to optimize a series to find a long acting compound,

- in pharmacology, the preparative biosynthesis of metabolites by cultured hepatocytes permits us to test their activity using other in vitro models, like radioreceptor assay. This approach gives a better understanding of the profile of new principles and by different routes of administration. It was for example particularly useful to study ergot derivatives which can't be given at high doses to animals or man, because their high activity, and for which metabolites can't be isolated from urine, because high hepatic clearance and biliary elimination,

- in toxicology, to help to the selection or validation of the animal models, as well as in depth investigation of some toxicological events, appropriate inter-species comparison in metabolism has to be performed,

- in clinical pharmacology to study, and in some cases anticipate, drug interactions which could modify the in vivo hepatic clearance. For example, in vitro investigations suggested different potentials of macrolide antibiotics for drug interactions, depending on their ability to induce and form an inactive complex with cytochrome P 450 (19). We have recently confirmed this by an in vivo pharmacokinetic study in Rhesus monkeys showing, when coadministered, troleandomycin or erythromycin dramatically increased plasma levels of dihydroergotamine (factor 6 to 10) (15), spiramycin did not show any interaction.

THE USE OF CULTURED HEPATOCYTES IN TOXICOLOGY

Beside the use in drug metabolism studies, cultured hepatocytes could also be useful in toxicology, at a very early stage of R and D, during the screening, or latter to study the mechanism of an hepatotoxicity observed in vivo.

This topic will be presented in the following presentations, and we would like only ask the question which still remain opened : what are the more relevant "end point" parameters to assess hepatotoxicity in vitro ?

- microscopic examination ?
- enzyme leakage ? intracellular measurements ? which enzymes ?
- proteins synthesis, metabolism of glycogen, albumin synthesis/ secretion, RNA synthesis, ureogenesis, glycerolipid biosynthesis ?

. functional monooxygenase activity measurement ?
. covalent binding measurement using radiolabelled drug ?

Another very interesting use of cultured hepatocytes in toxicology, which could be described as a test of screening, is the use in the mutagenicity assessment.

Mutagenicity potential of several carcinogens has been detected on cultured rat hepatocytes by measuring unscheduled DNA synthesis (17,20,27,28).

Several groups have shown certain rat hepatoma cell lines retain liver specific functions in culture (4, 5) and are capable of expressing the cytochrome P 450-dependant monooxygenases. Using these dedifferentiated cell lines, it has been shown possible to detect genotoxic potential, by the appearance of alkaline labile DNA sites (12,13).

More recently, cultured human hepatocytes have been used to demonstrate unscheduled DNA synthesis stimulated by a number of carcinogens such as aflatoxin B_1, 2 acetylamino fluorene, diethylnitrosamine or by tripelennamine (22, 25).

CONCLUSION

The use of cultured animal and human hepatocytes has given proof to be a useful tool in drug metabolism study and more generally in the safety evaluation of new drugs. Some problems or ideas have still to be discussed to progress more :

. qualitative validation in hepatotoxicity assessment and selection of "end point" parameters ?
. availability of hepatocytes from human origin, cryopreservation methods have been improved ; inter-individual variability ; human liver cell line, quid ?
. ethical considerations concerning the use of human material.

Naturally, cultured hepatocytes will not totally replace the in vivo investigations or other in vitro models using organs like isolated perfused liver for example. Nevertheless, by giving early information useful in medicinal chemistry, toxicology and pharmacology, the use of cultured hepatocytes would probably contribute to get faster and to improve the relevance and predictivity of our R and D.

REFERENCES

1. Berde, B. (1981) : The experimental biologist and the medical scientist in the pharmaceutical industry. Swiss Pharma 3, 29-35.
2. Bojar, H., Basler, M., Fuchs, F., Dreyfurst, R., Staib, W., Broelsch, Ch. (1976) : Preparation of parenchymal and non-parenchymal cells from adult human liver - morphological and biochemical characteristics. J. Clin. Chem. Clin. Biochem 14, 527-532.

3. Cano, J.P., Fabre, G., Rahmani, R., Bertault-Peres, P., DeSousa, G., Arnoux, P., Boré, P., Richard, B., Fabre, I., Lacarelle, B., Placidi, M., Coulange, C., Ducros, M., Rampal, M. (1988) : This volume.
4. Deschatrette, J., Weiss, M.C. (1974) : Characterization of differentiated and dedifferentiated clones from a rat hepatoma. Biochimie 56, 1603-1611.
5. Deschatrette, J., Moore, E.E., Dubois, M., Cassio, D., Weiss, M.C. (1979) : Dedifferentiated variants of a rat hepatoma : analysis by cell hybridization. Somatic Cell Gen. 5, 697-718.
6. Guerret, M., Julien-Larose, C., Lavène, D. (1981) : Application de la chromatographie en phase gazeuse - colonnes capillaires à l'élucidation du métabolisme du kétotifène chez le singe et l'homme. In : Premier Congrès Européen de Biopharmacie et Pharmacocinétique, 1,2,3 Avril 1981, Technique et Documentation, volume 2, 317-321.
7. Guguen-Guillouzo, C., Campion, J.P., Brissot, P., Glaise, D., Launois, B., Bourel, M., Guillouzo, A. (1982) : High yield preparation of isolated human adult hepatocytes by enzymatic perfusion of the liver. Cell. Biol. Int. Rep. 6, 625-628.
8. Houssin, D., Capron, M., Celier, C., Cresteil, T., Demaugre, F., Beaune, P. (1983) : Evaluation of isolated human hepatocytes. Life Sci. 33, 1805-1809.
9. Kiechel, J.R., Niklaus, P., Schreier, E., Wagner, H. (1975) : Metabolites of pindolol in different animal species. Xenobiotica 5, 741-754.
10. Kiechel, J.R., Schreier, E. (1977) : Ketotifen (HC 20-511) ADME studies in animals and man. Registration dossier SANDOZ.
11. Le Bigot J.F., Begue, J.M., Kiechel, J.R., Guillouzo, A. (1987) : Species differences in metabolism of ketotifen in rat, rabbit and man : demonstration of similar pathways in vivo and in cultured hepatocytes. Life Sci. 40, 883-890.
12. Loquet, C., Wiebel, F.J. (1982) : Geno- and cytotoxicity of nitrosamines, aflatoxin B_1, and benzo [a] pyrene in continuous cultures of rat hepatoma cells. Carcinogenesis 3, 1213-1218.
13. Loquet, C., Engelhardt, U., Schaefer-Ridder, M. (1985) : Differentiated genotoxic response of carcinogenic and non-carcinogenic benzacridines and metabolites in rat hepatoma cells. Carcinogenesis 6, 455-457.
14. Maekubo, H., Ozaki, S., Mitmaker, B., Kalant, N. (1982) : Preparation of human hepatocytes for primary culture. In Vitro 18, 483-491.
15. Martinet, M., Kiechel, J.R. (1983) : Interaction of dihydroergotamine and triacetyloleandomycin in the minipig. Eur. J. Drug. Metab. Pharmacokin. 8, 261-267.
16. Guillouzo, A. et al. (1987) : Manuscript submitted to Xenobiotica.
17. Mitchell, A.D., Casciano, D.A., Meltz, M.L., Robinson, D.E., San, R.H.C., Williams, G.M., Von Halle, E.S. (1983) : Unscheduled DNA synthesis tests. A report of the U.S. environmental protection agency gene-tox program. Mut.Res 123, 363-410.
18. Miyazaki, K., Takaki, R., Nakayama, F., Yamauchi, S., Koga, A., Todo, S. (1981) : Isolation and primary culture of adult human hepatocytes. Ultrastructural and functional studies. Cell Tissue Res, 218, 13-21.
19. Pessayre, D. (1983) : Effects of macrolide antibiotics on drug metabolism in rats and in human. Int. J. Clin. Pharm. 3, 449-458.

20. Probst, G.S., McMahon, R.E., Hill, L.E., Thompson, Ch. Z., Epp, J.K., Neal, S.B. (1981) : Chemically-induced unscheduled DNA synthesis in primary rat hepatocyte cultures : a comparison with bacterial mutagenicity using 218 compounds. Environm. Mutagen. 3, 11-32.
21. Reese, J.A., Byard, J.L. (1981) : Isolation and culture of adult hepatocytes from liver biopsies. In Vitro 17, 935-940.
22. Robbiano, L., Gazzaniga, G.M., Martelli, A., Pino, A., Brambilla, G. (1986) : DNA-damaging activity of tripelennamine in primary cultures of human hepatocytes. Mut. Res. 173, 229-232.
23. Seidl, G. (1983) : Cost of drug research. In : Decision making in Drug Research, ed Gross J. Raven Press, pp. 193.
24. Strom, S.C., Jirtle, R.L., Jones, R.S., Novicki, D.L., Rosenberg, M.R., Novotny, A., Irons, G., McLain, J.R., Michalopoulos, G. (1982) : Isolation, culture, and transplantation of human hepatocytes. J. Natn. Canc. Inst. 68, 771-778.
25. Strom, S.C., Novicki, D.L., Novotny, A., Jirtle, R.L., Michalopoulos, G. (1983) : Human hepatocyte - mediated mutagenesis and DNA repair activity. Carcinogenesis 4, 683-686.
26. Tee, L.B.G., Seddon, T., Boobis, A.R., Davies, D.S. (1985) : Drug metabolising activity of fresly isolated human hepatocytes. Brit. J. Clin. Pharmacol. 19, 279-294.
27. Williams, G.M. (1977) : Detection of chemical carcinogens by unscheduled DNA synthesis in rat liver primary cell cultures. Canc. Res. 37, 1845-1851.
28. Williams, G.M., Laspia, M.F., Dunkel, V.C. (1982) : Reliability of the hepatocytes primary culture/DNA repair test in testing of coded carcinogens and noncarcinogens. Mut. Res. 97, 359-370.

ACKNOWLEDGMENTS : We thank Mrs A. D'Amario and B. Corbier for her technical assistance in the preparation of the manuscript.

Résumé

La recherche et le développement pharmaceutiques sont un processus long, complexe et coûteux, et les échecs ont souvent des origines "biologiques". Pour ces raisons, l'intêret de différents modèles alternatifs d'étude in vitro a été évalué.
L'utilisation d'hépatocytes de rat, de lapin et d'hépatocytes humains adultes en culture a permis de montrer une excellente corrélation in vitro v.s. in vivo des voies métaboliques et des vitesses de métabolisation avec plusieurs médicaments. Ainsi, en fournissant des informations précoces, utiles en chimie (prodrogues), pharmacologie (interactions médicamenteuses) et toxicologie (comparaisons inter-espèces, hépatotoxicité, mutagénèse), les hépatocytes en culture sont un outil précieux dans la recherche et le développement pharmaceutiques.

The use of primary cultures of postnatal rat hepatocytes to investigate carbon tetrachloride-induced cytotoxicity

Kenneth S. Santone, Daniel Acosta[1], Salomon A. Stavchansky, James V. Bruckner

Department of Pharmacology and Toxicology (DA, KSS) and Department of Pharmaceutics (SAS), College of Pharmacy, The University of Texas at Austin, Austin, TX 78712, USA. Department of Pharmacology and Toxicology, College of Pharmacy, University of Georgia, Athens, GA 30602 (JVB), USA

ABSTRACT

Primary cultures of postnatal rat hepatocytes were utilized to investigate the cell injury caused by carbon tetrachloride. A rapid and considerable decrease in initial CCl_4 concentration in the treatment medium resulted after equilibration of CCl_4 between the aqueous and vapor phases of the closed treatment flask. CCl_4 was metabolized to a reactive intermediate that covalently bound to cellular proteins in a dose-dependent manner. Trypan blue dye exclusion and lactate dehydrogenase (LDH) leakage were used to measure CCl_4-induced changes in membrane integrity. Loss of membrane integrity occurred in a dose-dependent manner, with LDH leakage being the more sensitive indicator. Cellular adenosine triphosphate (ATP) content was an early and sensitive marker of intracellular damage with decreases in ATP levels paralleling changes observed in membrane integrity. Microsomal glucose-6-phosphatase activity was also a sensitive cytotoxic indicator of CCl_4-induced injury. ATP-dependent microsomal calcium uptake was quickly and dramatically inhibited following both 2 mM and 4 mM CCl_4 treatment to the cultured hepatocytes. ATP-dependent mitochondrial calcium uptake was only significantly inhibited with 4 mM CCl_4. The results indicate that changes in intracellular calcium dynamics may be an important aspect in the pathological consequences of CCl_4-induced hepatotoxicity.

KEYWORDS

Carbon tetrachloride, cultured hepatocytes, intracellular calcium dynamics

---

[1]Author to Whom Correspondence and Reprint Requests Should be Addressed. DA is presently the recipient of the Burroughs Wellcome Scholar in Toxicology Award.

INTRODUCTION

Calcium and calcium-protein complexes are important in the regulation of many cellular enzymes and processes (Cheung, 1980). Hepatocytes maintain an intracellular concentration of free calcium of approximately 0.2 µM, while extracellular calcium concentration reaches 1 mM (Murphy et al., 1980). The redistribution of calcium across the plasma membrane and the changes in calcium between intracellular storage sites may well play a determinate role in cytotoxin-induced cell injury (Trump et al., 1984). Previous studies have shown that cell injury followed by cell death can be directly linked to the influx of extracellular calcium (Casini and Farber, 1981; Fariss et al., 1985). Alternatively, there have recently been reports that an increase in cytosolic calcium arising from intracellular compartments may be a more important step in the cell injury process following toxic insult (Bellomo et al., 1984; Long and Moore, 1986; Trump et al., 1984).

Primary cultures of rat hepatocytes have been used to evaluate the potential injurious effects of xenobiotics at the cellular level, thereby avoiding neural, endocrine and hemodynamic factors which may complicate the interpretation of results in vivo. Such preparations make it possible to expose uniform cell populations to precise concentrations of toxicants, and to accurately monitor the ensuing dynamic sequence of functional and structural alterations (Acosta et al., 1985; Grisham, 1979; Stammati et al., 1981). The use of cultured cells enables species- and organ-specific toxicity to be studied. The nature of the cultured cell system and the ease of its manipulation may enable an insight into a chemical mechanism that underlies toxicity by measuring a modification of a subcellular macromolecule, enzymatic reaction, or organelle as a sensitive and specific indicator of toxicity (Acosta et al., 1985).

A relationship between calcium and CCl_4-induced hepatotoxicity was first developed by Reynolds (1963), who noted an increase in cellular calcium within 15 min of CCl_4 intoxication. Judah (1969) postulated a change in intracellular calcium stores as a potential important step in CCl_4 hepatotoxicity. Importantly, Moore et al. (1976) showed that immediately following CCl_4 ingestion, ATP-dependent calcium uptake in liver microsomes was severely inhibited. Finally, Long and Moore (1986) have measured a rise in cytosolic calcium following CCl_4 treatment to cultured hepatocytes. We have investigated the cell injury process following CCl_4 treatment in our postnatal rat cultured hepatocyte test system. We have utilized sensitive, early indicators of cell damage which allow us to evaluate cell injury occurring prior to irreversible cell death. We have also correlated CCl_4-induced hepatocyte damage with changes in intracellular calcium dynamics.

MATERIALS AND METHODS

The isolation and primary culture of parenchymal hepatocytes from 10-12 day old Sprague-Dawley rats was based on the method of Acosta et al. (1980). Briefly, rat livers were dissociated following an in situ perfusion with Hank's Ca^{++}-free balanced salt solution which contained .05% collagenase Type IV (Sigma Chemical Co., St. Louis, MO) and .5% bovine serum albumin fraction V (Sigma Chemical Co.). Isolated hepatocytes were plated in 25 cm^2 culture flasks (Falcon Labware #3013, Oxnard, CA) at a concentration of 5.5×10^6 cells in 3 ml of culture medium. The culture medium used was Dulbecco-Vogt's modification of Eagle's minimum essential medium (DMEM, Grand Island Biological Co., Grand Island, NY), deficient in arginine but supplemented with 1×10^{-4} M ornithine to inhibit non-parenchymal cell overgrowth (Leffert and Paul, 1973). The culture medium was also supplement with 10% (v/v) newborn bovine serum (Grand Island Biological

Co.), 1% bovine serum albumin, 0.01 g/L insulin, 0.05 g/L hydrocortisone sodium succinate and 0.3 g/L nicotinamide (all from Sigma Chemical Co.) to maintain differentiated hepatocyte function in primary culture (Santone and Acosta, 1982). Additionally, the culture medium contained 200 units/ml potassium penicillin G, 4 µg/ml amphotericin B (both from E.R. Squibb and Sons Inc., Princeton, NJ) and 200 µg/ml of streptomycin sulfate (Pfizer Lab, Groton, CT) to inhibit microbial contamination. Cell cultures were maintained in a humidified environment of 5% CO_2 - 95% air at 37°C.

CCl_4 experiments were performed exclusively on hepatocyte cultures which had been allowed to recover for a 24 hour period after isolation. The desired amount of CCl_4 (HPLC grade, Fisher Scientific, Pittsburg, PA) was added directly to a sealed serum bottle containing culture medium minus albumin and serum to preclude any CCl_4 nonspecific binding. The bottle was mechanically shaken for 15 min to dissolve the CCl_4. Treatments were performed by removing all old culture medium from the flask, rinsing each flask twice with 3 ml of treatment medium minus CCl_4, and replacing it with 3 ml of treatment medium containing CCl_4 at the desired concentration. Treatment medium contained 1.8 mM calcium.

Actual CCl_4 concentration was measured in the treatment medium at two different time intervals. First, CCl_4 concentration was determined at the start of the treatment period. These initial treatment levels were adjusted to be at 2, 3 and 4 mM CCl_4. The concentration of CCl_4 was also measured in the medium at the end of the treatment period. CCl_4 was analyzed by a modification of the method described by Watanabe et al. (1977). Ten ml of culture medium containing CCl_4 was placed in a teflon-lined screw-capped serum test tube. To this 1 ml of a solvent/internal standard mixture (100 ml carbon disulfide/50 µl trichloroethylene) was added and the cap screwed tight. The tube is shaken vigorously for 120 seconds, then centrifuged in a table top centrifuge for 10 min at 1150 x g. The aqueous layer was removed with a Pasteur pipet and 1 µl of lipid layer injected into a Hewlett-Packard No. 5710A gas chromatograph equipped with a hydrogen/air flame ionization detector. An OV-17 column was used with nitrogen as the carrier gas. Actual CCl_4 concentrations were determined by comparison of peak height ratios with those from a known CCl_4 standard curve.

The covalent binding of $^{14}C-CCl_4$ metabolites to cellular macromolecules was measured after incubating hepatocytes with either 2 or 4 mM $^{14}C-CCl_4$ (0.061 mCi/mmol, New England Nuclear, Boston, MA). Preparation of treatment medium and cell treatments were performed exactly as previously discussed except that $^{14}C-CCl_4$ binding utilized the technique of Sipes et al. (1977) in which following $^{14}C-CCl_4$ treatment, the medium was removed and cellular macromolecules precipitated with 10% w/v trichloroacetic acid. Methanol washes were used to remove any non-covalently bound $^{14}C-CCl_4$.

The method of Acosta and Sorenson (1983) was used to determine cellular viability via trypan blue dye exclusion. Following staining of the cells with 0.1% trypan blue in phosphate buffer (pH 7.4), the average number of nonviable cells to total cells was determined in five randomly selected areas of approximately 100 cells/area using phase contrast microscopy (200 x). Leakage of cytoplasmic lactate dehydrogenase into the treatment medium was used as a sensitive indicator of changes in plasma membrane integrity, and has been described in detail elsewhere (Mitchell et al., 1980).

The methods of Debetto et al. (1982) and George et al. (1982) were modified to determine the adenosine triphosphate (ATP) levels in cultured hepatocytes. The assay utilized a luciferin-luciferase mixture (Firefly lantern extract, Sigma Chemical Co.), which was diluted in H_2O and combined in a 1:4 ratio with a buffer containing 50 mM KH_2AsO_4 in 20 mM $MGSO_4$ (pH 7.4). The assay conditions were as follows: 20 µl of ice cold sample/standard, 100 µl of room temperature 0.1 M MOPS buffer (pH 7.4) and the reaction started with 100 µl of room temperature luciferin-luciferase complex. An ATP integrating photometer (New Brunswick, Model L 3000, New Brunswick, NJ) was used to measure the enzymatic reaction for 10 sec following a 10-sec delay, which allowed the reaction tube to be vortexed and placed in the machine. Results were compared to values of samples generated from reaction mixtures of known ATP concentration. The final amount of ATP reported was corrected for the amount of total protein present in the hepatocyte sample.

The isolation of cellular organelle fractions was achieved by differential centrifugation following disruption of the cultured hepatocytes in 0.25 M sucrose as described by Hogeboom (1955). Usually, homogenates from four flasks (22×10^6 hepatocytes) were necessary to add to each centrifuge tube in order to obtain enough protein in both the mitochondrial (12,000 x g) and the microsomal (100,000 x g) fractions.

Glucose-6-phosphatase activity was determined in the microsomal fraction of cells following CCl_4 treatment to the cultured hepatocytes. The method of Baginski et al. (1974) was utilized which measured the amount of inorganic phosphate liberated from glucose-6-phosphate in the presence of glucose-6-phosphatase from the sample after complexation with ammonium molybdate. Final values were corrected for protein concentration in the microsomal fraction.

A modification of the procedure described by Moore et al. (1976) was utilized to measure mitochondrial and microsomal fraction calcium uptake following CCl_4 treatment to the cultured hepatocytes. Mitochondrial and microsomal fractions were gently resuspended in 30 mM imidazole-histidine buffer and kept on ice until assayed. ^{45}Calcium uptake was carried out in 2.0 ml incubation medium (pH 7.0) consisting of the following: 30 mM imidazole-histidine buffer, 100 mM KCl, 5 mM $MgCl_2$, 10 µM $CaCl_2$, 5 mM ammonium oxalate, 0.8 µCi ^{45}calcium (Amersham, Arlington Heights, IL), 5 mM ATP and either 1.0 mg mitochondrial protein or 0.2 mg microsomal protein. Microsomal uptake was performed with the addition of 5 mM sodium azide to the incubation medium which has been found to inhibit mitochondrial contamination uptake without affecting microsomal uptake (Moore et al., 1976). Temperature of the incubation medium was maintained at 37°C in a Dubnoff metabolic shaker. Uptake was always initiated by the addition of the subcellular fraction, with a 30-min incubation/uptake period being used. Nonspecific binding of ^{45}calcium was determined using the same conditions as described above: however, ATP was replaced with 30 mM imidazole-histidine buffer in the incubation medium. Following the 30-min incubation period, 5 ml of ice-cold 0.25 M sucrose was added to the samples. This mixture was then filtered through Whatman GF/B glass microfiber filters which had been presoaked in ice cold 0.2 M sucrose and placed in a 10-sample Hoffer filtration manifold. The sample tube and filter were immediately washed with an additional 5 ml of sucrose. Filters were transferred to scintillation vials, 15 ml of scintillation cocktail was added, and ^{45}calcium was determined with liquid scintillation counting. Counting efficiency was determined to be 95 percent. Sample values were corrected for blank ^{45}calcium binding to filters in the absence of subcellular fraction and for non ATP-dependent bound ^{45}calcium. Final values reflected the concentration of protein in the corresponding mitochondrial or microsomal sample.

All protein values were determined by the microbiuret method (Bailey, 1967). Bovine serum albumin was used as the protein standard. This was always dissolved in the same solution the samples were placed in, to avoid potential interference problems.

Analysis of variance and Student-Newman-Keuls comparisons were used to assess the statistical significance of the differences observed, P < 0.05 (Snedecor and Cochran, 1967). All values represent the mean ± S.E.M.

RESULTS

Culture hepatocytes plated in 25 cm^2 plastic flasks were exposed to either 2 mM or 4 mM CCl_4 for 15, 30, 45 or 60 min time periods. Independent of initial concentration, at the end of the 15 min treatment period, approximately 9 percent of the initial CCl_4 remained in the culture medium (Table 1). Following the 30 min treatment periods and beyond, the amount of CCl_4 that remained in the culture medium reached an equilibrium of around 3.5 percent of initial value. The large difference between initial and latter CCl_4 concentrations was postulated to occur due to the high volatility of CCl_4 at 37°C, and its subsequent presence in the vapor phase of the closed culture flask system (Watanabe et al., 1977).

Table 1. Equilibration of carbon tetrachloride in culture medium

Initial CCl_4 Dosing Concentrations	Percent of Initial CCl_4 Remaining in Culture Medium			
	15 min	30 min	45 min	60 min
2 mM	8.9 ± 0.4	3.5 ± 0.2	3.5 ± 0.2	3.1 ± 0.7
4 mM	8.5 ± 0.4	3.6 ± 0.8	3.5 ± 0.2	3.7 ± 0.6

Culture medium containing CCl_4 was removed from sealed culture flasks following the various treatment periods and analyzed for CCl_4 levels. Results represent the percentage (mean ± S.E.M., n = 4) of CCl_4 remaining in the culture medium at the various treatment times in comparison to the initial CCl_4 concentration used to treat the cells at time 0.

An index of halomethane activation was obtained by measuring the covalent binding ^{14}C-CCl_4 to hepatocyte cellular macromolecules. When the cultured hepatocytes were exposed to 2 mM ^{14}C-CCl_4, 1.70 ± 0.12 nmoles (mean ± S.E.M., n = 4) ^{14}C-CCl_4 bound per mg of cellular protein was measured after a 15 min treatment period. Covalent binding in the cultured hepatocytes was dependent on CCl_4 concentration with an approximate two-fold increase in binding to 3.32 ± 0.24 nmole (mean ± S.E.M., n = 4) ^{14}C-CCl_4 bound per mg cellular protein seen after a 15 min treatment with 4 mM ^{14}C-CCl_4. No significant increase (P < 0.05) in ^{14}C-CCl_4 binding was found if treatment periods were increased to 60 min with either 2 or 4 mM ^{14}C-CCl_4 (results not shown).

The percent of viable cells remaining after exposure to CCl_4 for durations of 15, 30, 45 or 60 min is shown in Table 2. The viability of 2 mM and 3 mM CCl_4 treated cells was similar to that of untreated controls. It was only after a 60 min treatment that 3 mM CCl_4 was able to produce a slight 11 percent decrease in viability versus control. The 4 mM CCl_4 concentration was able to reduce hepatocyte viability, although not for a 15 min treatment period. Viability was reduced a maximum of 20 percent following a 4 mM CCl_4 treatment for 60 min.

Lactate dehydrogenase leakage from cultured hepatocytes following CCl_4 treatment is shown in Fig. 1. The lowest dose tested, 2 mM CCl_4, produced similar LDH

Table 2. Percentage of viable cells as a function of dose and duration of exposure to carbon tetrachloride

Treatment	Viable Cells (%)			
	15 min	30 min	45 min	60 min
Control	92 ± 2	91 ± 2	91 ± 2	92 ± 3
2 mM CCl$_4$	90 ± 2	90 ± 3	87 ± 4	84 ± 3
3 mM CCl$_4$	90 ± 2	89 ± 2	87 ± 4	82 ± 2*
4 mM CCl$_4$	89 ± 3	83 ± 3*	80 ± 3*	75 ± 4*

Parenchymal hepatocyte viability as determined by in situ trypan blue dye exclusion tests. Control cultures contain no CCl$_4$.

*Indicates significant decrease in viability in comparison to controls, $P < 0.05$. Results represent the mean ± S.E.M. (n = 4).

leakage to that of control cultures until the 60 min treatment. Following the 60 min treatment, 2 mM CCl$_4$ produced a slight 15 percent increase in LDH leakage over control values. The 3 mM CCl$_4$ treatment produced significant increases in LDH leakage also only after a 60 min treatment. This value represented an increase of 34 percent in leakage versus untreated controls. The highest CCl$_4$ concentration tested, 4 mM, produced marked increases in LDH leakage versus control values. These increases ranged from 67 percent over control for the 15 min treatment to 172 percent increase over control for the 60 min treatment. A similar pattern of toxicity was measured when hepatocyte potassium content was substituted for LDH leakage as a sensitive marker of plasma membrane integrity (results not shown).

The dose-dependent effects of CCl$_4$ on the adenosine 5'-triphosphate (ATP) concentration of cultured hepatocytes following various treatment periods are shown in Fig. 2. The 2 mM CCl$_4$ treatment produced similar ATP values as those found in untreated controls, up to the 60 min treatment. At 60 min, 2 mM CCl$_4$ produced a 13 percent decrease in the hepatocyte ATP content versus control. The 3 mM CCl$_4$ treatment produced approximately a 20 percent decrease in ATP levels at all four time periods. The highest CCl$_4$ concentration, 4 mM, produced a marked decrease in hepatocyte ATP content, reaching 64 percent of the ATP levels found in untreated controls.

The dose-dependent effects of CCl$_4$ on glucose-6-phosphatase activity for various time periods are shown in Fig. 3. The 2 mM CCl$_4$ concentration caused little change in microsomal glucose-6-phosphatase activity, although an 18 percent decrease versus control was noted at the 60 min treatment period. Hepatocytes treated with 3 mM CCl$_4$ showed larger decreases in glucose-6-phosphatase activity at the 45 and 60 min time points, with an approximate 26 percent decrease in activity versus untreated controls observed. The 4 mM CCl$_4$ treatments caused marked reduction in microsomal glucose-6-phosphatase activity. The decreased activity versus untreated controls ranged from a 30 percent decrease at 15 min to an approximate 45 percent decrease seen after 45 min, with the 4 mM treatment.

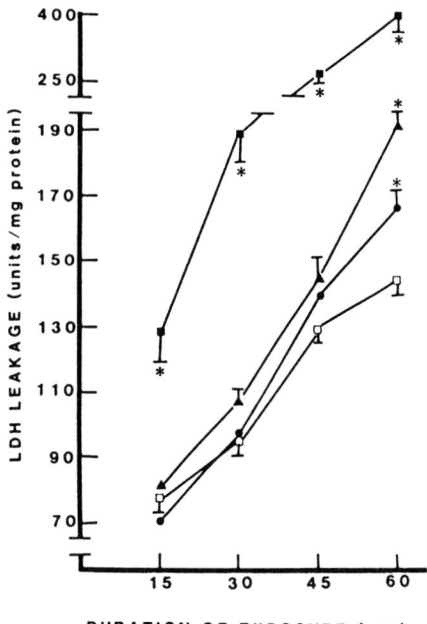
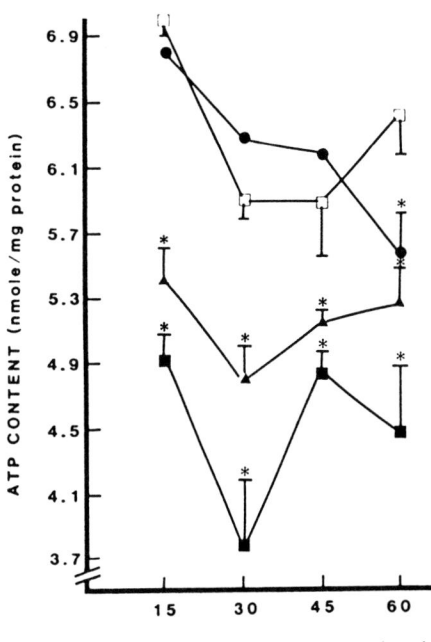

Fig. 1. Leakage of LDH in culture medium following CCl_4 treatment. Values represent the mean + S.E.M. (n = 8). *Significantly different from their respective controls, P < 0.05. (Some error bars omitted for clarity.) (□) Untreated control, (●) 2 mM CCl_4, (▲) 3 mM CCl_4 and (■) 4 mM CCl_4.

Fig. 2. Dose-dependent decrease in ATP content following CCl_4 treatment. Values represent the mean + S.E.M. (n = 6). *Significantly different from their respective controls, P < 0.05. (Some error bars omitted for clarity.) (□) Untreated controls, (●) 2 mM CCl_4, (▲) 3 mM CCl_4 and (■) 4 mM CCl_4.

ATP-dependent calcium uptake in mitochondrial and microsomal fractions following CCl_4 treatment to primary cultured hepatocytes is shown in Fig. 4. Mitochondrial calcium uptake was not significantly altered with 2 mM CCl_4. The 4 mM concentration of CCl_4 significantly decreased mitochondrial calcium uptake by 50 percent when compared to untreated control (0 mM CCl_4) fractions. ATP-dependent microsomal calcium uptake was signficantly reduced, 62 percent decrease from untreated control, when the low (2 mM) CCl_4 concentration was administered. With 4 mM CCl_4, microsomal calcium uptake was reduced to only 18 percent of untreated control values.

DISCUSSION

Although toxic effects of CCl_4 have been known since the 1920s, the exact mechanism leading to the cellular pathological consequences remains to be fully elucidated (Recknagel, 1983). Recently, emphasis on changes in calcium homeostasis has been implicated as a key step in the CCl_4-induced cell injury process.

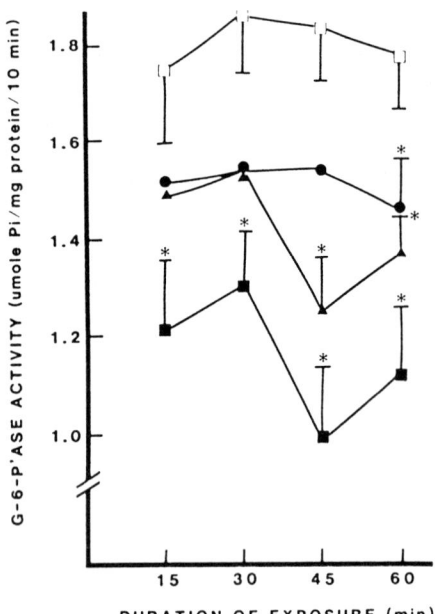
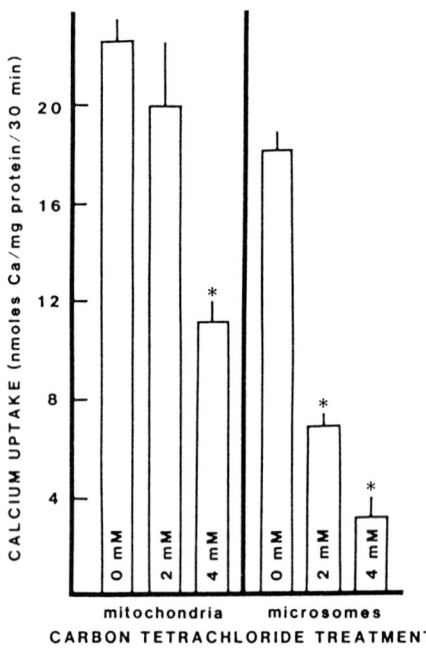

Fig. 3. Dose-dependent decrease in microsomal glucose-6-phosphatase activity following CCl_4 treatment to cultured hepatocytes. Values represent the mean ± S.E.M. (n = 4). *Significantly different from their respective controls, $P < 0.05$. (Some error bars omitted for clarity.) (□) Untreated control, (●) 2 mM CCl_4, (▲) 3 mM CCl_4 and (■) 4 mM CCl_4.

Fig. 4. ATP-dependent calcium uptake in rat liver mitochondrial and microsomal fractions from cultured rat hepatocytes treated with various concentrations of CCl_4 for 30 min. Non-ATP-dependent binding equaled 0.68 nmoles for mitochondrial fraction, 1.5 nmoles for microsomal fraction. Each value represents the mean ± S.E.M. (n = 4). *Significantly different from respective controls, $P < 0.05$.

These changes include either the influx of large amounts of extracellular calcium into the cell (Casini and Farber, 1981; Chenery et al., 1981) or changes in intracellular organelle calcium dynamics (Long and Moore, 1986; Moore, 1980; Moore et al., 1975). In the present study, primary cultures of postnatal rat hepatocytes were used as a model to investigate CCl_4-induced cell injury. An important aspect of the present study was the measurement of the actual CCl_4 in the treatment medium while utilizing a closed-flask system. A closed-flask treatment system was utilized to best control for CCl_4's volatility at 37°C. It was found that the concentration of CCl_4 in the culture medium decreased rapidly and considerably from the initial concentration following closure of the flask. This rapid equilibration of CCl_4 in closed in vitro test systems has previously been shown by Watanabe et al. (1977) with culture flasks, and also by Tyson et al. (1983) in their isolated hepatocyte test system. The decrease of CCl_4 concentration in the culture medium most likely results from the equilibration of

CCl_4 in the aqueous (medium) phase with the that found in the vapor phase of the culture flask (Watanabe et al., 1977).

Following the administration of ^{14}C-CCl_4 to our cultured hepatocytes, we were able to measure the covalent binding of ^{14}C-CCl_4 to cellular proteins. The covalent binding occurred in a dose-dependent manner at low nmole/mg protein levels, consistent with previous in vitro CCl_4 studies (Casini and Farber, 1981; Chenery et al., 1981). Since covalent binding is a measure of the activation of CCl_4 to a reactive intermediate (Gillette, 1981), this measurement has been used to indicate the capability of our cultured hepatocytes to metabolize CCl_4. In the intact animal, hepatocyte damage is dependent upon the metabolism of CCl_4 (Glende et al., 1976). Therefore, we have shown a similarity between what occurs in our in vitro system to what has been found in vivo concerning the metabolism and potential hepatotoxicity of CCl_4.

CCl_4-induced changes in membrane integrity were shown both by measurements of trypan blue cell viability and cytoplasmic LDH leakage. Cellular viability, as measured by the uptake or exclusion of trypan blue dye, was shown to be a less sensitive indicator of membrane toxicity in our cultured hepatocyte system (Table 2). This finding is consistent with previous findings from our laboratory (Mitchell and Acosta, 1981; Santone et al., 1982) as well as others (Bhuyan et al., 1976; Salocks et al., 1981). The loss of the ability for hepatocytes to exclude trypan blue dye is thought to indicate damage occurring at a late, irreversible stage (Bhuyan et al., 1976). Casini and Farber (1981), while exclusively utilizing trypan blue viability as a cytotoxic marker for CCl_4-induced hepatocyte damage, found it necessary to treat their cultures 2 to 10 hours before significant damage was measurable at equivalent concentrations of CCl_4.

It has been shown in this study, as well as by other laboratories (Chenery et al., 1981; Stacey and Priestly, 1978), that by using more sensitive indicators of membrane integrity CCl_4 damage can be found to occur within minutes. Loss of the intracellular enzyme, LDH, was shown to be a sensitive indicator of membrane toxicity induced by CCl_4 (Fig. 1). Our laboratory has previously shown the sensitivity of this cytotoxic marker (Mitchell and Acosta, 1981; Santone et al., 1982). Chenery et al. (1981) have shown LDH leakage to be a sensitive indicator of CCl_4-induced damage in their adult hepatocyte system. A question arises over whether loss of intracellular enzyme from chemically-damaged cells represents reversible or irreversible injury. Although there has been a good deal of conjecture on this point, a firm answer remains elusive (Judah et al., 1965; Trump et al., 1974). However, Grice et al. (1971) have shown that large serum enzyme changes, corresponding to the LDH leakage seen with the high 4 mM CCl_4 concentration in this study, generally occur only when cellular necrosis is present. Dose-dependent decreases in cellular ATP content were observed following CCl_4 treatment to cultured hepatocytes (Fig. 2). The decrease in ATP levels paralleled the changes observed in membrane integrity. It is known that increased ionized calcium present in the cytosol could result in a decrease in cellular ATP levels by creating an increased demand for ATP by the sodium (Judah et al., 1964) and calcium pumps (Moore et al., 1975). Also, increased cytosolic free calcium can be sequestered by the mitochondria (Reynolds, 1964). Higher levels of mitochondrial calcium have been shown to inhibit mitochondrial oxidative phosphorylation (Bygrave, 1977) therefore decreasing the ATP levels. George et al. (1982) have shown a correlation between LDH leakage and ionophore A23187-induced ATP decreases in the presence of calcium. Long and Moore (1986) have shown that cytosolic calcium does increase within 15 min following CCl_4 exposure to cultured hepatocytes. However, if an increased free cytosolic calcium is implicated in CCl_4-induced ATP decrease, it remains unclear whether cytosolic free calcium is elevated via influx of extracellular calcium interference in intracellular calcium sequestering sites or both.

CCl_4-induced changes in microsomal glucose-6-phosphatase activity occur rapidly in a dose-dependent manner (Fig. 3). This decrease in activity has been shown to be intimately related to the metabolic activation of CCl_4 and subsequent peroxidation of microsomal macromolecules (Glende et al., 1976). These changes in glucose-6-phosphatase activity in our cultured hepatocyte system parallel the changes observed following CCl_4 ingestion by rats (Moore, 1980).

CCl_4 was able to produce marked inhibition of ATP-dependent calcium uptake in microsomes following both 2 mM and 4 mM treatment to cultured hepatocytes, and in mitochondria following 4 mM CCl_4 (Fig. 4). Previously, the inhibition of microsomal calcium uptake following CCl_4 exposure has been shown both in vivo (Moore et al., 1976) and in cultured hepatocytes (Long and Moore, 1986). This is the first report of CCl_4-induced inhibition of mitochondrial calcium uptake, which only occurred at the highest CCl_4 concentration, 4 mM. It is thought that the 4 mM treatment in our test system represents a lethal, non-recoverable dose of CCl_4. The 2 mM concentration of CCl_4 caused significant inhibition of microsomal calcium uptake at time points where damage was not observed with other cytotoxic indicators. Also, the relative amount of inhibition of calcium uptake activity versus control was far greater than any other CCl_4-induced change observed, for the time periods measured. Therefore, it is felt that changes in microsomal calcium pump activity are an early, sensitive marker of CCl_4-induced hepatocyte injury that may precede other CCl_4-induced damage in the cell.

The inhibition of intracellular organelle calcium pump activity interferes with the normal pathways of calcium metabolism and homeostasis in the liver. The inhibition of calcium pump activity should increase the level of free cytoplasmic calcium. This increase in calcium may be responsible for changes seen following CCl_4-induced cell injury. It has been shown that CCl_4-induced inhibition of microsomal calcium pump activity elevates cytosolic calcium in cultured hepatocytes (Long and Moore, 1986). Lamb and Schwartz (1982) have shown that CCl_4 may activate calcium-dependent hepatic phospholipase C activity, increase diacylglycerol content, and cause a rapid degradation of structural phosphoglycerides. These phospholipid changes may be important in CCl_4-induced changes in plasma membrane permeability. Jewell et al. (1982) have related chemical-induced plasma membrane blebbing to increased cytoplasmic calcium lost from intracellular calcium sequestering sites. The above reports, combined with our present results, indicate that early changes in intracellular calcium dynamics may play a large role in CCl_4-induced cytotoxicity.

REFERENCES

Acosta, D., Anuforo, D.C., Smith, R.V. (1980): Preparation of primary monolayer cultures of postnatal rat liver cells. J. Tissue Cult. Meth. 6, 35-37.
Acosta, D., Sorensen, E.M. (1983): Role of calcium in cytotoxic injury of cultured hepatocytes. Ann. N.Y. Acad. Sci. 407, 78-92.
Acosta, D., Sorensen, E.M.B., Anuforo, D.C., Mitchell, D.B., Ramos, K., Santone, K.S., Smith, M.A. (1985): An in vitro approach to the study of target organ toxicity of drugs and chemicals. In Vitro Cell. Develop. Biol. 21, 495-504.
Baginski, E.S., Foa, P.P., Zak, B. (1974): Glucose-6-phosphatase. In Methods of Enzymatic Analysis, ed. I. Gutmann and H.U. Bergmeyer, pp 1794-1797. New York: Academic Press.
Bailey, J.L. (1967): Estimation of protein. In Techniques in Protein Chemistry, pp 341, New York: Elsevier Publishing Co.
Bellomo, G., Thor, H., Orrenius, S. (1984): Increase in cytosolic Ca^{2+} concentration during t-butyl hydroperoxide metabolism by isolated hepatocytes involves NADPH oxidation and mobilization of intracellular Ca^{2+} stores. FEBS Lett. 168, 38-42.

Bhuyan, B.K., Loughman, B.E., Fraser, T.J., Day, K.J. (1976): Comparison of different methods of determining cell viability after exposure to cytotoxic compounds. Exp. Cell Res. 97, 275-280.

Bygrave, F.L. (1977): Mitochondrial calcium transport. In Current Topics in Bioenergetics, Volume 6, ed. by D.R. Sanadi, pp 259-318. New York: Academic Press.

Casini, A.F., Farber, J.L. (1981): Dependence of the carbon tetrachloride-induced death of cultured hepatocytes on the extracellular calcium concentration. Am. J. Pathol. 105, 138-148.

Chenery, R., George, M., Krishna, G. (1981): The effect of ionophore A23187 and calcium on carbon tetrachloride-induced toxicity in cultured rat hepatocytes. Toxicol. Appl. Pharmacol. 60, 241-252.

Cheung, W.Y. (1980): Calmodulin plays a pivotal role in cellular regulation. Science 207, 19-27.

Debetto, P., Dal Toso, R., Varotto, R., Bianchi, V., Luciani, S. (1982): Effects of potassium dichromate on ATP content of mammalian cells cultured in vitro. Chem. Biol. Inter. 41, 15-24.

Fariss, M.W., Pascoe, G.A., Reed, D.J. (1985): Vitamin E reversal of the effect of extracellular calcium on chemically-induced toxicity in hepatocytes. Science 227, 751-754.

George, M., Chenery, R.J., Krishna, G. (1982): The effect of ionophore A23187 and 2,4-dinitrophenol on the structure and function of cultured liver cells. Toxicol. Appl. Pharmacol. 66, 349-360.

Gillette, J.R. (1981): An integrated approach to the study of chemically reactive metabolites of acetaminophen. Arch. Int. Med. 141, 375-379.

Glende, E.A., Hruszkewycz, A.M., Recknagel, R.O. (1976): Critical role of lipid peroxidation in carbon tetrachloride-induced loss of aminopyrine demethylase, cytochrome P-450 and glucose-6-phosphatase. Biochem. Pharmacol. 25, 2163-2170.

Grice, H.C., Barth, M.L., Cornish, H.H., Foster, G.V., Gray, R.H. (1971): Correlation between serum enzymes, isozyme patterns and histologically detectable organ damage. Food Cosmet. Toxicol. 9, 847-855.

Hogeboom, G. (1955): Fractionation of cell components of animal tissues. In Methods of Enzymology, Volume 1, ed. by S. Colowick and N. Kaplan, pp 16-19. New York: Academic Press.

Jewell, S.A., Bellomo, G., Thor, H., Orrenius, S., Smith, M.T. (1982): Bleb formation in hepatocytes during drug metabolism is caused by disturbances in thiol and calcium ion homeostasis. Science 217, 1257-1259.

Judah, J.D. (1969): Biochemical disturbances in liver injury. Brit. Med. Bull. 25, 274-277.

Judah, J.D., Ahmed, K., McLean, A.E. (1964): Possible role of ion shifts in liver injury. In Ciba Symposium on Cellular Injury, ed. by A.V. de Rebuck and J.P. Knight, pp 187-205. London: Churchill.

Judah, J.D., Ahmed, K., McLean, A.E. (1965): Pathogenesis of cell necrosis. Fed. Proc. 24, 1217-1221.

Lamb, R.G., Schwertz, D.W. (1982): The effects of bromobenzene and carbon tetrachloride exposure in vitro on the phospholipase C activity of rat cells. Toxicol. Appl. Pharmacol. 63, 216-229.

Leffert, H., Paul, D. (1973): Serum dependent growth of primary cultured differentiated fetal rat hepatocytes in arginine-deficient medium. J. Cell. Physiol. 81, 113-124.

Long, R.M., Moore, L. (1986): Elevated cytosolic calcium in rat hepatocytes exposed to carbon tetrachloride. J. Pharmacol. Exp. Ther. 238, 186-191.

Mitchell, D.B., Acosta, D. (1981): Evaluation of the cytotoxicity of tricyclic antidepressants in primary cultures of rat hepatocytes. J. Toxicol. Environ. Hlth. 7, 83-92.

Mitchell, D.B., Santone, K.S., Acosta, D. (1980): Evaluation of cytotoxicity in cultured cells by enzyme leakage. J. Tissue Cult. Meth. 6, 113-116.

Moore, L. (1980): Inhibition of liver-microsome calcium pump by in vivo administration of CCl_4, CHl_3 and 1,1-dichloroethylene. Biochem. Pharmacol. 29, 2505-2511.

Moore, L., Chen, T., Knapp, H.R., Landon, E.J. (1975): Energy-dependent calcium sequestration activity in rat liver microsomes. J. Biol. Chem. 250, 4562-4568.

Moore, L., Davenport, G.R., Landon, E.J. (1976): Calcium uptake of a rat liver microsomal subcellular fraction in response to in vivo administration of carbon tetrachloride. J. Biol. Chem. 251, 1197-1201.

Murphy, E., Coll, K., Rich, T.L., Williamson, J.R. (1980): Hormonal effects on calcium homeostasis in isolated hepatocytes. J. Biol. Chem. 255, 6600-6608.

Recknagel, R.O. (1983): Carbon tetrachloride hepatotoxicity: Status quo and future prospects. Trends Pharmacol. Sci. 4, 129-131.

Reynolds, E.S. (1963): Liver parenchymal cell injury: I. Initial alterations of the cell following poisoning with carbon tetrachloride. J. Cell. Biol. 19, 139-157.

Reynolds, E.S. (1964): Liver parenchymal cell injury: II. Cytochemical events concerned with mitochondrial dysfunction following poisoning with carbon tetrachloride. Lab. Invest. 13, 1457-1470.

Salocks, C.B., Hsieh, D.P., Byard, J.L. (1981): Butylated hydroxytoluene pretreatment protects against cytotoxicity and reduces covalent binding of aflatoxin B_1 in primary hepatocyte cultures. Toxicol. Appl. Pharmacol. 59, 331-345.

Santone, K.S., Acosta, D. (1982): Measurement of functional metabolic activity as a sensitive parameter of cytotoxicity in cultured hepatocytes. J. Tissue Cult. Meth. 7, 137-142.

Santone, K.S., Acosta, D., Bruckner, J.V. (1982): Cadmium toxicity in primary cultures of rat hepatocytes. J. Toxicol. Environ. Hlth. 10, 169-177.

Sipes, G., Krishna, G., Gillette, J.R. (1977): Bioactivation of carbon tetrachloride, chloroform and bromotrichloromethane: Role of cytochrome P-450. Life Sci. 20, 1541-1548.

Snedecor, G.W., Cochran, W.G. (1967): In Statistical Methods, pp 273-275. Ames, IA: Iowa State University Press.

Stacey, N., Priestly, B.G. (1978): Dose-dependent toxicity of carbon tetrachloride in isolated rat hepatocytes and the effects of hepatoprotective treatments. Toxicol. Appl. Pharmacol. 45, 29-39.

Trump, B.F., Berezesky, I.K., Sato, T., Laiho, K.U., Phelps, P.C., DeClaris, N. (1984): Cell calcium, cell injury, cell death. Environ. Hlth. Perspect. 57, 281-287.

Trump, B.F., Laiho, K.A., Mergner, W.J., Arstila, A.U. (1974): Studies on the subcellular pathophysiology of acute lethal cell injury. Beitr. Path. 152, 243-271.

Tyson, C.A., Hawk-Prather, K., Story, D.L., Gould, D.H. (1983): Correlations of in vitro and in vivo hepatotoxicity for five haloalkanes. Toxicol. Appl. Pharmacol. 70, 289-302.

Watanabe, S., Hioki, M., Mohri, T., Kitagawa, H. (1977): Transaminases of hepatic tissue culture cells and the effect of carbon tetrachloride on their leakage. Chem. Pharm. Bull. 25, 1089-1093.

Résumé

Des cultures primaires d'hépatocytes de rat nouveau-né ont été utilisées pour étudier les lésions cellulaires provoquées par le tétrachlorure de carbone. Une diminution rapide et importante de la concentration initiale en CCl_4 dans le milieu traité est observée après équilibre entre les phases aqueuse et gazeuse du flacon fermé. Le CCl_4 est métabolisé en un métabolite réactif qui se fixe de manière covalente sur les protéines cellulaires. Cette fixation est dose-dépendante. Le test d'exclusion au bleu trypan et la sortie de lacticodeshydrogénase (LDH) ont été retenus pour mesurer les altérations de l'intégrité membranaire induite par le CCl_4. La perte de celle-ci est dose-dépendante, la sortie de LDH étant l'indicateur le plus sensible. Le contenu en ATP intracellulaire est un marqueur précoce et sensible de lésions intracellulaires ; une baisse en ATP est parallèle aux modifications de l'intégrité membranaire. L'activité de la glucose 6 phosphatase microsomale est également un indicateur sensible de la cytotoxicité induite par le CCl_4. Le captage de calcium dans les microsomes ATP-dépendant est rapidement et fortement inhibé par traitement d'hépatocytes en culture par 2 mM et 4 mM de CCl_4. En revanche, la captage de calcium ATP-dépendant dans les mitochondries est seulement faiblement réduit en présence de 4 mM de CCl_4. Ces résultats indiquent que des variations dans les teneurs intracellulaires en calcium peuvent constituer un aspect important des conséquences pathologiques d'une hépatotoxicité induite par le CCl_4.

Drug metabolism and cytotoxicity in long-term cultured hepatocytes

André Guillouzo, Jean-Marc Bégué, Damrong Ratanasavanh, Christophe Chesné, Bernard Meunier*, Christiane Guguen-Guillouzo

*INSERM, U.49, Unité de Recherches Hépatologiques and *Clinique Chirurgicale B Hôpital Pontchaillou, 35033 Rennes Cedex, France*

Keywords : Hepatocytes, long-term culture, drug metabolism, drug cytotoxicity.

ABSTRACT

Isolated hepatocytes from various species, either in suspension or in culture, have been widely used for pharmacological and toxicological studies in recent years. However, since the cells exhibit rapid phenotypic changes in culture, they have been mainly used for short-term investigations, i.e. identification of metabolic pathways and acute toxicity assessment. Co-culturing hepatocytes from various species with undifferentiated rat liver epithelial cells makes it possible to design long-term experiments since in these conditions parenchymal cells retain the capability of expressing phase I and phase II drug reactions for several days or weeks. For various drugs the same metabolites as in vivo have been demonstrated for several days and chronic toxicity studies have been devised based on daily addition of a given drug for 2-3 weeks. All the results emphasize the interest of this model system and underline the importance of several parameters, i.e. culture conditions and the choice of cytotoxicity endpoints for predicting metabolic pathways and cytotoxicity of new drugs. Cultured hepatocytes represent a unique system for various studies on drugs, including pharmacokinetics, identification and production of metabolites, demonstration of drug interactions, and screening of new molecules.

INTRODUCTION

With the current trend of reducing laboratory animal experimentation for both ethical and financial reasons there is an increasing interest in alternative model systems for studying drug metabolism and cytotoxicity. These models include perfused organs, tissue slices, isolated cells, subcellular fractions and purified enzymes. Since the liver is the primary organ involved in drug metabolism a number of studies have already been performed with in vitro liver models. Intact hepatocytes either in suspension or in culture are more easily characterized and therefore more reproducible than organ cultures or organ slices. In addition cultured cells are theorically a suitable model for long-term investigations.

Most of the studies have been carried out with rodent cells (Fry and Bridges, 1979 ; Sirica and Pitot, 1981 ; Guillouzo, 1986). However, in view of the qualitative and quantitative interspecies differences which commonly exist in hepatic metabolism of xenobiotics, the validity of such extrapolation is open to question. The recent development of experimental conditions for the isolation of large yields of viable human hepatocytes should overcome these major shortcomings (Guguen-Guillouzo et al., 1986). However, losses in the most differentiated functions are well documented in hepatocyte cultures from various species (Guguen-Guillouzo and Guillouzo, 1983). In particular, monooxygenase activities rapidly decline. In conventional culture conditions, the cytochrome P-450 level falls to less than 20-40 % after 2 days in rodent hepatocytes (Guzelian et al., 1977 ; Fahl et al., 1979 ; Lake and Paine, 1982). By contrast human hepatocytes are more stable, containing 50-60 % of their initial cytochrome P-450 content after 5-6 days (Guillouzo et al., 1985). This observation is of particular importance since a number of factors may influence functional activities of human hepatocytes during the first hours following cell isolation. These factors, listed in Table I include not only those related to the donor but also those related to the conditions of cell isolation. Taking into account these shortcomings which may lead to the retention of functional values which can be quite variable from one cell population to another, we have attempted to define which culture conditions should allow the use of hepatocyte cultures for long-term studies on both drug metabolism and cytotoxicity. Recently, we have developed a co-culture system in which hepatocytes are associated with another liver cell type, probably derived from primitive biliary cells and which allows parenchymal cells from various species including man to survive much longer than in conventional culture (1-3 months versus 2-3 weeks) and to maintain various specific functions at high levels (Guguen-Guillouzo et al., 1983, 1986). As an example, the production of various plasma proteins, including albumin, hemopexin and haptoglobin remain relatively constant for several weeks (Guillouzo et al., 1984). The expression of these specific functions was found to be coupled with the maintenance of transcription activity of the corresponding genes (Fraslin et al., 1985). This model can be maintained in a serum-free medium but the presence of corticosteroids is required (Guguen-Guillouzo et al., 1983). Its interest for long-term studies on both drug metabolism and cytotoxicity is discussed here.

TABLE I : FACTORS WHICH MAY INFLUENCE FUNCTIONAL ACTIVITY OF FRESHLY ISOLATED HEPATOCYTES (From Guillouzo et al., 1987b).

Factors related to the donor
- Physiologic : age, sex
- Genetic
- Pathological : liver diseases
- Environmental : premedication, duration of coma, nutritional status.

Factors related to the isolation process
- Time between liver removal and dissociation
- Conditions of liver preservation before perfusion (temperature, washing with a buffer...)
- Cell viability.

DRUG METABOLISM

A number of studies have demonstrated the usefulness of isolated hepatocytes either in suspension or in short-term culture for analyses of drug metabolism and pharmacokinetics (Dumont et al., 1985 ; Guillouzo, 1986 ; Rogiers et al., 1987 ; Grislain et al., 1988 ; Rogiers et al., 1986 ; Ratanasavanh et al., 1988b). Species differences can be demonstrated (Chenery et al., 1987 ; Le Bigot et al. 1987). As an example Le Bigot et al. (1987) have shown that ketotifen was metabolized by different pathways in primary cultures of rat, rabbit and human hepatocytes. These pathways were the same as those found in vivo in the corresponding species. However after 2 days metabolic activity was markedly decreased in rodent hepatocytes indicating profound phenotypic changes in these cells. These observations together with others (Guguen-Guillouzo and Guillouzo, 1983) clearly indicate that pure hepatocyte cultures do not represent an appropriate system for studying drug induction and interactions.

Several studies performed in our laboratory during recent years support the idea that the co-culture system could be a model candidate for studies requiring long-term incubation of drugs with liver cells. Indeed when maintained in co-culture both rat and human hepatocytes retain a high cytochrome P-450 content for more than one week (Bégué et al., 1984 ; Guillouzo et al., 1985). Moreover, we have shown that cytochrome P-450 isozymes which are representative of the two major cytochrome P-450 families in human liver remain expressed in co-culture. One form, which oxidizes nifedipine and is preferentially located in centrilobular and mediolobular hepatocytes, was detected only in a fraction of cultured cells suggesting that there was no cell selection during the isolation process and maintenance of the functional heterogeneity in vitro (Ratanasavanh et al., 1986). Cytochrome P-450 responds to drugs. After 3 daily treatments with 3.2 mM sodium phenobarbital a 2-fold increase in the total cytochrome P-450 level was demonstrated in 9 days old human hepatocyte co-cultures (Guillouzo et al., 1985). Similarly after 3 daily treatments with erythromycin estolate, co-cultured rat hepatocytes were found to contain complexed cytochrome P-450 as previously described in vivo after administration of this antibiotic (Villa et al., 1985).

TABLE II : Relative percentage of unchanged ketotifen and metabolites found after a 24 hours incubation with adult human hepatocytes maintained either in pure or in co-culture for various times.

Culture	Age of the culture	Unchanged Ketotifen	Reduced Ketotifen	N-glucuronide
Pure culture	4 hours	25	48	25
	4 days	13	61	26
	6 days	50	50	0
Co-culture	4 days	13	43	44
	7 days	6	29	65
	21 days	29	59	12

The results are from Bégué et al., 1983.

In parallel with a prolonged maintenance of cytochrome P-450, co-cultured hepatocytes exhibit a longer capability of metabolizing drugs. Thus, ketotifen, which is converted to two major metabolites in humans, namely reduced ketotifen and a glucuronide, in humans was also found to give these two products in primary culture of human hepatocytes. However, the glucuronide was formed only during the first 4 days in pure culture while it still represented 12 % of the total metabolites formed in 21 days co-culture (Bégué et al., 1983) (Table II). More recently, we found that metabolism of pindolol and fluperlapine was also well maintained in 8 day human hepatocyte co-culture (Guillouzo et al., 1988). Interestingly metabolism of this latter involved various pathways including oxidation, demethylation, glucuronidation and sulphation which were all demonstrated in vitro even after 8 days.

Similarly, biotransformation of paracetamol was found to be maintained for a much longer period in rat hepatocyte co-culture. Oxidation and glucuronidation pathways remained high in co-culture over a 15 days study while in pure culture they declined markedly after 3-4 days. The sulphation pathway was also demonstrated ; it decreased in both cultures although at a lower extent after 3-5 days (Chesné et al., 1988).

In most cases, the major metabolites found in vivo were identified in vitro. However, it must be remembered that in vivo drugs can also be transformed in extrahepatic tissues and that in culture the drug metabolizing enzyme profile undergoes more or less marked qualitative and quantitative changes. Some enzymes or isozymes are more sensitive to culture conditions. Vandenberghe et al. (1988) have recently demonstrated that glutathione transferase activity may greatly change with subtle modifications in the composition of the nutrient medium.

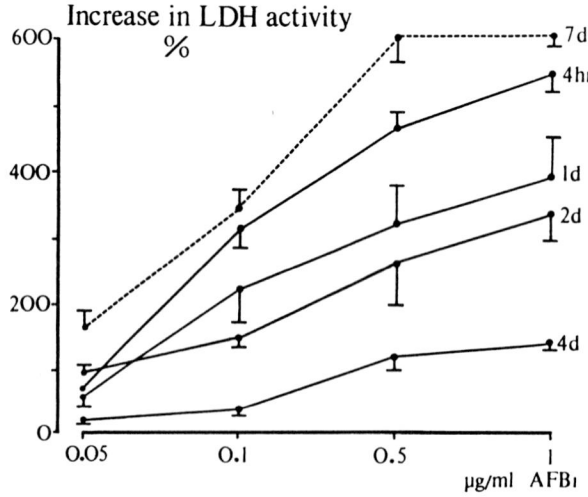

Figure 1 : Cytotoxicity of aflatoxin B_1 to rat hepatocytes maintained either in pure culture or in co-culture.
The mycotoxin was added to the medium of 4, 24, 48 and 96 h pure culture (——) and 7 days co-culture (- - -) and lactate dehydrogenase leakage was measured 24 h later. Each point and vertical bar represent the mean ± S.E. of four separate experiments (From Bégué et al., 1984).

DRUG CYTOTOXICITY

Most studies on xenobiotic cytotoxicity have dealt with the effect of a single dose added for a short period ranging between 1 and 24 hours and the effects have been monitored by numerous endpoints which measure membrane integrity or cellular functions. The most commonly used indicators of toxicity are trypan blue exclusion, leakage of lactate dehydrogenase, cell survival, cell morphology and protein synthesis level. The sensitivity and usefulness of each endpoint depend on the chemical tested. It has been suggested to select at least two endpoints (Vonen and Morland, 1984) and our experience agrees with this conclusion. Parameters which assess liver function are usually more sensitive than those which measure membrane integrity. In addition, it must be emphasized that cell injury can be greatly influenced by the environment and the ability of the cells to take up the compound. The composition of the medium (presence or absence of exogenous proteins, calcium concentration...) may be critical. Nevertheless, it is now well established that toxicity testing represents a simple and appropriate way to screen new molecules.

However, such a short-term assay does not reflect the common <u>in vivo</u> situation in which drugs often induce liver damage after only several days or months. Hepatotoxicity may be related to enzyme induction or drug interactions. This led us to use the co-culture system as an <u>in vitro</u> model for long-term drug toxicity assessment. A first study was performed with aflatoxin B_1. This mycotoxin is known to induce toxic effects after biotransformation by the cytochrome P-450-dependent system. While its toxicity decreased strongly with age in pure rat hepatocyte culture it remained high when 7 day co-cultures were used suggesting that the cytochrome P-450 isozyme involved in the formation of reactive metabolites was still active (Fig. 1).

Usually a typical study is conducted as follows. A series of drug concentrations (10^{-7} M to 10^{-2} M, if the drug is still soluble at this concentration) is tested over a 24 h period on 4 h rat hepatocyte cultures. Morphological changes visible under phase-contrast microscopy and lactate dehydrogenase leakage are used as endpoints. For long-term analyses, 3 or 4 concentrations are selected, the highest giving only minor morphological changes and/or increased lactate dehydrogenase activity in the medium after 24 h of treatment. The drug is first added to co-cultures after cell confluency is reached, i.e. 24-48 h after hepatocyte seeding and daily thereafter for 2-4 weeks (Ratanasavanh et al., 1988a). Depending on the drug tested, four situations can be observed : 1 -no cytotoxicity to both cell types is observed ; 2 - only hepatocytes are damaged ; 3 - only rat liver epithelial cells are damaged ; 4 - both cell types are sensitive to the drug. As found in acute toxicity testing major differences in the sensitivity of endpoints depending on the chemical tested may be noticed. As an example high concentrations of dantrium ($10^{-4} - 10^{-3}$ M) strongly inhibited albumin production while they had no obvious effect on lactate dehydrogenase leakage in adult rat hepatocyte co-cultures (Delval C., Rissel M. and Guillouzo A., unpublished observations) (Fig. 2).

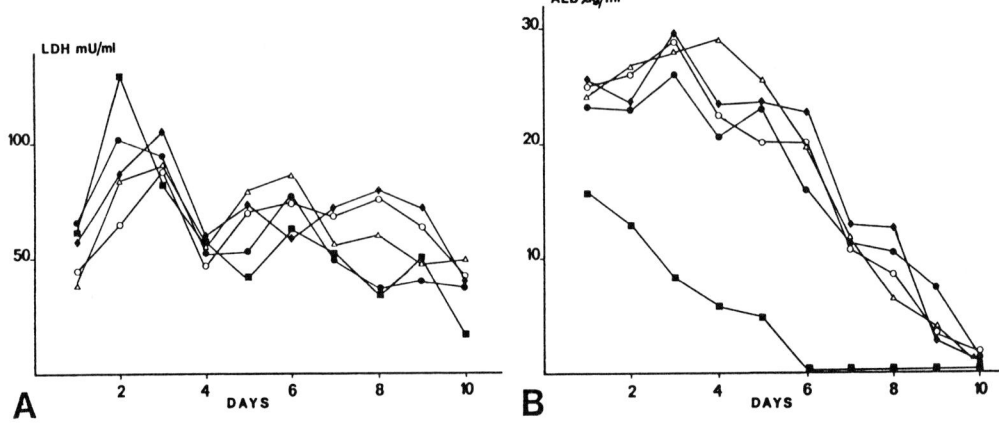

Figure 2 : Cytotoxicity of dantrium to rat hepatocyte co-cultures.
Dantrium dissolved in 1,2 propandiol was added daily at various concentrations. Lactate dehydrogenase activity (A) and albumin secretion levels (B) were measured daily in the medium. Each point represents the mean of three dishes from a typical experiment.
[Co-cultures treated with 10^{-4} M (■), 10^{-5} M (♦), 10^{-6} M (●) dantrium or with the solvent alone (△) ; control co-cultures (○)].

CONCLUSIONS AND PERSPECTIVES

Although the use of isolated hepatocytes as a model system in pharmacology and toxicology suffers from the absence of well-defined experimental conditions making it difficult for interlaboratory comparisons, there is no doubt that this model has already brought major advances in the study of pharmacokinetics, metabolic pathways and mechanism of hepatotoxicity. It is conceivable that within a few years this model will be included in the battery of tests which are obligatory in the course of development of new drugs. This will come from further evaluation of in vivo/in vitro correlations and endpoints of cytotoxicity and from multicentric studies. Considerable money and time will be saved from screening of new drugs and analogs and from species comparisons of both metabolism and cytotoxicity. Long-term experiments are required for various studies including drug interactions and chronic toxicity. Our results suggest that co-culture could represent an appropriate system. It may be underlined that both immature and mature hepatocytes from various species are able to interact with undifferentiated rat liver epithelial cells (Guguen-Guillouzo et al., 1984, 1986 ; Lescoat et al., 1985). A recent study has shown that liver endothelial cells are also capable of interacting with hepatocytes (Morin et al., 1986). Other conditions have been proposed for the maintenance of adult hepatocytes in a differentiated state for prolonged periods including addition of dimethylsulfoxide to the culture medium (Isom et al., 1985) and the use of a laminin-rich gel as a support (Bissell et al., 1987).

A number of studies have reported differences in both the rates and the routes of drug metabolism particularly when comparisons involved experimental animals and man. Therefore there is an increasing need to perform experiments directly on human hepatocytes. However, although these cells may be obtained in large numbers from a single perfusion, availability of human samples is irregular and rare. Consequently a method for successfully storing cells in excess is highly desirable (Guillouzo et al., 1987a). Our recent studies on rat hepatocytes indicate that about 50 % of the cells which attach to plastic just after isolation are still able to attach after cryopreservation in liquid nitrogen (Chesné et al., 1988). Just after thawing the cells exhibit some functional damage which requires several hours for repair. This can be achieved only when the cells are set up in co-culture. The same observations have been made with rat and human hepatocytes. This suggests that we have now the conditions to establish a bank of frozen hepatocytes from various donors, making possible analysis of genetic polymorphism in vitro.

Liver cell cultures are suitable for studying direct (predictable) toxicity. However, it is well known that several drugs are hepatotoxic only in a few percentage of treated patients, often related to a immunoallergic phenomenon. The design of appropriate culture conditions for the detection of such drugs would be a major progress and represents a new step in the development of safe and efficent drugs.

ACKNOWLEDGMENTS

The authors thank Mrs Annie Vannier for typing the manuscript. Personal work was funded by INSERM, MRES and the Fundation for Medical Research.

REFERENCES

Bégué, J.M., Le Bigot, J.F., Guguen-Guillouzo, C., Kiechel, J.R. and Guillouzo, A. (1983): Cultured human adult hepatocytes : a new model for drug metabolism studies. Biochem. Pharmacol. 32, 1643-1646.

Bégué, J.M., Guguen-Guillouzo, C., Pasdeloup, N. and Guillouzo, A. (1984): Prolonged maintenance of active cytochrome P-450 in adult rat hepatocytes co-cultured with another liver cell type. Hepatology 4, 839-842.

Bissell, D.M., Arenson, D.M., Maher, J.J. and Roll, F.J. (1987): Support of cultured hepatocytes by a laminin-rich gel. J. Clin. Invest. 79, 801-812.

Chenery, R.J., Ayrton, A., Oldham, H.G., Standring, P., Norman, S.J., Seddon, T. and Kirby, R. (1987) : Diazepam metabolism in cultured hepatocytes from rat, rabbit, dog, guinea pig and man. Drug Metab. Dispos. 15, 312-317.

Chesné, C., Gripon, P. and Guillouzo, A. (1988): Primary culture of cryopreserved rat hepatocytes. In Liver Cells and Drugs, ed. Guillouzo A. INSERM : Paris, John Libbey Eurotext : London (this volume).

Dumont, M., De Couet, G., Le Bigot, J.F., Erlinger, S. (1985): Mechanism of uptake of dihydroergotamine by isolated rat hepatocytes : effect of troleandomycin. J. Pharmacol. Exp. Ther. 234, 239-243.

Fahl, W.E., Michalopoulos, G., Sattler, G.L., Jefcoate, C.R., Pitot, H.C. (1979): Characteristics of microsomal enzyme controls in primary cultures of rat hepatocytes. Arch. Biochem. Biophys. 192, 61-72.

Fraslin, J.M., Kneip, B., Vaulont, S., Glaise, D., Munnich, A. and Guguen-Guillouzo, C. (1985): Dependence of hepatocyte-specific gene expression on cell-cell interactions in primary culture. EMBO J. 4, 2487-2491.

Fry, J.R. and Bridges, J.W. (1979): Use of primary hepatocyte cultures in biochemical toxicology. Rev. Biochem. Toxicol. 1, 201-247.

Grislain, L., Ratanasavanh, D., Mocquard, M.T., Raquillet, L., Bégué, J.M., du Vignaud, P., Genissel, P., Guillouzo, A. and Bromet, N. (1988): Primary cultures of rat and human hepatocytes as a model system for the evaluation of cytotoxicity and metabolic pathways of a new drug : S-3341. In Liver Cells and Drugs, ed. Guillouzo A. INSERM : Paris, John Libbey Eurotext : London (this volume).

Guguen-Guillouzo, C. and Guillouzo, A. (1983): Modulation of functional activities in cultured rat hepatocytes. Mol. Cell. Biochem. 53/54, 35-56.

Guguen-Guillouzo, C., Clément, B., Baffet, G., Beaumont, C., Morel-Chany, E., Glaise, D. and Guillouzo, A. (1983): Maintenance and reversibility of active albumin secretion by adult rat hepatocytes co-cultured with another liver epithelial cell type. Exp. Cell Res. 143, 47-54.

Guguen-Guillouzo C., Clément, B., Lescoat, G., Glaise, D. and Guillouzo, A. (1984): Modulation of human fetal hepatocyte survival and differentiation by interactions with a rat liver epithelial cell line. Develop. Biol. 105, 211-220.

Guguen-Guillouzo, C., Bourel, M. and Guillouzo, A. (1986): Human hepatocyte cultures. In Progress in Liver Diseases, eds. Popper H. and Schaffner F., Grune & Stratton, New York, vol. 8, pp. 33-50.

Guillouzo, A. (1986): Use of isolated and cultured hepatocytes for xenobiotic metabolism and cytotoxicity studies. In Isolated and cultured hepatocytes, eds. Guillouzo A. and Guguen-Guillouzo C. INSERM : Paris, John Libbey Eurotext : London pp. 313-332.

Guillouzo, A., Delers, F., Clément, B., Bernard, N. and Engler, R. (1984): Long-term production of acute-phase proteins by adult rat hepatocytes co-cultured with another liver cell type in serum-free medium. Biochem. Biophys. Res. Commun. 120, 311-317.

Guillouzo, A., Beaune, P., Gascoin, M.N., Bégué, J.M., Campion, J.P., Guengerich, F.P. and Guguen-Guillouzo, C. (1985): Maintenance of cytochrome P-450 in cultured adult human hepatocytes. Biochem. Pharmacol. 34, 2991-2995.

Guillouzo, A., Chesné, C., Ratanasavanh, D., Campion, J.P. and Guguen-Guillouzo, C. (1987a): Preservation of human liver cells and their function. In Drug metabolism from molecules to man. Benford D.J., Bridges J.W., Gibson G.G. Taylor & Francis, London, pp. 423-435.

Guillouzo, A., Ratanasavanh, D., Bégué, J.M. and Guguen-Guillouzo, C. (1987b): Utilisation des hépatocytes isolés pour l'évaluation de l'hépatotoxicité des médicaments. In Développement et Evaluation du Médicament. 3ème Colloque INSERM-DphM : INSERM Paris. Vol. 157, 163-174.

Guillouzo, A., Bégué, J.M., Maurer, G. and Koch, P. (1988): Identification of metabolic pathways of pindolol and fluperlapine in adult human hepatocyte cultures. Xenobiotica (in press).

Guzelian, P.S., Bissell, D.M., Meyer, U.A. (1977): Drug metabolism in adult rat hepatocytes in primary monolayer culture. <u>Gastroenterology 72</u>, 1232-1239.

Isom, H.C., Secott, T., Georgoff, I., Woodworth, C. and Mummaw, J. (1985): Maintenance of differentiated rat hepatocytes in primary culture. <u>Proc. Natl. Acad. Sci. USA 82</u>, 3252-3256.

Lake B.G., Paine, A.J. (1982): The effect of hepatocyte culture conditions on cytochrome P-450-linked drug metabolizing enzymes. <u>Biochem. Pharmacol. 31</u>, 2141-2144.

Le Bigot, J.F., Bégué, J.M., Kiechel, J.R. and Guillouzo, A. (1987): Species differences in metabolism of ketotifen in rat, rabbit and man : demonstration of similar pathways in vivo and in cultured hepatocytes. <u>Life Sci. 40</u>, 883-890.

Lescoat, G., Thézé, N., Clément, B., Guillouzo, A. and Guguen-Guillouzo, C. (1985): Modulation of fetal and neonatal rat hepatocyte functional activity by glucocorticoids in co-culture. <u>Cell Diff. 16</u>, 259-268.

Morin, O. and Normand, C. (1986): Long-term maintenance of hepatocyte functional activity in co-culture : requirements for sinusoïdal endothelial cells and dexamethasone. <u>J. Cell. Physiol. 129</u>, 103-110.

Ratanasavanh, D., Beaune, P., Baffet, G., Rissel, M., Kremers, P., Guengerich, F.P. and Guillouzo, A. (1986): Immunocytochemical evidence for the maintenance of cytochrome P-450 isozymes, NADPH cytochrome c reductase and epoxide hydrolase in pure and mixed primary cultures of adult human hepatocytes. <u>J. Histochem. Cytochem. 34</u>, 527-533.

Ratanasavanh, D., Baffet, G., Latinier, M.F., Rissel, M. and Guillouzo, A. (1988a) : Use of hepatocyte co-cultures in the assessment of drug toxicity from chronic exposure. <u>Xenobiotica</u> (in press).

Ratanasavanh, D., Bégué, J.M., Gelé, P., Grislain, L., Bromet, N., du Vignaud, P., Defrance, R., Mocaer, E. and Guillouzo, A. (1988b): Cytotoxicity and metabolism study of amineptine (S-1694-1) in cultured adult rat and human hepatocytes. In Liver Cells and Drugs, ed. Guillouzo A. INSERM : Paris, John Libbey Eurotext : London (this volume).

Rogiers, V., Paene, G., Sonck, W. and Vercruysse, A. (1987): Metabolism of procyclidine in isolated rat hepatocytes. Xenobiotica (in press).

Sirica, A.E and Pitot, H.C. (1980): Drug metabolism and effects of carcinogens in cultured hepatic cells. <u>Pharmacol. Rev. 31</u>, 205-228.

Vandenberghe, Y., Ratanasavanh, D., Glaise, D. and Guillouzo, A. (1988): Influence of various soluble factors on glutathione S-transferase activity in adult rat hepatocytes during culture. <u>In Vitro Cell Develop. Biol.</u> (in press).

Villa, P., Bégué, J.M. and Guillouzo, A. (1985): Erythromycin toxicity in primary cultures of rat hepatocytes. <u>Xenobiotica 15</u>, 767-773.

Résumé

Des hépatocytes préparés à partir d'espèces très diverses, y compris l'homme, ont été largement utilisés, en suspension ou en culture, pour des études pharmacologiques et toxicologiques au cours des dernières années. Toutefois, l'apparition de changements phénotypiques rapides et importants en a limité l'utilisation à des études de courte durée : par exemple l'identification de voies métaboliques ou l'évaluation de la toxicité aiguë. La possibilité de conserver des hépatocytes de différentes espèces capables d'exprimer les réactions de phase I et de phase II pendant plusieurs jours voire quelques semaines, en les cultivant avec des cellules épithéliales hépatiques de rat, a permis d'envisager des expériences de longue durée. Les métabolites de nombreux xénobiotiques, identifiés in vivo ont été retrouvés pendant plusieurs jours dans ce modèle de co-culture et des études de toxicité chronique ont été réalisées par addition quotidienne du composé testé pendant deux à trois semaines. Il faut néanmoins souligner que le choix de certains paramètres, par exemple la composition du milieu nutritif et les critères d'évaluation de la cytotoxicité est essentiel. Bien que les hépatocytes en culture représentent une approche réductioniste par rapport à l'organisme, il n'en demeure pas moins vrai qu'ils constituent un outil unique pour des études pharmacocinétiques, pour l'identification et la production de métabolites, la détermination d'interactions médicamenteuses et le criblage de nouvelles molécules potentiellement hépatotoxiques.

Drug metabolism and cytotoxicity in cultured fetal hepatocytes

P. Kremers

Université de Liège, Laboratoire de Chimie Médicale et de Toxicologie, Institut de Pathologie, Bâtiment B 23, B-4000 Sart Tilman, Liège 1, Belgium

ABSTRACT

Primary fetal rat hepatocytes in culture constitute an useful alternative model for the study of drug toxicity and drug metabolism.
In culture, these hepatocytes display several monooxygenase activities which can be induced by several chemical compounds. Moreover, the expression of cytochrome P-450 isozymes and dependent monooxygenase activities can be modified by appropriate treatment and culture conditions.
In the presence of corticoïds, these cells can be maintained functionnal for several weeks and should therefore constitute an interesting model for studies needing long term culture systems.

KEYWORDS

Fetal hepatocytes, cytochrome P-450, monooxygenase, drug metabolism, induction, drug toxicity.

INTRODUCTION

The main purpose of experimental Toxicology and Pharmacology is to provide scientific evidence for the assessment of the toxic potential of a substance and its metabolites. The substances concerned are not only drugs used for their therapeutic effects, but almost every chemical to which living organism and specially man may be exposed : namely, air and water pollutants, food additives and cosmetics. The toxicological study is supposed to furnish valuable informations about the various factors concerning the safe use of the product by man.

Procedures for estimating safety levels are largely based on animal experiments. Nevertheless animal experiments present a number of shortcomings: number of parameters involved, extrapolation of the results to the human situation is not always easy, governmental regulations ....

Consequently *in vitro* systems have become increasingly attractive alternatives (Stammati et al, 1981). Cells and more particularly hepatocytes in culture are one of the most promising *in vitro* models, and have been the subject of numerous studies during the last few years (Guillouzo and Guguen-Guillouzo, 1986).

Different types of hepatocytes and culture conditions have been described during this meeting. Our laboratory has been involved since several years with the primary culture of fetal rat hepatocytes (Kremers, 1986).
These cells divide in culture and express drug metabolizing enzyme activities. Their enzymatic activities are inducible by several compounds like polycyclic hydrocarbons and phenobarbital. Since the pioneer work of Nebert (Nebert and Gelboin, 1968), these cells have been largely used for the study of drug metabolizing enzymes. In an appropriate culture medium, these cells are able to express several cytochrome P-450 linked monooxygenase activities, namely those induced in adult animals by phenobarbital (Kremers et al, 1981).

Moreover we are now able to cultivate these fetal hepatocytes for longer periods. When treated with dexamethasone, the cultured hepatocytes are able to maintain their cytochrome P-450 levels and the dependent monooxygenases during at least 30 days (Bollinne et al, 1987). This experimental model will be particularly useful for the study of acute and chronic toxicity.

MATERIAL AND METHODS

Preparation of cell cultures

Livers of 18 days old fetuses are used to prepare the primary culture. The livers are removed, rinsed and minced under aseptic conditions. The tissue is dissociated after a short incubation with 0.2 % trypsin solution. The isolated cells are seeded at a density of 10^6 cells in 3 ml eagle's minimum essential medium supplemented with 10 % inactivated (30 minutes at 56°C) fetal calf serum in 6 cm diameter polystyrene petri dishes. The medium was removed 24 hours after hepatocyte seeding and then replaced every two days with fresh treatment medium. Hepatocytes are cultivated in an humidified incubator at 37°C under 5 % CO_2 in air (Van Cantfort et al, 1979).

At the end of the culture cells are scraped off the dishes, washed with a Dulbecco buffer and kept as dry pellet at -20°C. Just before enzymatic activity determinations they were suspended in 0.05 M Tris buffer at pH 7.6 and homogenized by sonication.

Measure of enzymatic activities

Enzymatic activities were measured on whole homogenates. Benzopyrene hydroxylase (AHH) was measured by the spectrofluorimetric assay (Nebert and Gelboin, 1968), ethoxycoumarin deethylase activities according to Greenlee et al (1978) and aldrin epoxidase according to Wolff et al (1979) using 1,1,1-trichloro-2,2-bis(p-chlorophenyl) ethane as internal standard.

Cytochrome P-450 concentrations were measured by the spectrophotometric method of Omura and Sato (1964) on microsomal preparation.

Lactate dehydrogenase (LDH) leakage is measured in the cell free medium by a standard enzymatic procedure (Cartier et al 1967).

In vivo measure of monooxygenase activity : aldrin (or ethoxycoumarin) were introduced in the culture medium at a final concentration of 5 µM and culture was continued for two hours in the presence of the substrate. The culture medium was then collected, extracted and the amount of dieldrin (or 7-hydroxycoumarin) determined according to the above mentionned methods. The hepatocytes could be further cultivated in the presence of a fresh medium.

RESULTS AND DISCUSSION

To illustrate some characteristics of the fetal rat hepatocytes in culture and their usefulness as a model for pharmacological and toxicological purposes we will shortly describe the results of a few typical experiments.

1) Modification of cytochrome P-450 expression in cultured cells by dexamethasone

Fetal hepatocytes in culture are known to express only P_1-450 dependent monooxygenase activities (Owens and Nebert, 1975). The presence of dexamethasone in the culture medium modifies this expression (table I). Aldrin epoxidase activity becomes inducible and AHH activity can be inhibited in vitro by metyrapone as in adult phenobarbital-treated rat liver microsomes. This is further confirmed by the immunological determination of the P-450 isozymes. The PCN-E and PB-B isozymes are respectively induced by dexamethasone and dexamethasone plus phenobarbital. In the absence of dexamethasone, phenobarbital induces P_1-450 like benzanthracene.

Table I. Enzymatic activities and P-450 isozymes in fetal liver cells after 96 hours of culture in the presence of inducers and dexamethasone

Inducer	Dexa 10^{-6}M	Aldrin epoxidase	A.H.H.	In vitro inhibition α-NF	MTR	Cytochrome P-450 Total	PB-B	PCN-E
		pmol.min^{-1}.mgr prot^{-1}		(% of non inhibited sample)		pmol/mgr prot		
-	-	0.72	14	73	91	40	< 2	<2
-	+	44.1	32.5	138	35	ND	9	55
PB 2.10^{-3}M	-	7.0	344.0	36	92	-	< 2	<2
PB 2.10^{-3}M	+	59.4	59	110	54	92	15	64
BA 5.10^{-5}M	-	2.1	41	46	110	-	< 2	<2
BA 5.10^{-5}M	+	41.5	96	73	85	123	20	55

2) Long term culture

The presence of dexamethasone in the culture medium allows to maintain the cells alive in culture for several weeks. Fig. 1 illustrates that, in these conditions, the hepatocytes continue to metabolize aldrin into dieldrin. In this case, enzymatic activities were determined on cells scraped off the dish and homogenized. The enzymatic activities may also be measured in vivo, without interrupting the culture, the substrate (ethoxycoumarin or aldrin) being directly added to the culture medium for a short period of time. The substrate is metabolized by the cells and the products of the reaction accumulate in the culture medium where they can be measured (table II). This method allows to control the activity of the cells during the treatment with an inducer or a potentially toxic agent.

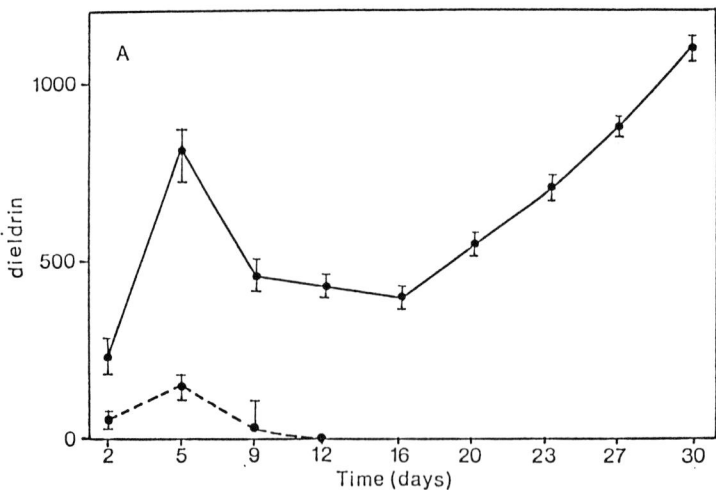

Figure 1. Aldrin epoxidase activity in cells cultivated in the presence of 10^{-6}M dexamethasone (full line) or in control medium (dashed line). The enzymatic activity is expressed in pmoles of dieldrin formed per hour and per mgr of total homogenate proteins.

Table II. Ethoxycoumarin-deethylase activity measured in vivo on cells in culture.

Treatment	Culture age (days)		
	7	9	15
DEXA 10^{-6}M	/	/	1.0
PB 2.10^{-3}M + DEXA 10^{-6}M	17	19	5.0

Results are expressed as nmoles of hydroxycoumarin formed per dish and per hour.

3) Primary culture for toxicological studies

Primary hepatocytes may be used to evaluate the dose dependent toxicological effects of a given compound in perfectly controlled conditions. Toxic effects were not only monitored by morphological parameters like microscopic examination and trypan blue exclusion test but also by more selective biochemical parameters namely lactate dehydrogenase (LDH) release into the culture medium, DNA and protein content of the hepatocytes, protein synthesis and production. Table III illustrates the dose dependent release of LDH after treatment with a toxic compound, cannabinol, as well as the correlated DNA and protein depletion of the cells.

Table III. Toxic effect of cannabinol on fetal liver cells in culture.

Cannabinol	LDH	Proteins	DNA
0	100	100	100
10^{-5}M	180	100	100
5×10^{-5}M	190	80	25
10^{-4}M	229	53	20

LDH release into the medium, DNA and protein content of the cells was evaluated after 96 hours of culture in the presence of cannabinol. Results are expressed as % of control.

4) Induction of drug metabolizing enzymes

It is often necessary to evaluate if a given drug is able to induce the drug metabolizing enzymes and eventually its own metabolism. This is easely done, using cells in culture. These may be treated with known amounts of a substance for a defined period of time in completely controlled conditions. The enzymatic activities as well as the cytochrome P-450 content of the cells can be evaluated and compared to that of hepatocytes treated with reference compounds. Table IV illustrates the effect on drug metabolizing enzymes of mebendazole, an anthelmintic drug. Mebendazole at high dosage was suspected to be an inducer in vivo. The experiment confirmed that it was able to induce AHH and ethoxycoumarin deethylase. No significant effect was observed on aldrin epoxidase. Furthermore, an immunological study by Western blot confirmed that this product was able to induce cytochrome P-450 BNF-B, the isozyme induced by polycyclic hydrocarbons.

Table IV. AHH, aldrin epoxidase and ethoxycoumarin deethylase activity in fetal rat hepatocytes after treatment for 46 hours with different inducers.

Treatment	AHH	Ethoxycoumarin deethylase	Aldrin epoxidase
		$pmol.min^{-1}.mgr\ prot^{-1}$	
Control	1,0	< 1,0	< 1,0
DEXA 10^{-6}M	1,3	3,8	6,7
PB 2.10^{-3}M	61	133	4,8
MBZ 10^{-7}M	1,3	< 1,0	< 1,0
MBZ 10^{-7}M + DEXA	2,5	4,5	3,0
MBZ 10^{-6}M	3,2	< 1,0	< 1,0
MBZ 10^{-6}M + DEXA	2,8	4,5	3,0
MBZ 10^{-5}M	14,4	19,7	< 1,0
MBZ 10^{-5}M + DEXA	24,5	45,1	3,0

CONCLUSIONS

This report illustrates that fetal rat liver cells in culture constitute an interesting approach for the study of drug metabolism and drug toxicity. In addition, this experimental model offers the possibility to investigate the qualitative and quantitative alterations in drug metabolism produced by xenobiotics. Cytochrome P-450 content and monooxygenase activities were maintained at a high level in cultured fetal hepatocytes for several weeks. By an appropriate treatment, the cytochrome P-450 expression of the hepatocytes can be modified so that regulation studies can be undertaken.

From the toxicological point of view, this experimental model offers the possibility to investigate acute as well as chronic hepatotoxicity in perfectly controlled conditions.

BIBLIOGRAPHY

Bollinne, A. (1987) : Long term maintenance of monooxygenases activities in cultured fetal hepatocytes. Cell Differentiation (in press).

Cartier, P., Leroux, J.P., Temkine, H. (1967) : Techniques de dosage des intermédiaires de la glycolyse dans les tissus. Ann. Biol. Clin. 25, 791-813.

Greenlee, W.F., Poland, A. (1978) : An improved assay for 7-ethoxycoumarin-o-deethylase activity. J. Pharmacol. Exp. Therap. 205, 596-605.

Guillouzo, A., Guguen-Guillouzo, Ch. (1986) : Research in isolated and cultured hepatocytes J. Libbey Eurotext Ltd - INSERM.

Kremers, P., Goujon, Fr., De Graeve, J., Van Cantfort, J., Gielen, J. (1981) : Multiplicity of cytochrome P-450 in primary fetal hepatocytes in culture. Eur. J. Biochem. 116, 67-72.

Kremers, P. (1986) : Drug metabolism in cultured fetal hepatocytes in Research in isolated and cultured hepatocytes, eds Guillouzo, A., Guguen-Guillouzo, Ch., J. Libbey Eurotext Ltd - INSERM, pp 285-312.

Nebert, D.W., Gelboin, H.V. (1968) : Substrate inducible microsomal aryl hydrocarbon hydroxylase in mammalian cell culture. J. Biol. Chem. 243, 6242-6249.

Omura, R.A., Sato, R. (1964) : The carbon monoxide binding pigment of liver microsomes. Evidence for its hemoprotein nature. J. Biol. Chem. 239, 2370-2385.

Stammati, A.P., Silano, V., Zucco, F. (1981) : Toxicology investigations with cell culture systems. Toxicology 20, 91-153.

Van Cantfort, J., Goujon, Fr., Gielen, J. (1979) : Benzopyrene metabolism in rat fetal hepatocytes in culture. Improved methodology and effect of substrate concentration. Chem. Biol. Interactions 28, 147-160.

Wolff, T., Deml, E., Wanders, H. (1979) : Aldrin epoxidation, a highly sensitive indicator specific for cytochrome P-450 dependent monooxygenase activities. Drug Metab. Disp. 7, 301-305.

Résumé

Pour les études de pharmacotoxicologie, il s'avère de plus en plus nécessaire de pouvoir disposer de modèles expérimentaux in vitro capables de répondre rapidement aux questions de sécurité et santé publique posées par l'utilisation d'un nombre de plus en plus élevé de produits de synthèse dans la vie quotidienne.

Parmi les nombreuses approches expérimentales proposées, la culture de cellules offre de multiples possibilités. Les hépatocytes en culture permettent notamment d'aborder efficacement les problèmes liés au métabolisme d'un produit et à l'effet sur ce métabolisme de facteurs tant endogènes qu'exogènes.

Contrairement aux hépatocytes de rats adultes, les hépatocytes foetaux se divisent et prolifèrent en culture. S'ils sont cultivés dans des conditions bien choisies (en présence de glucocorticoïdes par exemple). Ces hépatocytes sont à même d'exprimer plusieurs isoenzymes du cytochrome p-450 ainsi que les activités enzymatiques correspondantes. De plus, il est possible de les maintenir fonctionnels en culture pendant plusieurs semaines. Par un traitement approprié, il est possible de moduler l'expression des enzymes du métabolisme des médicaments dans ces cellules et d'étudier l'impact de ces modifications sur le métabolisme d'un médicament par exemple.

Cet article illustre certaines caractéristiques de ces cellules en culture primaire et décrit, au moyen de quelques exemples, les possibilités offertes par ce modèle expérimental. Ces hépatocytes foetaux en culture primaire permettent d'effectuer des mesures d'hépatotoxicité aussi bien aiguë que chronique. Ils nous ont également permis de caractériser l'effet inducteur d'un produit.

Ces quelques exemples démontrent l'intérêt d'un tel modèle non seulement pour les études pharmacologiques et toxicologiques mais aussi pour aborder les problèmes liés à la régulation des enzymes du métabolisme des médicaments.

Liver Cells and Drugs. Ed. A. Guillouzo. Colloque INSERM/John Libbey Eurotext Ltd. © 1988. Vol. 164, pp. 253-257.

In vitro models : liver microsomes and isolated perfused liver ; a comparison with *in vivo* metabolism (i.e. pefloxacin)

Françoise Collignon, Pierre Gires, Yves Vedrine, Véronique Piguet, Sylvie Martin, Jean Gaillot

Rhône-Poulenc Santé, Institut de Biopharmacie, 92160 Antony, France

KEY WORDS

In vivo - in vitro metabolism, isolated perfused liver, liver microsomes, pefloxacin

INTRODUCTION

The in vitro models of liver microsomes and isolated perfused liver may represent useful tools for the early metabolic screening of xenobiotics undergoing hepatic biotransformation. The fact that these models are simple, easy to develop and to standardize ensures the reproducibility of a great number of tests at a lower cost than studies conducted on whole animals. The unequivocal characteristics of the metabolic and kinetic responses facilitate the interpretation of their biological contents.

A comparative in vitro/in vivo biotransformation study of pefloxacin, an antimicrobial structurally related to quinolones, was carried out in research phase in 2 animals species, the rat and the rabbit, to evaluate the predictive value of the data supplied by these models and to define their role in pharmacological and toxicological research in industry.

MATERIALS AND METHODS

^{14}C pefloxacin (CEA France) was used as an aqueous solution in the various experiments conducted on Sprague Dawley rats and New Zealand White rabbits. Pefloxacin and its metabolites were synthesized by Laboratoire Roger Bellon (Alfortville, France).

Models of isolated and perfused rat and rabbit liver

The perfusion systems with recycling medium were developed according to Miller (1973) and Brauer (1951). The organ viability during the perfusions was controlled by physicochemical (temperature, pH, pressure, bile flow) and biochemical monitoring (Na^+, K^+, ALT, LDH). Pefloxacin was rapidly injected into the tank. The initial concentration (40 ug/ml) corresponded to the C_{Max} values observed in vivo following oral administration.

Models of rat and rabbit liver microsomes
These models consist in incubating pefloxacin (0.054 mM, 5 uCi) in the presence of a regenerative system of NADPH and microsomal proteins (2 mg/ml) for 3 hr at 37°C.

In vivo studies
In parallel, animals were treated by the oral route at the dosage of 100 mg/kg for the rat and 75 mg/kg for the rabbit. The excreta were collected over 0-24 hr.

HPLC analysis
The samples including microsomal incubating media, bile, perfusion fluid and urine were directly injected into a C8 column and analyzed by HPLC with reverse phase using a gradient elution system (^{14}C on line detection). The feaces were previously extracted with MeOH, HCl (0.25 %) mixture.

RESULTS

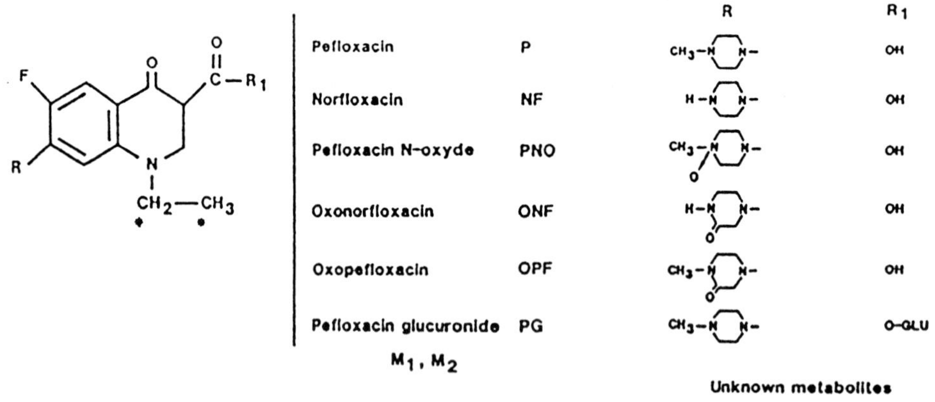

Fig. 1 - Chemical structure of pefloxacin and its derivatives

Five metabolites resulting from functionalization of the molecule by N-demethylation (NF), N-oxidation (PNO), ketoreduction (ONF, OPF) or from conjugation with glucuronic acid (PG) and 2 structurally unknown derivatives (M_1 and M_2) were detected and quantified in the various media or excreta. From the comparative analysis of the perfusion fluids (bile, perfusate), urines and feaces it is concluded that :

i) all the metabolites isolated in vitro - except M_2 detected only in rabbit bile - are found in vivo (fig. II),

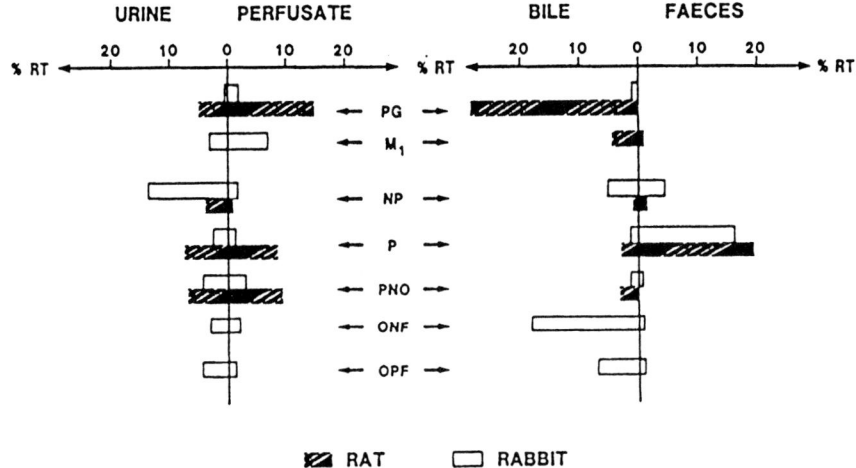

Fig. II - Comparative % amounts of pefloxacin and its metabolites found in the bile and perfusate of rat and rabbit liver isolated after 3 hr perfusion and in 0-24 hr urines and feaces of rats and rabbits.

ii) some metabolites are predominantly eliminated in the bile (M_2, ONF, OPF in rabbits) ; for others, higher amounts are found in the perfusate (e.g. PNO rat).

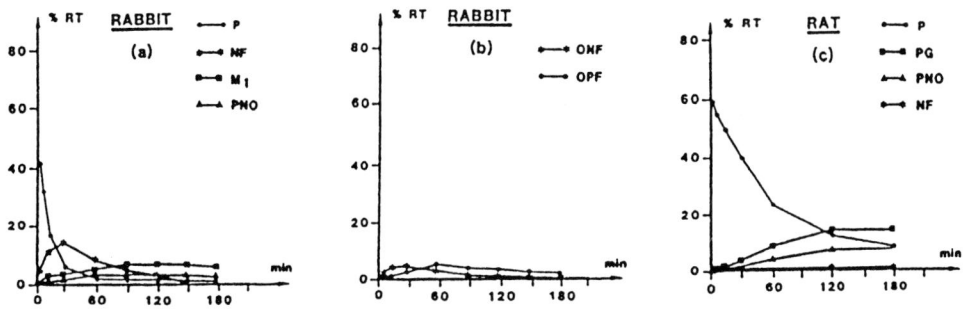

Fig. III - Time course of ^{14}C pefloxacin metabolism in isolated perfused liver of rabbit (a, b) or rat (c) experiments.

iii) the hepatic clearance of pefloxacin is higher in rabbits than in rats (fig. III). The metabolites can be separated into 2 groups depending on the kinetic profile of their concentrations in the perfusate : for one group, NF, ONF, OPF (rabbit), the concentrations attain a peak and for the other, PNO and M_1 (rabbit) or PNO, NF, PG (rat), the concentrations increase exponentially.

Such a kinetic difference suggests that the former derivatives (NF, ONF and OPF) could be labile intermediates in the overall biotransformation process of pefloxacin.

iv) the interspecies differences observed with the perfusion models are found in whole animals. Thus, glucuronic conjugaison is the major metabolic pathway in the rat, whereas oxidation into M_1 and M_2 is essentially characteristic of the rabbit species.

The metabolism of pefloxacin by liver microsomes (Fig.IV) results in the formation of PNO, NF (rat, rabbit) and M_1 (rabbit) which are found in urines in vivo. This slow biotransformation process, less marked in rats than in rabbits, predominantly leads to the production of PNO in both animal species.

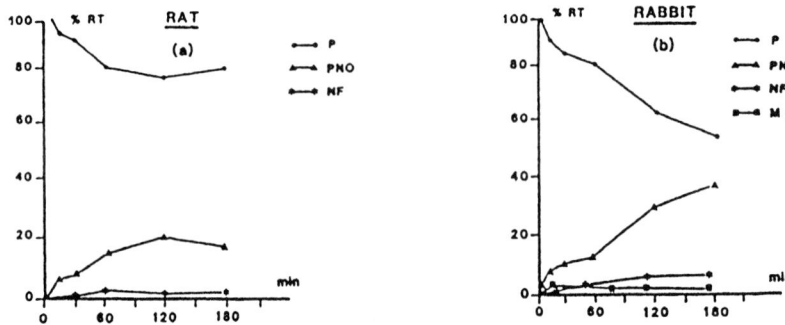

Fig. IV - Time course of ^{14}C pefloxacin metabolism by rat (a) or rabbit (b) liver micromes.

DISCUSSION

The objective of the comparative in vivo - vitro analysis of the metabolism of pefloxaxin used as tracer in these experiments, is to demonstrate the worthwhile potential and to determine the specific value of the biotransformating models, the liver microsomes and the isolated perfused liver.

The experimental results emphasize the excellent predictive value of the 2 models and the complementarity of the in vitro data they supply.

The liver microsome model gives an evaluation of the biotransformation potential of the hepatic tissue in a given species and is used to follow the formation of derivatives resulting from the direct interaction of the xenobiotic (or one of its metabolites) with the cyt. P-450 dependent monooxygenase system. This analysis may include a more detailed study of the potentially reacting intermediates. Such an evaluation, conducted during the research process on microsomal fractions of different origin (animal species or man) may contribute, at a very early stage, to the selection, in a chemical series, of the most promising molecule from the metabolic and toxicological points of view as well as to the choice of the animal species which are best appropriate for toxicology. Besides, the use of human microsomal fractions offers promising alternatives for the assessment of genetic factors on the metabolism of new substances.

The model of isolated perfused liver in which the liver parenchyme remains intact leads to more comprehensive studies of the metabolic pathways. Thus, all the metabolites of pefloxacin generated *in vivo* by phase I and II enzymes are produced during the perfusion. This model facilitates the analysis and isolation of metabolites and may contribute to the synthesis of radiolabelled reference derivatives. These characteristics are of particular interest in the case of substances with potent pharmacological activity for which a metabolic analysis *in vivo* is difficult on account of the very low dosage of administration, or even to study the fate or the potential toxicity of a bioformed derivative. The analogy between the urines and the perfusate indicates that this medium may be quite representative of the circulating metabolites *in vivo*. The rapid and early identification of these potentially active derivatives is promising in pharmacology and pharmacodynamics as it may help to explain the activity and guide the selection of metabolites for pharmacokinetic studies.

In addition, the isolated organ system supplies further information on :
 i) the capacity of hepatic extraction (suggesting an enterohepatic recycling process),
 ii) the distribution of the substance and its metabolites in the perfusion medium and the bile (implication of biliary excretion in the elimination process),
 iii) the impact of the biotransformation process on the total clearance of the molecule.

Thus, it appears as the single *in vitro* model enabling an unambiguous evaluation of the role of hepatic metabolism in the overall transport of a xenobiotic in the body. The variety of the inducing or inhibiting treatment which can be applied to the animal strongly suggests that it may also be used to control some limiting metabolism reactions. This model, which seems appropriate for the early study of the metabolic pathways of a new active substance in research may supply further valuable information, at the kinetic level, on the transport and the excretion of the molecule. It may be useful for interspecies comparisons but nevertheless remains limited to small species currently used in the laboratory (mouse, rat, guinea-pig, rabbit) for routine assays.

The *in vitro* models of liver microsomes and isolated perfused liver, even if they imply, as all *in vivo* experiments, a heavy analytical environment, rapidly generate data with predictive value on the metabolism and/or the kinetics of substances and thus contribute to the more rational selection of new molecules in the early phases of the pharmaceutical research and development process.

REFERENCES

Miller, L.L. (1973) : Technic of isolated rat liver perfusion. In "Isolated Liver Perfusion and its Applications", Raven Press N.Y., pp. 11-51

Brauer, R.W. Pessotti, R.L. and Pizzolato, R. (1951) : Isolated rat liver preparation, Bile production and other basic properties Proc. Soc. Exp. Biol. N.Y. 78, 174-198

In vivo fluorine-19 NMR study of 5-fluorouracil metabolism in isolated perfused mouse liver

Marie C. Malet-Martino, Sophie Cabanac, Jean-Pierre Vialaneix, Maryse Bon, Robert Martino

Laboratoire des IMRCP, Université Paul Sabatier, 118, route de Narbonne, 31062 Toulouse Cedex, France

KEY WORDS

5-fluorouracil, ^{19}F NMR, isolated perfused mouse liver

INTRODUCTION

5-fluorouracil (5FU) is a fluoropyrimidine widely used to treat advanced solid tumors, especially of the digestive tract. The cytotoxic activity of 5FU is the consequence of the intracellular formation of fluoronucleotides via the anabolic pathway of 5FU. There is also a competitive catabolic pathway for 5FU that leads sequentially to 5,6-dihydro-5-fluorouracil (5FUH$_2$), α-fluoro-β-ureidopropionic acid (FUPA), α-fluoro-β-alanine (FBAL) and fluoride ion, and occurs primarily in the liver.

We have already used ^{19}F NMR to monitor the metabolism of 5FU in tumor cells (Malet-Martino, 1986) and to demonstrate the quantitative importance of the catabolic route when 5FU was injected to cancer patients (Bernadou, 1985). The isolated perfused liver model can lead to an improved knowledge of the catabolic pathway of 5FU and especially to a better understanding of the recent trials developed to enhance 5FU activity with modulating agents interacting with 5FU metabolism.

MATERIALS AND METHODS

Liver perfusion
The livers were from 25-30 g Swiss mice fed at libitum. After the mice were anesthetized with sodium pentobarbital (60 mg/kg) intraperitoneally, the abdominal cavity was opened, the portal vein was rapidly catheterized and perfused. After the gallblader was incised, the liver was quickly dissected out of the abdominal cavity and placed into a 15 mm diameter NMR tube. The recirculating perfusate (70 ml) was pumped through a membrane oxygenator gassed with 95 per cent air, 5 per cent carbon dioxide, and then infused into the liver, through a water-jacketed tube, at constant temperature (37° C) and flow rate (2.5 ml/min). The perfusate which exits from the liver through the vena cava was allowed to bathe the liver and pumped from the bottom of the NMR tube at a rate slightly below the perfusion rate. Another suction line, positionned above the liver, draw off

excess perfusate, thus preventing overflow. The perfusate was a Krebs-Henseleit buffer + 7 per cent human erythrocytes + 2 per cent bovine serum albumin (pH = 7.3 - 7.4).

Liver viability assessment

Different tests were used. The pH of the perfusate was monitored continuously and did not change more than 0.1 unit during the 150 min of perfusion. Lactic deshydrogenase, alanine aminotransferase and aspartate aminotransferase activities were tested from the exiting perfusate by periodic sampling (each 30 min). These activities increased slightly with time but lay in the normal range. The potassium concentration of the perfusate was also periodically measured. An increase with time (certainly due to the lysis of erythrocytes) was noticed.

^{19}F NMR analysis

The 19F NMR spectra were recorded at 282.4 MHz on a Bruker AM-300 spectrometer. After a 30 min period of liver equilibration, the spectra were acquired in 5-min intervals (300 scans) for 2 hrs. The chemical shifts (δ) were reported relative to the chemical shift of trifluoroacetic acid (5 per cent (w/v) aqueous solution).

RESULTS AND DISCUSSION

For the low dose of 5FU (30 mg/kg body weight (b.w.), twice the dose clinically used), or 5FU + thymidine (30 and 180 mg/kg b.w. respectively), 5FU was never detected in the liver, since it was rapidly catabolized leading to FUPA (-110.8 ppm) in 5-10 min after the addition of 5FU, and FBAL (-112.5 ppm). 5FUH2 was not detected.

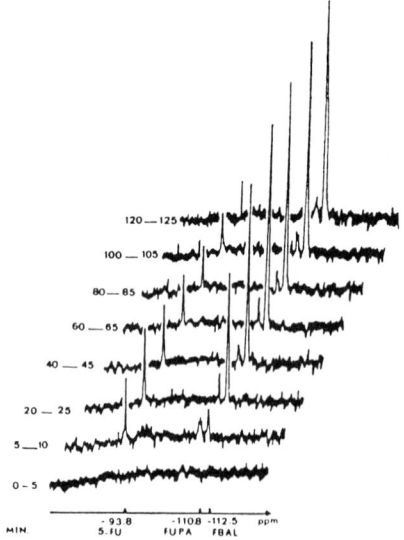

Fig. 1. ^{19}F NMR stack plots of isolated perfused mouse liver showing 5FU metabolic profile in eight spectra obtained in 5 min (300 scans) during the 125 min post-5FU addition into the perfusate. The dose of 5FU was 180 mg/kg b.w..

For the high dose of 5FU (180 mg/kg b.w.), 5FU (-93.8 ppm), FUPA and FBAL were observed in the liver (Fig. 1). The two catabolites FUPA and FBAL were detected as soon as 5FU appeared in the liver (5-10 min after the addition of 5FU to the perfusate); FBAL was rapidly (20-25 min after 5FU addition) by far the major catabolite. FBAL concentration increased and 5FU concentration decreased concomitantly with time. 5FUH2 was not detected. A signal at -88.8 ppm was detected after ≃60 min of perfusion. This low signal was only observed when accumulating 3000 scans.

For the high dose of 5FU + thymidine (180 mg/kg b.w. for each compound), 5FU, FUPA and FBAL were immediately observed (Fig. 2). After ≃30 min, two other signals (X, -88.8 ppm, and Y, -89.5 ppm) were detected; they increased with time and respectively reached ≃8 per cent and ≃4 per cent of the total fluorinated metabolites in the spectrum resulting from 1800 scans during the period 90-120 min after the addition of 5FU to the perfusate. All these signals were also detected in liver perchloric acid extracts, whereas all but the signal at -88.8 ppm were detected in the perfusate recorded at the end of the experiments. As 5-fluoro-2'-deoxyuridine (FUdR) was found in biofluids of patients treated with 5FU + thymidine (Woodcock, 1980), and a spectrum of the perfusate spiked with FUdR showed a net increase of the signal at -89.5 ppm, the most probable assignment for the -89.5 ppm peak was therefore FUdR. Moreover, when rat hepatocytes were incubated with high doses of 5FU or 5FU + thymidine, an intracellular 5FU glucuronide that was retained within the hepatocytes has been reported (Sommadossi, 1985). The signal at -88.8 ppm, only present in the liver, could therefore correspond to a 5FU glucuronide. Work is continuing to confirm these hypotheses.

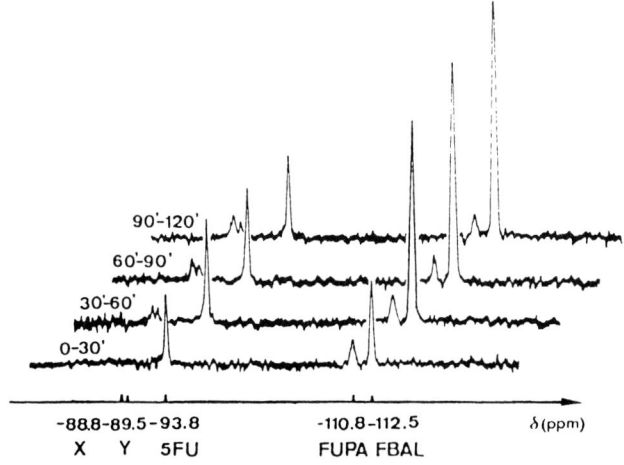

Fig. 2. ^{19}F NMR stack plots of isolated perfused mouse liver showing 5FU metabolic profile in four spectra obtained in 30 min (1800 scans) during the 120 min after the addition of 5FU+thymidine into the perfusate. The doses of 5FU and thymidine were 180 mg/kg b.w..

In conclusion, this work indicated that ^{19}F NMR of the isolated perfused liver is a convenient tool to follow the metabolic pathways of fluoropyrimidines, and probably of other fluorinated drugs.

REFERENCES

Bernadou, J. (1985): Complete urinary excretion profile of 5-fluorouracil during a six-day chemotherapeutic schedule, as resolved by 19F nuclear magnetic resonance. Clin. Chem. 31, 846-848.
Malet-Martino, M.C. (1986): Noninvasive fluorine-19 NMR study of fluoropyrimidine metabolism in cell cultures of human pancreatic and colon adenocarcinoma. Cancer Chemother. Pharmacol. 18, 5-10.

Sommadossi, J.P. (1985): Modulation of 5-fluorouracil catabolism in isolated rat hepatocytes with enhancement of 5-fluorouracil glucuronide formation. Cancer Res. 45, 116-121.

Woodcock, T.M. (1980): Combination clinical trials with thymidine and fluorouracil: a phase I and clinical pharmacologic evaluation. Cancer 45, 1135-1143.

Microsomal aldrin epoxidase activity in liver of diabetic (insulin deficient) rats and studies of its regulation by glucagon in isolated hepatocytes

Evelyne Rouer*, Patricia Rouet, Jean-Paul Leroux

*INSERM U.75, 156 rue de Vaugirard, 75730 Paris Cedex 15, France. * INSERM U.15, 24 rue du Faubourg St-Jacques, 75674 Paris Cedex 14, France*

KEY WORDS

Aldrin epoxidase, Glucagon, Liver microsomes, Isolated hepatocytes, Diabetic rats

INTRODUCTION

Biotransformation of xenobiotics in liver is mainly supported by the mixed-function oxidase system in which the terminal oxidase is cytochrome P-450 (Estabrook et al., 1963). Multiple isozymes of cytochrome P-450 have been isolated and enzymatic studies have shown that each of them possesses a substrate specificity relatively tight towards a few substrates and a broader one for numerous others (Ryan et al., 1979). Besides the diversity of its isozymes, another remarkable property of cytochrome P-450 isozyme is their ability to be specifically induced by various compounds such as barbiturates, polycyclic aromatic hydrocarbons, steroids and alcohol (Snyder and Remmer, 1979). As a consequence, the quantitative and qualitative aspects of drug metabolism depend on the amount of each isozyme (Guengerich et al., 1982). Recently attention has been focused on the possible regulation of some cytochrome P-450 isozymes by phosphorylation-dephosphorylation, without modification of their concentration (Pyerin et al., 1983, Janson et al., 1987), as that undergone by several key-enzymes of the energy metabolism (Cohen, 1984). By means of the catalytic subunit of cyclic AMP-dependent protein kinase these autors have realized the phosphorylation of purified cytochrome P-450 LM_2(the main phenobarbital inducible isozyme in rabbit liver) and they have noticed a decreased monooxygenase activity (Pyerin et al., 1984).

Drug metabolism is modified in the liver of diabetic insulin-deficient animals (Reinke et al.,1978, Rouer and Leroux, 1980) and the variations of certain monooxygenase activities could be ascribed to modified concentrations of some cytochrome P-450 isozymes (Rouer et al., 1986) perhaps as a result of the hyperglucagonemic state. However, hyperglucagonemia might also regulate monooxygenase activities by phosphorylation of cytochrome P-450 isozymes mediated by cAMP dependent protein kinase: thus the aim of the present work was to study aldrin epoxidase in the liver of diabetic rats, and to search for rapid modifications of that monooxygenase activity induced by glucagon in hepatocytes isolated from normal rat.

MATERIALS AND METHODS

Liver microsomal membranes and isolated hepatocytes were prepared from male Sprague Dawley rats (10 weeks old) as respectively reported by Cresteil et al. (1974) and Demaugre et al. (1978). Insulin deficiency was realized by a unique iv injection of streptozotocin (60 mg/kg freshly dissolved in saline solution pH 4,5). Glucosuric animals were killed two weeks later. Aldrin epoxidase activity was assayed as indicated by Wolff et al. (1979). Microsomal and cellular cytochrome P-450 was assayed as indicated respectively by Omura and Sato(1964) and Greim (1970). ATP and glycogen levels in hepatocytes were determined as described respectively by Cartier et al. (1967) and Chan and Exton (1976).

RESULTS AND DISCUSSION

Liver microsomal aldrin epoxidase, either expressed as specific or molecular activity, is two-fold lower in diabetic than in normal rats (Table 1).

Table 1: Aldrin epoxidase activity and cytochrome P-450 content in liver microsomes from normal or diabetic rats.

	Cytochrome P-450 $nmol \times mg^{-1}$ proteins	Specific activity $nmol \times min^{-1} \times mg^{-1}$ proteins	Molecular activity $nmol \times min^{-1} \times nmol^{-1}$ cyt. P-450
Normal rats	0.87 ± 0.03	1.88 ± 0.37	2.68 ± 0.44
Diabetic rats	1.20 ± 0.04	0.69 ± 0.35	1.14 ± 0.42

We have previously reported (Rouer et al., 1982) that the activity of epoxide hydrolase (tested with styrene oxide as substrate) is increased in streptozotocin-induced diabetic mice. Epoxide hydrolase is one of the phase II enzymes of the drug metabolism, which converts the primary metabolites produced by the cytochromes P-450 into more hydrophylic compounds by means of conjugation. In the present case, aldrin is firstly metabolized to dieldrin which is a very stable epoxide: its conjugation with water to produce a diol metabolite is very low (Ichinose and Kurihara, 1985). Thus the lower amount of dieldrin measured in diabetic rats cannot result from a more active secondary biotransformation. In contrast this may be explained by a decreased enzyme activity and/or a decreased amount of the cytochrome P-450 isozyme(s) supporting aldrin epoxidase activity. However the low activity can be only apparent and result from a dilution effect by the increase of the total amount of cytochrome P-450 assayed by spectrophotometry (Table 1). It is now demonstrated that diabetes induces new species of cytochrome P-450 (Past and Cook, 1982) and enhances the level of some pre-existing cytochromes (Rouer et al., 1985). In liver of streptozotocin-induced diabetic mice, we have noticed that total microsomal proteins are increased (Rouer, unpublished data), so the lower expression of aldrin epoxidase when related to microsomal proteins, might also be explained by this dilution effect. It is why rapide effects of glucagon on the aldrin epoxidase activity of isolated hepatocytes have been investigated.

Isolated liver cells have been prepared and their viability tested by measurements of their ATP and glycogen levels (Table 2). Their high levels indicate that the metabolic integrity has been maintained and that hepatocytes may be used in metabolic studies. Level of cytochrome P-450 is in agreement with report by Moldeus et al. (1978) and hepatocytes effectively epoxidize aldrin as previously shown by Kurihara et al.(1984). Addition of glucagon (10^{-7} M) to the incubation medium leads to a 30% inhibition of aldrin epoxidase (Table 2). On the other hand the metabolic response of cells to the hormone is probed by its glycogenolytic effect: the glycogen consumption is 1.6 fold stimulated by glucagon (Table 2).

Thus, isolated hepatocytes stimulated by glucagon are able to modify their metabolizing activity towards a xenobiotic. The total cytochrome P-450 is not significantly modified so, the decrease aldrin epoxidase activity cannot be explained by the dilution effect discussed above.
The action of glucagon on the isolated hepatocytes leads to the same result (a

decreased aldrin epoxidation) as compared to the activity in liver microsomes from diabetic rats (in which glucagon level is high). Pyerin et al.(1984) have shown that the in vitro phosphorylation of a purified cytochrome P-450 decreases its monooxygenase activity, so we may postulate that in intact hepatocytes some isozymes of cytochrome P-450 undergo a phosphorylation-dephosphorylation process which rapidly modulates their activities.

Table 2 : Aldrin epoxidase activity, cytochrome P-450 and glycogen levels in isolated hepatocytes incubated in presence or in absence of 10^{-7} M glucagon.

Incubation time	0 min	5min	
	- glucagon	- glucagon	+ glucagon
Glycogen (1)	2216	1852	1633
Cytochrome P-450 (2)	0.25	0.22	0.27
Aldrin epoxidase (3)	-	155	110

(1) expressed in nmol of glucose equivalent/10^6 cells.
(2) expressed in nmol/10^6 cells.
(3) expressed in pmol of dieldrin formed/min/nmol cyt. P-450.
Results are the means of 2 individual experiments.
At time 0 min, the ATP content was 19.3 µmol/10^9 cells.
Addition of aldrin (in 10µl ethanol) or ethanol alone does not affect it.
Vehicle of glucagon (10 µl Hcl 0.1N) does not affect any of the parameters assayed.

REFERENCES

CARTIER, P., LEROUX, J.P. and TEMKINE, H. (1967). Techniques de dosage des inmédiaires de la glycolyse dans les tissues .Ann. Biol. Clin., 25 , 791-813.
CHAN, T.M., and EXTON, H. (1976). A rapid method for the determination of glycogen content and radioactivity in small quantities of tissue or isolated hepatocytes .Anal. Biochem., 71 , 96-105 .
COHEN, P. (1984). Hormones, second messengers and the reversible phosphorylation of proteins: an overview. Bio. Essays., 2 ,63-68 .
CRESTEIL, T., FLINOIS, J.P., PFISTER, A. and LEROUX, J.P. (1979). Effect of microsomal preparations and induction on Cytochrome P-450 dependent monooxygenases in fetal and neonatal rat liver.Biochem.Pharmacol., 28 , 2057-2063.

DEMAUGRE, F. LEROUX, J.P. and CARTIER, P. (1978). The effects of pyruvate concentration, dichloroacetate and ∝-cyano-4 hydroxycinnamate on gluconeogenesis, ketogenesis and 3-hydroxybutyrate/3-oxobutyrate ratios in isolated hepatocytes. Biochem. J., 172, 91-96.

ESTABROOK, R.W., COOPER, D.Y. and ROSENTHAL, O. (1963). The light reversible carbon monooxide inhibition of the steroid C 21-hydroxylase system of the adrenal cortex. Biochem. Z., 338, 741-755.

GREIM, H. (1970). Synthesesteigerung und Abbauhemmung bei der Vermehrung der mikrosomalen Cytochrome P-450 und b-5 durch phenobarbital. Naunyn-Schmiedeberg's Arch. Pharmak., 266, 261-275.

GUENGERICH, F.P., DANNAN, G.A., WRIGHT, S.T. MARTIN, M.V. and KAMINSKY, L.S. (1982). Purification and characterization of liver microsomal cytochromes P-450. Biochemistry, 21, 6019-6030.

ICHINOSE, R. and KURIHARA, N. (1985). Uptake of dieldrin, lindane and DDT by isolated rat hepatocytes. Pestic. Biochem. Physiol., 23, 116-122.

JANSSON, I., EPSTEIN, P. and SCHENKMAN, J. (1987). Inverse relationship between cytochrome P-450 phosphorylation and complexation with cytochrome b5. Fed. Proceed., 46, 1955.

KURIHARA, N., HORI, N. and ICHINOSE, R. (1984). Cytochrome P-450 content and aldrin epoxidation to dieldrin in isolated rat hepatocytes. Pestic. Biochem. Physiol., 21, 63-73.

MOLDEUS, P., HOGBERG, J. and ORRENIUS, S. (1978). Isolation and use of liver cells, in "Methods in Enzymology" (Fleischer, S. and Packer, L. Eds). Acad. Press. New York, 52, 60-65.

OMURA, T. and SATO, J. (1964). The carbon monoxide binding pigment of liver microsomes. I. Evidence for its hemoprotein nature. J. Biol. Chem., 239, 2370-2378.

PAST, M.R. and COOK D.E. (1982). Drug metabolism in a reconstitued system by diabetes-dependent hepatic cytochrome P-450. Res. Commun. Chem. Pathol. Pharm. 37, 81-90.

PYERIN, W., WOLF, C.R., KINZEL, V. KUBLER, D. and OESCH, F. (1983). Phosphorylation of cytochrome P-450 dependent monooxygenase components. Carcinogenesis, 4, 573-576.

PYERIN, W., TANIGUCHI, H., STIER, A., OESCH, F. and WOLF C.R. (1984). Phosphorylation of rabbit liver cytochrome P-450 LM_2 and its effect on monooxygenase activity. Biochem. Biophys Res. Commun. 122, 620-626.

REINKE, L.A., STOHS, S.J. and ROSENBERG H. (1978). Altered activity of hepatic mixed-function monooxygenase enzymes in streptozotocin-induced diabetic rats. Xenobiotica, 8, 611-619.

RYAN, D.E., THOMAS, P.E., KORZENIOWSKI, D. and LEVIN W. (1979). Separation and characterization of hightly purified form of liver microsomal cytochrome P-450 from rats treated with polychlorinated biphenyls, phenobarbital and 3-methylcholanthrene. J. Biol. Chem., 254 , 1365-1374.

ROUER, E.and LEROUX, J.P. (1980). Liver microsomal cytochrome P-450 and related monooxygenase activities in genetically hyperglycemic (ob/ob and db/db) and lean streptozotocin-treated mice .Biochem. Pharmacol., 29 , 1959-1962.

ROUER, E., MAHU, J.L., COLUMELLI, S., DANSETTE, P., and LEROUX J.P. (1982). Induction of drug metabolizing enzymes in the liver of diabetic mice. Biochimie, 64 , 961-967.

ROUER, E., BEAUNE, P., AUGEREAU, C. and LEROUX, J.P. (1985). The effect of different hyperglucagonemic states on monooxygenase activities and isozymic pattern of cytochrome P-450 in mouse .Bioscience Rep., 5 , 335-341.

ROUER, E., BEAUNE, P. and LEROUX J.P. (1986). Immunoquantitation of some cytochrome P-450 isozymes in liver microsomes from streptozotocin-diabetic rats. Experientia, 42 , 1162-1163.

SNYDER, R. and REMMER, M. (1979). Classes of hepatic microsomal mixed-function oxidase inducers. Pharm. Ther., 7 , 203-244.

WOLFF, T., DEML, E. and WANDERS, H. (1979). Aldrin epoxidation, a highly sensitive indicator specific for cytochrome P-450 dependent monooxygenase activities. Drug. Metab. Dispos., 7 , 301-305 .

Metabolism of caffeine and three of its tri-deuteromethyl isotopomers

Bruno Ribon, Youssef Benchekroun, Michel Désage, Jean-Paul Riou*, Jean-Louis Brazier

*Laboratoire d'Etudes Analytiques et Cinétiques du Médicament, Faculté de Pharmacie, 8, Avenue Rockefeller 69373 Lyon Cedex 08, France. * INSERM U.197, Laboratoire de Médecine Expérimentale, Faculté de médecine Alexis-Carrel, Rue G. Paradin, 69372 Lyon Cedex 08, France*

KEYWORDS

Caffeine, metabolism, isotope effects, hepatocytes

INTRODUCTION

For about 15 years, growing interest has been devoted to stable isotope techniques using ^{2}H (D), ^{13}C, ^{15}N and ^{18}O labeled compounds as tracers for pharmacokinetic and metabolic studies (Baillie, 1981). More recently, the field of applications of these tracers has been extended to more specific problems such as isotope effects (Brazier, 1987). These effects consist of alterations in the behaviour of molecules on substitution by stable (or radioactive) isotopic atoms affecting both physicochemical and biological parameters (Foster, 1985 ; Hanzlik, 1983 ; Pohl, 1984 ; El Tayar, 1984). Caffeine (1,3,7-trimethylxanthine) is extensively cleared and eliminated by animals and man through liver metabolism to a series of partially demethylated xanthines and uric acids (Bonati, 1984-85). The detectable primary metabolites correspond to caffeine N-demethylation (Theophylline, Theobromine and Paraxanthine) and C- oxydation (trimethyluric acid). Horning (1976, 1979) showed that substitution of a CD_3 group for a CH_3 group as in 1-CD_3-caffeine, for example, enhances demethylation at position 7 making this reaction the major metabolic pathway. This author have called this phenomenon, which occurs when compounds are metabolized by multiple alternate rather than sequential pathways, "metabolic switching".

In recent years, isolated hepatocytes became an increasingly popular system for the study of drug metabolism and hepatotoxicity (Guillouzo, 1986).

In the following study, we examine the ability of freshly isolated rat hepatocytes to biotransform caffeine and three of its trideuteromethyl isotopomers : 1,3,7-$(CD_3)_3$-caffeine ; 1,7-$(CD_3)_2$-caffeine ; 3,7-$(CD_3)_2$-caffeine and to demonstrate qualitative and quantitative isotope effects on the formation rate of their 4 organic extractable metabolites : 1,3-dimethylxanthine (theophylline) ; 1,7-dimethylxanthine (paraxanthine) ; 3,7-dimethylxanthine (theobromine) and trimethyluric acid .

MATERIALS AND METHODS

Chemicals

Chemicals were obtained from the following sources :
1,3,7-trideuteromethylcaffeine (1,3,7-TDMX) ; 1,7-trideuteromethylcaffeine
(1,7-TDMX) and 3,7-trideuteromethylcaffeine (3,7-TDMX) were provided by
Dr. Falconnet (1986).
1,3,7-trimethylxanthine (1,3,7-TMX) ; 3-isobutyl-1-methylxanthine (3-IBMX) and
3-methylcholanthrene (3-MC) from Sigma Chemical Co. $(1,3-^{15}N , 2-^{13}C)$-trimethyl-
xanthine from C.E.A. (Saclay, France). Collagenase (Clostridiopeptidase) from
Boehringer. Sodium pentobarbital 6 % from Clin-Midy (Paris, France). All others
chemicals and solvents were of analytical grade and obtained from local commercial
sources.

Animals

Hepatocytes were isolated from adult male Wistar rats of 250-300 g body weight.
A 12 h light cycle was maintained automatically and animals were provided ad lib.
with standard laboratory food and water. Rats were induced by one i.p. injection
of 30 mg/kg body weight of 3-MC dissolved in corn oil 24 h before isolation
(Aldridge, 1977). Animals were anesthetized with sodium pentobarbital 6 %
(1 mg/kg body weight, i.p.) at the same time a day (10 h a.m.).

Hepatocytes preparation and caffeine incubation

Isolated hepatocytes were prepared essentially by the collagenase perfusion
technique of Berry and Friend (1969) as previously described by Riou (1976). After
isolation, liver cells were suspended in a Krebs-Ringer bicarbonate buffer supplemented with 1 % bovine serum albumin, 20 mM glucose and 10 mM pyruvate.
Three stock solutions of unlabeled caffeine associated with each of its deuterated
isotopomers were prepared in the same medium. The reaction was started by the
addition of the drug solution to the cell suspension. The final drug concentrations
were 0.016 to 0.022 mM for each caffeine analogues and the final cell concentrations were 1.6 to 4.1 x 10^6 cells/ml (12-32 mg/ml ; wet weight). The incubation
medium containing the pair of caffeines was distributed (4 ml) in six 25 ml
erlenmeyer flasks, continuously shaken and oxygenated (O_2 95 %, CO_2 5 %). One
flask without drugs was incubated in the same manner.

At zero time and at the following incubation times : 15, 30, 45, 60 and 90 min,
flasks were removed. 0.8 ml of cold perchloric acid (12 % V/V) was added, kept
on ice for 10 min and centrifugated. The supernatant fraction was neutralized
and stored at - 20°C.

Trypan blue exclusion test as well as ATP content measurement were routinaly performed as a control of cell viability. All preparation used in the present experiments had a viability equal or better than 85 %. ATP was measured in neutralized
liver cell perchloric extract with a standard enzymatic method (mean $\pm$ SD, n = 9,
2.7 $\pm$ 0.1 umol/g at 0 min and 2.3 $\pm$ 0.2 umol/g at 90 min).

Metabolism results are presented as the mean of triplicate incubations with
hepatocytes obtained from a single rat.

Caffeine and metabolites assay

Following incubation, caffeine analogues and metabolites concentrations were
determined by mean of GC-MS according to a method derived from theophylline
assay (Désage, 1984).

500 ul of each incubated sample were added with 50 ul internal standard solution and extracted with 2 x 2 ml of a chloroform : isopropanol mixture (85:15 V/V) at pH = 1 (HCl 0.1 M). Internal standard is either $(1,3-^{15}N, 2-^{13}C)$ caffeine for unlabeled and trideuteromethyl caffeines assay or 3-IBMX for metabolites assay. After extraction, derivatization (butylation) of the NH groups of both theophylline, paraxanthine, theobromine, trimethyluric acid and internal standard (3-IBMX) was performed according to the alkylation procedure described by Greeley (1974) for barbiturates. The dry residue was dissolved in 100 ul of a toluène : ethyl acetate (5:2 V/V) mixture and one ul of the subsequent solution injected into the chromatograph : HP 5790 ; OV 1701 capillary column ; splitless mode ; injection port temperature 215°C ; single column temperature ramp 100°C to 220°C, 12°C/min.

A HP 5990 A quadripolar Mass Selective Detector permitted quantitation of selected ions corresponding to the various caffeine analogues and their metabolites (Fig. 1).

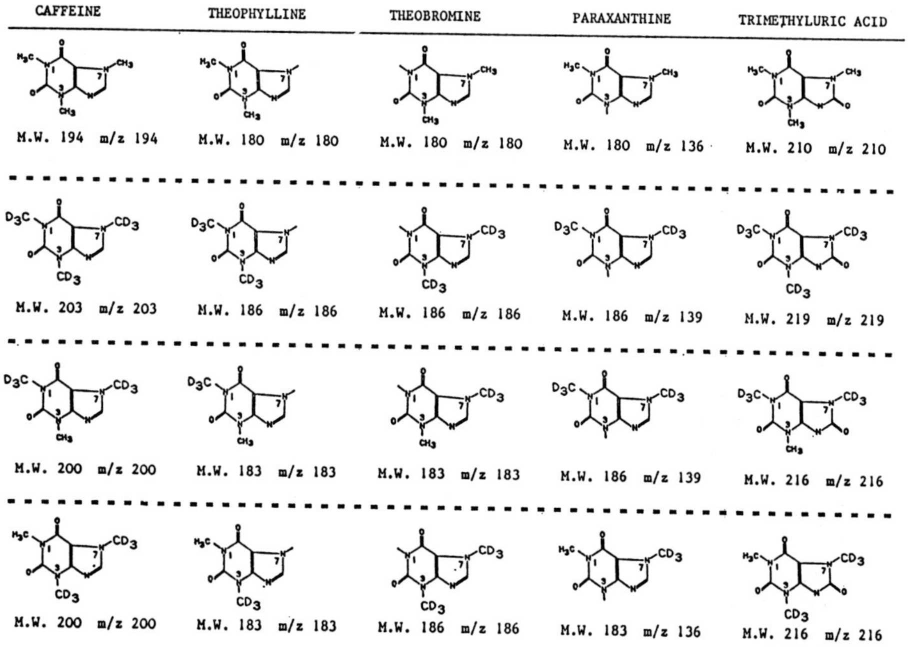

Fig. 1 : Various caffeines analogs and their potential N-demethylated and C-oxidized metabolites.
(name - structure - molecular weight (M.W.) - selected ions (m/z) monitored)

RESULTS

The apparent half-lives of caffeine and its 3 deuterated isotopomers are summarized in Table 1.

Table 1 - Apparent half-lives of caffeine and its 3 deuterated isotopomers. Importance of the isotope effect.

Couples of caffeine analogues	Apparent half-lives min (mean ± S.D.)	Isotope effect $t1/2_D / t1/2_H$
unlabeled caffeine	31,4 ± 6,3	
$1,3,7-(CD_3)_3$-caffeine	57,3 ± 3,1	1,8
unlabeled caffeine	16,6 ± 0,9	
$1,7-(CD_3)_2$-caffeine	18,3 ± 4,8	1,1
unlabeled caffeine	24,7 ± 4,1	
$3,7-(CD_3)_2$-caffeine	33,0 ± 6,1	1,3

It can be seen that the calculated differences between caffeine and both di-trideuteromethylcaffeine half-lives is smaller than that calculated between caffeine and its tri-trideuteromethyl analogue. In this molecule, the CH_3 groups are substituted by CD_3 groups and all sites of N-demethylation are affected by isotope effect. As a consequence the metabolism rate of each pathway from caffeine is reduced (experiment 1 in Fig. 2).

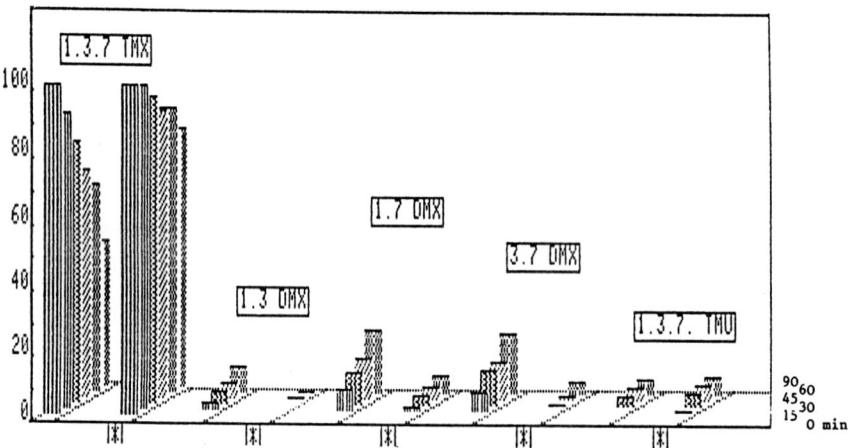

Fig. 2 : Proportions of caffeines and metabolites .
Experiment 1 : UNLABELED CAFFEINE and $1,3,7-(CD_3)_3$-CAFFEINE
(Values are expressed as the percent of the total molecules at each time of incubation. 1,3,7-TMX=caffeine ; 1,3-DMX= theophylline ; 3,7-DMX=theobromine ; 1,7-DMX=paraxanthine and 1,3,7-TMU=trimethyluric acid.
(*) indicate labeled analogues.)

On the contrary, in 1,7-$(CD_3)_2$-caffeine and in 3,7-$(CD_3)_2$-caffeine, the metabolism is preferably switched toward the remaining unlabeled methyl group, which is more easily oxidized. Results clearly show that 1,7-$(CD_3)_2$-caffeine demethylations at position 1 and 7 are depressed (experiment 2 in Fig. 3) and that 1,7-$(CD_3)_2$-paraxanthine becomes the major metabolite. Neither 1-(CD_3)-theophylline nor 7-(CD_3)-theobromine were found in incubation medium after 90 min. 3,7-$(CD_3)_2$-caffeine demethylations at 3 and 7 positions are also depressed (experiment 3 in Fig. 4). 3,7-$(CD_3)_2$-theobromine becomes the major metabolite and neither 3-(CD_3)-theophylline nor 7-(CD_3)-paraxanthine were found.

No isotope effect could be observed in the formation of trimethyluric acid, since oxidation takes place at C8 position which is not directly affected by isotope substitution.

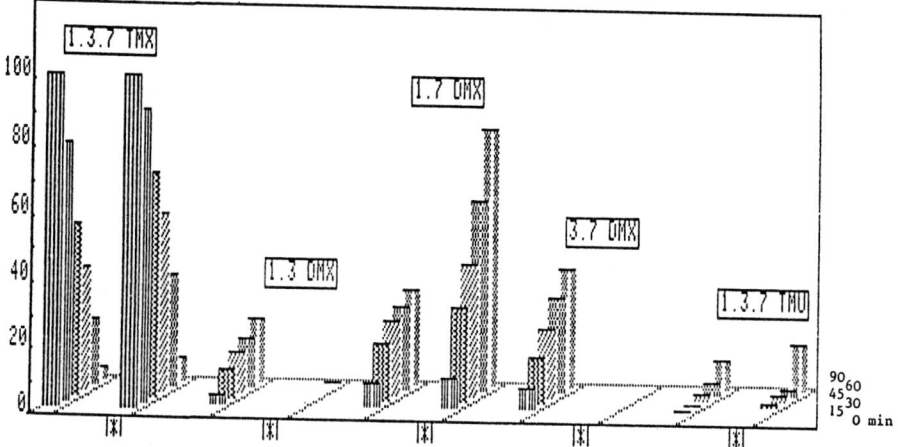

Fig. 3 : Experiment 2 : UNLABELED CAFFEINE and 1,7-$(CD_3)_2$-CAFFEINE.

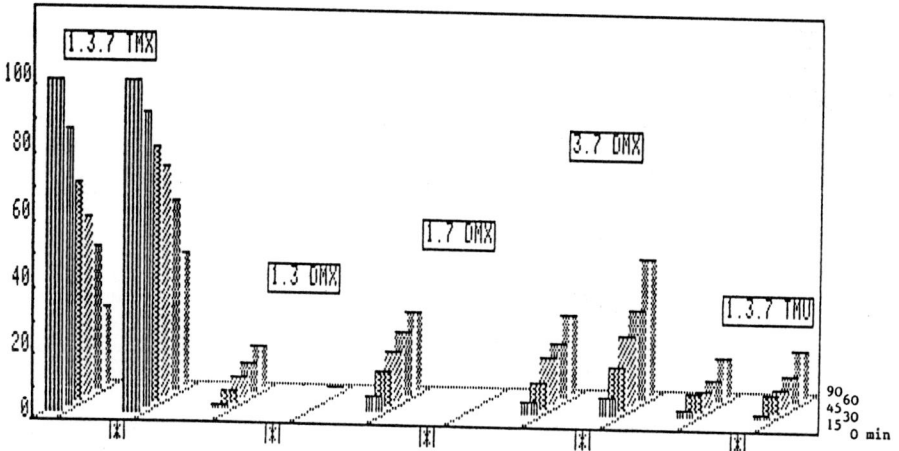

Fig. 4 : Experiment 3 : UNLABELED CAFFEINE and 3,7-$(CD_3)_2$-CAFFEINE.

CONCLUSION

The ability of isolated rat hepatocytes to metabolize caffeine is clearly demonstrated. N.demethylation and C-oxidation reactions occur as described in vivo or in liver microsomes.

Moreover this system is able to reveal isotope effects on metabolic pathways as a consequence of deuterium substitution on the molecular sites of metabolism. Considering how large the incidence of isotopic substitution on kinetic and metabolic processes may be, deuterium labelling associated with hepatocytes use may constitute very usefull tools for mechanisms investigations in molecular pharmacology and toxicology.

Acknowledgments

We are grateful to M. Odeon for excellent technical assitance and to C. Dufour for expert secretarial assistance.

REFERENCES

Aldridge A., Parsons W.D., Neims A.H. (1977) : Stimulation of caffeine metabolism in the rat by 3-methylcholanthrene. Life Sci. 21, 967-974.
Baillie T.A. (1981) : The use of stable isotopes in pharmacological research. Pharm. Rev. 33, 81-132.
Berry M.N. and Friend D.S. (1969) : High yield preparation of isolated rat liver parenchymal cells. J. Cell Biol. 43, 506-520.
Bonati M., Latini R., Tognoni G., Young J.F., Garattini S. (1984-85) : Interspecies comparaison of in vivo caffeine pharmacokinetic in man, monkey, rabbit, rat and mouse. Drug Metab. Rev. 15, 1355-1383.
Brazier J.L., Ribon B., Falconnet J.B., Cherrah Y., Benchekroun Y. (1987) : Etude et utilisation des effets isotopiques en pharmacologie. Thérapie (in press).
Désage M., Soubeyrand J., Soun A., Brazier J.L., Georges Y. (1984) : Automated theophylline assay using gas chromatography and a mass-selective detector. J. Chromatogr. 336, 285-291.
El Tayar N., Van de Waterbeemd H., Gryllaki M., Testa B., Trager W.F. (1984) : The lipophilicity of deuterium atoms. A comparaison of shake-flask and HPLC methods. Int. J. Pharm. 19, 271-281.
Falconnet J.B., Brazier J.L., Désage M. (1986) : Synthesis of seven deuteromethyl-caffeine analogues. Observation of deuterium isotope effects on CMR analysis. J. Label. Compound. Radiopharm. 23, 267-276.
Foster A.B. (1985) : Deuterium isotope in the metabolism of drugs and xenobiotics : implications for drug design. In Advances in drug research, ed. B. Testa, pp 1-40. London : Academic Press.
Greeley R.H. (1974) : Rapid esterification for gas chromatography. J. Chromatogr. 88, 229-233.
Hanslik R.P. (1983) : Effect of substituents on reactivity and toxicity of chemically reactive intermediate. Drug Metab. Rev. 13, 207-234.
Horning M.G., Haegele K.D., Sommer K.R., Nowlin J., Stafford M., Thenot J.P. (1976) : Metabolic switching of drugs pathways as a consequence of deuterium substitution. In Proceedings of the Second International Conference on Stable Isotopes, ed. E.R. Klein and P.D. Klein, pp 41-54, Springfield : Conf 751027 Ntis.
Horning M.G., Nowling J., Thenot J.P., Bouwsna O.J. (1979) : Effect of deuterium substitution on the rate of caffeine metabolism. In Stables Isotopes : Proceedings of the third international conference, ed. E.R. Klein and P.D. Klein, pp 379-384, Oak Brook, Academic Press.
Riou J.P., Claus T.H., Pilkis S.J. (1976) : Control of pyruvate kinase activity by glucagon in isolated hepatocytes. Biochem. Biophys. Res. Commun 73, 591-599.

Isolated hepatocytes as a model to study the disposition of carcinogenic benzo(a)pyrene metabolites

Maria Jonsson, Margareta Martinez, Lennart Dock[1], Bengt Jernström

Department of Toxicology, Karolinska Institutet. [1] National Institute of Environmental Medicine, Stockholm, Sweden

KEY WORDS

Benzo(a)pyrene diol epoxide, glutathione conjugation, carcinogen disposition, isolated cells.

INTRODUCTION

The tumourigenicity of benzo(a)pyrene (BP) is correlated with the formation of (+)-anti-BP-7,8-dihydrodiol-9,10-epoxide (BPDE) and its subsequent binding to the exocyclic nitrogen of deoxyguanosine in DNA (Cooper et al., 1983). Processes, enzymic or non-enzymic, tending to inhibit the intracellular accumulation of BPDE are thus likely to restrict DNA-damage and biological consequences thereof.

In the present study we have used freshly isolated hepatocytes from non-treated or 3-methylcholanthrene(MC)-treated rats (control- and MC-cells, respectively) as models to investigate the disposition of BPDE in intact cells.

METHODS

Freshly isolated hepatocytes (5×10^6/ml, viability >90 per cent as judged by trypan blue exclusion, for details see Moldéus et al., 1978) were suspended in Krebs-HEPES buffer, pH 7.4, and incubated at 37° C with unlabelled or tritium-labelled BPDE (obtained from Chemsyn Science Labs., Lenexa, Kansas, USA). In some experiments the cells were preincubated with diethylmaleate (0.5 mM) for 5 min in order to reduce the intracellular level of glutathione (GSH). Aliquots (100 μl) of the incubation mixture were removed at various time points and the reaction terminated by addition of 400 μl methanol and 25 μl 2 M mercaptoethanol in 0.4 M NaOH (Michaud et al., 1983, Dock et al., 1986). Cellular proteins were precipitated by the method of Wessel and Flügge (1984) prior to analysis by high performance liquid chromatography (HPLC). The extent of protein binding of BPDE was determined by using tritiated BPDE. The protein pellet was dissolved in 5 per cent sodium dodecyl sulfate and an aliquot analyzed by liquid scintillation counting.

A rapid and convenient reverse phase HPLC method was developed for the separation of the various products of BPDE in the cells. By using a Waters associates Z-module fitted with a 5µ C-18 analytical column and a solvent system of acetonitrile in 25 mM ammonium acetate, pH 3.5, delivered at a flow rate of 6 ml/min, it was possible to separate glutathione (GSH)-conjugates of BPDE as well as tetrols, pentols and mercaptoethanol derivatives of BPDE in a single run. The fluorescence of the eluate was monitored using a Shimadzu fluorometer equipped with a 12 µl flow through cell. The quantum yield of the various products at the wavelengths chosen ($\lambda ex=350$ nm, $\lambda em=400$ nm), was determined by using tritiated BPDE. The experimental data points were fitted to first-order rate equations by using a computer program for nonlinear least square regression analysis. The correlation coefficients were generally >0.995.

RESULTS AND DISCUSSION

Figure 1 shows HPLC separation of products derived from BPDE after incubation with hepatocytes obtained from non-treated (1A and 1B) or MC-treated rats (1C). The identities of the products and their relative quantum yields are presented in Table 1.

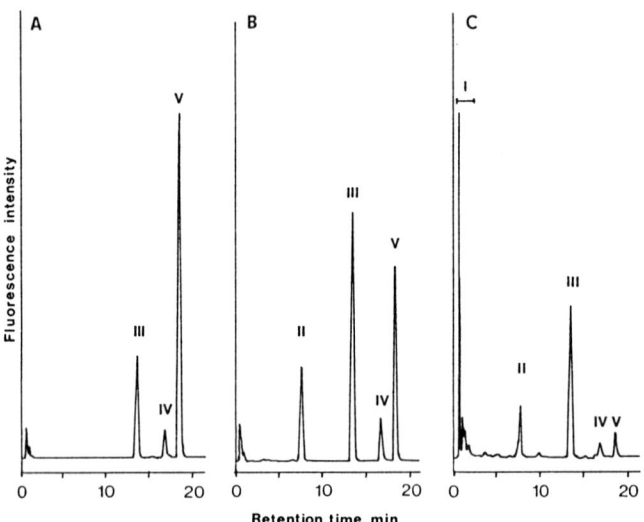

Fig. 1. HPLC separation of products derived from BPDE in isolated hepatocytes. A: control-cells, zero-time; B: control-cells, 5 min; C: MC-cells, 5 min. See Table 1 for peak identities.

Figure 2 shows representative patterns of BPDE disposition in control-cells (Fig. 2A) and control-cells partially depleted of GSH (2B). The intracellular halflife of BPDE in control-cells was generally 1-3 min, depending on the actual cell preparation. Depletion of GSH increased the intracellular halflife of BPDE ~3-fold. Accordingly, the presence of a high cellular level of GSH is essential to allow a rapid and efficient removal of BPDE. The conjugation of BPDE with GSH is likely to be catalyzed by different GSH transferase isoenzymes (Jernström et al., 1985). Protein binding of BPDE in both cell types was estimated to be less than 2 per cent of added substrate. Figure 2C shows a representative pattern of

Table 1. HPLC peak identities and relative quantum yields

Peak(s)	I	II	III	IV	V
R_t (min)	<2	7.5	13.7	17	18.5
Product(s)	n.i.[1]	BPDE-GSH	Tetrol	Tetrol	BPDE-HSEtOH[2]
Rel. quantum yield	n.d.[3]	1	16	16	1

[1] not identified - probably contain BP triol epoxide-adducts
[2] BPDE-mercaptoethanol-conjugate
[3] not determined

BPDE disposition in MC-cells. The halflife of BPDE in MC-cells was comparable to that in control-cells although the pathways of elimination differed. The extent of BPDE-GSH conjugate formation is less than 50 per cent of that in control-cells. In part this is accounted for by the formation of pentols, formed by hydrolysis of triol epoxides derived from BPDE (Gräslund et al., 1986), and an increased protein binding. Moreover, several highly polar products (R_t<2 min), were observed. These have not yet been fully identified but most probably include GSH-derivatives of the BP triol epoxides (Jernström et al., 1984). Depletion of GSH in MC-cells decreased the rates of GSH-conjugate formation and BPDE disappearance but substantially increased the binding of BPDE-derived products to cellular proteins (3- to 5-fold, data not shown).

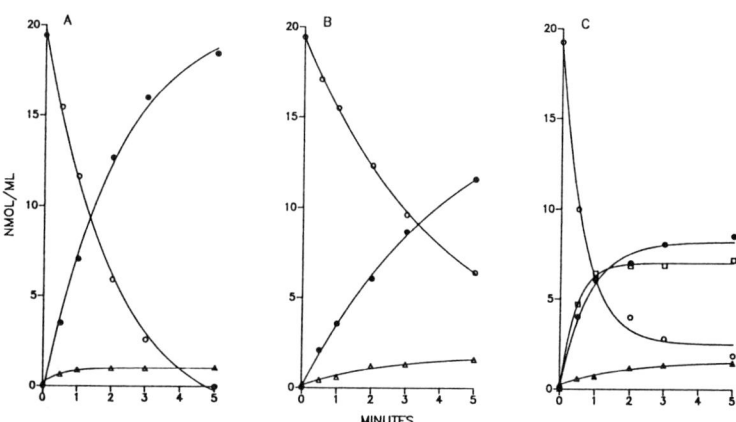

Fig. 2. Disposition of BPDE in isolated hepatocytes as a function of time.
A: control-cells; B: control-cells, partially depleted of GSH; C: MC-cells.
Symbols: -o-: BPDE; -•-: BPDE-GSH conjugates; -△-: tetrols; -▲-: protein adducts; -▫-: not identified.

CONCLUSION

The halflife of $_6$BPDE in isolated hepatocytes from non-treated rats, at a cell density of 5×10^6/ml, is in the order of 1-3 min. The main route of BPDE elimination and detoxication in these cells is via conjugation with GSH (>95 per cent) whereas intracellular hydrolysis of BPDE to tetrols and covalent binding of BPDE to cellular proteins seem to be minor pathways. A 80 per cent reduction of the intracellular GSH level significantly increases the halflife of BPDE and slightly stimulates the formation of tetrols.

Pretreatment of rats with MC induces the cytochrome P-448-linked monooxygenase activity and hepatocytes from these animals show a shift in the pathway of elimination. The dominating route in these cells is via further oxidation of BPDE to triol epoxides and covalent binding of these reactive intermediates to various cellular nucleophiles including proteins and GSH.

These experiments demonstrate two major pathways for the elimination of carcinogenic BPDE from intact cells (Fig. 3), one which should be considered purely detoxifying and one which may be of importance in restricting DNA-damage and tumour initiation but could have severe side-effects due to extensive protein binding.

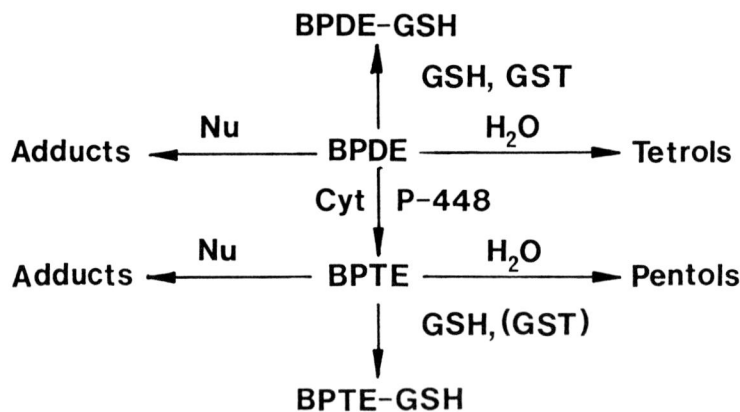

Fig. 3. Pathways of BPDE disposition in isolated hepatocytes.
Nu: nucleophiles; GST: GSH transferase; BPTE: BP triol epoxide.

REFERENCES

Cooper, C.S., Grover, P.L. and Sims, P. (1983): The metabolism and activation of benzo(a)pyrene. Prog. Drug Metab. 7, 295-396.
Dock, L., Waern, F., Martinez, M., Grover, P.L. and Jernström, B. (1986): Studies on the further activation of benzo(a)pyrene diol epoxides by rat liver microsomes and nuclei. Chem.-Biol. Interact. 58, 301-318.
Gräslund, A., Waern, F. and Jernström, B. (1986): Studies by fluorescence and NMR spectroscopy of the major product formed after further metabolism of (±)-7β,8α-dihydroxy-9α,10α-oxy-7,8,9,10-tetrahydrobenzo(a)pyrene. Carcinogenesis 7, 167-170.
Jernström, B., Martinez, M., Meyer, D.J. and Ketterer, B. (1985): Glutathione conjugation of the carcinogenic and mutagenic electrophile (±)-7β,8α-dihydroxy-9α,10α-oxy-7,8,9,10-tetrahydrobenzo(a)pyrene catalyzed by puri-

fied rat liver glutathione transferases. Carcinogenesis 6, 85-89.

Jernström, B., Martinez, M., Svensson, S.-Å. and Dock, L. (1984): Metabolism of benzo(a)pyrene-7,8-dihydrodiol and benzo(a)pyrene-7,8-dihydrodiol--9,10-epoxide to protein-binding products and glutathione conjugates in isolated rat hepatocytes. Carcinogenesis 5, 1079-1085.

Michaud, D.P., Gupta, S.C., Whalen, D.L., Sayer, J.M. and Jerina, D.M. (1983): Effects of pH and salt concentration on the hydrolysis of benzo-(a)pyrene-7,8-diol-9,10-epoxide catalyzed by DNA and polyadenylic acid. Chem.-Biol. Interact. 44, 41-52.

Moldéus, P., Högberg, J. and Orrenius, S. (1978): Isolation and use of liver cells. Methods Enzymol. 51, 60-71.

Wessel, D. and Flügge, U.I. (1984): A method for the quantitative recovery of protein in dilute solution in the presence of detergents and lipids. Anal. Biochem. 138, 141-143.

ACKNOWLEDGEMENTS

This study was supported by the Swedish Cancer Society.

The metabolism of ^{14}C-loxtidine by isolated rat and dog hepatocytes

Martin K. Bayliss, J.A. Bell, A. Bradbury, K. Wilson*

*Glaxo Group Research Limited, Ware, Herts., UK * Hatfield Polytechnic, Hatfield, Herts., UK*

KEYWORDS

Loxtidine, Rat, Dog, Hepatocyte, N-dealkylation, Glucuronylation, Drug Metabolism.

INTRODUCTION

Loxtidine hemisuccinate is a potent, long acting histamine H_2-receptor antagonist. In laboratory animals ^{14}C-loxtidine undergoes metabolism by several routes (Bell et al., 1983) (Fig. 1) and shows important species differences.

In the rat, the major route is N-dealkylation to produce the propionic acid metabolite (IV). The extent of N-dealkylation is saturable <u>in vivo</u>. In the dog, phase 1 metabolism is limited and the compound at both high and low doses is extensively conjugated to form loxtidine glucuronide (II).

Figure 1 METABOLIC PATHWAYS OF LOXTIDINE

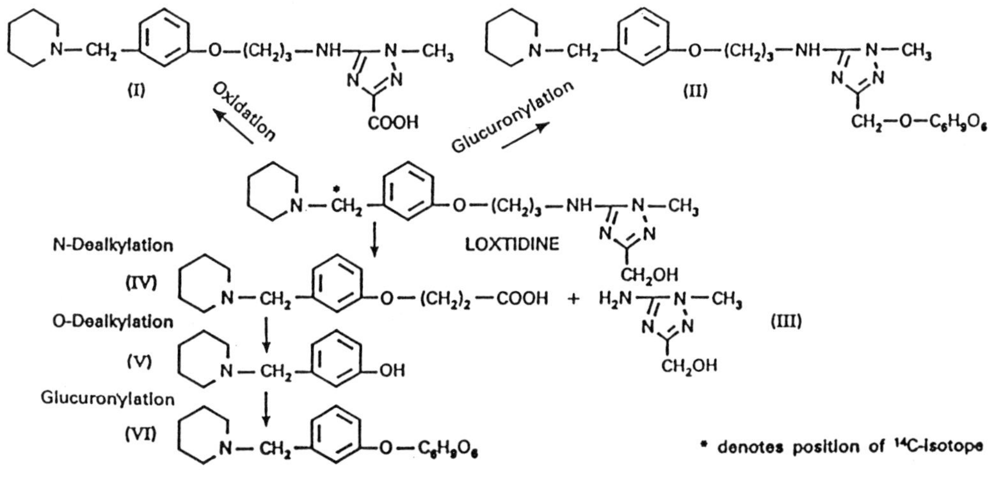

* denotes position of ^{14}C-isotope

These species differences make loxtidine an ideal model compound for the evaluation of the use of isolated hepatocytes in the prediction of drug metabolism in vivo.

METHODS

Hepatocyte Preparation

Hepatocytes from a male AH random hooded rat and a male beagle dog were prepared by a three stage perfusion with collagenase according to the method of Oldham et al., (1985). Washed isolated hepatocytes were suspended in Williams Medium E containing L-glutamine (4mM) at a final concentration of approximately 2×10^6 cells/ml.

Cell viability (87-91%) was determined by trypan blue (0.8%) exclusion and lactate dehydrogenase leakage.

Metabolic Studies

Isolated rat and dog hepatocytes (2×10^6 cells/ml) were incubated with ^{14}C-loxtidine hemisuccinate (0.06 MBq/mg) at concentrations of 5, 10, 25, 50 and 100µM (2ml total incubate volume) in Williams Medium E at 37 C for up to 3 hours under a water saturated atmosphere of oxygen/carbon dioxide (95%:5%). Control (non-viable) hepatocytes were prepared by heat treatment (10 mins at 100 C) before the addition of ^{14}C-loxtidine. Samples were withdrawn at various times and placed in acetone to stop the reaction.

Metabolites produced from dog hepatocytes were incubated with β-glucuronidase (280 Fishman Units) and sulphatase (12 Units) in 0.05M sodium acetate buffer (pH5) at 37 C for 18 hours to hydrolyse conjugates.

Metabolites from hepatocyte and enzyme incubates were analysed by radio thin layer chromatography on silica G60 using

Ethyl acetate	:	Propan-2-ol	:	Water	:	0.88 Ammonia
(25		15	:	8	:	2,by vol.)

Radioactive areas on the thin layer chromatography plates were recorded and integrated by use of a Isomess IM 3000 linear analyser (Raytest, Sheffield, U.K.) linked to Apple IIe data system.

RESULTS

No break down of ^{14}C-loxtidine occured in control (non-viable) incubations with either rat or dog hepatocytes.

Rat Hepatocytes

When ^{14}C-loxtidine was incubated with viable rat hepatocytes several metabolites (I, II, IV and V) were detected (Fig. 2).

The major radioactive metabolite produced from ^{14}C-loxtidine by rat hepatocytes at all concentrations was the propionic acid metabolite (IV). The extent of metabolism of ^{14}C-loxtidine was saturable, being greatest at the lowest concentration (Fig. 2 and 3).

Figure 2: THE METABOLISM OF ^{14}C-LOXTIDINE BY ISOLATED RAT HEPATOCYTES

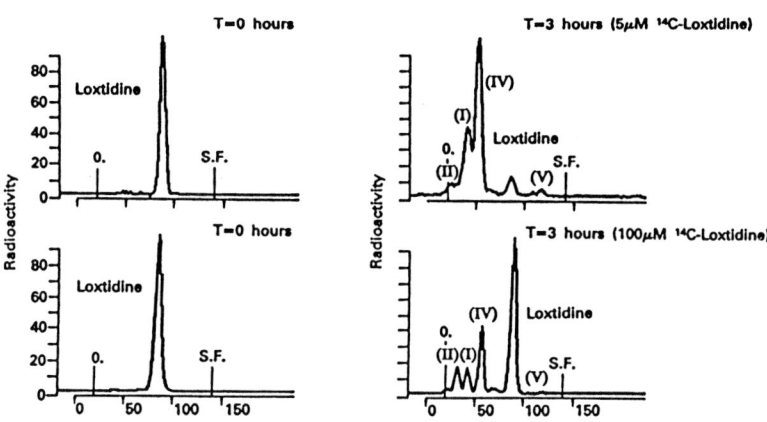

Dog Hepatocytes

When ^{14}C-loxtidine was incubated with dog hepatocytes only two metabolites (I and II) were detected (Fig. 4). The major radioactive metabolite at all concentrations was metabolite (II).

Incubation of metabolite (II) with β-glucuronidase showed it to be the glucuronide conjugate of ^{14}C-loxtidine (Fig. 5).

The extent of metabolism of ^{14}C-loxtidine was saturated at the highest concentration studied (100μM) (Fig. 4 and 6).

DISCUSSION

All the previously identified metabolites of ^{14}C-loxtidine produced in vivo by rat and dog were formed by rat and dog hepatocytes. As in the whole animal the major route for the metabolism of ^{14}C-loxtidine in rat hepatocytes was N-dealkylation. This metabolic pathway has been shown to be saturated in the isolated hepatocyte system. This effect was also seen in vivo (1-50mg ^{14}C-loxtidine base/kg).

As seen in the whole animal the major metabolic route for ^{14}C-loxtidine by dog hepatocytes was glucuronylation of loxtidine. Only trace amounts of the carboxylic acid metabolite (I) were detected in vitro. At concentrations of 5-50μM ^{14}C-loxtidine glucuronylation was not saturable in dog hepatocytes. However, saturation of ^{14}C-loxtidine glucuronylation was evident at loxtidine concentrations above 50μM.

This study has demonstrated that the metabolism of loxtidine in isolated hepatocytes shows the same species differences and dose relationships as those seen in vivo. These results, therefore, illustrate the usefulness of isolated hepatocytes in the prediction of drug metabolism in vivo.

Figure 3: THE EFFECT OF CONCENTRATION ON THE N-DEALKYLATION OF ^{14}C-LOXTIDINE BY ISOLATED RAT HEPATOCYTES

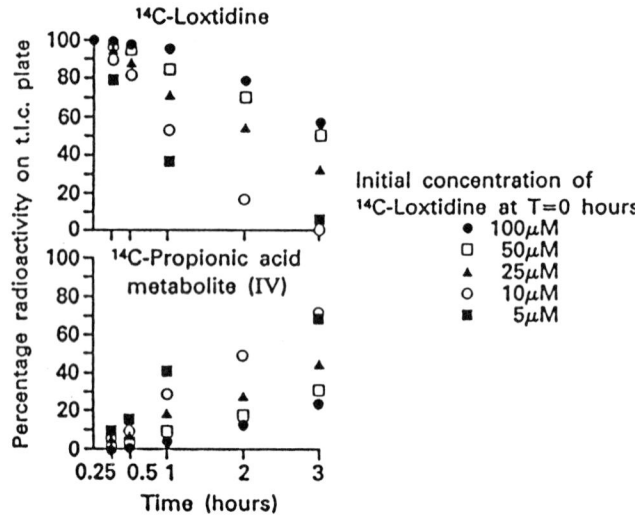

Figure 4: THE METABOLISM OF ^{14}C-LOXTIDINE BY ISOLATED DOG HEPATOCYTES

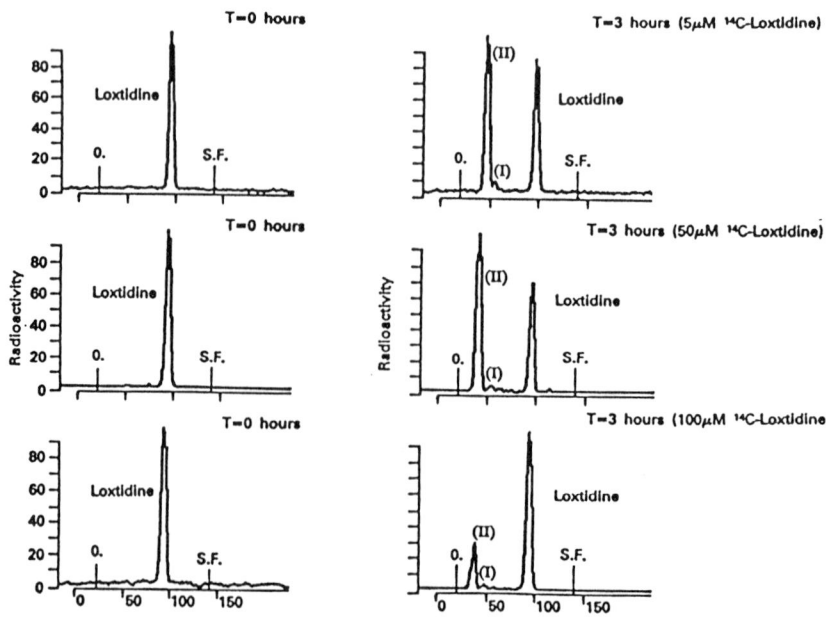

Figure 5: INCUBATIONS OF METABOLITE (II) FROM DOG HEPATOCYTES WITH ß-GLUCURONIDASE

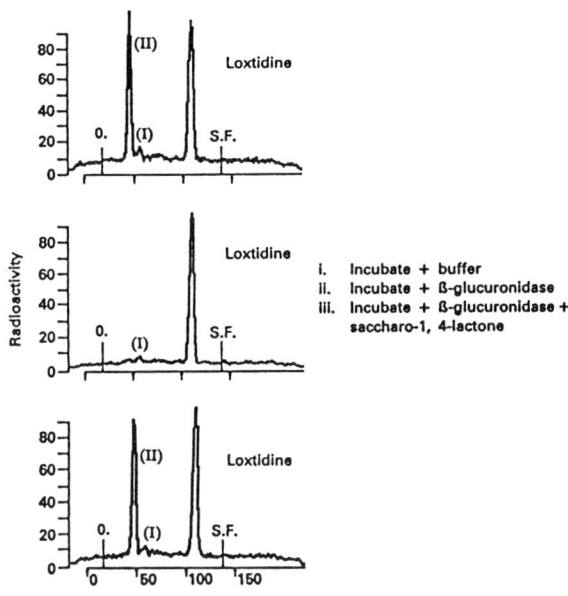

i. Incubate + buffer
ii. Incubate + ß-glucuronidase
iii. Incubate + ß-glucuronidase + saccharo-1, 4-lactone

Figure 6: THE EFFECT OF CONCENTRATION ON THE GLUCURONYLATION OF ^{14}C-LOXTIDINE BY ISOLATED DOG HEPATOCYTES

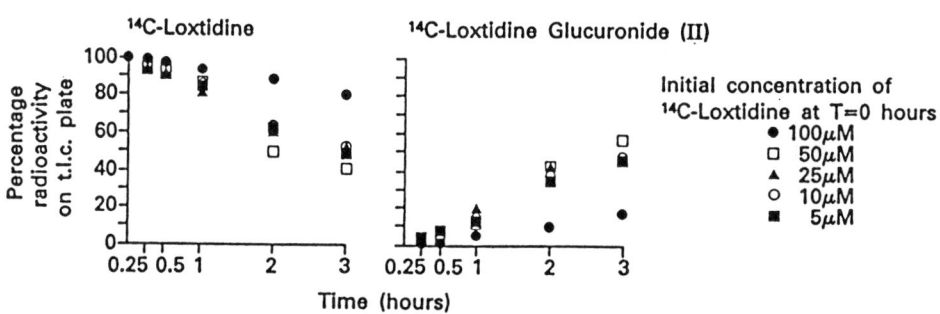

Initial concentration of ^{14}C-Loxtidine at T=0 hours
- 100 μM
- 50 μM
- 25 μM
- 10 μM
- 5 μM

REFERENCES

Bell, J.A., Bradbury, A., Jenner, W.N., Manchee, G.R., and Martin, L.E. (1983): The metabolism of loxtidine in rat and dog. Biochem. Soc. Trans. 11, 715.

Oldham, H.G., Norman, S.J., and Chenery, R.J. (1985): Primary cultures of adult rat hepatocytes - model for the toxicity of histamine H_2-receptor antagonists. Toxicology, 36, 215-229.

Caffeine metabolism by human and rat hepatocytes in primary culture

François Berthou*, Damrong Ratanasavanh**, Christian Riché*, André Guillouzo**

*Laboratoires de Biochimie-Pharmacologie, Faculté de Médecine, 29285 Brest Cedex, France,
**INSERM U.49, Hôpital de Pontchaillou, 35033 Rennes Cedex, France

KEY WORDS

Caffeine - Metabolism - Hepatocyte culture - Rat - Human - Monooxygenase activities.

INTRODUCTION

Caffeine is a pharmacologically active alkaloid which is widely used in beverages and as a drug. It is extensively metabolized in-vivo into a wide number of metabolites (Arnaud, 1984). Its biotransformation principally occurs in the liver via the microsomal mixed-function monooxygenases containing cytochromes P-450 (Aldridge et al., 1977 ; Wietholtz et al., 1981). Accordingly, caffeine has been proposed as a model compound for measuring liver function (Renner et al., 1984).

While caffeine is known to be almost totally metabolized in-vivo, many studies have demonstrated that its metabolic rate is dramatically decreased in in-vitro models including liver microsomes (Arnaud and Welsch, 1980; Bonati et al., 1980 ; Ferrero and Neims, 1983 ; Grant et al., 1987). As noted by these authors this discrepancy, as yet, remains unexplained. Since only short-term In - vitro systems have been tested , it may be postulated that intact hepatocytes could represent a more appropriate model for studying hepatic metabolism of caffeine. Indeed parenchymal cells from various species, including man, at different ages can be easily prepared and cultured for periods of days or weeks depending on the culture conditions tested.

MATERIAL and METHODS

Chemicals
Methylxanthines were purchased from Sigma (St Louis, MO, USA). The purity of caffeine was checked by HPLC and exceeded 99.9% with respect to its possible metabolites.

Liver samples
Human livers were obtained from three post-mortem neonates (1 to 3 weeks old) and eight kidney transplantation donors (20-40 years old). Dietary habits and exposure to environmental chemicals before death were not known. All the livers were histologically normal. All these samples were obtained according to the recommandations of the local ethical committee.
Rat livers were obtained from 200-300g male Sprague-Dawley animals.

Activity of liver microsomes
Liver microsomes from 6 human adults were prepared by the method of Meier et al. (1983). Microsomal ethoxyresorufin 0-deethylase (EROD) activity was determined by method of Prough et al. (1978). Protein content was determined by the method of Lowry et al. (1951).

Cell isolation and culture
Adult and newborn human hepatocytes were prepared by collagenase perfusion according to Guguen-Guillouzo et al. (1982). The cells were seeded at the density of 2.5×10^6 cells per 28 cm^2 Petri dish in 4 ml of nutrient medium. This latter consisted of a mixture of 75% minimum essential medium and 25% medium 199 containing 10 ug/ml bovine insulin, 0.2% bovine serum albumin and 10% foetal calf serum. The medium was changed 8-16 h later and the fresh medium was supplemented with 3×10^{-6} M hydrocortisone hemisuccinate.
Rat hepatocytes were isolated by the two-step collagenase perfusion method (Guguen-Guillouzo and Guillouzo, 1986). The cells were seeded and cultured according to the conditions described for human cells. The medium to which 3×10^{-6} M hydrocortisone hemisuccinate was added was renewed 4 h after cell seeding.

Metabolic studies
Cultured hepatocytes were incubated with caffeine dissolved in the culture medium at concentrations ranging between 10^{-4} M and 10^{-3} M. No cell toxicity was detected at these concentrations. Some experiments were carried out using [8^{14}C]-caffeine (specific activity 1.8 m Ci/mmole) purchased from Amersham, UK.
Media and cells were collected after a 24 h incubation. Metabolites were extracted from media and sonicated cells by a chloroform/isopropanol mixture (85/15, v/v) after saturating aqueous phase with ammonium sulfate.

Quantification of metabolites by HPLC
Metabolites were separated by HPLC - reversed phase on Nucleosil C-18 with a mobile phase consisting of a quaternary mixture of water/tetahydrofuran/acetic acid/acetonitrile with a linear elution gradient. They were identified by their retention times with reference to pure standards. They were quantified with respect to their relative UV - 280 nm - response factor.

RESULTS

Overall metabolism
Caffeine was shown to be a poor substrate for monooxygenases of hepatocytes in primary culture. In human adults important inter-individual variations regarding the overall metabolism were observed. Two groups could be characterized according to their metabolic capacity. Hepatocytes from two human adults (Group A) metabolized up to 9.5 and 15.5% of 10^{-3} M caffeine respectively while those of the six other adults (Group B) metabolized only about 0.8% ($\pm$ 0.6 ; n = 3) and 5.1% ($\pm$ 3.6 ; n = 3) of substrate at 10^{-3} and 10^{-4} M respectively. This very low metabolic capacity is in agreement with the results obtained with microsomes although the incubation

time is different: 24 h for hepatocytes versus about 15 min for microsomes. Despite their great apparent dispersion when expressed by percent of substrate transformed at different concentrations, the data appeared more homogeneous when they were expressed by the metabolic rate (Table 1). Low metabolic activity was also found with both newborn hepatocytes and adult rat hepatocytes (Table 1).

Table 1. Caffeine metabolism rate (expressed as nmole / 10^6 cells /24 h)

Hepatocytes	Number of subjects	Range
Human newborn	3	16 - 20
Human adult		
group A	2	152 - 248
group B	6	5 - 24
Adult rat	3	8 - 13

In order to attempt to explain this very low metabolism of caffeine, adult rat hepatocytes were incubated for 24 h with a substrate mixture containing [8-^{14}C]-caffeine at 10^{-4} M and the three cold dimethylxanthines (DMX), namely theobromine, paraxanthine and theophylline, at 1.5×10^{-6} M each, i.e. at the concentration close to that obtained after 24 h incubation with pure caffeine 10^{-4} M. Although the three DMX were present in culture medium at the beginning of incubation, 8.5% of caffeine was metabolized at a rate of 13.4 nmoles/10^6 cells/24 h. Therefore the metabolic capacity was not inhibited by metabolites released in the culture medium.

This low metabolic capacity of cultured hepatocytes to transform caffeine, as also demonstrated with liver microsomes from rat (Arnaud and Welsch, 1980 ; Bonati et al., 1980), mouse (Ferrero and Neims, 1983) and human (Grant et al.,1987; Berthou et al, unpublished observation), did not reflect the in-vivo situation. Indeed, it has been shown that only 2% of a plasma concentration of 0.5×10^{-4} M caffeine was found unmetabolized in urine of humans (Arnaud, 1984). Such a discrepancy remains unclear. Since the drug is also extensively metabolized in the isolated perfused liver (less than 5% of unchanged caffeine after a 3 h perfusion (Arnaud et Welsch, 1980), it may be postulated that these differences could be related to the different experimental models used. It is assumed that the half-life time $t_{1/2}$ can be calculated according to the expression derived from first-order kinetics: $t_{1/2} = 0.693 V_d / C_l$, where V_d is the distribution volume and C_l the metabolic clearance. Assuming that the metabolic rate was 26 nmoles/24 h/4 ml incubation dish (see above) the metabolic clearance was estimated to be 0.26 ml/24 h. Accordingly the half-life time of caffeine in our in-vitro experiments would be 10 days. This result must be compared to 5 h, the half-life time determined in-vivo. This working hypothesis can be applied to the perfused rat liver model. Arnaud and Welsch (1980), found that 42% and 95% of 1 umole caffeine in 100 ml of perfused liquid was metabolized in 30 min and 3 h respectively. Accordingly the half-life time was determined to be 0.65 h, i.e. very close to 0.88 h determined in-vivo (Bonati and Garattini, 1984). However further studies are needed to validate this hypothesis which could correlate in-vivo and in-vitro determinations of drug metabolism rates.

Metabolic profiles of caffeine

The metabolic profile characterized in-vivo (Arnaud and Welsch, 1981) was qualitatively recovered in hepatocyte cultures. However only the primary metabolites were obtained. The major metabolites were dimethylxanthines resulting from oxidative demethylation. The other minor metabolic pathways consisted of oxidation giving 1,3,7-trimethyluric acid (1,3,7-TMU) and hydratation on the same position giving after ring opening 6-amino-5[N-formylmethylamino] 1,3-dimethyluracil (1,3,7-DAU). Figure 1 summarizes the pathways leading to the three dimethylxanthines, the uric acid and the diaminouracil derivative.

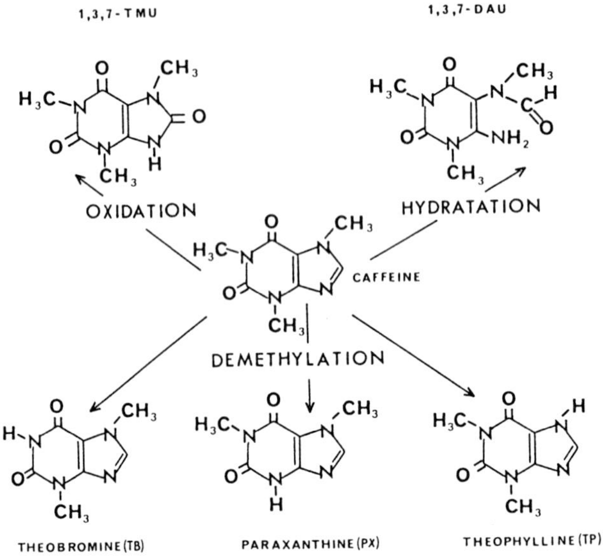

Fig.1 Metabolites produced directly from caffeine in cultured adult rat and human hepatocytes.

Metabolic profiles were different according to species, development stage and environmental factors. Fig. 2 shows comparative patterns of the three DMX. The loss of the 3-methyl group from caffeine to produce paraxanthine was the preferential path of metabolism in human adults of group B. This result is in agreement with in-vivo previous studies (Arnaud and Welsch, 1981; Bonati and Garattini, 1984). In contrast to human adult hepatocytes, each demethylation pathway was of similar importance in adult rat hepatocytes, giving a nearly equal proportion of the three DMX. Such a finding is in agreement with in-vivo studies where relatively low doses of caffeine were administred (Wietholtz et al., 1981). On the other hand caffeine was only demethylated at the 7-methyl group to form theophylline in newborn human hepatocytes. Although caffeine metabolism in the newborn child was studied by Aldridge et al.(1979) by analysing urinary metabolites, but without separation of theophylline and paraxanthine, their results make comparison difficult. However our results are in agreement with the findings of Bada et al. (1979). who demonstrated that only theophylline could be quantified in plasma of human newborns receiving caffeine.

The metabolic profiles of human adult hepatocytes from group A were nearly similar to those obtained in human newborns so that theophylline accounted for up to 97% of total DMX. As such a profile was associated with a very high metabolic rate, it can be suggested that differences between groups A and B

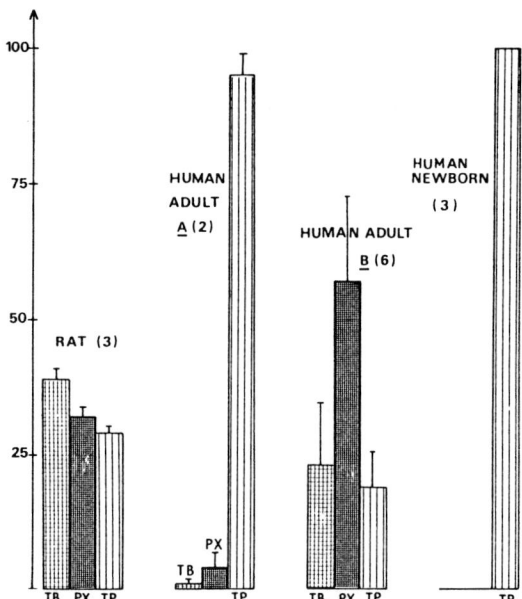

Fig. 2 Relative ratio of the three dimethylxanthines formed from caffeine.
TB = theobromine;   PX = paraxanthine;   TP = theophylline

could be explained by a previous induction of livers by environmental compounds including polyaromatic hydrocarbons (PAH) of tobacco smoke. Indeed stimulation of caffeine metabolism by PAH (Wietholtz et al.,1981; Aldridge et al., 1977) and smoking (Parsons et al., 1978) is well documented. Moreover it was demonstrated by using a caffeine breath test (Wietholtz et al.,1981) that the 7-demethylation to form theophylline clearly discriminated between smokers and non-smokers. In order to validate our hypothesis, the ethoxyresorufin deethylation (EROD) activity, which is inducible by cigarette smoking (Williams et al., 1986), was measured in liver microsomes of two groups A and B of human adults. The EROD activity was 185 ($\pm$ 66) pmoles/min/mg microsomal protein for five subjects of group B whereas it was 675 for the one subject of group A whose microsomes could be obtained. Therefore it can be suggested that the apparently abnormal behaviour of hepatocytes from group A could be due to the fact that these donors were heavy smokers.
These results are thought to provide an adequate basis for the study of cytochrome P-450 isoenzymes involved in caffeine metabolism.

ACKNOWLEDGEMENTS

This study was supported by INSERM (CRE 86 7002)

REFERENCES

Aldridge, A., Parsons, W.D., Neims, A.H. (1977) : Stimulation of caffeine metabolism in the rat by 3-methylcholanthrene. Life Sci., 21 , 967-974.
Aldridge, A., Aranda, J.V., Neims, A.H.(1979) : Caffeine metabolism in the newborn. Clin. Pharmacol. Ther., 25 , 447-453.

Arnaud, M.J., Welsch, C. (1980) : Comparison of caffeine metabolism by perfused rat liver and isolated microsomes. In **Microsomes, drug oxidations and chemical carcinogenesis**,eds R.W. Estabrook, H.V. Gelboin, J.R. Gilette, P.J. O'Brien, pp. 813-816. New - York : Academic Press.

Arnaud, M.J. , Welsch, C. (1981) : Theophylline and caffeine metabolism in man. In **Theophylline and other methylxanthines; methods in clinical pharmacology**, eds N. Rietbrock, B.G. Woodcook, A.H. Stalb, vol. 3, pp. 135-148. Braunschweig Wiesbaden: Vieweg.

Arnaud, M.J. (1984) : Products of metabolism of caffeine. In **Caffeine, perspectives from recent research**, ed P.B. Dews. pp. 3-38, Berlin : Springer-Verlag.

Bada, H.S., Khanna, N.N., Somani, S.M.(1979) : Interconversion of theophylline and caffeine in newborn infants. **J. Pediatr.**, 94 , 993-995.

Bonati, M., Latini, R., Marzi, E., Cantoni, R., Belvedere, G. (1980) : [2-^{14}C] caffeine metabolism in control and 3-methylcholanthrene induced rat liver microsomes by high pressure liquid chromatography. **Toxicol. Lett.**, 7 , 1-7.

Bonati, M., Garattini, S. (1984) : Interspecies comparison of caffeine disposition. In **Caffeine , perspectives from recent reseach** ed P.B. Dews, pp. 48-56, Berlin: Springer-Verlag.

Ferrero, J.L., Neims, A.H. (1983): Metabolism of caffeine by mouse liver microsomes : GSH or cytosol causes a shift in produts from 1,3,7-trimethylurate to a substitued diaminouracil. **Life Sci.**, 33 , 1173-1178.

Grant, D.M., Campbell, M.E., Tang, B.K., Kalow, W. (1987) : Biotransformation of caffeine by microsomes from human livers : kinetics and inhibition studies. **Biochem. Pharmacol.**, 36 , 1251-1260.

Guguen-Guillouzo, C., Campion, J.P., Brissot, P., Glaise, D., Launois, B., Bourel, M., Guillouzo, A. (1982) : High yield preparation of isolated adult human hepatocytes by enzymatic perfusion of the liver. **Cell. Biol. Int. Rep.**, 6 , 625-628.

Guguen-Guillouzo, C., Guillouzo, A. (1986) : Méthodes de préparation d'hépatocytes adultes et foetaux. In **Hépatocytes isolés et en culture**, eds A. Guillouzo, C. Guguen-Guillouzo, pp. 1-12, Paris:INSERM and John Libbey Eurotext.

Lowry, O.H., Rosebrough, N.G., Farr, A.L. , Randall, R.J. (1951). Protein measurement with the Folin phenol reagent.**J. Biol.Chem.**, 193 , 265-275

Meier, P.J., Mueller, H.K., Dick, B., Meyer, U.A. (1983) : Hepatic monooxygenase activities in subjects with a genetic defect in drug oxidation. **Gastroenterology**, 85 , 685-692.

Prough, R.A., Burke, M.D., Mayer, R.T. (1978) : Direct fluorometric methods for measuring mixed-function oxidase activity. In **Methods in enzymology**, eds S. Fleischer, L. Packer. LII , pp. 372-340, Academic Press: New York

Parsons, W.D., Neims, A.H. (1978): Effect of smoking on caffeine clearance. **Clin. Pharmacol. Ther.**, 24 , 40-45.

Renner, E., Wietholtz, H., Huguenin, P., Arnaud, M.J., Preisig, R.,(1984) : Caffeine : a model coumpound for measuring liver function **Hepatology**, 4 , 38-46.

Wietholtz, H., Voegelin, M., Arnaud, M.J., Bircher, J., Preisig, R. (1981) : Assessment of the cytochrome P-448 dependent liver enzyme system by a caffeine breath test. **Eur. J. Clin. Pharmacol.**, 21 , 53-59.

Williams, F.M., Mutch, E., Woodhouse, K.W., Lambert, D. , Rawlins, M.D. (1986): Ethoxyresorufin O-deethylation by human liver microsomes. **Br. J. Clin. Pharmac.**, 22 , 263-268.

Cytotoxicity and metabolism study of amineptine (S-1694-1) in cultured adult rat and human hepatocytes

Damrong Ratanasavanh*, Jean-Marc Bégué*, Patrick Gelé**, Luc Grislain**, Norbert Bromet**, Pierre du Vignaud**, Rémi Defrance***, Elisabeth Mocaer***, André Guillouzo*

*INSERM, U.49, Unité de Recherches Hépatologiques, Hôpital Pontchaillou, 35033 Rennes Cedex, France. ** Technologie Servier, Division de Pharmacocinétique et Métabolisme, 45007 Orléans, France. *** Institut de Recherches Internationales Servier, 92205 Neuilly-sur-Seine, France

Keywords : Amineptine - metabolism - hepatotoxicity - rat-human - hepatocytes - in vivo - primary culture.

INTRODUCTION

Hepatocytes in suspension or in culture have been widely used to evaluate drug cytotoxicity and drug metabolism (Guillouzo, 1986). However, the studies have been performed mainly on rodent hepatocytes and it is well known that major differences may exist between human and experimental animals in the response to drugs. Concerning drug cytotoxicity studies, up to now, most of the investigations have been limited to the assessment of toxic effects of a single dose, over a short period, not exceeding a few hours or one day. The aim of this work was to determine whether cultured hepatocytes could be used as a model system to investigate species differences in metabolism as well as in long-term toxicity of new drugs. To answer this question we have used primary cultures of rat and human hepatocytes. Long-term studies were performed with hepatocyte co-cultures. Indeed, in this condition, hepatocytes survive longer and maintain specific functions for several days or weeks (Guguen-Guillouzo et al., 1983). As a reference we have selected amineptine (S 1694-1) a new antidepressant agent, and its effects were compared to those obtained with amitriptyline, an analog drug.

MATERIAL AND METHODS

Isolation and culture of hepatocytes.

Rat hepatocytes : The cells were isolated from the liver of 200-300 g Sprague-Dawley rats by perfusion with 0.025 % collagenase as previously described (Guguen-Guillouzo et al., 1983). They were seeded at a density of 5×10^5 cells per 10 cm^2 petri dish in 2 ml of Ham F12 medium containing 0.2 % bovine serum albumin, 10 µg/ml bovine insulin and 10 % fetal calf serum. A part of the cultures was set up as pure cultures, the other was set up as co-cultures by adding an equivalent number of rat liver epithelial cells (Guguen-Guillouzo et al., 1983). The medium was supplemented with 3×10^{-6} M hydrocortisone hemisuccinate after 4 h and 24 h in pure culture and co-culture respectively, and renewed daily thereafter.

Human hepatocytes : The livers were obtained from kidney transplantation donors and the cells were isolated by collagenase perfusion as previously described (Guguen-Guillouzo et al., 1982). The cells were seeded at the density of 5×10^5 cells per 10 cm^2 petri dish in 2 ml of medium. The following steps were those described for rat hepatocytes except that rat liver epithelial cells were added only 16-18 h after cell seeding.

Metabolism studies.
Only pure rat and human hepatocyte cultures were used. ^{14}C-S-1694-1 (10 µCi /flask) was incubated with hepatocyte cultures for 24 h. Then, media and cells were collected and stored separately at -80°C until analysis. They were extracted and analysed by GC-MS and HPLC linked to U.V. and radioactivity detectors according to the methods described by Du Vignaud et al. (this volume).

Cell treatment.
A first series of experiments was performed with pure cultures to determine the maximum non toxic concentration of each drug after a 24 h incubation. The drugs were added at various concentrations to 4 h cultures (rat hepatocytes) or 16 h cultures (human hepatocytes).
A second series of experiments was performed with co-cultures for long-term ("chronic") drug toxicity assessment. Various concentrations were selected, the highest scoring + in the acute cytotoxicity test. They were added 24 h after rat liver epithelial cell seeding for the first time and then every day with medium renewal for 10 to 13 days.

Morphological examination.

Light microscopy : living cultures were examined daily under phase-contrast microscopy. The degree of cytotoxicity was evaluated by giving a score graded from 0 (controls) to +++ (Ratanasavanh et al., 1987).
+ : corresponded to appearance of a few dense or refringent intracytoplasmic granules and/or slight alteration of the cell shape ; ++ : to the presence of many intracellular granules and shrinking of some cells ; +++ : to accumulation of a number of intracytoplasmic granules and/or disruption of the cell monolayer. A toxic effect was retained for ++ and +++.

Electron microscopy : at the end of experiments, hepatocyte cultures were fixed by 2.5 % glutaraldehyde in sodium cacodylate buffer 0.1 M, pH 7.4 for 5 min. at 4°C, then post-fixed by 1 % O_SO_4 in sodium cacodylate buffer for 30 min, dehydrated and embedded in Epon.

Biochemical assays
Albumin secretion rate was measured daily in the culture medium by laser immunonephelometry (Guguen-Guillouzo et al., 1983) as an index of specific hepatocyte function. Lactate dehydrogenase (LDH) leakage was determined daily as an index of cell toxicity using the M.A.-Kit Roche, LDH opt. DGKC (ref. 1431-3) and a Cobas Bio apparatus.

RESULTS.

Metabolism.
Figure 1 shows metabolic pathways of amineptine obtained from in vivo studies in rat and in man. These results are presented in details elsewhere (Du Vignaud et al., this volume).

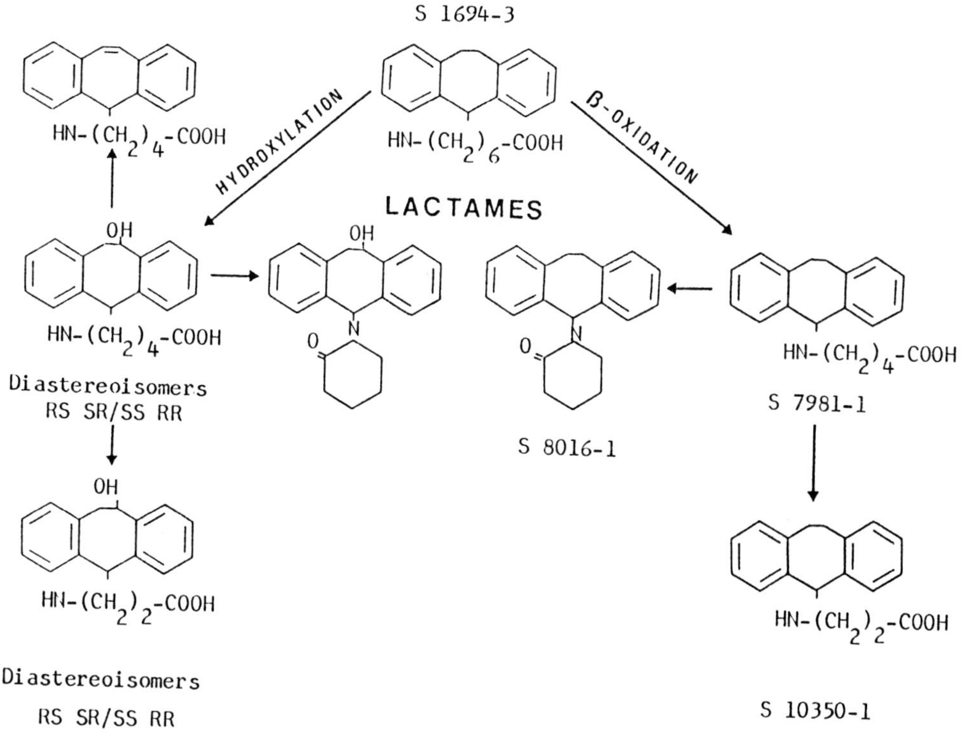

Fig. 1 : In vivo metabolism pathways of amineptine in rat and in man.

Briefly, amineptine was transformed either by β-oxidation of the amino heptanoic chain or by hydroxylation of the 10 position of the dibenzocyclobenzyl ring which when combined with β-oxidation, resulted in the formation of two diastereoisomers. These primary metabolites can be further transformed by a second β-oxidation. Conjugated metabolites were detected in man but not in rat. All major metabolites found in vivo were characterized in extracts from media of rat and human hepatocyte cultures (Fig. 2). In addition, species differences were found. S-7981, a metabolite resulting from the first β-oxidation of the parent compound, was formed in higher amounts in human hepatocytes than in rat hepatocytes. By contrast, as in vivo, more hydroxylated metabolites were produced by rat hepatocytes than by human hepatocytes.

Cytotoxicity

Short-term treatment.
A short-term treatment of pure cultures of rat and human hepatocytes was performed to determine the maximum non toxic concentration of amineptine and amitriptyline, the reference drug. This last compound was found to be cytotoxic to rat and human hepatocytes at concentrations about 10-fold lower than those of amineptine (Table I).

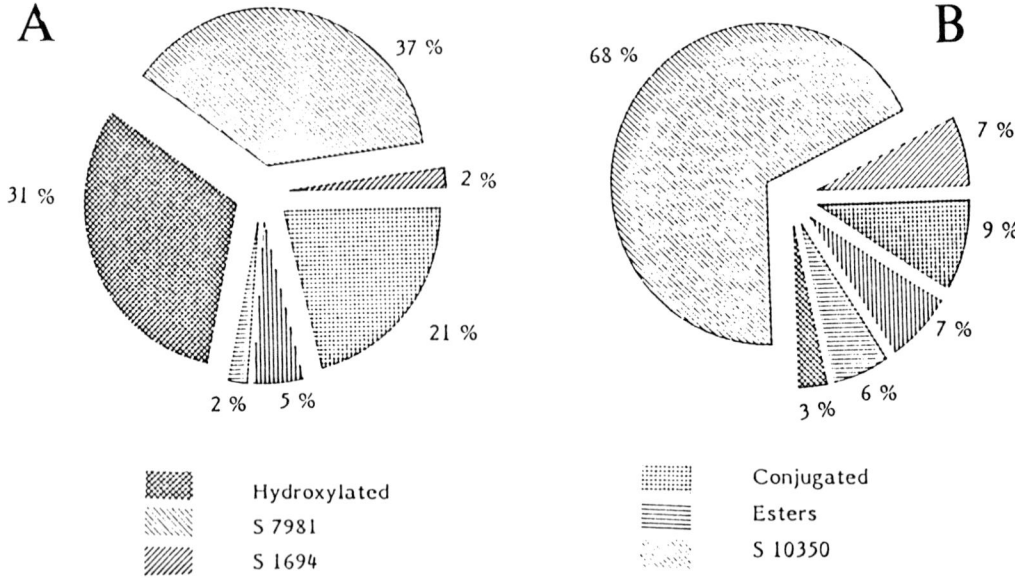

Figure 2 : Metabolites produced from amineptine in rat (A) and human (B) hepatocyte cultures.

TABLE I : Assessment of short-term cytotoxicity of amineptine and amitriptyline to rat and human hepatocytes in pure culture by light microscopic examination.

Species	Days of treatment	Drug concentration (Mol.)					
		Amineptine			Amitriptyline		
		1.5×10^{-5}	3×10^{-4}	6×10^{-4}	2×10^{-5}	4×10^{-5}	8×10^{-5}
Rat	1	0	0	+++	+	++	+++
	2	0	+	+++	+	++	+++
Human	1	0	0	+++	+	++	+++
	2	0	+	+++	+	+++	+++

The degree of toxicity was graded from 0 (controls) to +++ (see the methods section).

At concentrations lower than or equal to 300 µM, amineptine did not provoke any obvious morphological and LDH leakage changes in rat and human hepatocytes. At 600 µM cell detachment and LDH leakage were observed after 24 and 48 h in rat and human hepatocyte cultures respectively (Table II).

TABLE II : Effect of amineptine on LDH release in pure cultures of rat and human hepatocytes.

Species	Days of treatment	Control	Drug concentration (Mol.)		
			1.5×10^{-4}	3×10^{-4}	6×10^{-4}
Rat	1	100	85.9 ± 9.5	99.3 ± 9.5	262.0 ± 199.3
	2	100	57.0 ± 10.6	82.8 ± 31.9	152.7 ± 27.4
Human	1	100	N.D.	105.0 ± 0.1	119.02 ± 5.5
	2	100	N.D.	121.4 ± 30.3	235.7 ± 50.5

The results are expressed as percentages of controls. N.D. : not determined.

TABLE III : Assessment of long-term cytotoxicity of amineptide to co-cultured human hepatocytes by light microscopic examination.

Days of treatment	Drug Concentration (Mol.)			
	0	7.5×10^{-5}	1.5×10^{-4}	3×10^{-4}
1	0	0	0	+
3	0	0	0	++
5	0	0	+	++
7	0	0	+	++
9	0	0	+	++
11	0	0	+	++
13	0	0	+	++

The degree of toxicity was graded from 0 (controls) to +++ (see methods section).

Long-term treatment

Chronic toxicity was assessed with hepatocyte co-cultures. The results obtained with amitriptyline have already been partially reported elsewhere (Ratanasavanh et al. , 1988). This drug induced morphological alterations and accumulation of secondary lysosomes in rat and human hepatocyte co-cultures, at a concentration as low as 2 µM. Amineptine at 75 µM, did not provoke any morphological changes in human hepatocyte co-cultures, even after 13 days of treatment (Table III). In contrast, at this dose amineptine induced alterations of cell structure in rat hepatocytes as soon as on day 5 of treatment. These results were confirmed by electron microscopic examination (Fig. 3). At 150 μM, a slight alteration of the cell structure was observed after 5 days in human hepatocyte co-cultures and at higher doses, the presence of many intracellular granules was observed after 2 or 3 days of treatment. LDH leakage was slightly increased during the treatment but not in a significant manner (Fig. 4). In contrast, albumin production was markedly decreased (Fig. 5).

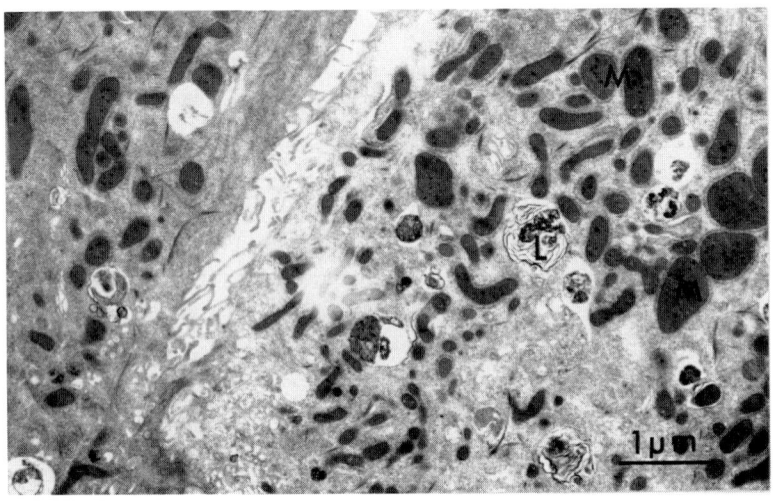

Figure 3 : Electron microscopic appearance of a rat hepatocyte co-cultured for 13 days in the presence of 75 μM amineptine. (L : lysosome ; M : mitochondria).

DISCUSSION

Amineptine is extensively metabolized in vivo in both rats and humans (Du Vignaud et al, this volume). Less than 2 % of the parent compound was found unchanged in urine. When amineptine was incubated with rat and human hepatocytes in primary culture, the results were similar to those observed in vivo in many aspects. S-7981 which represents a major metabolite observed in humans, was found also to be the major metabolite formed in vitro. On the other hand, the hydroxylated metabolites which were predominantly formed in the rat, were found also to be the most abundant in cultured rat hepatocytes and in higher amounts than in cultured human hepatocytes. Amineptine was cytotoxic to rat and human hepatocytes in conventional cultures only at high doses (about 100 times more than the maximum plasma concentration after standard therapeutic dosage). The concentrations which induced LDH leakage and morphological changes were 10 fold higher than those of amitriptyline, an analog drug. It may be assumed that a short-term treatment of hepatocytes in pure culture does not always reflect the in vivo toxicity of many compounds. Indeed a number of drugs, including amineptine (Stricker and Spoelstra, 1985), can induce hepatic injury at therapeutic doses but only after weeks or months. As reported previously (Ratanasavanh et al., 1988) hepatocytes in co-culture make the possibility of investigating the effects of drugs after several daily additions. The maximum non toxic drug concentration can be lowered or not depending on the compound tested.

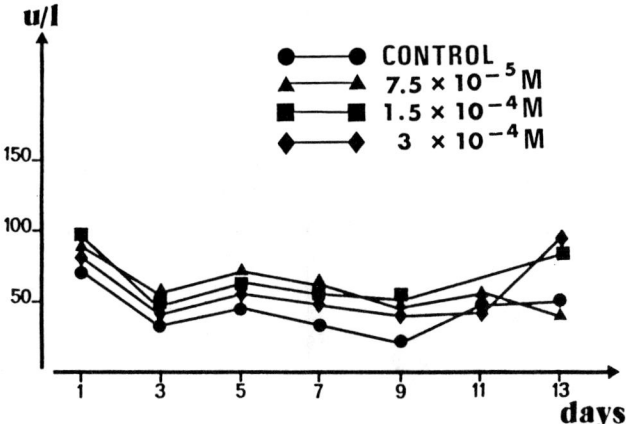

Figure 4 : Effect of long-term amineptine treatment of human hepatocyte co-cultures on LDH leakage.

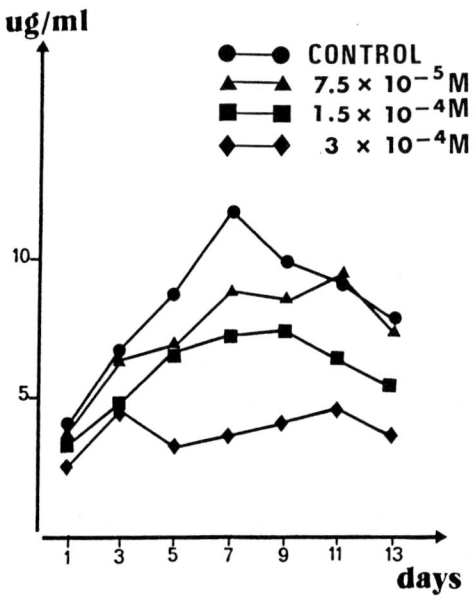

Figure 5 : Effect of long-term amineptine treatment of human hepatocyte co-cultures on albumin production.

Thus the threshold of toxic concentration of amineptine was lowered by 8 and 4 fold in rat and human hepatocyte co-cultures respectively. When compared to amitriptyline amineptine was found to be much less cytotoxic as assayed by light and electron microscopy which was found to represent sensitive indices of cytotoxicity after short-term and, especially, long-term drug treatment. Measurement of LDH leakage showed that the integrity of cell plasma membrane was not affected during 10-12 days of amineptine treatment. The increase in LDH activity was observed only at the end of experiment. In contrast, amineptine inhibited albumin secretion into the medium as a function of drug concentrations and this inhibition was observed on the first day of treatment. Amitriptyline induced the same effect at a concentration 10 times lower. These results suggest that amineptine can be considered as a non hepatotoxic drug.
Obviously more than one endpoint must be used to assess drug in vitro cytotoxicity. Albumin production and daily morphological examination by light microscopy are, compared with LDH leakage, sensitive indices for assessing time- and concentration-related effects of the tested drugs in long term cytotoxicity studies. Other endpoints, such as synthesis of intracellular and secreted proteins after incorporation of radioactive amino-acids or inhibition of glycerolipid secretion (Boelsterli et al., 1987) can also be useful and sensitive tests.

ACKNOWLEDGMENTS

We thank Mrs A. Vannier for typing the manuscript. This work was partly supported by the Ministère de l'Industrie et de la Recherche.

REFERENCES

Boelsterli, U.A., Bouis, P. and Donatsh, P. (1987). Psychotropic drugs as inhibitors of glycerolipid biosynthesis and secretion in primary rat hepatocyte cultures. Toxic. In Vitro 1, 127-132.

Du Vignaud, P., Gele, P., Delbos, J.M., Bromet, N. and Mocaer, E. (1988): Metabolism of ^{14}C-S 1694-1 in rat, dog and man (this volume).

Guguen-Guillouzo, C, Campion, J.P., Brissot, P., Glaise, D., Launois, B., Bourel, M. and Guillouzo, A. (1982): High yield preparation of isolated human adult hepatocytes by enzymatic perfusion of the liver. Cell Biol. Int. Rep. 6, 625-628.

Guguen-Guillouzo, C., Clément, B., Baffet, G., Beaumont, C., Morel-Chany, E., Glaise, D. and Guillouzo, A. (1983): Maintenance and reversibility of active albumin secretion by adult rat hepatocytes co-cultured with another liver epithelial cell type. Exp. Cell Res. 143, 47-54.

Guillouzo, A. (1986): Use of isolated and cultured hepatocytes for xenobiotic metabolism and cytotoxicity studies. In Isolated and cultured hepatocytes eds A. Guillouzo and C. Guguen-Guillouzo, pp 327-346, Paris : INSERM, London : John Libbey.

Ratanasavanh, D. Baffet, G., Latinier, M.F., Rissel, M., Guillouzo, A. (1988): Use of hepatocyte co-cultures in the assessment of drug toxicity from chronic exposure. Xenobiotica, in press.

Stricker, B.H.C.H., Spoelstra, P. (1985): In Drug-induced disorders : drug induced hepatic injury, ed. M.N.G. Dukes pp. 278-279. Amsterdam, Elsevier.

Human hepatocytes as an alternative model to the use of animal in experiments

J.P. Cano, R. Rahmani, G. Fabre, B. Richard, B. Lacarelle, P. Boré, P. Bertault-Peres, G. de Sousa, I. Fabre, M. Placidi, C. Coulange*, M. Ducros*, M. Rampal*

*INSERM U.278, 13385 Marseille Cedex 5, France. *Service d'Urologie et de Greffe Rénale, La Timone, Marseille, France*

KEY WORDS:
Human hepatocytes, Transport, Metabolism, Midazolam, Vinca alkaloids, Mitoxantrone.

INTRODUCTION

The liver plays a major role in the metabolism of drugs and other exogenous compounds. For this reason, an attractive model for the assessment of the metabolic process potentially involved in the pharmacokinetic behaviour and overall pharmacological and toxicological response consists of isolated and cultured hepatocytes from various species -including man-.(Shull, 1987). This model also provides an interesting approach to the understanding of metabolic interactions observed in clinical practice (drug-drug or drug-endogenous compounds interactions). However, the major drawback of this model consists in the qualitative and quantitative interspecies differences in the hepatic metabolism of drugs (Guillouzo, 1985). Hence the extrapolation to humans of the results obtained with animal hepatocytes remains hazardous. Thus, the use of human hepatocytes constitutes an interesting alternative method for surmonting these problems.

Viable human hepatocytes are difficult to obtain due to ethical problems, size of the organ and adequate surgical sampling procedure. Few research groups have developed techniques for isolating human hepatocytes either from liver biopsies or a portion of the left lobe of liver (Reese, 1982; Strom, 1982; Guguen-Guillouzo, 1982). In this article, we report an efficient procedure for obtaining several milliards of viable hepatocytes (20×10^9 hepatocytes) from a whole human liver. Metabolic characteristics of freshly isolated hepatocytes, were studied both in suspension and in primary-culture.

I/ FRESHLY ISOLATED HEPATOCYTES IN SUSPENSION

1/ Isolation of hepatocytes from whole human livers :

Whole human livers were taken under strict ethical conditions

shortly after death from kidney and/or heart transplantation donors. Organs were first thoroughly washed "in situ" with 5 to 10 liters of 4°C cold sterile Collin's solution.
The organ was placed in a perfusion apparatus, equipped with a peristaltic pump, a recirculating water heater, and a membrane oxygenator. The liver was washed via the portal vein with an oxygenized HEPES (20 mM), NaCl (120 mM), KCl (5 mM) buffer (pH 7.5, containing 0.5 % glucose (w/v)), at ambiant temperature. Following this, the organ temperature was progressively raised to 37-38°, by perfusion under a recirculating mode of 2.5 l of the same HEPES buffer.
Subsequently a collagenase solution (0.05 % in HEPES buffer, pH : 7.5, 37°C), was added into the perfusion system, and the organ maintained under a constant warmed, humidified and oxygenated atmosphere. We observed -following numerous animal experiments (dog, pig...)- that the kinetics of hepatic enzymes leakage (ALAT, ASAT, LDH...), together with the liver macroscopic aspect, were precise indicators of the tissue dissociation stage.

Throughout the course of the experiment, these parameters were continuously monitored in the recirculating medium, and collagenase action stopped when a dramatic increase of the enzyme activity was noticed in the perfusate. Fig 1 illustrates the kinetic of the enzyme's appearance in this medium. In this specific case, the recirculation of the enzymatic solution has to be stopped at 25 minutes, following addition of the collagenase.

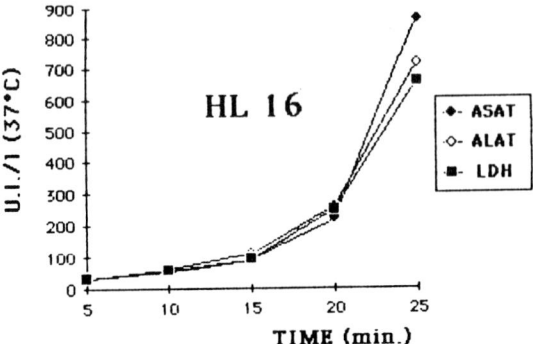

Fig. 1: Release of hepatic enzymes during the perfusion

2/ Preparation of cell suspension
The organ was placed in an ice-chilled receptacle. Glisson's capsule was then disrupted, the liver gently minced, and the liberated cells diluted in a buffer consisting of HEPES (10 mM), NaCl (120 mM), KCl (6.2 mM), CaCl2 (0.9 ml) and BSA (1 % w/v) (pH : 7.4) (washing buffer).
The cellular suspension was centrifuged twice after filtration (50 x g for 2 min) in ice cold washing buffer. The final sediment of this low-speed centrifugation, consisting mainly of parenchymal liver cells, was resuspended in the incubation medium, until being used either as hepatocyte in suspension or in culture. The cell population consisted almost exclusively of morphologically intact, free parenchymal cells. The viability of the purified hepatocytes, assessed by trypan blue staining, ranged between 85 and 95 %.

3/ Incubation procedure and metabolic studies
Freshly isolated hepatocytes were suspended at a final density of 2.5 to 5 x 10^6 cells/ml and were incubated at 37°C in Ham F12 medium . The pH was maintained at 7.4 by passing over the cell suspension a warm and humidified 95% O_2, 5 % CO_2 . The cell preparation was gently stirred by a teflon paddle throughout the incubation.
The experiments were initiated with the addition of radiolabelled

drug, in the incubation medium. For the transport and metabolism kinetic studies, 0.5 ml of the cell suspension were layered on 400 ul of inert silicone oil (density : 1.03), at selected times (from 30 sec to 2 hrs) (Reed, 1984). The tubes were centrifuged at 15 000 x g for 30 seconds. Portions of the extracellular and/or intracellular medium were analyzed using specific HPLC methodologies.

II/ PRIMARY-CULTURES OF HEPATOCYTES

Human hepatocytes were resuspended in HAM F12 medium supplemented by: 10 % fetal calf serum, insulin, glucagon, L-thyroxin, transferrine, linoleic acid and antibiotics. Cells (2.5×10^6) were plated on 60 mm-diameter plastic dishes in 4 ml of medium. After a 4 to 8-hours adhesion period, medium was removed and supplemented with 10^{-6} M dexamethasone.

A representative illustration of characteristic primary human hepatocyte cultures is shown in Fig. 2.

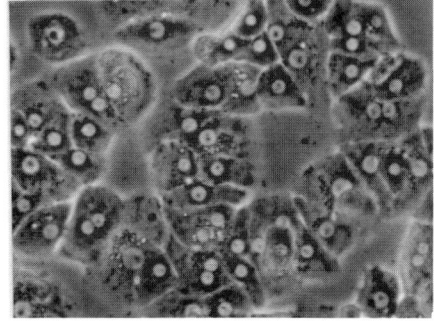

Fig. 2: Phase contrast microscope photograph of human hepatocytes

III/ CRYOPRESERVATION

After being washed, human hepatocytes, were resuspended in HAM F12 supplemented with 10 % DMSO, and 20 % fetal calf serum. The final hepatocyte concentration ranged usually between 20 and 40 x 10^6 cells/ml. The cell suspension -placed in sterile polypropylene tubes (1.8 ml for 12 x 35 mm tubes - Nunc Ltd)-, was equilibrated at 4°C for periods of time never exceeding 20 minutes. Cell freezing was performed with a NICOOL ST 20. Samples were transferred into liquid nitrogen when a temperature of - 150° C was attained. Hepatocytes were stored at - 196°C for periods of up to one year.

IV/ DRUG METABOLISM IN HUMAN HEPATOCYTES

FRESHLY ISOLATED HEPATOCYTES IN SUSPENSION

1/ Metabolism of midazolam

Midazolam is a watersoluble imidazobenzodiazepine which exhibits hypnotic effects with a short duration of action (Gerecke, 1983). Its biotransformation includes oxidative pathways (1-hydroxy-4-hydroxy- and di-hydroxy-derivatives) as well as glucuronidation. Metabolism of this molecule, which is well known in man, was checked as a test of the enzyme hepetocytes activity since i/ its biotranformation involves phase I and phase II reactions; ii/ all metabolites are already known and available as standards and, iii/ its pharmacokinetic as well as that of its 1-hydroxylated derivative were intensively studied for many years in our laboratory.

The extracellular kinetic (from 5 min to 2 hr) of biotransformation of midazolam has been studied following exposure of freshly isolated human hepatocytes to 1 ug/ml ^{14}C-midazolam (Fig 3). The extracellular level of midazolam decreased by one-half within 5 min and only very low amounts of unchanged drug were detectable after 45 min. Concomitantly several metabolites appeared in this medium. 1-hydroxy-midazolam rapidly formed reaching a maximum value between the 30th and the 45th minute. The 4-hydroxylated derivative was also detected in the extra-cellular compartment, but its level remained low throughout the entire period of observation. After a 1.5 hr incubation period, low amounts of 1,4-dihydroxy-midazolam were also found. Moreover a highly polar derivative - the 1-hydroxy-midazolam glucuronide - was present in significant amount after a 2 hr exposure.

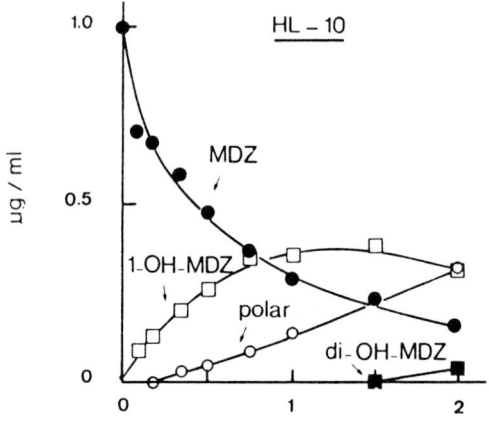

Fig. 3: Kinetics of midazolam metabolism

2/ Uptake and metabolism of Vinca alkaloïds

Vindesine (VDS) and Navelbine (NVB) are two semisynthetic Vinca alkaloïds (V.A) related to vinblastine. They are currently undergoing clinical trials in Europe. "In vivo" and "in vitro" studies in humans and animals have been conducted for several years in our laboratory (Rahmani 1986 and 1987) with the aim of arriving at a better understanding of the important interindividual and interdrug variabilities of V.A. in terms of toxicity and efficacy. Indeed, the almost complete ignorance of their metabolic fate stands, to some extent, in the way of their rational therapeutic use, and also in all probability, in the way of the development of new analogues with better therapeutic index. For this reason, hepatocytes freshly isolated from animal or human liver were used to investigate VDS and NVB accumulation and metabolism. Cells (5×10^6 cells/ml) were exposed to various concentrations of each drug (from 10^{-8} M to 10^{-6} M)) over periods of from 1 min to 2.5 hrs. Intracellular and extracellular media were then analyzed by a sensitive and specific HPLC method. Although cellular captation and metabolism of V.A. were significant in rat hepatocytes, strong quantitative (VDS) and/or qualitative (NVB) interspecies differences were demonstrated for both processes (Fig. 4). These results stress the importance of using the more predictive and appropriate tool, for a correct screening of transport and metabolic events at the liver site.
Human hepatocytes, accumulate both molecules rapidly and to a great extent (35 % to 75 % of total radiolabel incorporated in 15 min for VDS and NVB respectively) resulting in high transmembrane gradients (up to 150 to 200). Moreover unchanged V.A. represented the major intracellular form, whereas metabolites rapidly crossed the cell membrane and accounted for more than 75 % of the total extracellular radioactivity at the end of the experiment (Fig. 5). However, under the same experimental procedure, these two molecules exhibited significantly different influx and metabolism kinetic profiles. NVB was shown to be more avidly taken up by the cells, presumably due to its greater hydrophobicity, which could facilitate its diffusion in plasma membranes. This fact, may at least in part, explain the higher distribution volume of NVB (Vd = 28.6 ± 11.7 l/kg) compared to VDS (Vd = 8.8

± 5 l/kg)) as estimated after I.V bolus injection of these anticancer drugs in patients. Human hepatocytes also provide the opportunity to advance the idea that the large interindividual variations observed for VDS plasmatic clearances in cancer patients, may result from the important inter-liver differences in VDS metabolism.

These results bring out the importance of performing "in vitro" research in human cells, as soon as possible at a preclinical stage during a new drug's development.

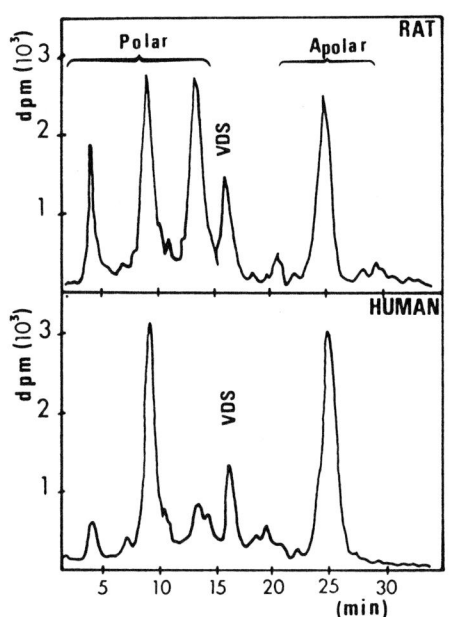 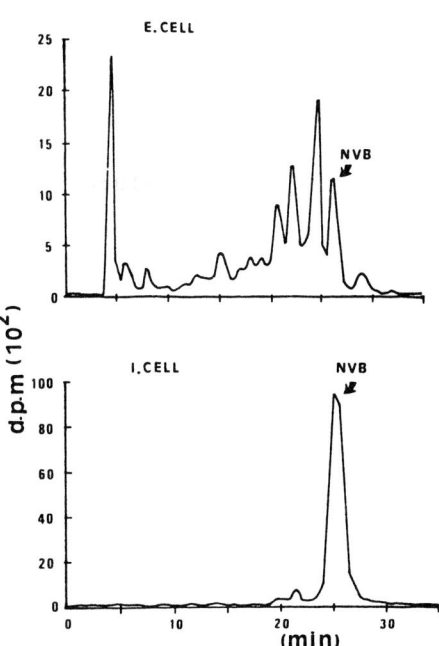

Fig. 4: Interspecies variability in VDS metabolism

Fig. 5: Radiochromatogram of NVB and its metabolites in extracellular and intracellular media

HEPATOCYTES IN PRIMARY-CULTURE

Metabolism of Mitoxantrone

Mitoxantrone or 1,4-dihydroxy-5,8-bis-((2-((2-hydroxyethyl)-amino)-ethyl)-amino-9,10-anthracenedione dihydrochloride is an anticancer drug with significant clinical activity (Shenkenberg, 1986). Savaraj et al. (1982) compared two groups of patients ; a group with hepatic impairment and another group without any liver dysfunction. The average total plasmatic clearance for mitoxantrone in the first group was decreased to less than one-half of that in patients in the latter group, whereas the terminal half life value of the drug was almost doubled.

Could this phenomenon have been predicted on the basis of preclinical in vitro experiments?

We therefore analyzed the metabolism of mitoxantrone using

freshly isolated hepatocytes from human liver in primary cultures (Richard, 1987). Hepatocytes were incubated in the presence of ^{14}C-Mitoxantrone concentrations ranging from 1 to 20 uM over a period of 24 hours. Extracellular medium was analyzed by a HPLC methodology which permitted the quantification of the unchanged drug and its metabolites (Fig. 6 inset). The very rapid decrease of extracellular mitoxantrone (Fig. 6) is due to its accumulation within the cells and its subsequent metabolism. Indeed two metabolites appeared in the extracellular compartment and were identified as the mono- and di-carboxylic acid derivatives of mitoxantrone.The dicarboxylic acid derivative represented the main extracellular metabolite as found in patient urines.
The metabolism of mitoxantrone was linear over the range concentrations used: 30 % of the initial drug were metabolized after 24 hours of incubation (Fig. 7).
These data demonstrate that mitoxantrone is slowly but intensively metabolized to various derivatives which rapidly efflux in the extracellular compartment. This study shows the important role of the liver in the metabolism of mitoxantrone in humans without using any in vivo animal experiments.

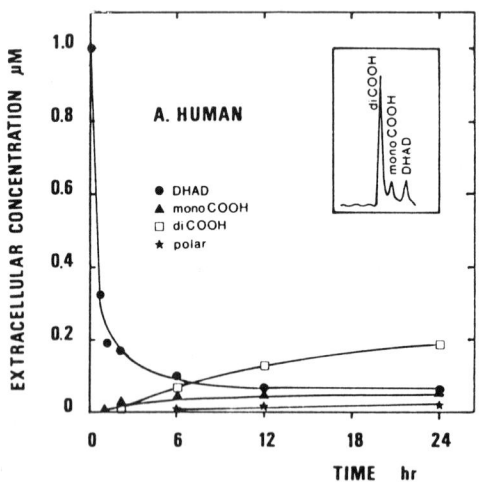 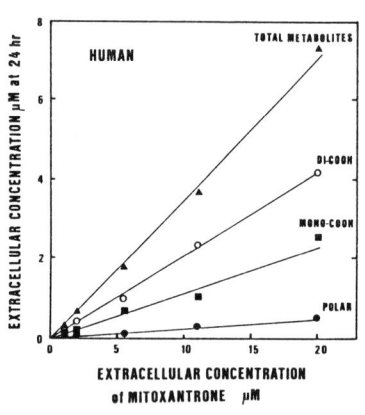

Fig. 6: Metabolism of mitoxantrone in human hepatocytes. Inset represents the extracellular metabolic profile (24th hr)

Fig. 7: Dose-dependance study of mitoxantrone metabolism in hepatocytes in primary culture.

CONCLUSION

Human hepatocytes model at a preclinical stage of drug development is a potentially powerful tool in :
1/ selecting the animal species most closely related to humans on the basis of metabolic pattern,
2/ assessing the duration of pharmacological response, particularly of those drugs exhibiting different metabolic

clearances (eg. benzodiazepines),
3/ predicting the pharmacological behaviour of analogues belonging to the same family (eg. Vinca alkaloïds),
4/ the understanding and prediction of drug interactions,
5/ explaining the metabolic origins of interindividual variabilities in drug response.
The design of Phase I clinical trials could be improved by the use of data generatered by this human hepatocytes model.

REFERENCES:

Fabre, G., Rahmani, R., Placidi, M., Covo, J., Cano J. and Coulange, C., Ducros, M., Rampal, M. (1987) : Isolation and metabolic characterization of human hepatocytes from a whole adult human liver, using midazolam as a substance probe. Submitted for publication in Drug Metab. Dispos.

Gerecke, M. (1983): Chemical structure and properties of midazolam compared with other benzodiazepines. Br. J. Clin. Pharmacol. 16, 11S-16S.

Guillouzo, A., Begue J.M., Campion J.P., Gascoin M.N. and Guguen-Guillouzo C. (1985) : Human hepatocyte cultures : a model of pharmaco-toxicological studies. Xenobiotica, 15, 635-641.

Guguen-Guillouzo, C., Campion, J.P., Brissot, P., Glaie, D., Launois, B., Bourel, M. and Guillouzo, A. (1982) : High yield preparation of isolated human adult hepatocytes by enzymatic perfusion of the liver. Cell Biol. Int. Rep., 6, 625-628

Rahmani, R., Bruno, R., Iliadis, A., Just, S., Barbet, J., and Cano, J.P. (1987) : Clinical pharacokinetics of the antitumor drug navelbine (5'-noranhydrovinblastine). Cancer Research.
In press

Rahmani, R., Gueritte, F., Martin, M., Cano, J.P., and Barbet, J. (1986) : Comparative pharmacokinetics of antitumor vincaalkaloïds. Cancer Chemother. Pharmacol., 16, 223-228

Reese, J.A. and Byard, J.L. (1982) : Isolation and culture of adult hepatocytes from liver biopsies. In vitro, 17, 935-941

Richard, B., Fabre, G., DeSousa, G., Cano, J.P. (1987): Metabolism of mitoxantrone by hepatocytes in primary culture isolated from different species including man. Proc. Amer. Assoc. Cancer Res. , 28, 422.

Savaraj, N., Lu, K., Manuel, V., Loo, T.L. (1982): Pharmacology of mitoxantrone in cancer patients. Cancer Chemother. Pharmacol. 8, 113-117.

Shenkenberg, T.D. and Von Hoff, D.D. (1986) : Mitoxantrone : a new anticancer drug with significant activity. Annals Intern. Medicine, 105, 67-81

Shull, L.R., Kirsch, D.G., Lohse, C.I. and Wisniewski, J.A. (1987) : Application of isolated hepatocytes to studies of drug metabolism in large food animals. Xenobiotica, 17, 345-363.

Comparative penetration of free and polymethacrylic nanoparticle-bound doxorubicin in cultured rat hepatocytes

Alain Rolland, Jean-Marc Bégué*, François Chevanne, Roger Le Verge, André Guillouzo*

*Laboratoire de Biopharmacie, UER Médicament, 2, Avenue du Pr Léon Bernard, 35033 Rennes Cedex, France. * INSERM, U.49, Unité de Recherches Hépatologiques, Hôpital de Pontchaillou, 35033 Rennes Cedex, France*

Keywords : Polymethacrylic nanospheres, cultured rat hepatocytes, doxorubicin, doxorubicin-loaded nanoparticles, endocytosis, drug targeting.

INTRODUCTION

Several drug carriers have been designed to target drugs to specific organs or cells. The purpose of these new drug delivery systems is to lower parenteral administered doses and consequently to attenuate side-effects (Couvreur et al., 1982 ; Illum and Davis, 1982 ; Kreuter, 1983 ; Puiseux and Delattre, 1984 ; Al Khouri et al., 1986). Among these delivery systems poly-alkylcyanoacrylate nanoparticles were thought to be promising ; however, their surface is rapidly degraded making difficult long-term covalent binding of drugs such as doxorubicin (Couvreur et al., 1982). Recently, polymethacrylic nanoparticles (0.3 µm in diameter) with low degradation were designed as a new drug-carrier (Rolland et al., 1986a, 1987a, 1987b, ; Le Verge and Rolland, 1987). Since in vivo experiments demonstrated that after intravenous injection the nanospheres were mainly removed by the liver (Rolland, 1987), the penetration of free and nanoparticle-bound doxorubicin (DX) was compared in adult rat hepatocytes maintained in primary culture. Indeed, doxorubicin is one of the most important drugs usually used in the field of cancer chemotherapy, for the treatment of various tumors, such as hepatocarcinoma, however, its therapeutic use is limited by various side-effects, such as acute hematologic disorders and dose-dependent cardiac toxicity (Rinehart et al., 1974).

MATERIALS and METHODS

Polyalkylmethacrylate nanoparticle preparation

The nanospheres were prepared by aqueous emulsion copolymerization of methacrylic monomers (methyl methacrylate, 2-hydroxypropyl methacrylate, methacrylic acid, ethylene glycol dimethacrylate) as previously described (Rolland et al., 1986b, 1986c). The nanoparticle size (0,3 µm in diameter) was assessed using a Coulter^R Nano-Sizer and their morphology was observed by scanning electron microscopy (Fig. 1) as described by Rolland et al. (1986c).

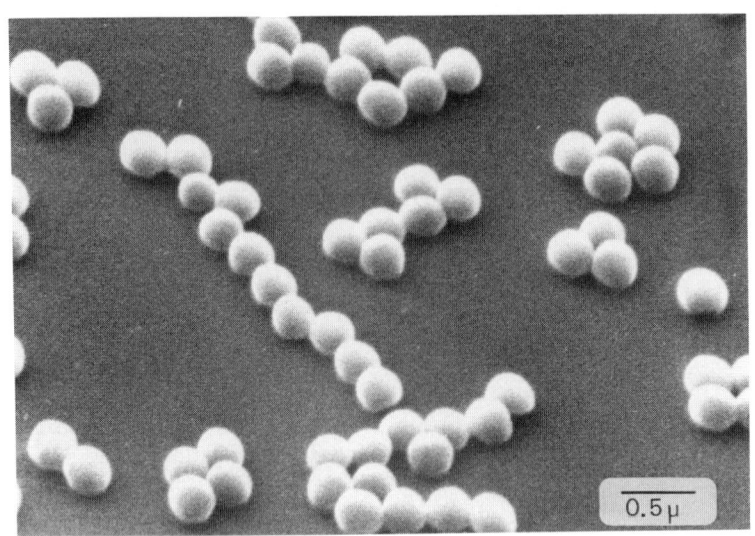

Figure 1 : Scanning electron microscopic micrograph of polymethacrylic nanoparticles (diameter = 0.3 µm).

Free and nanoparticle-bound doxorubicin
DX (adriblastine[R], R. Bellon Laboratory) was dissolved in distilled water (1 mg/ml). This aqueous solution of DX was dropped with stirring to the nanoparticle suspension previously adjusted to pH 8.4 to give either a final concentration of either 0.1 or 1 mg DX/ml of nanoparticle suspension. The absorption yield was about 100 %.

Primary cultures of rat hepatocytes
Rat hepatocytes were obtained by enzymatic dissociation of rat liver (Guguen et al., 1975). They were seeded at a density of 5×10^5 cells/10 cm^2 petri dish with 2 ml of medium. The medium consisted in a mixture of 75 % minimum essential medium and 25 % medium 199 (Gibco - USA) supplemented with 200 µg per ml bovine serum albumin, 10 µg per ml bovine insulin, 10 % fetal calf serum and buffered at pH 7.4 with carbonate under a 5 % CO_2-95 % air humidified atmosphere. Four hours after hepatocyte seeding and, prior to experimentation the medium, now containing 7×10^{-5} M hydrocortisone hemisuccinate, was renewed.

Incubation procedure
Twenty four hours after cell seeding, cultures were incubated for 24 h at 37°C in darkness with either free or nanoparticles-bound DX at concentrations ranging from 50 to 500 ng DX/ml of culture medium. DX was bound to the initial suspension of nanoparticles (2.4×10^{12} nanoparticles/ml) at two concentrations, A : 0.1 ng DX/ml and B : 1 mg DX/ml. After dilution the number of nanoparticles was 10-fold higher in the A than in the B suspension.

DX toxicity
Free or bound DX-induced cytotoxicity was assessed by examination of cultures under light microscopy and quantified by measurement of lactate dehydrogenase (LDH) leakage in the culture medium.

Quantitative determination of DX in hepatocytes
DX concentrations were measured in both medium and cell extracts by reversed phase high performance liquid chromatography as described elsewhere (Rolland, 1987).

Electron microscopic examination
To visualize the penetration of nanoparticles into hepatocytes, part of the petri dishes was set up for transmission electron microscopic examination. Cell cultures were briefly washed with PBS, then fixed in situ for 30 min. with a 2.5 % glutaraldehyde solution buffered with 0.1 M sodium cacodylate (pH 7,4). Thereafter, the samples were post-fixed in a 1 % osmium tetroxide solution in sodium cacodylate buffer for 30 min, dehydrated in graded ethanol and embedded in epon.

RESULTS

Toxicity of free and bound DX
Whatever the concentrations of free and bound DX, neither morphological alteration nor LDH leakage were observed (not shown).
Nanoparticle endocytosis
Endocytosis of the nanospheres by cultured rat hepatocytes and their intracytoplasmic accumulation are shown in Fig. 2 and 3 respectively.

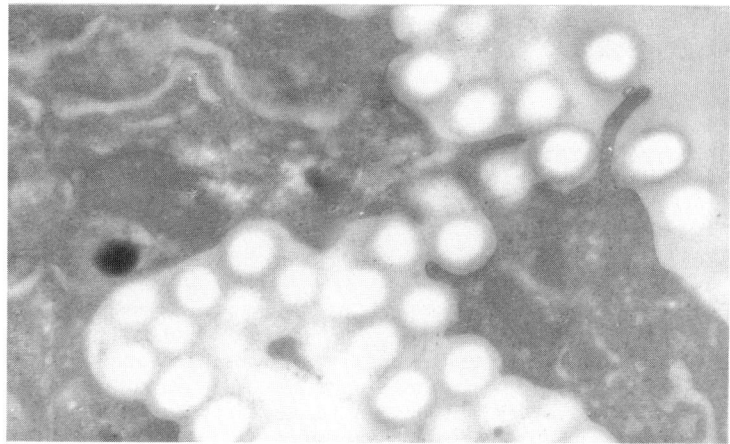

Figure 2 : Endocytosis of nanospheres by cultured rat hepatocytes. (x 48,000).

Intracellular DX concentrations
When DX was bound to the nanoparticles (Table I), intracellular DX concentrations were markedly enhanced (from 11 % to 64 %)

Initial DX concentrations (ng/ml)	Intracellular DX concentrations (ng/ml)		
	Free DX	Bound DX (A)	Bound DX (B)
50	16.34	26.82 (+64%)	26.37 (+61%)
100	42.76	54.41 (+27%)	56.67 (+33%)
250	121.13	144.43 (+19%)	134.42 (+11%)
500	210.89	260.59 (+24%)	264.15 (+25%)

Table I : Intracellular concentrations of DX in rat hepatocytes incubated with various concentrations of free or bound DX. The number of nanoparticles was 10 fold higher in the A than in the B suspension.

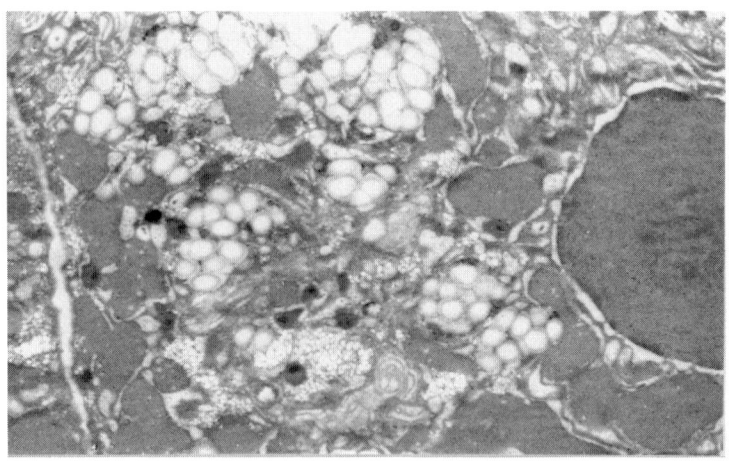

Figure 3 : Intracytoplasmic accumulation of nanoparticules in cultured rat hepatocytes. (x 12,000).

CONCLUSION

The results emphasize the usefulness of polymethacrylic nanoparticles as a new drug-carrier. This delivery system, of which synthesis is simple and reproducible, markedly enhances intracellular concentrations of drugs such as doxorubicin by endocytosis of the whole particle. Nanoparticle-bound DX could be hopefully used to increase the therapeutic activity of this anthracycline in cancer chemotherapy, especially in hepatocarcinoma treatment. Our findings also suggest that cultured rat hepatocytes should be of a great help to understand mechanisms of such specific penetration.

ACKNOWLEDGMENTS

The authors thank A. Vannier for typing the manuscript.

REFERENCES

Al Khouri, F., Roblot-Treupel L., Fessi H., Devissaguet J.P. and Puisieux F. (1986): Development of a new process for the manufacture of polyisobutyl-cyanoacrylate nanocapsules. Int. J. Pharm. 28, 125-132.

Couvreur, P., Roland, M. and Speiser, P. (1982): Biodegradable particles containing a biologically active substance, U.S. Patent n° 4, 329-332.

Couvreur, P., Kante, B., Grislain, L., Roland, M. and Speiser, P. (1982): Toxicity of polyalkylcyanoacrylate nanoparticles. II : Doxorubicin-loaded nanoparticles. J. Pharm. Sci. 71, 790-792.

Guguen, C., Guillouzo, A., Boisnard, M., Le Cam, A. and Bourel, M. (1975): Etude ultrastructurale de monocouches d'hépatocytes de rat adulte cultivés en présence d'hémisuccinate d'hydrocortisone. Biol. Gastroenterol. 8, 223-231.

Illum, L. and Davis, S.S. (1982): The targeting of drugs parenterally by use of microspheres. J. Parent. Sci. Techn. 36, 242-248.

Kreuter, J. (1983): Evaluation of nanoparticles as drug delivery systems. I : Preparation methods. Pharm. Acta Helv. 58, 196-209.

Le Verge, R. and Rolland, A. (1987): Nanoparticules à base de polymères méthacryliques, procédé de préparation et application comme vecteur de médicament. Eur. Patent, n° 87400695.

Puisieux, F. and Delattre, J. (1984): Les liposomes. Applications thérapeutiques, Techniques et Documentation, ed. Lavoisier, Paris, France.

Rinehart, J.J., Lewis, R.P. and Baleerzak, S.P. (1974): Adriamycin cardiotoxicity in man. Ann. Intern. Med. 81, 475-478.

Rolland, A., Gibassier, D., Sado, P. and Le Verge, R. (1986a): Méthodologie de préparation de vecteurs nanoparticulaires à base de polymères acryliques. J. Pharm. Belg. 41, 83-93.

Rolland, A., Gibassier, D., Sado, P. and Le Verge, R. (1986b): Préparation, purification et propriétés des vecteurs nanoparticulaires à base de polymères méthacryliques. In : 4 th International Conference on Pharmaceutical Technology, Paris (APGI, Ed.), vol. 4, pp 183-192.

Rolland, A., Gibassier, D., Sado, P. and Le Verge, R. (1986c): Purification et propriétés physico-chimiques des suspensions de nanoparticules de polymères acryliques. J. Pharm. Belg. 41, 94-105.

Rolland, A. (1987): Mise au point et applications de nanosphères à base de copolymères méthacryliques. Intérêts pour la vectorisation d'agents cytostatiques (anthracyclines). Ph.D. Thesis n°1, Université de Rennes I, Faculté de Pharmacie, Rennes, France.

Rolland, A., Merdrignac, G., Gouranton, J., Bourel, D., Le Verge, R. and Genetet B. (1987a): Flow cytometric quantitative evaluation of phagocytosis by human mononuclear and polymorphonuclear cells using fluorescent nanoparticles. J. Immunol. Meth. 96, 185-193.

Rolland, A., Bourel, D., Genetet, B. and Le Verge, R. (1987b): Monoclonal antibodies covalently coupled to polymethacrylic nanoparticles : in vivo specific targeting to human T lymphocytes. Int. J. Pharm. 39, 173-180.

Metabolism of propranolol, lidocaine and antipyrine in hepatocytes isolated from rats with inflammation

B. Chindavijak, F.M. Belpaire, F. de Smet, N. Fraeyman, M.G. Bogaert

Heymans Institute of Pharmacology, University of Gent Medical School, De Pintelaan 185, B-9000 Gent, Belgium

Keywords
Inflammation, hepatocytes, drug metabolism, propranolol, lidocaine, antipyrine.

Introduction

In humans and in rats with inflammation, the plasma concentrations of propranolol and other drugs which are mainly bound to α_1-acid glycoprotein (α_1-AGP) are increased after their oral administration (Schneider and Bishop 1982). As for high extraction drugs such as propranolol, the area under the curve (AUC) after oral administration is inversely related to the free fraction of drug in plasma and to the intrinsic clearance (Wilkinson and Shand 1975), changes of both factors could be involved. The free fraction of propranolol is indeed decreased in inflammation, due to the increased α_1-AGP concentrations (Piafsky et al 1978). For some drugs, however, a decrease in intrinsic clearance could be present, as suggested e.g. by in vitro studies in rats with experimental inflammation (Whitehouse and Beck, 1973).

To evaluate more precisely the hepatic enzymatic activity of rats with turpentine-induced inflammation, we investigated the in vitro metabolism of propranolol and of lidocaine, another high extraction drug, and of antipyrine, a low extraction drug, using isolated hepatocytes. For comparative purposes, the influence of SKF 525A was also studied. For propranolol, serum levels were also measured after oral administration, in order to evaluate the influence of inflammation on the in vivo hepatic intrinsic clearance.

Methods

Animals

Male Wistar rats, 350-480g, were used. For the study in isolated hepatocytes, one group of rats served as controls and was not pretreated; in a second group, inflammation was induced by i.m. injection of turpentine oil, 0.5 ml in one hindlimb 48 hr, and 0.5

ml in the other hindlimb 24 hr before sacrifice. A third group of rats received SKF 525A 100 mg/kg I.P., 1 hr before sacrifice.

For the study of the serum concentrations of propranolol, catheters were inserted in control and turpentine-treated rats under short ether anaesthesia. Two hours later, propranolol (5 mg/kg) was administered orally, and blood samples were taken in function of time.

Preparation of isolated hepatocytes.

The hepatocytes were isolated by the perfusion technique described by Seglen (1972), with minor modifications. This includes a 10 min perfusion with non-recirculating calcium-free Krebs-bicarbonate buffer containing 0.5 mM EGTA, followed by perfusion for 20 min, with recirculation, with 100 ml Krebs-bicarbonate buffer containing 50 mg collagenase and 3.3 mM $CaCl_2$. After several washings, the cells were resuspended in Krebs-bicarbonate buffer at 4°C. Viability of the hepatocytes was assessed by trypan blue dye exclusion. Only preparations with more than 80% viable cells were used. For the metabolism study, incubations were done in a total volume of 3 ml at 37°C under an atmosphere of 95% O_2/5% CO_2. The final cell concentration was for antipyrine and propranolol 1.2×10^6 and for lidocaine 0.7×10^6 viable cells/ml. After preincubation for 5 min, the drug was added to give a final drug concentration in the incubation mixture of 0.5 mM for antipyrine (containing 0.54×10^5 cpm of N-methyl-C^{14}-antipyrine), 0.04 mM for lidocaine or 0.03 mM for propranolol. Incubation times were 30 min for antipyrine, 8 min for lidocaine and 15 min for propranolol. The concentrations of antipyrine metabolites, of lidocaine and of propranolol were measured as described by Chindavijak et al. (1987).

Determination of serum concentrations and protein binding

Serum concentrations of propranolol and antipyrine were measured with HPLC (Rosseel et al., 1981). Serum protein binding of propranolol was measured with equilibrium dialysis (Belpaire et al., 1982).

Calculations and statistical analysis

The AUCs for propranolol were calculated with the trapezoidal rule. Intrinsic clearance (Cl_{intr}) was calculated from the equation $Cl_{intr} = D/Fu \cdot AUC$, where Fu is the free fraction and D the dose.

The data were expressed as means ± S.E.M. and differences between groups were analysed using the Mann-Whitney U-test. P<0.05 was considered as the level of significance.

Results

The influence of administration of turpentine oil and SKF 525A on the metabolism of antipyrine, lidocaine and propranolol by the isolated hepatocytes is shown in Table 1. After turpentine treatment, the disappearance rates of antipyrine, lidocaine and propranolol were decreased markedly; SKF 525A also slowed down the disappearance rates.

Table 1: Metabolisme of antipyrine, lidocaine and propranolol determined in isolated hepatocytes of control rats, of rats treated with turpentine oil and of rats treated with SKF 525A. The metabolizing activity of isolated hepatocytes is expressed as nmol of drug disappearing per 10^6 viable cells per min. Data are given as means ± S.E.M.

	Control rats (n=7)	Turpentine-treated rats (n=7)	SKF 525A-treated rats (n=7)
Antipyrine	0.50±0.05	0.20±0.01***	0.13±0.02***
Lidocaine	1.97±0.19	0.65±0.09***	0.52±0.08***
Propranolol	0.61±0.05	0.43±0.03**	0.26±0.05***

** $p<0.02$, *** $p<0.001$ (Mann-Whitney U-test).

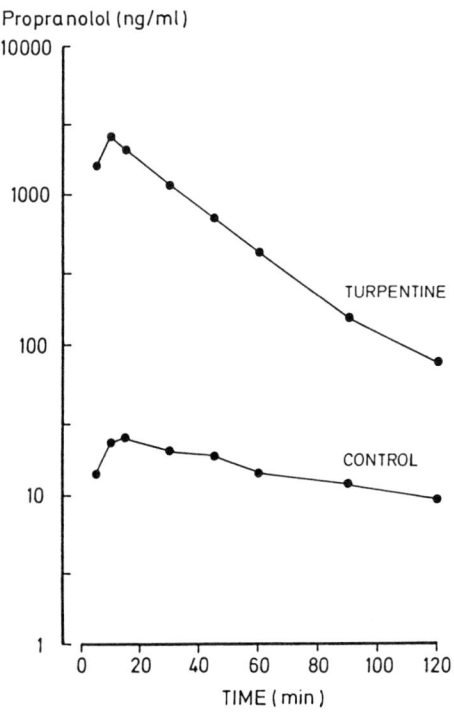

Fig.1. Serum concentrations of propranolol in function of time after oral administration (5mg/kg) in a control rat and a turpentine-treated rat.

Figure 1 shows a representative example of the plasma concentrations of propranolol after oral administration in a control rat and in a rat treated with turpentine oil. In the rats with inflammation the mean AUC after oral administration was more than 40 times higher than in the healthy rats (79758 ± 12071 vs 1733 ± 242 ng/ml.hr; $p<0.001$; n = 9 in each group); the free fraction of propranolol was approximately 5 times lower (2.47 ± 0.13 vs 11.47 ± 0.52 %; $p<0.001$; n = 9). The intrinsic clearance was decreased from 30.4 ± 4.7 to 3.2 ± 1.8 l/kg/min ($p<0.001$; n = 9).

Discussion

After oral administration of propranolol and other drugs that are bound to α_1-AGP, their serum concentrations are increased in patients with inflammatory diseases and in rats with Freund adjuvant arthritis (Schneider and Bishop 1982). In our rats with turpentine-induced inflammation an important increase in AUC after oral administration was observed, as compared to control rats. As the AUC after oral administration is inversely related to the fraction of unbound drug in serum and the hepatic intrinsic clearance (Wilkinson and Shand 1975), the decrease of hepatic intrinsic clearance which reflects hepatic drug metabolizing activity, might contribute to the increase of the drug serum concentrations. Indeed, intrinsic clearance, calculated from our in vivo results, is decreased 10 times in the turpentine-treated rats, and this decrease in drug metabolism was confirmed in our in vitro study using isolated rat hepatocytes.

For the three drugs, we found a decrease in metabolizing activity in hepatocytes of rats with inflammation. This effect was, however, less pronounced for propranolol than for the two other drugs, suggesting that turpentine treatment has a selective effect on certain cytochrome P-450 subpopulations or on conjugating enzymes. Our results with hepatocytes are largely in agreement with those obtained for different drugs in studies using hepatocytes, 9000xg supernatant fraction or microsomal fraction in rat with different models of inflammation (Beck and Whitehouse, 1974; Ishizuki et al., 1983; Kobusch et al., 1986; Chindavijak et al., 1987). In contrast, Barber et al. (1982) found in microsomes of rats with adjuvant-induced arthritis, only a slight, non-significant decrease in propranolol metabolism.

SKF 525A treatment slowed the disappearance rate of the three drugs studied more than turpentine. The inhibitory effect of SKF 525A was, like that of turpentine, less pronounced for propranolol, suggesting again a selective effect on drug metabolizing enzymes.

As turpentine does not reach the liver (Kaplan and Jamieson, 1977), the change in metabolizing activity probably reflects the influence of inflammation, and not a direct effect on drug metabolizing enzymes. Furthermore Kobusch et al. (1986), recently found that turpentine oil given orally led to induction, and not to inhibition of drug metabolizing enzymes.

The results with isolated hepatocytes demonstrate that the hepatic intrinsic clearance of both low and high extraction drugs is reduced as a result of inflammation; the in vivo results for propranolol confirm this finding. This decrease is one of the factors responsible for the increase of the plasma concentrations of propranolol in rats with turpentine-induced inflammation and could also be of importance in patients with inflammatory diseases.

References

Barber, H.E., Finlayson, J.R., Hawksworth, G.M., Poole,S., Steele, W.H. and Walker, K.A. (1982): Metabolism and serum protein binding of propranolol in rats with raised erythrocyte sedimentation rates. Br. J. Pharmacol. 76, 224P.

Beck,F.J. and Whitehouse, M.W. (1974): Impaired drug metabolism in rats associated with acute inflammation: a possible assay for anti-injury agents. Proc. Soc. Exp. Biol. Med. 145, 135-140.

Belpaire, F.M., Bogaert, M.G. and Rosseneu, M. (1982): Binding of ß-adrenoceptor blocking drugs to human serum albumin, to α_1-acid glycoprotein and to human serum. Eur. J. Clin. Pharmacol. 22, 253-256.

Chindavijak, B., Belpaire, F.M. and Bogaert, M.G. (1987): In-vitro biotransformation of antipyrine, lignocaine and propranolol in liver of rats with turpentine-induced inflammation. J. Pharm. Pharmacol. 39, in press.

Ishizuki, S., Furuhata, K., Kaneta, S., Fujihira, E. (1983): Reduced drug metabolism in isolated hepatocytes from adjuvant arthritic rats. Res. Comm. Chem. Path. Pharmacol. 39, 261-276.

Kaplan, H.A. and Jamieson, J.C. (1977): The effect of inflammation on rat liver ß-galactosidase and ß-N-acetylglucosaminidase. Life Sci. 21, 1311-1316.

Kobusch, A.B., Erill, S. and du Souich, P. (1986): Relationship between changes in seromucoid concentrations and the rate of oxidation or acetalytion of several substrates. Drug Metab. Dispos. 14, 663-667.

Piafsky, K.M., Borga, O., Odar-Cederlöf, I., Johansson, C. and Sjöqvist, F. (1978): Increased plasma protein binding of propranolol and chlorpromazine mediated by disease-induced elevations of plasma α_1-acid glycoprotein. N. Eng. J. Med. 299, 1435-1438.

Rosseel, M.T. and Bogaert, M.G. (1981): High-performance liquid chromatographic determination of propranolol and 4-hydroxypropranolol in plasma. J. Pharm. Sci. 70, 688-689.

Schneider, R.E. and Bishop, H. (1982): ß-blocker plasma concentrations and inflammatory disease: clinical implications. Clin. Pharmacokin. 7, 281-284.

Seglen, P.O. (1972): Preparation of rat liver cells. I. Effect of Ca^{2+} on enzymatic dispersion of isolated, perfused liver. Exptl. Cell Res. 74, 450-454.

Wilkinson, G.R. and Shand,D.G. (1975): A physiological approach to hepatic drug clearance. Clin. Pharmacol. Ther. 18, 377-390.

Whitehouse, M.W. and Beck, F.J. (1973):Impaired drug metabolism in rats with adjuvant-induced arthritis: a brief review. Drug Metab. Dispos. 1, 251-255.

Liver Cells and Drugs. Ed. A. Guillouzo. Colloque INSERM/John Libbey Eurotext Ltd. © 1988. Vol. 164, pp. 321-324.

Rat hepatocyte cultures and stereoselective biotransformation of disopyramide enantiomers

Pascal Le Corre[1], Damrong Ratanasavanh[2], Denis Gibassier[1], Anne-Marie Barthel[2], Pierre Sado[1], Roger Le Verge[1], André Guillouzo[2]

[(1)] Laboratoire de Pharmacie Galénique et Biopharmacie, Université de Rennes 1, 2 Avenue du Pr. Léon Bernard, Rennes, France. [(2)] Unité de Recherches Hépatologiques INSERM U.49, Hôpital Pontchaillou, Rennes, France

KEY WORDS

rat hepatocyte culture, disopyramide enantiomers, stereoselectivity,cytotoxicity, biotransformation.

INTRODUCTION

At present, a significant number of the drugs produced by organic synthesis exhibit chirality. Disopyramide, a class I_A antiarrythmic agent, is marketed as a racemate: R(-) and S(+) disopyramide, (R(-) DP and S(+) DP). Disopyramide metabolism displays important species differences. In the rat, biotransformation of disopyramide leads to mono-N-dealkylated and arylhydroxylated metabolites (Fig. 1), these metabolic pathways are stereoselective (Cook et al., 1982). The importance of drug enantiomers in pharmacotoxicology is now well established (Williams and Lee, 1985). Although disopyramide is widely used and is generally well tolerated, several cases of hepatic injury by this drug have been described (Stricker and Spoelstra, 1985). Among the various in vitro approaches for the study of drug metabolism are cultured hepatocytes, which express drug metabolizing enzyme activities for the longest period (Guillouzo, 1986).The aim of this work was to study the cytotoxocity of disopyramide enantiomers in primary cultures of adult rat hepatocytes and to determine wether this in vitro system is capable of biotransforming disopyramide stereoselectively. The results were compared with those obtained in vivo (Cook et al., 1982).

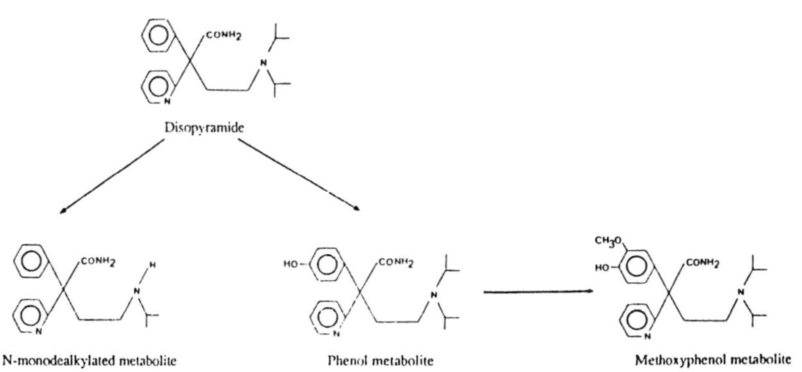

Fig. 1. Metabolic pathways of disopyramide in rat (Cook et al., 1982).

MATERIALS AND METHODS

Hepatocytes were obtained by collagenase perfusion of Sprague Dawley rat (2 months old) liver. The cells were seeded at a density of 2.5×10^6 cells per plate in 5 ml of Ham F12 medium containing 10 µg/ml bovine insulin, 0.2 % bovine serum albumin and 10 % foetal calf serum. The medium was changed 4 hours later and the fresh medium was supplemented with 3×10^{-6} M hydrocortisone hemisuccinate.
Cytotoxicity of R(-) DP and S(+) DP was estimated by lactate dehydrogenase (LDH) leakage and morphological changes in hepatocyte cultures according to Ratanasavanh et al.(1988).
Cultured hepatocytes were incubated separately with R(-) DP and S(+) DP, dissolved in the medium. At the end of the incubation cells and supernatants were separated and metabolism was stopped by freezing at -80°C.
Disopyramide enantiomers were obtained by optical resolution of the racemic according to the method described by Burke et al. (1980). The enantiomeric purity of R(-) DP and S(+) DP was determined by a liquid chromatographic method using a stereoselective column packed with human α_1- acid glycoprotein (Le Corre et al., 1987).The enantiomeric purity of R(-) DP and S(+) DP was 97.7 and 96.2 %, respectively.
Since we did not dispose of the arylhydroxylated metabolites, overall biotransformation of R(-) DP and S(+) DP was determined by the disappearance of the parent drug. Biotransformation by N-dealkylation was estimated by the formation of the mono-N-dealkylated metabolite.The chiral carbon centre is not involved in N-dealkylation (Cook et al., 1982); thus the metabolite formed is stereochemically related to the parent disopyramide enantiomer.
Assay of disopyramide and of mono-N-dealkylated metabolite, carried out in supernatant and cells which were sonicated, was performed by a reversed phase HPLC method with parachlorodisopyramide as internal standard. The mobile phase contained methanol and acetate buffer 0.1 M, pH 5.1 (35:65, v/v).The flow rate was 1 ml/min and the detection was set at 254 nm.

RESULTS

At low concentration (147.5 µmol/l), only S(+) DP increased LDH activity (138 %) in the medium (Fig. 2). At 295 µmol/l, both R(-) DP and S(+) DP provoked LDH leakage but the increase was more noticable with S(+) DP than with R(-) DP. At higher concentrations the cytotoxic effect of these two enantiomers was not significantly different. Light microscopic examination confirmed the biochemical study in the sense that S(+) DP, at concentrations of 147.5 to 295 µmol/l, induced more morphological changes than R(-) DP (results not shown). The cytotoxicity threshold of R(-) DP and S(+) DP was much higher than the substrate concentrations used for metabolism studies.

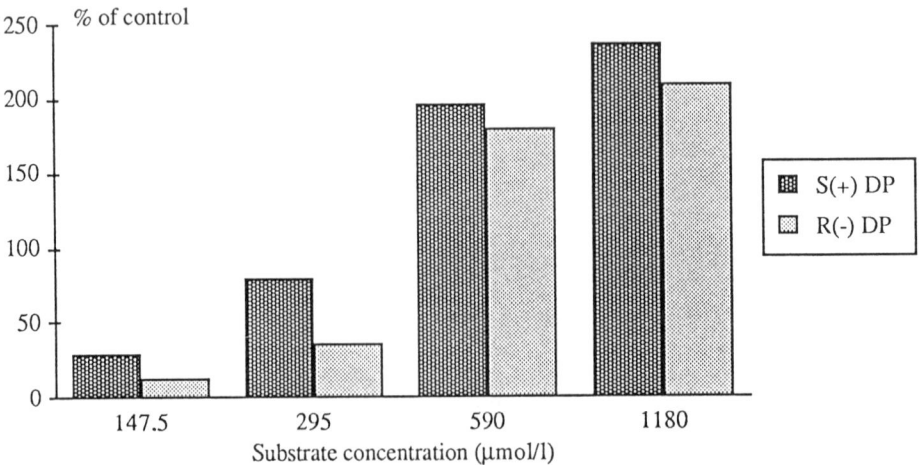

Fig. 2. LDH leakage versus concentration of R(-) DP and S(+) DP in hepatocyte cultures.

The precision of the study model was estimated in a statistic assay of overall biotrasformation of both enantiomers. The mean ± CV (n=10) overall biotransformation of R(-) DP and S(+) DP were 28.4 ± 7.8 % and 86.0 ± 3.0 %, respectively (Fig.3).

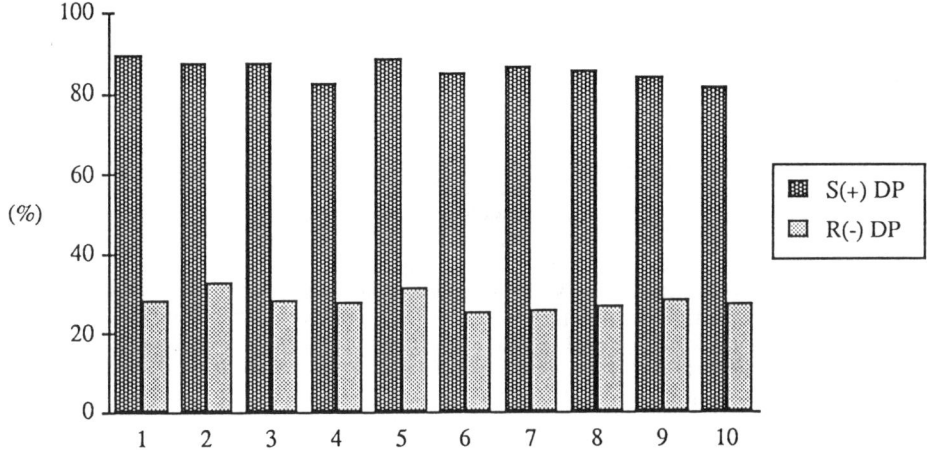

Fig. 3. Statistical determination (n=10) of overall biotransformation of R(-) DP and S(+) DP.

To determine an optimum incubation time, a kinetic assay of overall biotransformation of R(-) DP and S(+) DP was performed. The rate of overall biotransformation of both enantiomers reached a plateau 24 hours after the beginning of the incubation and was quite complete (95.6 %) for S(+) DP. Accordingly, all subsequent experiments were performed after a 24 hour incubating period. The rate of overall biotransformation of S(+) DP was, in the substrate concentration range studied, about 2.5 fold higher than that of R(-) DP (Fig.4.). At low concentrations, 2.95 and 5.9 µmol/l, S(+) DP was almost entirely metabolized : 98.5 % and 95.4 %, respectively while only 40.2 % and 39 % of R(-) DP were biotransformed. When higher substrate concentrations were incubated, the rates of overall biotransformation of both enantiomers decreased.

Inversely, N-dealkylation of S(+) DP was much lower than that of R(-) DP, especially at the lowest substrate concentrations. At 2.95 and 5.9 µmol/l, the rates of N-dealkylation of S(+) DP were 0.2 % and 0.5 % while 9.8 % and 10.6 %, respectively, of R(-) DP were biotransformed via N-dealkylation.

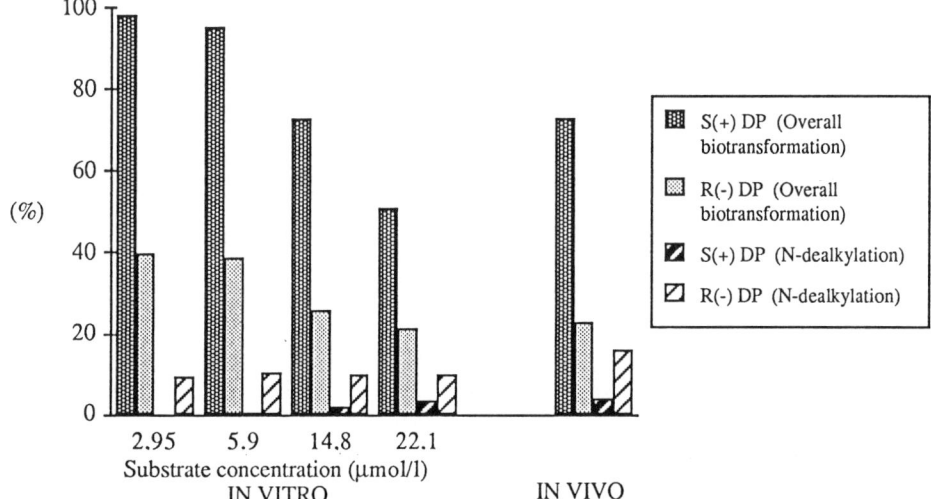

Fig. 4. Stereoselectivity in overall biotransformation and N-dealkylation of disopyramide. Comparison between in vitro data and in vivo data (Cook et al., 1982).

DISCUSSION

When rat hepatocytes in culture were used to assess the cytotoxicity of disopyramide enantiomers, S(+) DP was found to be more cytotoxic than R(-) DP, especially with the concentrations ranging from 147.5 to 295 µmol/l. With higher concentrations, no difference in cytotoxicity was observed between the two enantiomers. It is important to notice that the concentrations provoking the cytotoxicity in hepatocyte cultures were higher than the therapeutic plasma concentrations (10 to 25 fold). The exact mechanism of cytotoxic effect of disopyramide remains to be elucidated. But it was reported that the stereoselective toxic effect of some drugs is related to their stereoselective metabolism (Vermeulen, 1987). In the substrate concentration range studied, as well as for much higher concentrations (data not shown), the relative contribution of the N-dealkylation in the overall biotransformation of both enantiomers increased with the substrate concentration and was higher for R(-) DP but never became predominant. As the monodealkylated metabolite was cytotoxic in hepatocytes cultures at only very high concentrations (from 1180 µmol/l, results not shown), this suggests that arylhydroxylated metabolites should be responsible for the stereoselective cytotoxicity. The present study, carried out in rat hepatocyte cultures, provided information on both metabolite profile and extent of metabolism of disopyramide enantiomers. The in vitro metabolite profile agrees with in vivo data of the literature : overall biotransformation and N-dealkylation of disopyramide were stereoselective. Indeed, S(+) DP was extensively biotransformed while the monodealkylated metabolite formed from R(-) DP was higher. When the results were expressed not in percentage terms but per amount of substrate metabolized, the greater the substrate concentration, the greater the amount metabolized, thus, indicating a lack of metabolic saturation. The correlation between in vitro and in vivo approaches was not only qualitative but also quantitative. As indicated by the similar rates of overall biotransformation and N-dealkylation, cultured rat hepatocytes show a good predictive value for the study of the stereochemistry of the oxidative metabolic pathways of disopyramide (Fig. 4).

Hepatocytes in culture are largely used to investigate cytotoxic effects and metabolism of drugs (Guillouzo, 1986). In such system, a large concentration of drug is generally used and it is often difficult to extrapolate results from in vitro to in vivo because of this large concentration. It is interesting to note that the correlation observed in the rates of biotransformation were obtained with substrate concentrations (2.95 to 22.1 µmol/l) related to the mean disopyramide plasma concentrations measured in vivo (Cook et al., 1982). With higher concentrations (lower than the cytotoxicity threshold), the quantitative comparison with in vivo data became much less evident.

The good agreement between the results obtained with this non invasive model and in vivo data suggests that cultured rat hepatocytes are a suitable method for the study of hepatic metabolism of disopyramide enantiomers.

REFERENCES

Burke T.R., Nelson W.L., Mangion M., Hite G.J., Mockler C.M. and Ruenitz P.C. (1980) : Resolution, absolute configuration, and antiarrhythmic properties of the enantiomers of disopyramide, 4-(diisopropylamino)-2-(2-pyridyl)-2-phenylbutyramide. J.Med.Chim. 23, 1044 -1047.

Cook C.S., Karim A. and Sollman P. (1982) : Stereoselectivity in the metabolism of disopyramide

Guillouzo A. (1986) : use of isolated and cultured hepatocytes for xenobiotic metabolism and cytotoxicity studies. in Isolated and cultured hepatocytes, ed A. Guillouzo, C. Guguen - Guillouzo,pp 313-331. Paris : Editions Inserm, London : John Libbey.

Le Corre P., Gibassier D., Sado P. and Le Verge R. (1988) : Simultaneous assay of disopyramide and monodesisopropyldisopyramide enantiomers in biological samples by liquid chromatography. J. Chrom., in press.

Ratanasavanh D., Baffet G., Latinier M.F., Rissel M. and Guillouzo A. (1988) : Use of hepatocyte co-cultures in the assessment of drug toxicity from chronic exposure. Xenobiotica, in press.

Stricker B.H.C. and Spoelstra P. (1985) : in Drug-induced hepatic injury, ed M.N.G. Dukes. New-York : Elsevier.

Vermeulen, N.P.E. (1987) : Stereoselectivity in the enzymatic biotransformation of drugs and other xenobiotics. In Drug metabolism - From molecules to man, ed D.J. Benford, J.W. Bridges, G.G. Gibson, pp 615-639. London, New - York and Philadelphia : Taylor and Francis.

Williams K. and Lee E. (1985) : Importance of drug enantiomers in clinical pharmacology. Drugs 30, 330-354.

Metabolic profiling of the mutagenic heterocyclic amine IQ using rat isolated hepatocytes.

J.C. Peleran, M. Baradat, J.F. Sutra, G.F. Bories

INRA, Laboratoire des Xénobiotiques, BP 3, 31931 Toulouse Cedex, France

KEY WORDS

Metabolic profile, isolated hepatocyte, heterocyclic amine, IQ.

INTRODUCTION

2-amino-3-methylimidazo[4,5-f]quinoline (IQ) is one of a dozen mutagenic heterocyclic amines identified in protein pyrolysates and cooked food. It has been shown to be carcinogenic to mice (Ohgaki et al., 1984) and rat (Takayama et al., 1984) causing hepatocellular and intestinal adenocarcinoma.

Biochemical studies have shown that these heterocyclic amines are biotransformed to N-hydroxylated derivatives N-acetylation and conjugation with glutathione have been shown to occur when using subcellular systems.

The metabolic fate of IQ has been investigated in Rat using labelled IQ (Sjodin and Jagerstad, 1984 ; Tureski et al., 1986; Peleran et al., 1987).

Until now the results are limited to the identification of the N-acetylated and 3-N-demethylated IQ as minor free metabolites in the urine (Peleran et al., 1987), and to the N-sulfamate in urine and feces (Tureski et al., 1986).

An HPLC analysis of the IQ metabolites in the urine and bile has been performed in order to obtain complete metabolic profiles. Major and unidentified metabolites were separated. The preparation of small quantities of these metabolites for subsequent identification were envisaged, using conventional extraction and purification methods from the biological matrices, as well as rat isolated hepatocytes.

MATERIAL AND METHODS

Materials

Triatiated IQ (7.65 mCi/mM) was obtained from standard IQ synthesized in the laboratory by tritium exchange (Service des Molécules Marquées, CEA, Saclay, France) and subsequently purified by TLC. Radiochemical purity (<99 %) was checked by radio-TLC and radio-HPLC.

Animal experiments

Wistar rats (250 g, males) placed in metabolic cages received a single oral dose of 0.76 mg ^{3}H-IQ. The urines were collected for 24 h in glass bottles containing 5 ml toluene as preservative agent. Other animals were kept under anesthesia following dosage, the bile duct was catheterized and the bile collected for 2 h.

Isolated hepatocytes

Hepatocytes were prepared from non-induced 200 g male rats according to Seglen (1976). Trypan blue exclusion was better than 85%. Incubations were performed with 2.5 millions cells/ml HEPES buffer under normal atmosphere and shaking for 2 h, after addition of 200 µg (3.8×10^6 dpm) ^{3}H-IQ.

Metabolic profiling

The analysis was performed on the butanolic extract of the urines, on the methanolic dilution (1:1) of the bile and the methanolic dilution (1:1) on the hepatocyte incubation medium, using high performance liquid chromatography (HPLC). The chromatographic conditions retained were as follows : a ODS 2, 5 µm, 25 x 0.42 cm column ; a gradient elution (A : ammonium acetate solution 20 mM ; B : 80 % ammonium acetate plus 20 % acetonitrile) : 0-25 % B (25 min), 25 % B (10 min), 25-100 % B (15 min) at 1 ml/min flow ; fraction collection : 0.2 ml. Two millilitres of an aqueous counting scintillant (ACS II, Amersham Corp. Arlington Heights, Il) were added and the radioactivity measured in a liquid scintillation spectrometer.

RESULTS AND DISCUSSION

More than 90 % of the total radioactivity of the urine, bile and hepatocyte incubate was recovered as well resolved peaks on the corresponding chromatograms (Fig. 1A, 1B and 1C). Therefore it may be considered that this HPLC gradient analysis leads to reliable complete metabolic profiles of IQ. The radioactivity of the urinary profile (Fig. 1A) is distributed into seven main peaks plus unchanged IQ. The N-acetyl IQ and 3-N-demethyl IQ appear as very minor peaks as well as IQ, that confirms previous observations of Peleran et al. (1987). The other peaks correspond to more polar metabolites. Due to the lack of standard IQ sulfamate, this metabolite already identified as a minor metabolite (5%) of rat urine (Turesky et al., 1986) has not been positionned on the profile. The major peaks 1,2 and 3 on the profile corres-

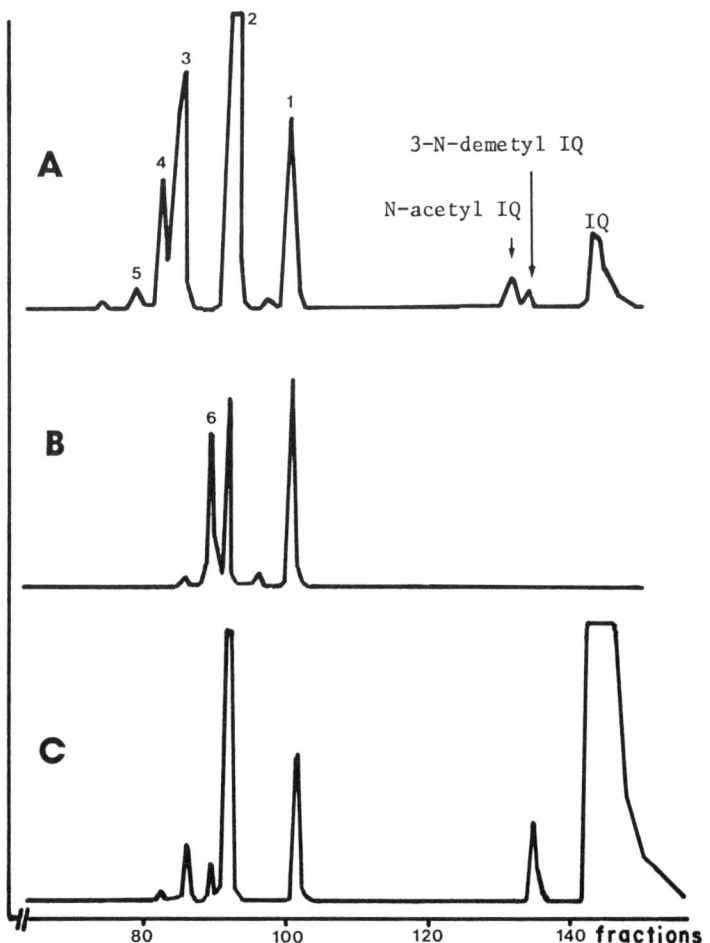

Fig.1 - HPLC metabolic profiles of ^{3}H-IQ in the urine (A), bile (B), and isolated hepatocyte incubates (C)

pond to 11, 45.6 and 21.0 % of the total radioactivity of the urine, respectively. The biliary profile (Fig. 1B) does not exhibit free IQ nor the acetylated or demethylated metabolites. However five metabolites with similar retention times as those of the urinary polar metabolites are present while an additional one (peak 3) appears.

The metabolic profile obtained from the isolated hepatocytes (Fig. 1C) shows that both the urinary biliary metabolites are produced, but at different extent. A major contribution of metabolites 1 and 2 is observed (5.4% and 85.0 % respectively).

Therefore this _in vitro_ technique could proved to be an efficient way to produce these metabolites in order to carry on further identification. The effect of the incubation time course on the biotransformation yield of ^{3}H-IQ (Fig. 2) indicates a practically linear increase of metabolite 2 synthesis ever a 6 h period, while production of metabolite 1 reached a steady state level. The UV (254 nm) detection (data not reported) indicates that the

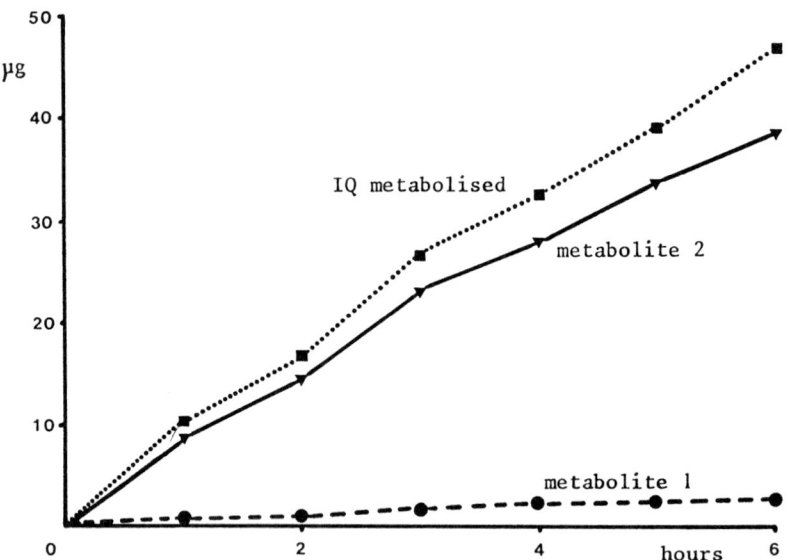

Fig.2 - Influence of the incubation duration on the production of IQ metabolites 1 and 2 from isolated hepatocytes incubated with ^3H-IQ

hepatocyte incubates contain considerably less interfering substances than the urinary or bile extracts, making the clean-up procedure and final purification much easier. Thus, the use of isolated hepatocytes seems to be a very efficient tool for further progress in the identification of IQ metabolic pathways.

REFERENCES

Ohgaki, H., Kusama, K., Matsukura, N., Morino, K., Hasegawa, H., Sato, S., Takayama, S. and Sugimura, T. (1984) : Carcinogenicity in mice of a mutagenic compound, 2-amino-3-methylimidazo[4,5-f]quinoline, from broiled sardine, cooked beef and beef extract. Carcinogenesis, 5, 921-

Peleran, J.C., Rao, D. and Bories, G. (1987) : Identification of the cooked food mutagen 2-amino-3-methylimidazo[4,5-f]quinoline (IQ) and its N-acetylated and 3-N-demethylated metabolites in rat urine. Toxicology, 43, 193-199.

Takayama, S., Nakatsaru, Y., Masuda, M., Ohgaki, H., Sato, S. and Sugimura, T. (1984) : Demonstration of carcinogenicity in F344 rats of 2-amino-3-methylimidazo [4,5-f]quinoline from broiled sardine, fried beef and beef extract. Gann, 75, 467-

Turesky, R.J., Skipper, P., Tannenbaum, S.R., Coles, B. and Ketterer, B. (1986) : Sulfamate formation is a major route for detoxification of 2-amino-3-methylimidazo[4,5-f]quinoline in the rat. Carcinogenesis, 7, 1483-

Seglen, P.O. (1976) : Preparation of isolated rat liver cells. In Methods in Cell Biology 13, ed D.M. Prescott, pp 29-83. New-York: Academic Press.

Sjodin, P. and Jagerstad, M. (1984) : a balance study of ^{14}C-Labelled ^3H-imidazo[4,5-f]quinoline-2-amines (IQ and MeIQ) in rats. Food Chem. Toxicol., 22, 207-210.

Biotransformation of sodium valproate in isolated rat hepatocytes

Vera Rogiers, André Callaerts, Walter Sonck, Antoine Vercruysse

Department of Toxicology, Free University Brussels (VUB), Laarbeeklaan 103, B-1090 Brussels, Belgium

KEYWORDS

Valproate, hepatocytes, liver cells, biotransformation.

INTRODUCTION

Sodium valproate (VP) is an effective and widely used anticonvulsant in adults and children.
Reversible and irreversible liver toxicity have been observed in children (Zimmerman, 1972). The mechanism, however, is unknown. In the literature, it is speculated that one or more of the unsaturated metabolites of VP could be responsible (Zimmerman, 1972; Schäfer, 1984).
Since the formation of these metabolites is cytochrome P-450 dependent, co-medication of potent enzyme-inducing anticonvulsants such as phenobarbital, phenytoin and carbamazepine could have broad implications with respect to the metabolic generation of unsaturated derivatives.

In order to be able to study the VP biotransformation under different, well-defined conditions, freshly isolated hepatocytes, kept for some hours in suspension, have been chosen as an in vitro model since the similarities in the metabolic profiles of VP in rat and man are striking.

METHODS

24 hr fasted adult male Wistar rats, weighing 200-250 g were used. Hepatocytes, isolated as previously described (Rogiers, 1984), were incubated for 4 hours. The medium consisted of Krebs Henseleit-buffer pH 7.4, supplemented with 2% (w/v) bovine serum albumin and 10 mM glucose. 500 µM VP was added to the medium, containing $5\ 10^6$ cells/ml. The incubations were carried out at 37°C in a shaking incubator (120 oscill./min) and the medium was gassed with 95% O_2 + 5% CO_2 every hour. Samples were taken at different time intervals.

Deconjugation, extraction and silylation were carried out according to Nau (1981).

Gas chromatographic/mass spectrometric analyses were conducted using a Hewlett-Packard 18947A fitted with a J & W on-column injector and a 50 m fused silica ov 1701 BP capillary column (0.25 mm int. diam.). A typical temp. programme was : (1) isothermal at 90°C for 5 min; (2) 90°-120°C at 2°C/min; (3) 120°-180°C at 5°C/min, followed by 10 min. isothermal at 180°C.
The mass spectrometer (Hewlett-Packard 5990 A) was operated in the selected ion-monitoring mode. The mass-to-charge ratio (m/z) is for every metabolite indicated in Fig. 2.
Reference samples of the various VP metabolites were synthesized in our laboratory or were a gift from Sanofi-Labaz. They were analysed under the same conditions as the samples.

During the whole experiment, cell damage was measured using the NADH penetration test described by Moldeus (1978).

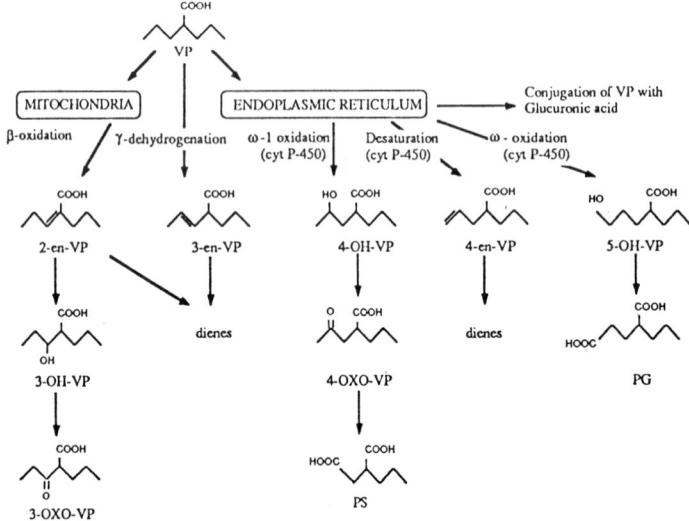

Fig. 1. : In vivo biotransformation of VP according to Granneman (1984) and corrected according to Rettie (1987)
VP : valproic acid; 2-en-VP : 2-propylpent-2-enoic acid; 3-en-VP : 3-propylpent-3-enoic acid; 4-en-VP : 4-propylpent-4-enoic acid; 3-OH-VP : 3-hydroxy-2-propylpentanoic acid; 4-OH-VP : 4-hydroxy-2-propylpentanoic acid; 5-OH-VP : 5-hydroxy-2-propylpentanoic acid; 3-oxo-VP : 2-propyl-3-oxo-pentanoic acid; 4-oxo-VP : 2-propyl-4-oxo-pentanoic acid; PG : 2-propylglutaric acid; PS : 2-propylsuccinic acid; IS : phenylbutyric acid as internal standard.

RESULTS AND DISCUSSION

- Separation of the various VP metabolites

From Fig. 2 it is clear that the various metabolites and their isomers are well separated so that quantitative determination is possible (even with a flame ionisation detector if higher amounts should be present).

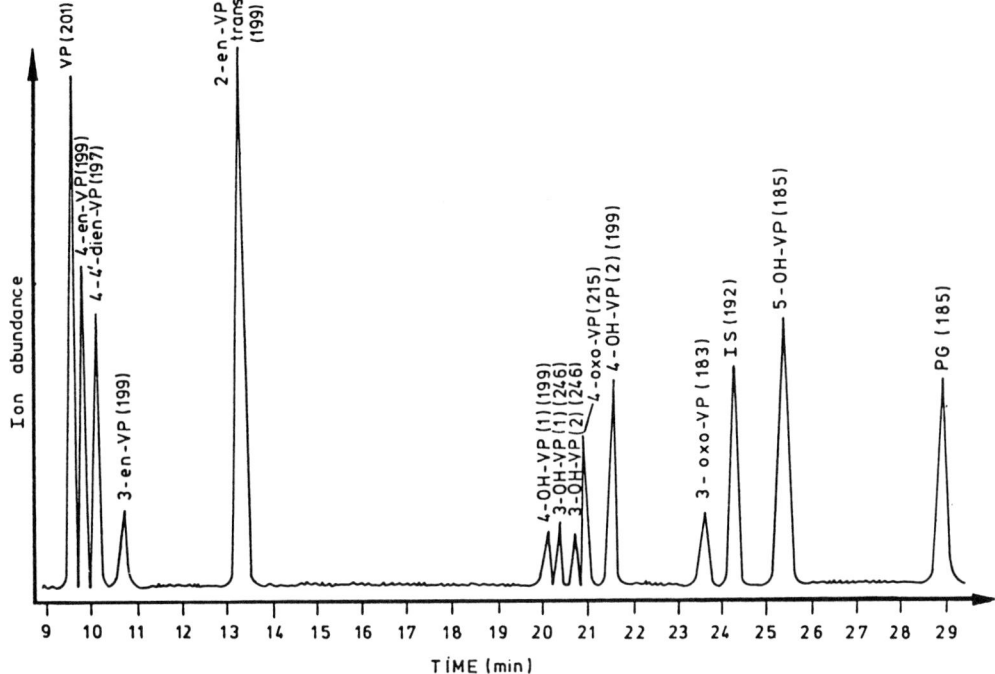

Fig. 2. : Separation of the various VP metabolites using GC/MS in SIM mode. m/z is indicated for every metabolite. The abbreviations are the same as indicated in Fig. 1.

- Biotransformation pattern of VP in rat hepatocytes

  a) free metabolites

  In Figs. 3 and 4, preliminary results concerning the disappearance of VP from the incubation medium in function of time and of the formation of metabolites are shown. Typical results for one experiment (out of three) are shown here.

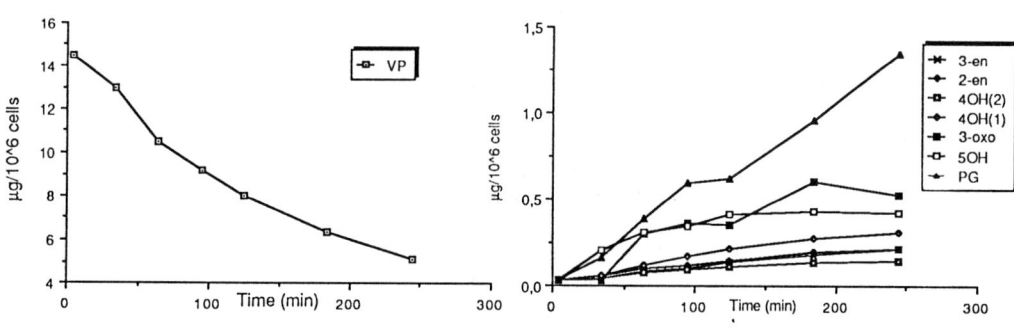

Fig. 3. : Disappearance of VP from the incubation medium.

Fig. 4. : Formation of free VP metabolites in freshly isolated rat hepatocytes. The abbreviations are as in Fig. 1.

331

VP has in the conditions described here a half-life of 152 min. (Fig.3).
When hepatocytes, derived from phenobarbital pretreated rats (i.p. injection
of 80 mg/kg/day for 3 days) were involved, its half-life decreased to 74
min., showing the pronounced effect that induction by co-medication might
have on VP metabolism (results not shown here). The major free metabolites
formed under control conditions (Fig. 4) consisted of PG, 3-oxo-VP and 5-OH-
VP. In terms of the given VP dosis it means that, after 4 hours of incubation, their concentrations represented 8,3 and 3% respectively.
Minor free metabolites were 4-OH-VP, 3-en-VP and 2-en-VP. Their formation
represented 2,1 and 1% of the initial VP dosis after 4 hours. 4-en-VP, a
suspected toxic metabolite, and diens were not formed during control conditions. Studies are underway now to define co-medication conditions under
which these metabolites could be formed. In our assays 4,4'dien-VP, 2,3-
dien-VP and 2,4-dien-VP formations have been checked using m/z = 197.

b) conjugated metabolites

The major conjugated metabolites were VP and PG, present after 4 hours in
concentrations of about 19% and 13% respectively of the initial VP dosis.
Minor conjugated derivatives were 5-OH-VP (2%), 4-OH-VP (2%) and only traces
of conjugated 4-en-VP and 2-en-VP were found back (both nearly 0,15% of the
VP dosis).

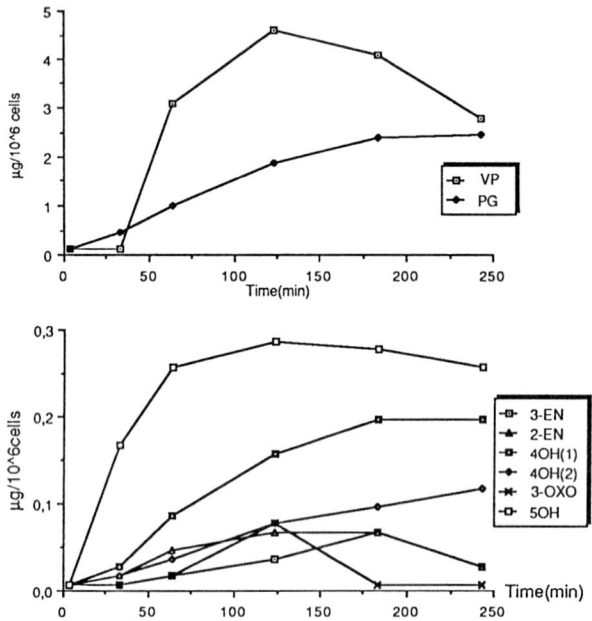

Fig. 5A, B. : Formation of conjugated VP metabolites in freshly
isolated rat hepatocytes.
The abbreviations are as indicated in Fig. 1.

For the different time intervals the total amount of metabolites found back
was 100% $\pm$ 8.

The cell viability, as measured by NADH penetration, was the same for the
control cells as for those with VP added. There was a linear decrease in
viability of about 8% per hour. The results of Figs. 3,4 and 5 were not
corrected for the changes in viability.

In the literature, data concerning the biotransformation of VP in isolated hepatocytes are not existing. As far as the metabolite pattern in rat urine is concerned, quantitative data have been reported by Granneman (1984). When these results were compared with our preliminary results, it seems that the "in vitro" biotransformation of VP in freshly isolated hepatocytes is very similar to the "in vivo" situation. The same metabolites are formed and their quantitative % pattern is very comparable. Thus, isolated rat hepatocytes could represent a suitable model for the study of VP biotransformation under well-defined conditions.

REFERENCES

Granneman, G.R., Wang, S.I., Machinist, J.M. and Kesterson, J.W. (1984) : Aspects of the metabolism of valproic acid. Xenobiotica, 14, 375-387.

Moldeus, P. (1978): Paracetamol metabolism and toxicity in isolated hepatocytes from rat and mouse. Biochem. Pharmacol. 27, 2859-2863.

Nau, H., Wittfoht, W., Schäfer, H., Jakobs, C., Rating,D. and Helge, H. (1981) : Valproic acid and several metabolites : quantitative determination in serum, urine, breast milk and tissues by GC-MS using selected ion monitoring. J. Chromatogr., 226, 69-78.

Rettie, A.E., Rettenmeier, A., Howald, W.N. and Baillie, T.A. (1987) : Cytochrome P-450 catalyzed formation of Δ^4-VPA, a toxic metabolite of valproic acid. Science, 235, 890-893.

Rogiers, V., Paeme, G., Vercruysse, A. and Bouwens, L. (1984) : Procyclidine metabolism in isolated rat liver cells. In Pharmacological, morphological and physiological aspects of liver aging. Ed. C.F.A. Van Bezooyen pp.121-126. Rijswijk : Eurage.

Schäfer, H. and Lührs, R. (1984) : Responsibility of the metabolite pattern for potential side effects in the rat being treated with valproic acid, 2-propylpenten-2-oic acid and 2-propylpenten-4-oic acid. In Metabolism of antiepileptic drugs. Ed. R.H. Levy pp. 73-83. New York : Raven Press.

Zimmerman, H.J. and Ishak, K.G. (1982) : Valproate-induced hepatic injury : analyses of 23 fatal cases. Hepatology 2, 591-597.

Effects of ciclosporin A on bile acid uptake, conjugation and release in cultured rat hepatocytes

Urs A. Boelsterli, Patrick Bouis, Peter Donatsch

Sandoz Ltd., Preclinical Research, Toxicology Department, CH-4002 Basel, Switzerland

KEY WORDS

Ciclosporin A, bile acids, hepatocytes, cytotoxicity

INTRODUCTION

Ciclosporin A (CsA), a cyclic endecapeptide of fungal origin, is widely used therapeutically as a potent immunosuppressant drug. Beside its nephrotoxic effects, impairment of hepatic function is one of the adverse reactions associated with CsA. High doses of CsA caused clinical hepatotoxicity, predominantly elevated serum bile acid levels, elevated serum bilirubin levels, and mild increases in serum aminotransferases activities (reviews: Cohen et al., 1984, and Mentha and Houssin, 1986; Lorber et al., 1987). A similar pattern of liver dysfunction has been reported in rats given CsA (Farthing and Clark, 1981; Ryffel et al., 1983; Stone et al., 1984; Yagisawa et al., 1986). The mechanism of CsA hepatotoxicity is not yet well understood, but several authors suggest that the inhibition of the bile acid dependent bile flow is a key event in the development of CsA-induced cholestasis. Whole animal studies (Stone et al., 1984) and *in situ* liver perfusion studies (Rotolo et al., 1986) demonstrated a decrease of bile flow and bile acid output as a consequence of CsA administration, followed by an increase in serum bile acid levels. Furthermore, Ziegler and Frimmer (1986) characterized the uptake kinetics of cholate in freshly isolated rat hepatocytes and demonstrated that CsA inhibited cholic acid uptake into hepatocytes in a non-competitive manner.

In view of the pivotal role of bile acid transport for the generation of bile flow and, consequently, for the excretion of bilirubin and other cholephilic compounds, *in vitro* studies on the effects of CsA on the hepatocellular handling of bile acids might help to determine if these effects play a role in the hepatobiliary dysfunction associated with CsA. The aim of this study was to investigate the effects of CsA on the uptake, conjugation and secretion of bile acids and to correlate these effects with the cytotoxicity endpoints, lactic dehydrogenase (LDH) leakage and cell morphology, in primary cultures of rat hepatocytes.

MATERIALS AND METHODS

Hepatocyte isolation and cultivation

Hepatocytes were isolated from young adult male Wistar rats (Kfm:WIST, Kleintierfarm Madörin, Füllinsdorf, Switzerland), as previously described (Boelsterli et al., 1987). The cells were suspended in WME supplemented with 10% FCS, insulin (10^{-7} M), dexamethasone (10^{-7} M), and penicillin/streptomycin (100 U/ml), and diluted to a final concentration of 5×10^5 cells/ml. The hepatocytes were seeded onto culture dishes at a final cell density of 7.5×10^4 cells/cm_2 and incubated at $37^\circ C$ in 95% air/5% CO_2. After an attachment period of 3 hr, the medium was aspirated and replaced with fresh WME, completed as described above, containing 1.6% FCS and various concentrations of CsA.

In vitro exposure to drugs

Stock solutions of CsA were freshly prepared by dissolving the drugs in DMSO (final DMSO concentration, 1.5%, v/v) which was then directly added to the culture medium. Control plates were incubated with the culture medium, both with and without the solvent.

Intracellular accumulation, conjugation and secretion of (14C)-cholate and (14C)-taurocholate

Following exposure to CsA for various time periods, the cell monolayers were incubated at $37^\circ C$ with 5 uM (carboxyl-14C)-cholic acid (52 mCi/mmol, Radiochemical Centre, Amersham, U.K.) in WME (completed) containing 1.6% FCS in the absence of CsA. The media were then collected and centrifuged (200xg/5 min) to remove detached cells. The hepatocytes were washed with 3x5 ml ice-cold 0.9% saline and subsequently scraped off into saline, using a rubber policeman, and ultrasonicated. The contents of radiolabelled unconjugated and conjugated cholic acid in the cells and in the extracellular medium were determined in order to estimate net uptake, conjugation and release of the bile acids. The samples were acidified with HCl, and the unconjugated cholic acid was extracted with ethyl acetate. The taurocholic acid was recovered in the aqueous phase. The results were expressed as nmol bile acid/mg cellular protein.

To identify the conjugated bile acids, cells and medium containing conjugated (14C)-cholate were extracted with chloroform/methanol (2:1,v/v), and the methanol/water phase was concentrated using a Minicon concentrator (Amicon, Danvers, MA, USA). The extracts were dried under nitrogen, dissolved in a small amount of methanol, and applied onto silica gel 60 TLC foils. The bile acids were separated according to Usui (1963).

Measurement of LDH release and cellular protein

LDH activity in the culture medium and in the cells was assayed spectrophotometrically using a Merckotest Kit (Merck, Darmstadt, FRG). Enzyme activity was expressed as the percentage of the total activity present in cells at the beginning of the incubation. Protein content was determined according to Bradford (1976).

RESULTS

Exogenously added (14C)-cholic acid (5 uM) was rapidly taken up by the hepatocytes (Fig. 1A). The cholic acid was readily conjugated to taurine (representing 93.4 % of conjugates) or glycine (5.6%) as demonstrated by TLC analysis. The intracellular content of taurocholate and the amount released into the extracellular medium increased as a linear function of time for at least 60 min, the duration used as standard incubation time for the subsequent studies with CsA (Fig.1B).

Exposure of the hepatocytes to CsA caused a marked, time and concentration-dependent inhibition of cholate net uptake (Figs. 1A, 2A), as well as an inhibition of taurocholate accumulation in the cells (Figs. 1B,2B). Similarly, taurocholate release into the medium was also decreased following incubation with 10^{-7} M and higher concentrations of CsA (Figs. 1B,2B). DMSO, which was used as a solvent for CsA, did not cause inhibitory effects on either intra- or extracellular bile acid contents at the concentration used in all culture dishes including the controls (1.5%, v/v).

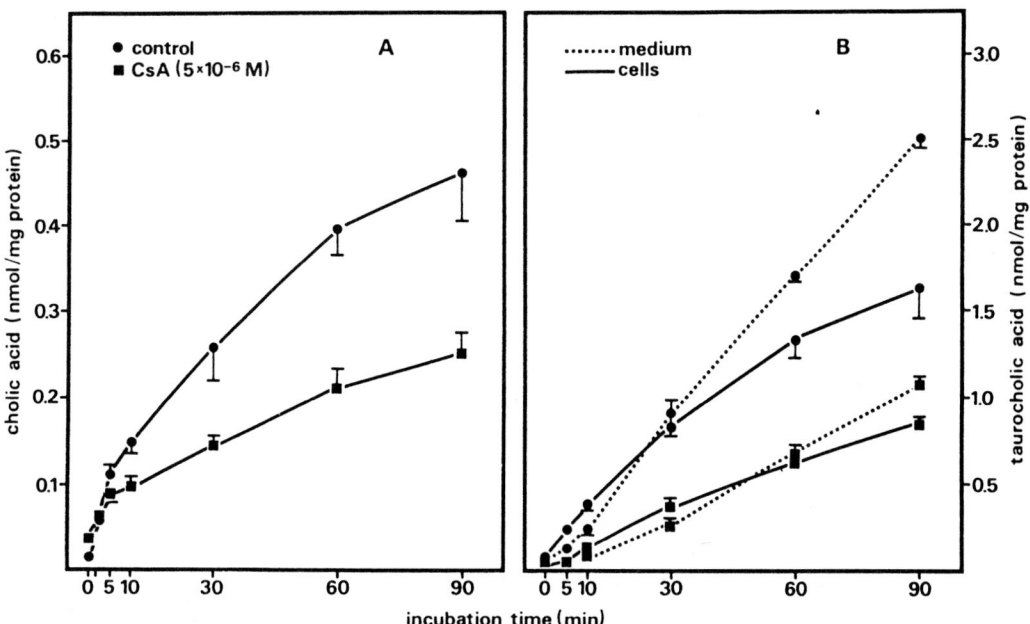

Fig. 1. Time-course of the inhibition by CsA of cholic acid uptake into hepatocytes (A), and accumulation of newly formed taurocholic acid in the cells and its release into the culture medium (B). Culture plates were preincubated with 5×10^{-5} M CsA or the vehicle alone for 2 hr. Subsequently, fresh medium without CsA but containing (14C)-cholic acid (5 uM) was added and the plates were incubated for the durations indicated. The symbols represent means ± SD (n=3). Values significantly different from the control values were assessed by the t-test (*, p<0.05; **, p<0.01).

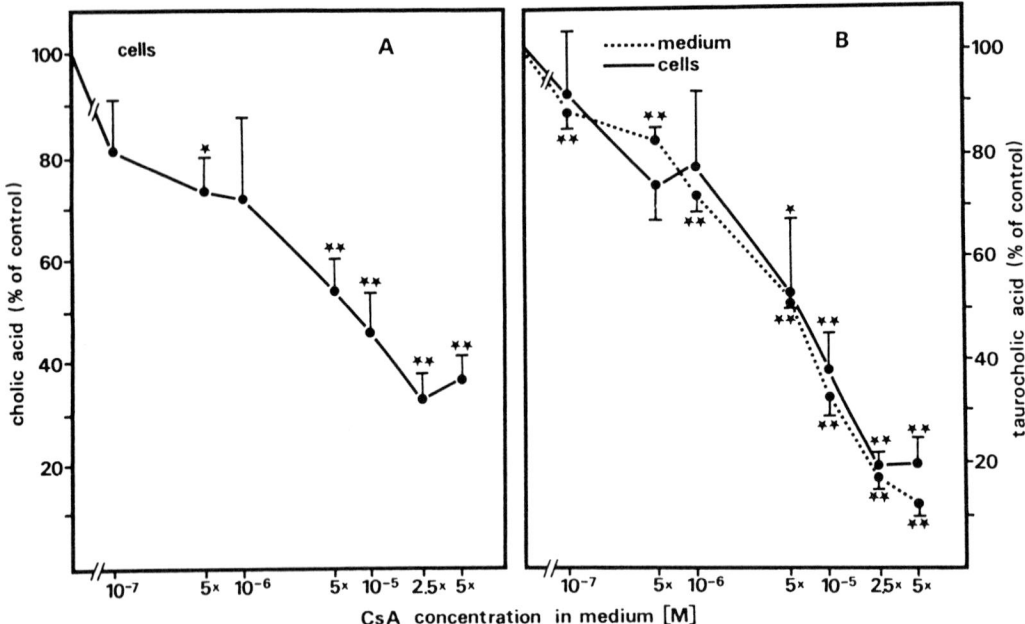

Fig. 2. Inhibition of cholic acid uptake (A), and of taurocholate formation and release (B) as a function of the CsA concentration. Hepatocytes were preincubated with various concentrations of CsA for 2 hr. Subsequently, fresh medium without CsA but containing (14C)-cholic acid (5 uM) was added, and the cultures were incubated for 60 min. The symbols represent means $\pm$ SD (n=3). Values significantly different from the control values were assessed by the t-test (*, $p<0.05$; **, $p<0.01$).

TABLE 1. LDH release from cultured hepatocytes exposed to CsA

CsA concentration (M)	LDH activity in medium (% of control)	
	2 hr exposure	17 hr exposure
0 (solvent control)	100 $\pm$ 3 [a]	100 $\pm$ 7 [b]
5.0×10^{-7}	108 $\pm$ 15	76 $\pm$ 24
1.0×10^{-6}	86 $\pm$ 5	89 $\pm$ 5
5.0×10^{-6}	96 $\pm$ 10	145 $\pm$ 45
1.0×10^{-5}	92 $\pm$ 4	241 $\pm$ 24 *
2.5×10^{-5}	100 $\pm$ 4	294 $\pm$ 6 *
5.0×10^{-5}	126 $\pm$ 3 *	440 $\pm$ 78 *

[a], Control (2 hr): 7.3 $\pm$ 0.2% of the total cell-associated LDH activity at the start of the experiment; [b], control (17 hr): 14.7 $\pm$ 1.1% of the total cell-associated LDH activity at the start of the experiment. The values are the means $\pm$ SD of 3 experiments. Values significantly different from the control value were assessed by the t-test (*, $p<0.01$).

The time and concentration-related effects of CsA on LDH release from hepatocytes are shown in Table 1. Whereas a 2 hr incubation period resulted in minimal LDH release without any morphological changes of the cells, prolonged incubation (17 hr) caused enzyme leakage at 10^{-5} M and higher concentrations of CsA. Correspondingly, morphological abnormalities (change of the cellular shape, intracellular lipid droplets, cell detachment) were evident at concentrations of 10^{-5} M and higher.

Table 2 summarizes the effects of CsA on LDH release and taurocholate secretion as a function of the duration of exposure. Whereas a 15 hr washout period (medium without CsA) following a 2 hr exposure to CsA had the same effect on LDH leakage as a continuous 17 hr incubation with CsA, the same treatment attenuated the drug's inhibitory effect on taurocholate secretion.

TABLE 2. Effects of toxic concentrations of CsA on LDH release or taurocholate secretion as a function of the duration of exposure

Endpoint of toxicity	Duration of exposure to CsA		
	2 hr	17 hr	2 hr+15 hr washout
LDH release	5×10^{-5} M	10^{-5} M	10^{-5} M
Taurocholate secretion	10^{-7} M	10^{-7} M	10^{-5} M

The above values show the CsA concentrations at which significant changes occurred. Taurocholate secretion is defined as the net taurocholate release into the culture medium after 60 min incubation with (14C)-cholic acid (5 uM).

DISCUSSION

Bile acid uptake, conjugation and secretion into bile are specific functions of the liver that have been maintained in vitro by using freshly isolated hepatocytes (Schwarz et al., 1975; Anwer et al., 1976; Anwer and Hegner, 1979; Schwenk, 1980) or primary cultures of rat hepatocytes (Schwarz et al., 1979; Scharschmidt and Stephen, 1981). The observation that such functions were altered in animals receiving CsA prompted us to investigate the effects of CsA on the hepatocellular handling of bile acids in rat hepatocyte cultures. The results of the present study demonstrate that CsA markedly inhibited net uptake and tauroconjugation of exogenously added cholate and its subsequent release into the culture medium as a function of the drug concentration. This functional impairment was evident using CsA concentrations as low as 10^{-7} M, a level at which the cells were still intact even after prolonged incubation with CsA, as judged by the lack of LDH release into the medium (Table 1). Since a scoring of morphological changes always paralleled the data obtained from measurements of LDH activity in the culture medium, the lack of any morphological abnormalities in the hepatocytes at low CsA concentrations confirmed the findings that the impairment of bile acid handling by far preceded the appearance of clear cytotoxicity. This impairment of a hepatocyte-specific function in the absence of general cytotoxic effects confirmed the results of an in vivo rat study with CsA (Stone et al., 1984).

It has been shown that CsA inhibits the initial uptake rate of cholate in freshly isolated hepatocytes in a non-competitive manner (Ziegler and Frimmer, 1986). From the present data it cannot be determined, however, whether the rate of tauroconjugation and the rate of bile acid secretion were also inhibited under the experimental conditions used. Thus, the impairment of the hepatocellular handling of bile acids was defined as the net release of newly formed taurocholate into the culture medium during incubation with cholic acid at a physiological concentration (5 uM). The inhibitory effect of CsA on (14C)-taurocholate secretion was not dependent on the total time during which CsA was present in the medium and was partly reversible upon removal of the drug from the medium (Table 2).

The in vitro concentrations of CsA causing impairment of the hepatocellular handling of bile acids were in the same range as the steady state CsA plasma concentrations in patients featuring hyperbilirubinemia and cholestasis (> 0.1 uM). LDH leakage, however, could only be induced in vitro using CsA concentrations that exceeded therapeutic trough plasma levels by a factor of at least 10.

In conclusion, primary cultures of rat hepatocytes provide a suitable model for the study of CsA-induced changes of bile acid uptake and tauroconjugation. They may also be useful to further analyze the underlying mechanisms of ciclosporin-induced cholestasis. In addition, this test may prove to be a useful endpoint for a comparative evaluation of the hepatotoxic potential of CsA and its congeners in vitro, since the release of tauroconjugated cholate from exogenously added (14C)-cholic acid can easily be monitored during the exposure of hepatocytes to xenobiotics.

REFERENCES

Anwer, M.S., Hegner, D. (1979): Study of cholic acid conjugation by isolated rat hepatocytes. Hoppe-Seyler's Z. Physiol. Chem. 360, 515-522.
Anwer M.S., Kroker R., Hegner D. (1976): Cholic acid uptake into isolated rat hepatocytes. Hoppe-Seyler's Z. Physiol. Chem. 357, 1477-1486.
Boelsterli U.A., Bouis P., Donatsch P. (1987): Psychotropic drugs as inhibitors of glycerolipid biosynthesis and secretion in primary rat hepatocyte cultures. Toxicol. In Vitro 1, (in press).
Bradford M.M.(1976): A rapid and sensitive method for the quantitation of microgram quantities of protein utilizing the principle of protein-dye binding. Anal. Biochem. 72, 248-254.
Cohen D.J., Loertscher R., Rubin M.F., Tilney N.L., Carpenter, C.B., Strom T.B. (1984): Cyclosporine: A new immunosuppresive agent for organ transplantation. Ann. Int. Med. 101, 667-682.
Farthing M.J.G., Clark M.L. (1981): Nature of the toxicity of cyclosporin A in the rat. Biochem. Pharmacol. 30, 3311-3316.

Lorber, M.I., Van Buren, C.T., Flechner, S.M., Williams, C., Kahan, B.D. (1987): Hepatobiliary and pancreatic complications of cyclosporine therapy in 466 renal transplant recipients. Transplantation 43, 35-40.

Mentha G., Houssin D. (1986): La ciclosporine: un immunosuppresseur sélectif en hépatologie. Gastroentérol. Clin. Biol. 10, 641-647.

Rotolo F.S., Branum G.D., Bowers B.A., Meyers W.C. (1986): Effect of cyclosporine on bile secretion in rats. Amer. J. Surg. 151, 35-40.

Ryffel B., Donatsch P., Madörin M., Matter B.E., Rüttimann G., Schön H., Stoll R., Wilson J. (1983): Toxicological evaluation of cyclosporin A. Arch. Toxicol. 53, 107-141.

Scharschmidt B.F., Stephens J.E. (1981): Transport of sodium, chloride and taurocholate by cultured rat hepatocytes. Proc. Natl. Acad. Sci. USA 78, 986-990.

Schwarz L.R., Barth C.A. (1979): Taurocholate uptake by adult rat hepatocytes in primary culture. Hoppe-Seyler's Z. Physiol. Chem. 360, 1117-1120.

Schwarz L.R., Burr R., Schwenk M., Pfaff E., Greim H. (1975): Uptake of taurocholic acid into isolated rat liver cells. Eur. J. Biochem. 55, 617-623.

Schwenk M. (1980): Transport systems of isolated hepatocytes. Arch. Toxicol. 44, 113-126.

Stone B.G., Udani M., Schade R.R. (1984): Cyclosporine cholestasis in the absence of hepatic toxicity: a rat model. Hepatology 4, 1047.

Usui T. (1963): Thin-layer chromatography of bile acids with special reference to separation of keto bile acids. J. Biochem. 54, 283-286.

Yagisawa T., Takahashi K., Teraoka S., Yamaguchi Y., Toma H., Agishi T., Ota K. (1986): Cyclosporine tissue levels and morphological and functional changes in organs of cyclosporine-treated rats. Transplant. Proc. 18, 1272-1277.

Ziegler K., Frimmer M. (1986): Cyclosporin A and a diaziridine derivative inhibit the hepatocellular uptake of cholate, phalloidin and rifampicin. Biochim. Biophys. Acta 855, 136-142.

Primary culture of cryopreserved rat hepatocytes

Christophe Chesné, Philippe Gripon, André Guillouzo

INSERM U.49, Unité de Recherches Hépatologiques, Hôpital Pontchaillou, 35033 Rennes Cedex, France

---

Keywords : rat hepatocytes, primary culture, cryopreservation, paracetamol.

INTRODUCTION

Isolated hepatocytes have been increasingly used in biochemical, pharmacological and toxicological studies over the last years (Sirica and Pitot, 1980 ; Guillouzo, 1986). Since the rates and routes of drug metabolism are often different in man and in animals, the need for experiments on human cells is evident. However, human samples are unfrequent and unpredictable. Moreover, cell yields from the perfusion of a large portion of the liver are usually too high to be used immediately after isolation. The only present ways to preserve isolated hepatocytes are culturing and freezing. In culture, human hepatocytes, which are functionnally more stable than their rat counterparts, retain the capability of expressing phase I and phase II drug reactions for several days or longer when they are co-cultured with rat liver epithelial cells (Guguen-Guillouzo et al., 1983).

For long-term preservation, only freezing can be envisioned. Many attempts have been made to freeze rodent and sometimes human hepatocytes. However, most have stressed the occurrence of impaired functions after thawing (Table I). A recent study in our laboratory has somewhat overcome these shortcomings. Indeed, we have shown that more than 50 % of rat hepatocytes which are able to attach and survive in culture when seeded just after isolation, still possess these properties after thawing (Chesné and Guillouzo, 1988). The main question is now to determine whether, after freezing, hepatocytes are able to repair cellular damage in culture. Preliminary results on rat hepatocytes maintained in both conventional culture conditions and co-culture are reported here.

MATERIAL AND METHODS

Hepatocyte isolation

Sprague-Dawley rats (male, 300 g weight) were anaesthetized and received 2000 IU heparin. The liver was first washed with a Ca^{++}-free hepes buffered solution and then perfused with the same buffer containing 0.025 % collagenase and 5 mM $CaCl_2$ (Guguen-Guillouzo and Guillouzo, 1986). The flow rates were 30 and 15 ml/min

TABLE I : SUMMARY OF THE MAIN RESULTS OBTAINED WITH FROZEN HEPATOCYTES.

Species	Cryoprotectant (v/v)	Cooling rate (°C/min)	Viability (Trypan blue test, %)	Attachment (%)	Functional activities	References
Rat	10 % DMSO	2 - 7	80	ND	Gluconeogenesis impaired just after thawing	Le Cam et al., 1976
Rat	9 % DMSO	0.5 - 10	70	ND	Strong decrease of protein synthesis just after thawing	Fuller et al., 1980
Rat	12 % DMSO	1 - 2	62	28	Strong decrease of protein synthesis after a 48 h culture	Nutt et al., 1980
Rat	10 % DMSO	1	66	ND	Metabolic activation of cyclophosphamide	Karlberg and Lindahl-Kiessling, 1981
Rat	10 % DMSO 20 % DMSO 10 % glycerol	1	80	23 - 28	Fast decrease of microsomal associated functions during a 24 h culture	Novicki et al., 1981
Rat	12 % DMSO	1 - 2	70	ND	Strong decrease of protein synthesis, bilirubin conjugation and gluconeogenesis just after thawing	Fuller et al., 1982, 1984, 1985
Rat	10 % DMSO	39	78	59	Protein synthesis, gluconeogenesis, ureogenesis and tyrosine aminotransferase induction preserved	Gomez-Lechon et al., 1984
Human	10 % DMSO	1	78	ND	Decrease of benzopyrene metabolism after a 24 h culture	Moore and Gould, 1984
Rat	10 % DMSO	1 - 2	42	37	Fast decrease of the cyt. P-450 content during a 24 h culture	Jackson et al., 1985
Human	10 % DMSO	1.5	57	31	Albumin secretion preserved during a 15 day culture	Rintjes et al., 1986
Woodchuck	20 % DMSO	ND	ND	weak	Ability to be infected by the human δ hepatitis virus	Taylor et al., 1987
Rat	16 % DMSO	2 - 3	65	33 - 47	Moderate decrease of protein secretion after a 24 h culture	Chesné and Guillouzo, 1988

ND : not determined

respectively. After several washings, the cells were suspended in the culture medium and counted in a 0.05 % trypan blue solution in phosphate buffered saline.

Hepatocyte culture
Cells (7×10^5) were seeded in 35 mm diameter Petri dishes in 2 ml of medium (MEM/199, 3/1 v/v) containing 10 % foetal calf serum (FCS), 20 µg/ml bovine insulin, 0.1 % bovine serum albumin (BSA), 50 IU/ml penicillin and 50 µg/ml streptomycin. The dishes were incubated at 37°C in an humidified atmosphere of air/CO_2 (95 %-5 %). The medium, supplemented with 7×10^{-5} M hydrocortisone hemisuccinate, was renewed after 4 h and daily thereafter.

Freezing and thawing
The conditions of freezing and thawing were those defined from preliminary experiments described in another paper (Chesné and Guillouzo, 1988). In outline, an equal volume of L15 medium with 0.2% BSA and containing dimethylsulfoxyde (DMSO) was added slowly to the cell suspension. The final proportions of DMSO and FCS were 16 and 20 % (v/v) respectively. After a 30 min incubation at room temperature, freezing vials containing hepatocytes were placed in a polystyrene pack and transferred to a -70°C freezer (cooling rate : -3°C/min). After one hour, the vials were plunged in liquid nitrogen. The storage lasted from one day to several weeks. The cells were thawed in a waterbath at 37°C and diluted in L15 medium containing 0.8 M glucose. After centrifugation, the cells were seeded as fresh cells.

Electron microscopic examination
Rat hepatocyte pure and co-cultures were fixed in situ by 2.5 % glutaraldehyde in sodium cacodylate buffer 0.1 M pH 7.4. Post-fixation was performed in a 1 % osmium tetroxide solution in sodium cacodylate and dehydratation in graded ethanol. The cultures were embedded in Epon and contrasted with uranyl acetate and lead citrate before examination.

Evaluation of functional activities
Albumin and transferrin secreted in the culture medium during each 24 h period, were determined by immunonephelometry (Guguen-Guillouzo et al., 1983).
Paracetamol was selected as a substrate for analysis of drug metabolism enzyme capacity. It was incubated in a complete culture medium during 4-16 hours at a non toxic concentration of 1 mM. The proteins of the incubates (0.2 ml) were then precipitated with 1 ml methanol containing the internal standard, 3-acetamidophenol. The supernatants were dried under vacuum and the residues were dissolved in 100 µl water. A 20 µl aliquote was injected on an HPLC column (Microbondapak C18 Waters). The elution was obtained with a gradient of 100 % A : sodium acetate 20 mM ajusted to pH 2.5 with acetic acid to 80 % A and 20 % B : methanol in 20 min at 1 ml/min. The conjugates of paracetamol with glucuronic acid, sulfate, glutathione, cysteine and mercapturic acid (kindly provided by Winthrop, Guilford, England), detected at 250 nm, were eluted respectively at 8, 9.5, 12, 15 and 18 min. The recovery of conjugates varied between 92 and 100 % and the coefficient of intra and interday variation was under 5 % at 10^{-5} M.

RESULTS

The viability of cryopreserved cells determined by the trypan blue exclusion test was around 65 % of the seeded cell population. When expressed as the percentage of cells attached after 16 h, the viable cells represented 40 % of the total population. Using both light and electron microscopy, the morphology of cultured frozen cells did not show any evident alteration after some days of culture when compared with cultures of unfrozen cells (Fig. 1).

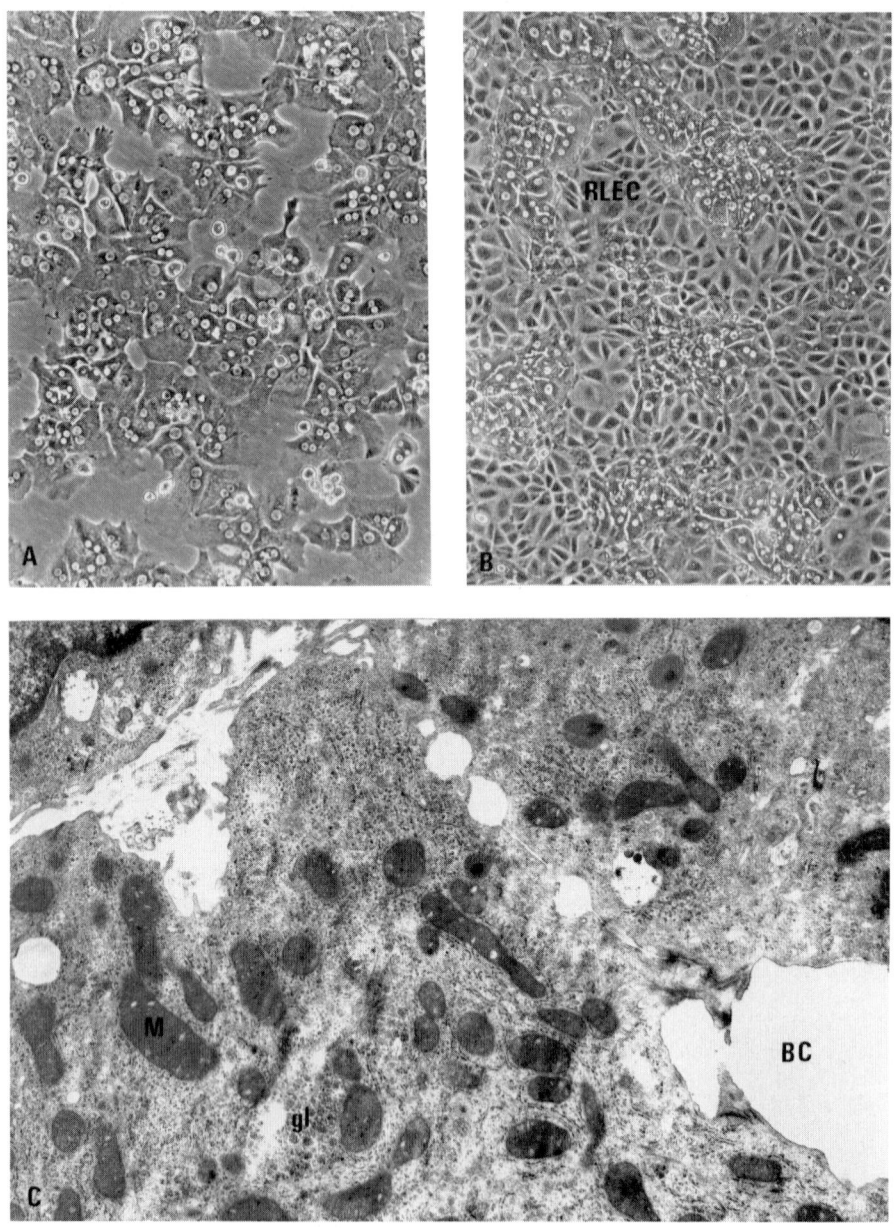

Figure 1 : **Morphology of cultured thawed rat cells.**
A and B : Light microscopy ; (A) pure culture after 24 h (x 225),
(B) co-culture with rat liver epithelial cells (RLEC) after 15 days
(x 225).
C : Electron microscopy ; co-culture after 10 days.
(M : mitochondrion ; GL : glycogen particles ; BC : bile canaliculus)
(x 8,900).

Protein secretion in the culture medium was also determined. Transferrin secreted by frozen cells reached elevated levels in co-culture, becoming comparable to those of fresh cells after 4-5 days (Fig. 2). The same curves were obtained for albumin secretion (results not shown). However, contrary to fresh cells, frozen cells maintained in pure culture were not able to maintain the same protein production rate during the first 48 hours ; the secretion rate dropped quickly and was very low by the third day.

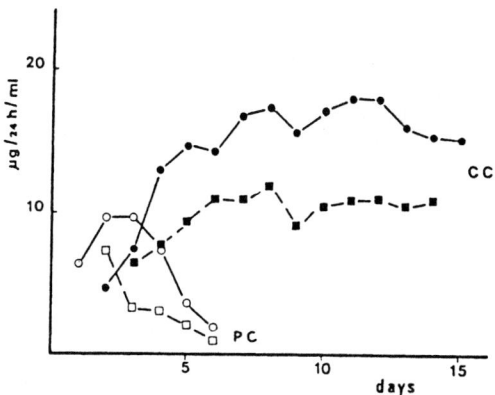

Figure 2 : Secretion of transferrin in the medium of rat hepatocyte pure (PC) and co-culture (CC).

Metabolism of paracetamol was used as another biochemical parameter of the functional capacity of frozen hepatocytes. This drug allowed assay of phase I and phase II reactions. The results are displayed in figure 3. Again, frozen cells behaved in co-culture as fresh cells. The oxidation pathway was preserved during the 2 weeks of culture ; it even increased after some days. By contrast, this activity declined rapidly in pure culture of both unfrozen and frozen cells. However, the decline was earlier and faster in the latter.
Phase II reactions were also well preserved in frozen cells. Cysteine and mercapturic acid conjugates derived from the glutathione conjugate were constantly detected during co-culture (results not shown), contrary to pure culture. Glucuronic conjugates were produced at a high rate and sulfation, though at a reduced rate, was always active. Interestingly the rates of conjugates with glutathione, sulfate and glucuronic acid formed were close to those found previously with hepatocyte suspensions (Moldeus, 1978) or during the first 48 h of culture (Emery, 1985).
Pure cultures of rat liver epithelial cells did not exhibit any production of transferrin and paracetamol metabolites (not shown).

CONCLUSION

Attachment to the culture substratum implies that the cells possess some functional activities and therefore represents a more valuable test of viability than the trypan blue exclusion test. However, the functional activity of frozen hepatocytes is impaired and is not restored in pure culture. Specific functions decrease very rapidly. By contrast, the co-culture model seems to represent a more suitable culture system allowing frozen cells to recover functional activities close to those found in unfrozen cells after a few days. This culture system together with improvement of freezing conditions should offer new perspectives for biochemical and pharmacological studies on hepatocytes from various species, including man.

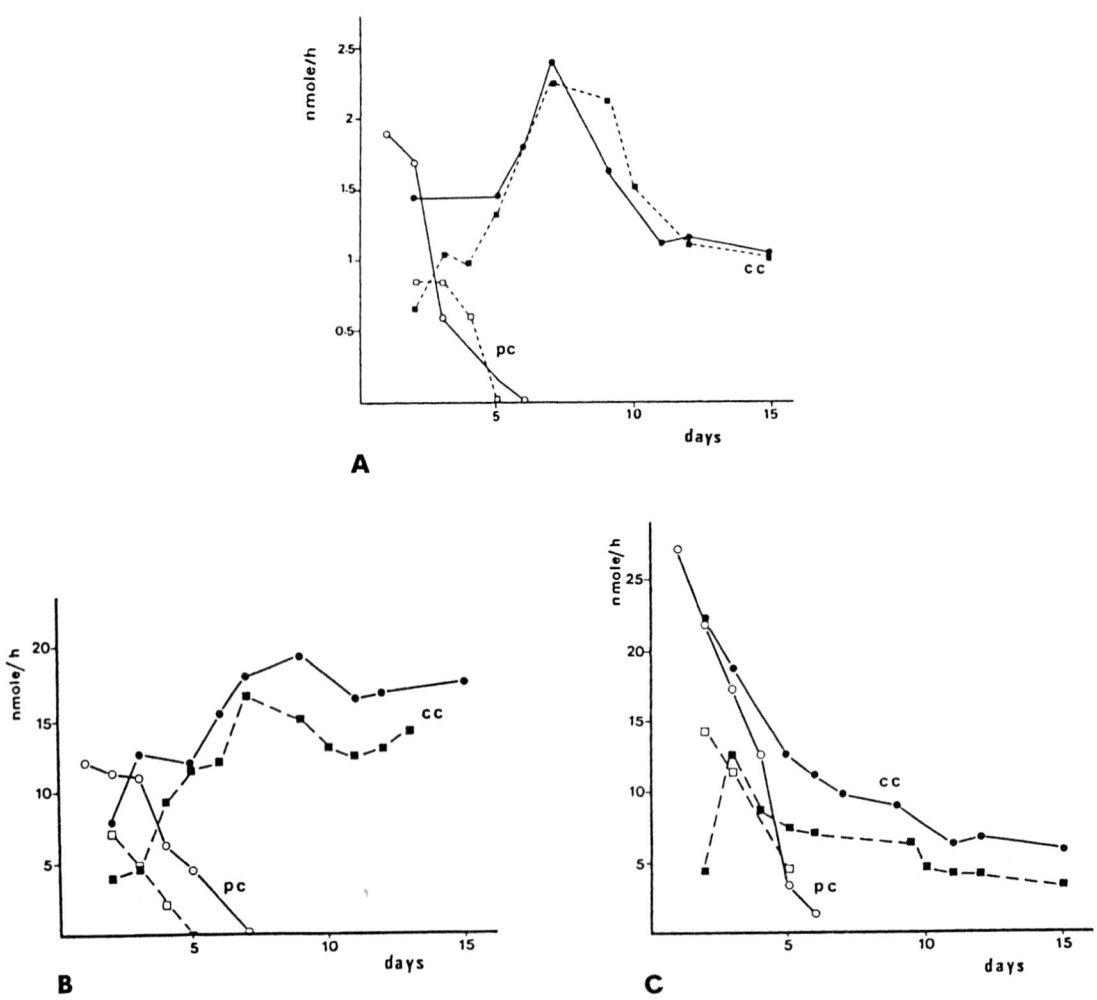

Figure 3 : Biotransformation of paracetamol in pure culture (PC) and co-culture (CC) of rat hepatocytes.
A) Oxidation pathway. This pathway includes oxidation by the cytochrome P-450-dependent monooxygenase system, then conjugation with glutathione. This conjugate can be hydrolysed to give a cysteine conjugate, which can be itself acetylated to form a mercapturic acid derivative. Oxidation is the sum of these three compounds.
B) conjugation with glucuronic acid ; C) conjugation with sulfate.

ACKNOWLEDGMENTS

C. Chesné was supported financially by IRIS (Institut de Recherches Internationales SERVIER). We are grateful to A. Vannier for typing the manuscript.

REFERENCES

Chesné, C. and Guillouzo, A. (1988): Cryopreservation of isolated rat hepatocytes : a critical evaluation of freezing and thawing conditions. Cryobiology (submitted).

Emery, S., Oldham, H.G., Norman S.J. and Chenery, R.J. (1985): The effect of cimetidine and ranitidine on paracetamol glucuronidation and sulphation in cultured rat hepatocytes. Biochem. Pharmacol. 34, 1415-1421.

Fuller, B.J., Morris, G.J., Nutt, L.H. and Attenburrow, V.D. (1980): Functional recovery of isolated rat hepatocytes upon thawing from -196°C. Cryo-Letters 1, 139-146.

Fuller, B.J., Grout, B.W. and Woods, R.J. (1982): Biochemical and ultrastructural examination of cryopreserved hepatocytes in rat. Cryobiology 19, 493-502.

Fuller, B.J. (1985): Cryopreservation of isolated rat hepatocytes in pellet form. Cryo-letters 6, 49-56.

Gomez-Lechon, M.J., Lopez, P. and Castell, J.V. (1984): Biochemical functionality and recovery of hepatocytes after deep freezing storage. In Vitro 20, 826-832.

Guguen-Guillouzo, C., Clément, B., Baffet, G., Beaumont C., Morel-Chany, E., Glaise, D. and Guillouzo A. (1983): Maintenance and reversibility of active albumin secretion by adult rat hepatocytes co-cultured with another liver epithelial cell type. Exp. Cell Res. 143, 47-54.

Guguen-Guillouzo, C. and Guillouzo, A. (1986): Methods for preparation of adult and fetal hepatocytes. In Isolated and cultured hepatocytes, eds A. Guillouzo and C. Guguen-Guillouzo, pp. 1-12.Paris : Les Editions INSERM, London: John Libbey Eurotext.

Guillouzo, A. (1986) : Use of isolated and cultured hepatocytes for xenobiotic metabolism and cytotoxicity studies. In Isolated and cultured hepatocytes, eds A. Guillouzo and C. Guguen-Guillouzo, pp. 313-331. Paris : Les Editions INSERM, London : John Libbey Eurotext.

Jackson, B.A., Davies, J.E. and Chipman, J.K. (1985): Cytochrome P-450 activity in hepatocytes following cryopreservation and monolayer culture. Biochem. Pharmacol. 34, 3389-3391.

Le Cam, A., Guillouzo, A. and Freychet, P.(1976): Ultrastructural and biochemical studies of isolated adult rat hepatocytes prepared under hypoxic conditions. Cryopreservation of hepatocytes. Exp. Cell Res. 98, 382-395.

Moldeus, P. (1978): Paracetamol metabolism and toxicity in isolated hepatocytes from rat and mouse. Biochem. Pharmacol. 27, 2859-2863.

Moore, C.J. and Gould, M.N. (1984): Metabolism of benzopyrene by cultured human hepatocytes from multiple donors. Carcinogenesis 5, 1577-1582.

Novicki, D.I., Irons, G.P., Strom, S.C., Jirtle, R. and Michalopoulos, G. (1982): Cryopreservation of isolated rat hepatocytes. In Vitro 18, 393-399.

Nutt, L.H., Attenburrow, V.D. and Fuller, B.J. (1980): Investigations into repair of freeze/thaw damage in isolated rat hepatocytes. Cryo Letters 1, 513-518.

Rijntjes, P.J.M., Moshage H.J., Van Gemert P.J.L., De Waal R. and Yap S.H. (1986): Cryopreservation of adult human hepatocytes. The influence of deep freezing storage on the viability, cell seeding survival, fine structures and albumin synthesis in primary cultures. J. Hepatol. 3, 7-18.

Sirica, A.E. and Pitot, H.C. (1980): Drug metabolism and effects of carcinogens in cultured hepatic cells. Pharmacol. Rev. 31, 205-228.

Taylor, J., Mason, W., Summers, J., Goldberg, G., Coates, L., Gerin, J. and Gowans, E. (1987): Replication of human hepatitis delta virus in primary cultures of woodchuck hepatocytes. J. Virol. 61, 2891-2895.

Biotransformation and cytotoxicity studies in primary hepatocyte cultures derived from different mammalian species

W.C. Mennes, B.J. Blaauboer, C.W.M. van Holsteijn

Institute of Veterinary Pharmacology, Pharmacy and Toxicology, University of Utrecht, PO Box 80176, Utrecht, The Netherlands

KEYWORDS

hepatocytes, primary culture, comparative study, aniline, cytochrome P-450, cytotoxicity, biotransformation

INTRODUCTION

Isolated hepatocytes have proven to be a suitable system to investigate biotransformation and cytotoxicity mechanisms (Sirica and Pitot, 1980). As compared with microsomes the environment of the enzymatic systems is in better agreement with the in vivo situation and results obtained with this cellular system are more easily extrapolated to in vivo. Suspension cultures have the disadvantage of short life and a stressed physiology due to the synthesis of biomatrix components (Blaauboer and Paine, 1979). This may be circumvented by the use of cells in primary culture. However, cells derived from rat liver rapidly lose their cytochrome P-450 content (Guzelian et al., 1977; Maslansky and Williams, 1983), making the results of biotransformation studies difficult to interpret. The behaviour of the cytochrome P-450 levels in primary cultures of hepatocytes derived from other mammalian species is less well investigated (Maslansky and Williams, 1983). The use of hepatocytes from an other mammalian species with a more stable mixed function oxygenase system would be a great advantage in the extrapolation from in vitro to in vivo, leading to a better understanding of mechanisms of toxicity of compounds of which toxicity depends on biotransformation. Furthermore, interspecies extrapolation of toxicological data may be carried out with more precision if in vitro comparisons of biotransformation and cytotoxicity can be made Eventually, this could result in a reduction in the use of animals in toxicological experiments.

The aim of this study was to describe the changes in total cytochrome P-450 concentration in primary cultures of hepatocytes derived from several mammalian species and to investigate the biotransformation of aniline in these cells. In vivo and in suspension cultures this compound is bioactivated to several products, among others 4-aminophenol and N-hydroxyaniline (Kiese, 1974; Blaauboer and van Holsteijn, 1983; Evelo et al., 1984), which both give rise to the formation of ferrihemoglobin, the latter being the more potent. N-hydroxylation products may also react with tissue macromolecules (Kiese and Taeger, 1976). As these biotransformation reactions are cytochrome P-450 dependent (Gorrod, 1978), changes in the levels of cytochrome P-450 may well be reflected in changes in the rate of formation of the metabolites.

METHODS

Animals
Male Wistar rats (200-250 g) and Syrian golden hamsters (80-100 g) were purchased from CIVO-TNO Zeist, The Netherlands and kept on a commercially available rodent chow. Dog, sheep, monkey (Maccaca fascialis) and human livers were obtained from the Faculty of Veterinary Sciences (Utrecht University), the Institute for Research of Animal Breeding (IVO Zeist, The Netherlands), the National Institute of Public Health and Environmental Hygiene (Bilthoven, The Netherlands) and a local hospital, respectively.

Cell isolation and culture
Hepatocytes were isolated by the two-step collagenase perfusion technique as described by Paine et al. (1979a) with minor modifications. Rat livers were perfused in situ via the portal vein with 400 ml Hank's Balanced Salt Solution (HBSS, Gibco) without Ca^{2+} and Mg^{2+}, followed by a collagenase (Boehringer) solution (0.05 per cent in HBSS) containing 2.5 mM $CaCl_2$. With hamster and monkey livers, this method did not yield enough cells with a sufficiently high viability. We treated these livers with 400 ml of 0.5 mM EGTA in HBSS. Of dog, sheep and human livers, only a 30 g portion of a lobe was used. As with hamster and monkey liver cells the isolation of hepatocytes of sheep was succesful only after the use of HBSS containing EGTA. Usually cell yields were about $5*10^8$ cells with a viability (determined by trypan blue exclusion) greater than 90 per cent. Cell preparations with a viability less than 85 per cent were discarded.

Cells were cultured in 9 cm plastic petri dishes in 10 ml serum free Waymouth MB 572/1 (Gibco) medium at a density of $5*10^6$ cells/dish. Media for cells that would stay in culture for periods longer than 2 hr were supplemented with insulin (10^{-6} M, Sigma), hydrocortisone (10^{-5} M, Sigma) and gentamycin (50 mg/l, Sigma). The cultures were incubated with aniline for 2 hr, after which cells and media were harvested separately.

Chemical analyses
Cytotoxicity was measured as leakage of LDH into the medium according to Bergmeyer et al. (1965). Cytochrome P-450 was determined according to Paine et al. (1979b). Protein was determined as described by Lowry et al. (1951), using bovine serum albumin (Sigma) as a standard. Disturbances due to aniline were prevented by washing proteins with 5 per cent trichloroacetic acid. Production of N-hydroxy-aniline was measured according to Blaauboer and Wit (1978). 4-Aminophenol production was determined as described by Evelo et al. (1984).

RESULTS AND DISCUSSION

In freshly isolated hepatocytes, total cytochrome P-450 levels varied from 72 pmoles/ mg protein in human cells to about 260 pmoles/ mg protein in monkey hepatocytes (table 1). The enzyme(s) appeared to be more stable in hepatocyte cultures from hamsters, sheep and humans than in cultures of rat, dog and monkey hepatocytes. The decline in cytochrome P-450 levels observed in the rat cells was similar to that reported by other authors (Guzelian et al., 1977; Maslansky and Williams, 1983).

Table 1. Cytochrome P-450 contents of hepatocytes derived from several mammalian species (mean ± s.d.; sheep and monkey: individual values).

SPECIES	N	FRESHLY ISOLATED (pmoles/ mg protein)	24 Hr. CULTURE (% retained)
RAT	4	181 ± 22	56 ± 18
HAMSTER	6	183 ± 26	80 ± 15
SHEEP	3	194 ± 52	70 ± 6
DOG	2	120 - 160	30 - 76
MONKEY	2	210 - 312	50 - 60
MAN	6	72 ± 26	89 ± 16

Aniline was not cytotoxic, even at very high concentrations (fig. 1). This means that during the incubations the normal intracellular circumstances remain more or less intact. Aniline was metabolised to the toxicologically active N-hydroxyaniline (fig. 2). Apparently, the levels of N-hydroxyaniline reached are not high enough to cause damage to the cells within 2 hours. It should be noted that in vivo the main target tissue in aniline intoxication is the blood (Kiese, 1974) and that N-hydroxyaniline in vivo is mainly associated with the hemoglobin in the erythrocytes (Kiese and Taeger, 1976). Surprisingly, in the 24 hr cultures of hamster hepatocytes the secretion of N-hydroxyaniline was greater than in cultures of freshly isolated hamster cells. In the 24 hr cultures, the level of cytochrome P-450 was reduced to about 80 per cent of the initial value. A decrease in metabolic activity was observed in rat hepatocytes but not in monkey hepatocytes. In the latter cells, however, the cytochrome P-450 level declined just as in the rat cells. As pointed out in the introduction, the conversion of aniline to its N-hydroxy metabolites is cytochrome P-450 dependent.

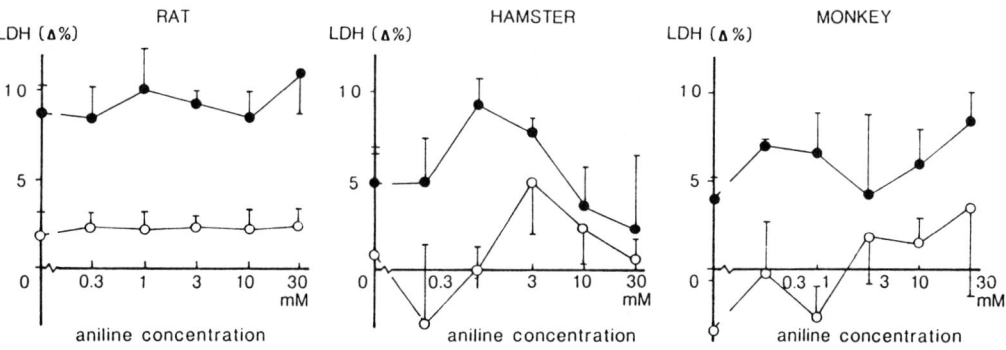

Fig. 1. Toxicity of aniline to primary cultures of rat, hamster and monkey hepatocytes after a 2 hr exposure (● freshly isolated, o 24 hr cultures, mean ± s.d. of triplicate incubations).

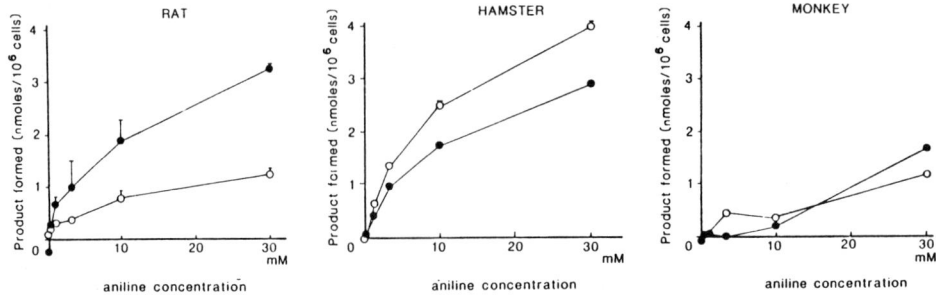

Fig. 2. Production of N-hydroxyaniline by rat, hamster and monkey hepatocytes during a 2 hr exposure to aniline (● freshly isolated, o 24 hr cultures, mean ± s.d. of triplicate incubations).

The observed discrepancies between the behaviour of the cytochrome P-450 concentration and the formation of aniline N-hydroxylation products indicates the presence of one or more cytochrome P-450 isozymes with different stabilities in the species mentioned.

In rat hepatocyte cultures, the formation of 4-hydroxylation products was also studied (fig. 3). 4-Aminophenol was secreted mainly as its glucuronic acid and sulfate conjugates at the lower substrate concentrations. At substrate concentrations greater than 1 mM the secretion of the conjugated metabolite was saturated. These findings are in good agreement with the results of Evelo et al. (1984) obtained with rat hepatocytes in suspension culture.

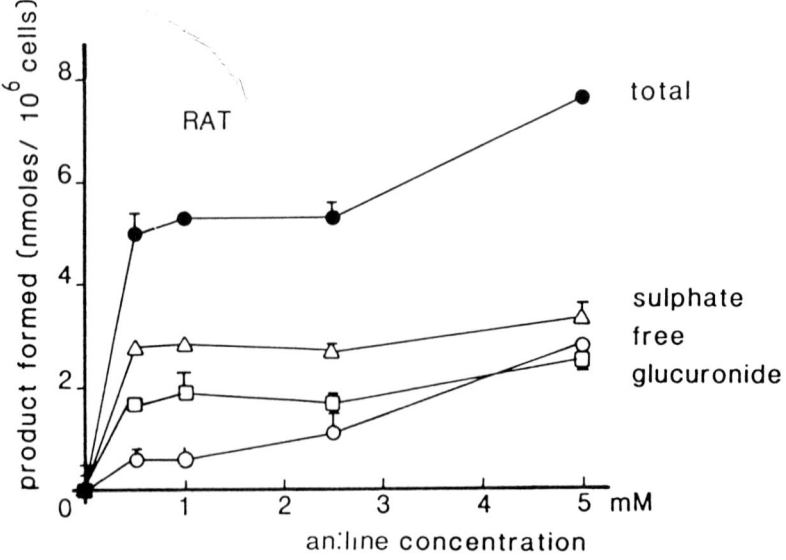

Fig. 3. Production of 4-aminophenol by 24 hr old rat hepatocyte cultures during a 2 hr exposure to aniline (mean ± s.d. of triplicate incubations).

REFERENCES

Bergmeyer, H.U., Bent, E., Hess, B. (1965): Lactic Dehydrogenase. In Methods of Enzymatic Analysis, ed H.U. Bergmeyer, pp 736-743. Weinheim: Verlag Chemie GmbH.

Blaauboer, B.J., van Holsteijn, C.W.M. (1983): Formation and disposition of N-hydroxylated metabolites of aniline and nitrobenzene by isolated rat hepatocytes. Xenobiotica 13, 295-302.

Blaauboer, B.J., Paine, A.J. (1979): Attachment of rat hepatocytes to plastic substrata in the absence of serum requires protein synthesis. Biochem. Biophys. Res. Commun. 90, 368-374.

Blaauboer, B.J. and Wit J.G. (1978): Aniline metabolism in birds in relation to ferrihemoglobin formation in avian erythrocytes. In Biological oxidation of nitrogen, ed J.W. Gorrod pp 369-374. Amsterdam, Elsevier Biomedical Press.

Evelo, C.T.A., Versteegh, J.F.M., Blaauboer, B.J. (1984): Kinetics of the formation and secretion of the aniline metabolite 4-aminophenol and its conjugates by isolated rat hepatocytes. Xenobiotica 14, 409-416.

Gorrod J.W. (1978): The current status of the pKa concept in the differentiation of enzymic N-oxidation. In Biological oxidation of nitrogen ed J.W. Gorrod pp 201-212. Amsterdam, Elsevier Biomedical Press.

Guzelian, P.S., Bissell, D.M., Meyer, U.A. (1977) Drug metabolism in adult rat hepatocytes in primary culture. Gastroenterology 72, 1232-1239.

Kiese, M. (1974): Methemoglobinemia: a comprehensive treatise, pp 98-101. Cleveland: CRC press.

Kiese, M., Taeger, K. (1976): The fate of phenylhydroxylamine in human red cells. Naunyn-Schmied. Arch. Pharmacol. 292, 59-66.

Lowry, O.H., Rosebrough, N.J., Farr, A.L., and Randall, R.J., (1951): Protein measurement with the folin phenol reagent. J. Biol. Chem. 193, 265-275.

Maslansky, C.J., Williams, G.M. (1983): Isolation and culture of primary hepatocytes derived from rat, mouse, hamster, guinea pig and rabbit. In Isolation, characterization and use of hepatocytes, eds R.A. Harris, N.W. Cornell. pp 87-92. Amsterdam: Elsevier Biomedical Press.

Paine, A.J., Williams, L.J., Legg, R.F. (1979a): In The Liver: Quantitative Aspects of Structure and Function, eds R. Preisig, J.Bircher. pp 215-263. Aulendorf: Editio Cantor.

Paine, A.J., Williams, L.J., Legg, R.F. (1979b): Apparent maintenance of cytochrome P-450 by nicotinamide in primary cultures of rat hepatocytes. Life Sci. 24, 2185-2192.

Sirica, A.E., Pitot, H.C. (1980): Drug metabolism and effects of carcinogens in cultured hepatic cells. Pharmacol. Rev. 31, 205-228.

Primary cultures of rat and human hepatocytes as a model system for the evaluation of cytotoxicity and metabolic pathways of a new drug S-3341

Luc Grislain*, Damrong Ratanasavanh**, Marie-Thérèse Mocquard*, Laurence Raquillet*, Jean-Marc Bégué**, Pierre du Vignaud*, Patrick Génissel***, André Guillouzo**, Norbert Bromet*

* Technologie Servier, Division de Pharmacocinétique et Métabolisme, 45007 Orléans, France.
** INSERM U. 49, Unité de Recherches Hépatologiques, Hôpital Pontchaillou, 35033 Rennes Cedex, France. *** Institut de Recherches Internationales Servier, 92205 Neuilly-sur-Seine, France

Key words : S-3341, Metabolism, Chronic cytotoxicity, Rat, Human, Hepatocyte culture.

INTRODUCTION

When put in culture adult hepatocytes exhibit rapid phenotypic changes leading to the loss of the most differentiated functions, including metabolizing enzyme activities (Guguen-Guillouzo and Guillouzo, 1983). However, they remain able to express phase I and phase II drug reactions for 24-48 hours in conventional culture (Le Bigot et al., 1987) and this capability is markedly improved when parenchymal cells are co-cultured with a rat liver epithelial cell line (Guillouzo, 1986). In this study, hepatocyte cultures were used to predict metabolic pathways and cytotoxicity of a new hypertensive agent S-3341 (Laubie et al., 1985) prior to its in vivo administration.

MATERIAL AND METHODS

Isolation and culture of hepatocytes.

Rat hepatocytes : The cells were isolated from the liver of 200-300 g Sprague-Dawley rats by perfusion with 0.025 % collagenase as previously described (Guguen-Guillouzo et al., 1983). They were seeded at a density of 5×10^5 cells per 10 cm^2 petri dish in 2 ml of Ham F12 medium containing 0.2 % bovine serum albumin, 10 µg/ml bovine insulin and 10 % fetal calf serum. A part of the cultures was set up as pure cultures, the other was set up as co-cultures by adding an equivalent number of rat liver epithelial cells (Guguen-Guillouzo et al., 1983). The medium was supplemented with 3×10^{-6} M hydrocortisone hemisuccinate after 4 h and 24 h in pure culture and co-culture respectively, and renewed daily thereafter.

Human hepatocytes : The livers were obtained from kidney transplantation donors and the cells were isolated by collagenase perfusion as previously described (Guguen-Guillouzo et al., 1982). The cells were seeded at the density of 5×10^5

cells per 10 cm² petri dish in 2 ml of medium. The following steps were those described for rat hepatocytes except that rat liver epithelial cells were added only 16-18 h after cell seeding.

Metabolism studies. Only pure rat and human hepatocyte cultures were used. T^4C-S 3341-3 (10 µCi/flask) was incubated with hepatocyte cultures for 24 h. Then, media and cells were collected and stored at -80°C separately until analysis. Extractions and analyses were carried out as previously described (Guillouzo et al., 1988). Briefly, liquid/liquid extraction was performed. The residues were examined by thin layer chromatography and structural analysis was carried out by mass spectometry linked to gas chromatography.

Cell treatment
A first series of experiments was performed with pure cultures to determine the maximum non toxic concentration of each drug after a 24 h incubation. The drugs were added at various concentrations to 4 h cultures (rat hepatocytes) or 16 h cultures (human hepatocytes).
A second series of experiments was performed with co-cultures for long-term ("chronic") drug toxicity assessment. Various concentrations were selected, the highest scoring + in the acute cytotoxicity test (see Ratanasavanh et al., this volume). They were added 24 h after epithelial cell seeding for the first time and then every day with medium renewal for 10 to 18 days.

Morphological examination

Light microscopy : living cultures were examined daily under phase-contrast microscopy. The degree of cytotoxicity was evaluated by giving a score graded from 0 (controls) to +++ (Ratanasavanh et al., this volume).

Electron microscopy : at the end of experiments, hepatocyte cultures were fixed by 2.5 % glutaraldehyde in sodium cacodylate buffer 0.1 M, pH 7.4 for 5 min at 4°C, then post-fixed by 1 % OsO_4 in sodium cacodylate buffer for 30 min, dehydrated and embedded in Epon.

Biochemical assays. Albumin secretion rate was measured daily in the culture medium by laser immunonephelometry (Guguen-Guillouzo et al., 1983) as an index of specific hepatocyte function.
Lactate dehydrogenase (LDH) leakage was determined daily as an index of cell toxicity using the M.A.-Kit Roche, LDH opt. DGKC (ref. 1431-3) and a Cobas Bio apparatus.

RESULTS

Metabolism : Figure 1 shows the possible metabolic pathways of S-3341 observed in vivo. S-3341 can be transformed by oxidation to give the metabolites S 11316 and S 11461, or by hydrolysis to give S 11460 and S 11459.
When S-3341 was incubated with rat hepatocytes for 24 h, only 31 % of the parent drug were found in culture media indicating a good biotransformation of the molecule. Four metabolites resulting from either oxidation (S 11316 and S 11461) or hydrolysis (S 11460 and S 11459) of S 3341 have been characterized (Fig. 2A).

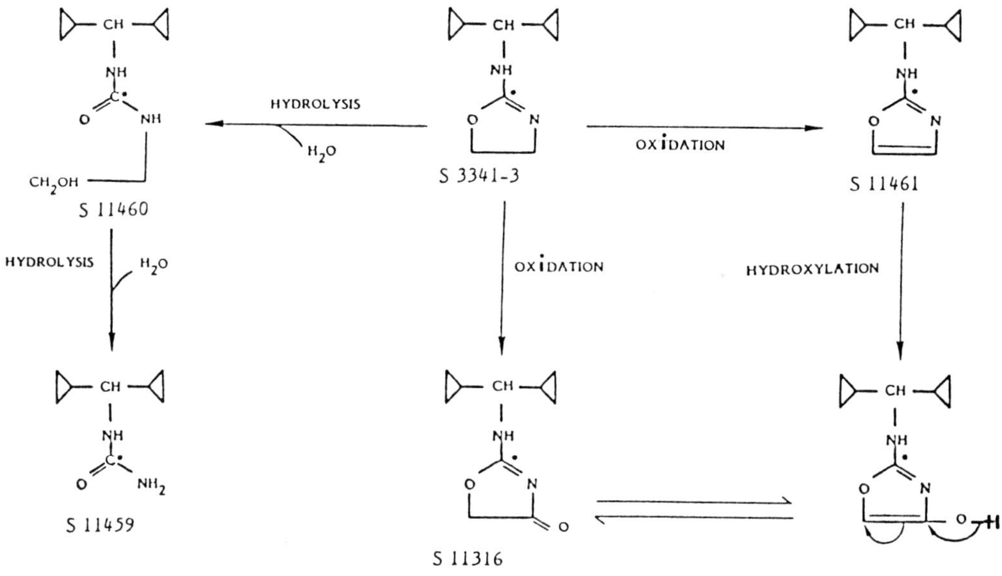

Figure 1 : Possible metabolic pathways of S 3341 in rat and humans.

Most of the metabolites found with the hepatocyte culture model have been identified in the rat (Fig. 2B). However, the percentage of unchanged S-3341 was much higher in vivo than in vitro.
After a 24 h incubation with human hepatocytes, 96 % of the total radioactivity S-3341 corresponded to unchanged S-3341. Traces of S 11459, S 11460 and S 11316 were detected (Fig. 2C). When S 3341 was administered to humans, also about 80 % of parent drug were found to be eliminated unchanged (Fig. 2D). The three metabolites found in vitro were demonstrated.

Cytotoxicity evaluation.
The results of short-term and long-term treatment by S 3341 in rat hepatocyte cultures have been already reported elsewhere (Guillouzo et al., 1987). In short-term treatment, S 3341 was found to be non cytotoxic to rat hepatocytes in pure culture at concentrations below 200 µg/ml. For long-term treatment, at 50 µg/ml, the drug induced morphological changes from the 8th day in rat heptocyte co-cultures (Guillouzo et al., 1987). In human hepatocyte co-cultures, at 25 µg/ml S 3341 did not affect cell morphology, LDH leakage and albumin production. At 50 µg/ml, no marked morphological alterations were observed until 12 days of treatment (Table 1) ; morphological changes appeared at the 18th day. However, LDH activity in the medium and albumin production remained unchanged. Only at the highest dose used in this experiment (200 µg/ml) S 3341 increased LDH leakage (Fig. 3), decreased albumin production (Fig. 4) and a cell detachment

was observed at the end of treatment (18th day). Electron microscopic analysis confirmed the results obtained by light microscopy. Indeed, 25 µg/ml S 3341 did not induce any change in hepatocyte fine structure while in the presence of 50 µg/ml secondary lysosomes containing membrane circular figures or amorphous material were observed (Fig. 5). At 100 and 200 µg/ml, S-3341-treated cells exhibited cytoplasmic lipid droplets, in addition to secondary lysosomes (not shown). The same observations were made on rat liver epithelial cells treated with S 3341 (not shown).

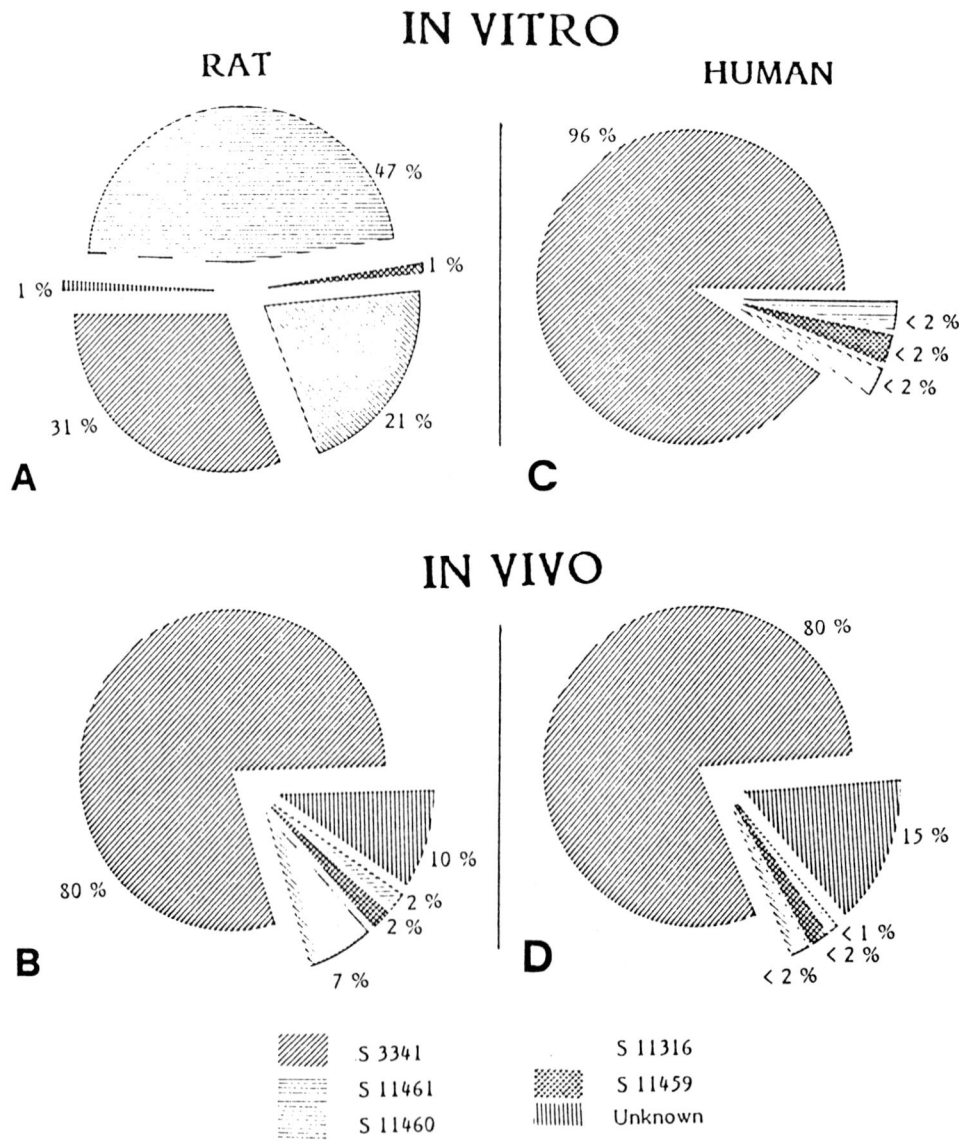

Figure 2 : Metabolites formed from S 3341 in rat (A) and human (C) hepatocyte cultures. The results obtained in rat (B) and human (D) are given for comparison.

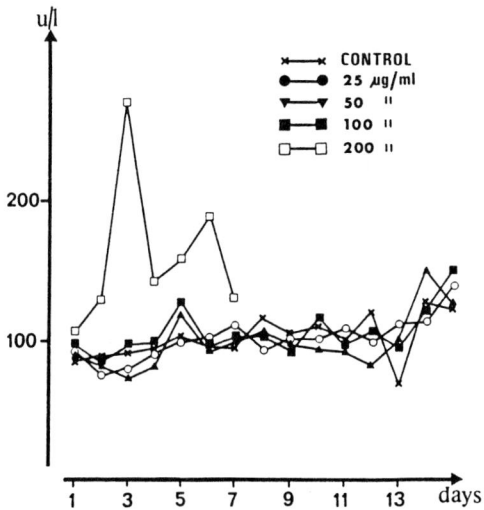

Figure 3 : Effect of long-term treatment of human hepatocyte co-cultures by S 3341-3 on LDH leakage.

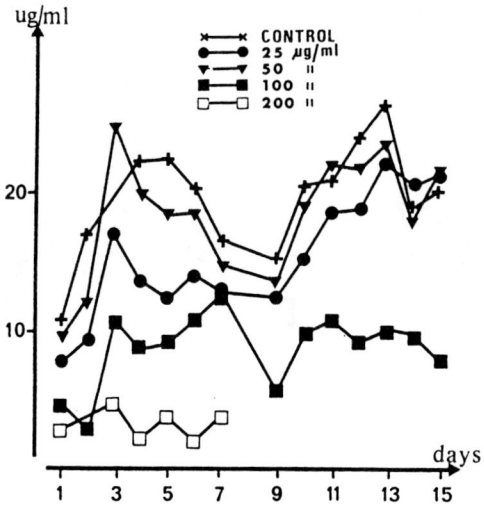

Figure 4 : Effect of long-term treatment of human hepatocyte co-cultures by S 3341-3 on albumin production.

TABLE I : Long-term cytotoxicity of S-3341 to co-cultured human hepatocytes. Light microscopic observation.

Days of treatment	Drug concentration (µg/ml)				
	0	25	50	100	200
4	0	0	0	+	++
6	0	0	+	++	++
12	0	0	+	++	+++
18	0	0	++	+++	X

Evaluation of toxicity was based on two independent experiments in triplicate. The degree of toxicity was graded from 0 (controls) to +++ (see the methods section).

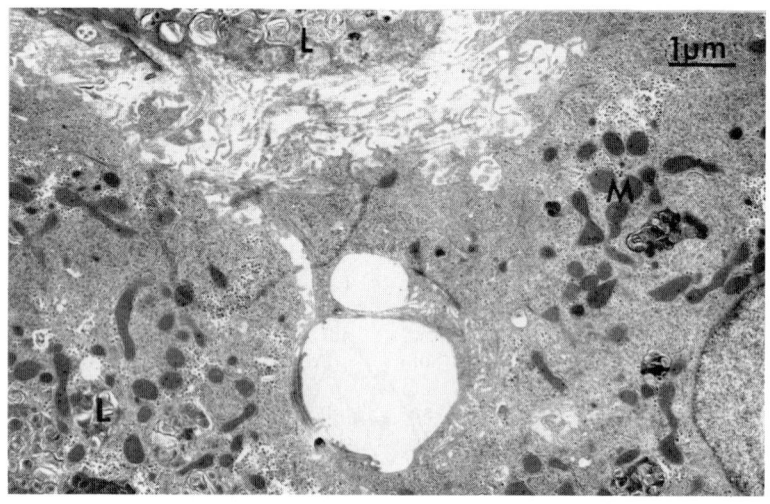

Figure 5 : Electron microscopic appearance of human hepatocyte co-cultured for 15 days in the presence of 50 µg/ml S-3341. (L : lysosomes ; M : mitochondria).

DISCUSSION

In human, S 3341 was poorly metabolized by cultured hepatocytes ; 90 % of the parent drug remained unchanged after a 24 h incubation. In vivo the same trend was confirmed, most of the molecule was excreted unchanged. In rat hepatocytes,

S 3341 was extensively metabolized, only 31 % of the parent drug remained unchanged (Guillouzo et al., 1987). A good in vivo/in vitro correlation was observed in the routes of S 3341 metabolism as shown in figure 2 suggesting that hepatocyte cultures represent a good model system to identify drug metabolites formed in vivo.

Cytotoxicity studies indicate that this new hypertensive agent is not hepatotoxic. Indeed, the maximum non-toxic concentration was approximately 3000 times the highest plasma concentration observed in clinical studies (unpublished results).

Since hepatocytes were not more sensitive than rat liver epithelial cells which do not express drug metabolizing enzymes it may be assumed that no toxic reactive metabolites were formed by liver parenchymal cells.

ACKNOWLEDGMENTS

We thank Mrs A. Vannier for typing the manuscript.

REFERENCES

Guguen-Guillouzo, C., Campion, J.P., Brissot, P., Glaise, D., Launois, B., Bourel, M. and Guillouzo, A. (1982): High yield preparation of isolated human adult hepatocytes by enzymatic perfusion of the liver. Cell Biol. Int. Rep. 6, 625-628.

Guguen-Guillouzo, C., Clément, B., Baffet, G., Beaumont, C., Morel-Chany, E., Glaise, D. and Guillouzo, A. (1983): Maintenance and reversibility of active albumin secretion by adult rat hepatocytes co-cultured with another liver epithelial cell type. Exp. Cell Res. 143, 47-54.

Guguen-Guillouzo, C. and Guillouzo, A. (1983): Modulation of functional activities in cultured rat hepatocytes. Mol. Cell. Biochem. 53/54, 35-56.

Guillouzo, A. (1986): Use of isolated and cultured hepatocytes for xenobiotic metabolism and cytotoxicity studies. In Isolated and cultured hepatocytes, eds. A. Guillouzo and C. Guguen-Guillouzo, pp 313-331, Paris: Les Editions INSERM, London : John Libbey Eurotext.

Guillouzo, A., Grislain, L., Ratanasavanh, D., Mocquard, M.T., Bégué, J.M., Du Vignaud, P., Bromet, N., Génissel, P. and Beau, B. (1988): Use of hepatocyte cultures for preliminary metabolism and cytotoxicity studies of a new anti-hypertensive agent : oxaminozoline, Xenobiotica, in press.

Laubie, M., Poignant, J.C., Scuvee-Moreau, J., Dabire, M., Dresse, A. and Schmitt, H. (1985): Pharmacological properties of (N-dicyclopropylmethyl)-amino-2-oxazoline S 3341, an α_2 adrenoreceptor agonist. J. Pharmacol. 16, 259-278.

Ratanasavanh, D, Bégué, J.M., Gelé, P., Grislain, L., Bromet, N., du Vignaud, P., Defrance, R., Mocaer, E. and Guillouzo, A. (1988): Cytotoxicity and metabolism study of amineptine (S-1694-1) in cultured adult rat and human hepatocytes (this volume).

Liver Cells and Drugs. Ed. A. Guillouzo. Colloque INSERM/John Libbey Eurotext Ltd. © 1988. Vol. 164, pp. 365-370.

Metabolism of doxorubicin, epirubicin and daunorubicin by human and rat hepatocytes in primary culture

Marie-Annick Le Bot*, Jean-Marc Bégué**, Dominique Kernaleguen*, Jacques Robert***, Damrong Ratanasavanh**, Yves Guédes*, Christian Riché*, André Guillouzo**

** Laboratoire de Pharmacologie, Faculté de Médecine, Brest, France. ** INSERM U.49, Unité de Recherches Hépatologiques, Hôpital de Pontchaillou, Rennes, France. *** Fondation Bergonié, Bordeaux, France.*

Keywords : Anthracyclines, human, rat, hepatocytes, primary culture.

INTRODUCTION.

Anthracycline antibiotics are widely used in the treatment of a large range of tumors (Young et al., 1981). However, severe side effects, particularly acute cardiotoxicity (Rinehart et al., 1974) limit their therapeutical usefulness. Whether these toxic effects could be related to the parent drug and/or its metabolites has not yet been established since metabolism of anthracyclines remains poorly understood. To gain more information on the metabolites formed from anthracyclines by the liver, human and rat hepatocyte cultures were compared in their abilities to metabolize doxorubicin, epirubicin and daunorubicin.

MATERIAL AND METHODS.

Chemicals

The structures of the three anthracyclines studied, namely doxorubicin, epirubicin and daunorubicin are given in Figure 1. Doxorubicin, daunorubicin and their respective standard 13-di-hydro metabolite doxorubicinol and daunorubicinol were kindly supplied by Roger Bellon laboratories (Neuilly, France). Epirubicin, a doxorubicin derivative obtained by replacing the natural aminosugar daunosamine by the corresponding 4'-epi-analog, epirubicinol and their respective glucuronides were a gift from Farmitalia-Carlo Erba (Milan, Italy).

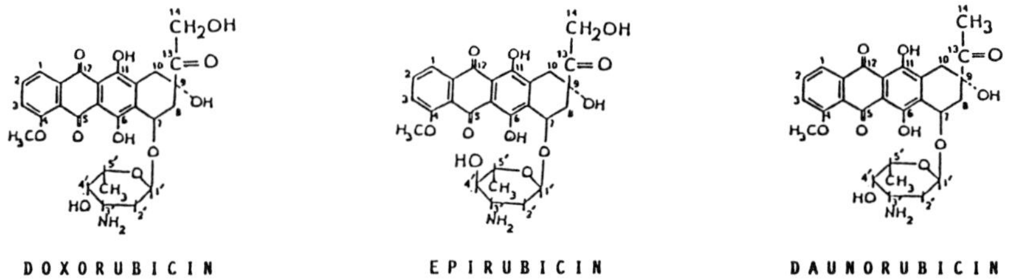

DOXORUBICIN EPIRUBICIN DAUNORUBICIN

Figure 1 : **Chemical structure of the three anthracyclines studied.**

Cell isolation and culture.
Human hepatocytes : Human hepatocytes were obtained from three male kidney donors aged between 17 and 31 years. Histological examination revealed normal liver. The dissociation procedure of the liver has been described elsewhere (Guguen-Guillouzo et al., 1982). Briefly, a selected area of the organ was first rapidly washed by perfusion through the left portal vein with HEPES (N-2-hydroxyethyl-piperazine-N'-2 ethane sulfonic acid) buffer, pH 7.4, then dissociated by perfusing an HEPES-buffered solution containing 0.05 % collagenase.
Isolated hepatocytes were seeded at a density of 8×10^6 cells per 75 cm^2 culture flask in 10 ml of medium. This medium was a mixture of 75 % minimum essential medium and 25 % medium 199 (Gibco, USA) supplemented with 200 μg/ml serum bovine albumin, 10 μg/ml bovine insulin and 10 % fetal calf serum. The cultures were maintained under a 5 % CO_2-95 % air humidified atmosphere. The medium added with 10^{-6} M hydrocortisone hemisuccinate was renewed after around 8 h and just before the beginning of the incubation period with anthracyclines which occurred between the 24th and the 48th hour.

Rat hepatocytes.
Rat hepatocytes were obtained from 4 male Sprague-Dawley animals weighing 180-200 g by perfusion of the whole liver, first with Hepes buffer then with a 0.025 % HEPES-buffered collagenase solution. Culture conditions were those described for human cells. Rat hepatocyte cultures were used 24 h after cell seeding.

Incubation with anthracyclines.
The three anthracyclines were directly dissolved in the culture medium just before the beginning of the 24 h incubation period at concentrations of 0.2, 0.15 and 0.5 μM for doxorubicin, epirubicin and daunorubicin respectively. At these concentrations the drugs were found to be non-toxic as judged by light microscopic examination and measurement of lactate dehydrogenase leakage. To prevent photolytic degradation of the molecules, all manipulations were performed under subdued light and cultures were incubated in total darkness. In order to evaluate chemical degradation and/or fixation of the drug on plastic, each molecule was incubated in the same conditions in the absence of hepatocytes.

Identification and quantification of metabolites.
Parent drugs and their metabolites were determined in culture medium. After 24 h of incubation with anthracyclines, the medium was harvested and immediately frozen (-20°C) until extraction of remaining parent drugs and metabolites.

Extraction procedures.
The extraction procedure from culture media was as described by Robert (1980). Media were run through C-18 bonded silica (Sep-Pak, Waters). After washing with phosphate buffer, anthracyclines and their metabolites were eluted by methanol. The resulting eluates were evaporated to dryness under a stream of nitrogen.

High pressure liquid chromatograhic (HPLC) analysis.
HPLC analysis was performed with a Spectra Physics ternary pump system on 5 μm C-18 bonded silica columns of 125 x 4 mm (Merck, Germany). Fluorescence detection was performed using a JASCO FP 210 spectrofluorimeter with an excitation wavelength of 467 nm and an emission wavelength of 550 nm. The solvent was a mixture of ammonium formate buffer (0.05 M, pH 4) and acetonitrile as described by Israel et al. (1978). The gradient mode was used for better characterization of metabolites. The ratio buffer/acetonitrile was maintained at 80/20 (v/v) for 5 min and then linearly raised to 40/60 in 10 min, and

maintained for 5 min, with a flow rate of 1.1 ml/min. Each sample was reconstituted with phosphate buffer (pH 7) and 50 µl were injected into the column.
Retention times were compared with those of standards of parent drugs and metabolites. Determination of fluorescent compound(s) from the medium which could interfere with anthracyclines in the analytic procedure was performed by incubating cells in the absence of drugs.
Each metabolite was expressed as the percentage of total fluorescence (100 %) which corresponded to unchanged drug and metabolites in the culture medium.

RESULTS

Whatever the drug tested, no interference with fluorescent compound from the incubated medium was observed in HPLC analyses.

Doxorubicin. After a 24 h incubation period in the culture medium about 50 % of doxorubicin was degraded. Both rat and human hepatocytes metabolized doxorubicin to its 13-dihydro-derivative doxorubicinol (Fig.2). However, marked quantitative differences were noticed since doxorubicinol, which accounted for 38 % in cultured human hepatocytes did not exceed 9 % in rat cells (Table I).

Epirubicin. When incubated in the culture medium epirubicin underwent a rapid degradation process since only 50 % of the parent drug was recovered after 24 h. During this incubation period about 92 % of the drug was metabolized by human hepatocyte cultures giving the 13-dihydro metabolite : epirubicinol (13 %) and glucuronides of both parent drug (51 %) and epirubicinol (27.6 %) (Fig. 2). Rat hepatocyte cultures which were unable to perform glucuronidation metabolized only 15 % of epirubicin in its 13-dihydro-derivative (Table I).

Daunorubicin. In contrast to doxorubicin, daunorubicin was not degraded during a 24 h incubation in the culture medium in the absence of hepatocytes. Rat and human hepatocyte cultures metabolized this molecule to a similar extent (86 %) (Table I). One and three unknown metabolites could be observed in the incubates from human and rat hepatocytes respectively (Fig. 2). They accounted for only 5 % of the total metabolites.

DISCUSSION

The results reported here clearly indicate marked variations in both the rates and the routes of metabolism between the three anthracyclines tested, namely doxorubicin, epirubicin and daunorubicin, as well as species differences.
A conspicuous degradation of two anthracyclines out of three was observed after a 24 h incubation in the absence of cells. About 50 % of the initial amount of added doxorubicin or epirubicin could no longer be detected as parent drug or metabolites. Such a chemical degradation has already been reported to occur in culture media but not in infusion fluids. This disappearance from the culture medium (Poochikian et al., 1981) could also be due, at least partly, to the fixation of these anthracyclines on plastic. The values of chemical degradatic were certainly lower when the drugs were incubated in the presence of hepatocytes since a fraction of them was metabolized.
Doxorubicin and epirubicin were more extensively transformed by human hepatocytes than by their rat counterparts while no species difference was evidenced for daunorubicin. For doxorubicin and daunorubicin the major metabolite formed in both cells resulted from the reduction of the parent drug giving a 13-dihydro-derivative by a non cell-specific NAPH-dependent aldoketo reductase system.

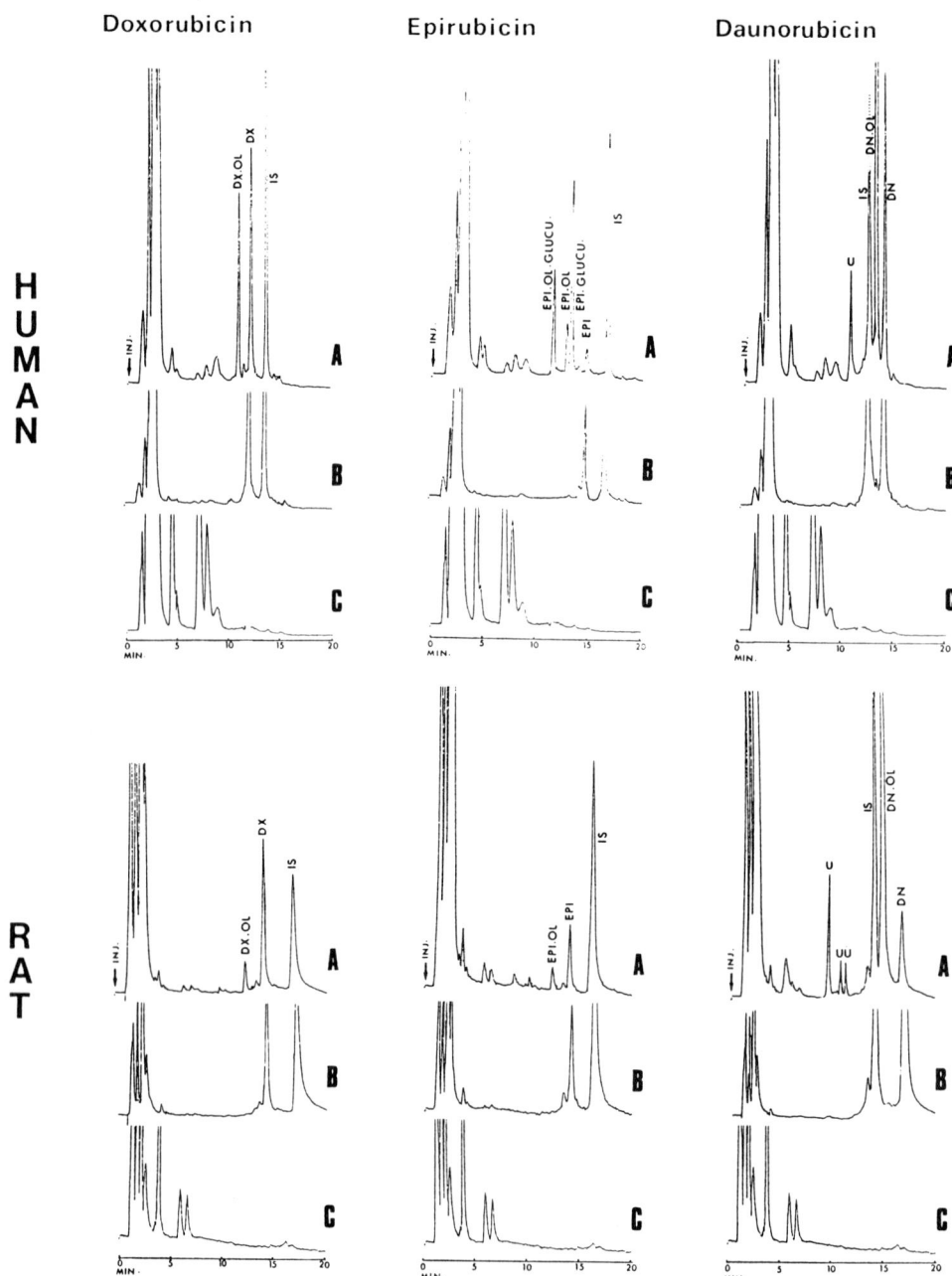

Figure 2 : HPLC chromatograms of medium extracts from human and rat hepatocyte cultures incubated with 0.2 µM doxorubicin, 0.15 µM epirubicin and 0.5 µM daunorubicin. A : cultures incubated with anthracycline ; B : medium with anthracycline in the absence of cells ; C : medium without anthracycline in the presence of cells.
IS : Internal Standard, U : Unidentified peak.

DOXORUBICIN

Cell origin	Parent drug	Doxorubicinol
Human	62 ± 2	38 ± 2
Rat	92 ± 9	9.1 ± 0.9

EPIRUBICIN

Cell origin	Parent drug	Epirubicinol	Glucuronide of epirubicin	Glucuronide of epirubicinol
Human	8 ± 3	13.6 ± 0.4	51 ± 2	27.6 ± 0.4
Rat	85 ± 5	15 ± 5	ND	ND

DAUNORUBICIN

Cell origin	Parent drug	Daunorubicinol	Unknown metabolites 1	Unknown metabolites 2	Unknown metabolites 3
Human	14 ± 1	81 ± 1	5.03 ± 0.06	ND	ND
Rat	15 ± 3	80 ± 2	1.0 ± 0.3	0.8 ± 0.4	2.9 ± 1

TABLE I : Comparative metabolism of anthracyclines in human and rat hepatocyte cultures.
Results expressed as percentages of total fluorescence (100 %) are mean ± SEM of 3 and 4 experiments in duplicate for human and rat hepatocytes respectively. (ND : not detected).

Species differences in metabolic pathways were found with epirubicin and daunorubicin. Indeed, while rat hepatocytes were capable of forming only a 13-dihydro-derivative from epirubicin, human cells were able to conjugate both the parent drug and the reduced derivative (epirubicinol) with glucuronic acid. These metabolic pathways are in agreement with in vivo data (Robert et al., 1985). By contrast additional unknown metabolites of daunorubicin were observed only with rat hepatocytes. These results present further evidence of the risk of extrapolation of results obtained on animal cells to the human situation.

In summary, the findings on the metabolism of anthracyclines by cultured human and rat hepatocytes reflect those obtained in vivo and suggest that primary cultures of hepatocytes from various species represent a suitable model system for identifying drug metabolism pathways in vivo in the corresponding species.

ACKNOWLEDGMENTS

The authors thank Mrs A. Vannier for typing the manuscript.

REFERENCES

Guguen-Guillouzo, Campion, J.P., Brissot, P., Glaise, D., Launois, B., Bourel, M. and Guillouzo, A. (1982): A high yield preparation of isolated human adult hepatocytes by enzymatic perfusion of the liver. Cell Biol. Int. Rep. 6, 625-628.

Israel, M., Pegg, N.J., Wilkinson, P.M. and Garnick, M.B. (1978): Liquid chromatographic analysis of adriamycin and metabolites in biological fluids. J. Liquid Chromatogr. 1, 759-809.

Poochikian, G.K., Cradock, J.C. and Flora, K.P. (1981): Stability of anthracycline antitumor agents in four infusion fluids. Am. J. Hosp. Pharm. 38, 483-486.

Rinehart, J.J., Lewis, R.P. and Baleerzak, S.P. (1974): Adriamycin cardiotoxicity in man. Ann. Intern. Med. 81, 475-478.

Robert, J. (1980): Extraction of anthracyclines from biological fluids for HPLC evaluation. J. Liquid Chrom. 3, 1561-1572.

Robert, J., Vrignaud, P., Nguguen-Ngoc, T., Iliadis, A., Mauriac, L. and Hurteloup, F. (1985): Comparative pharmacokinetics and metabolism of doxorubicin and epirubicin in patients with metastatic breast cancer. Cancer Treat. Rep. 69, 633-640.

Young, R.C., Ozols, R.F. and Myers, C.E. (1981): The anthracycline antineoplastics drugs. N. Engl. J. Med. 305, 139-153.

Predictive value of the *in vitro* test for hepatotoxicity of xenobiotics

M. José Gómez-Lechón, Amparo Larrauri, Teresa Donato, Pilar López, Angel Montoya, José V. Castell

Centro de Investigación del Hospital La Fe, Insalud, Avda. de Campanar 21, E-46009 Valencia, Spain

Key words: Hepatotoxicity, cultured hepatocytes, xenobiotics.

INTRODUCTION

Hepatocytes in monolayer culture retain most of the specific capabilities of liver (Castell et al. 1983; Guillouzo, 1986), reproduce to a large extent the biochemistry of the intact liver cells, and is an atractive model for studying the hepatic effects of xenobiotics. Several attempts have been made to establish experimental protocols for in vitro screening of hepatotoxicity of compounds (Acosta et al. 1985). In previous research only cytotoxic parameters (cell viability, cell survival, enzyme leakage etc.) were assessed. This certainly represents one possible approach to a general screening protocol but may leave out of consideration substances that impair cell function without causing cell death. Such an effect, although not critical for the hepatocyte itself, is of toxicological significance, since the general homeostasis of the organism can be indirectly altered as a consequece of the hepatocyte malfunction. The detection of this metabolic cell injury produced by xenobiotics and its reversibility is desirable but at the same time extremely difficult to assess "in vivo". An "in vitro" model aimed at evaluating the hepatotoxicity of xenobiotics has to take into consideration this possibility.

In our laboratory, a screening test consisting of an integrated series of experiments has been developed and used in several studies (Castell et al. 1985; 1986 a,b) to evaluate the action of a xenobiotic on the biology and biochemistry of hepatocytes. This screening uses cultured cells, instead of isolated cells, what allows the design of experiments with longer exposures to the xenobiotics. In developing the "in vitro" assay for hepatotoxicity, several facts were taken into consideration: first, the use of a biological system that should reproduce to a great extent the biochemistry of the liver; second, the choice of the most appropiate cytological/biochemical parameters for detecting and quantifying the hepatotoxic (cytotoxic or metabolic) effects of the xenobiotic in culture; and finally, the predictive value of the data obtained "in vitro" in relation to the expected and/or observed toxicity "in vivo".

MATERIAL AND METHODS

The "in vitro" hepatotoxicity screening protocol.

As summarized in Fig. 1, the strategy of the screening protocol involves exposing the hepatocytes in cultures to the xenobiotic at different concentrations for variable periods of time. The hepatocytes were obtained from 200-250 g S&D male rats fed ad libitum. The liver was perfused with collagenase as described in detail elsewhere (Gómez-Lechón et al.1984), and cultured on fibronectin-coated dishes in serum-free conditions (Gómez-Lechón and Castell, 1983; Castell et al. 1985). Xenobiotics are added to plates at different concentrations and then two types of effects are evaluated: 1) cytotoxic effects during the initial stages of culture prior to the formation of the confluent monolayer; this helps to determine the highest concentration of a xenobiotic compatible with hepatocyte survival, and 2) effects on the metabolism and specific liver cell functions of the xenobiotic treated cells at sub-lethal concentrations.

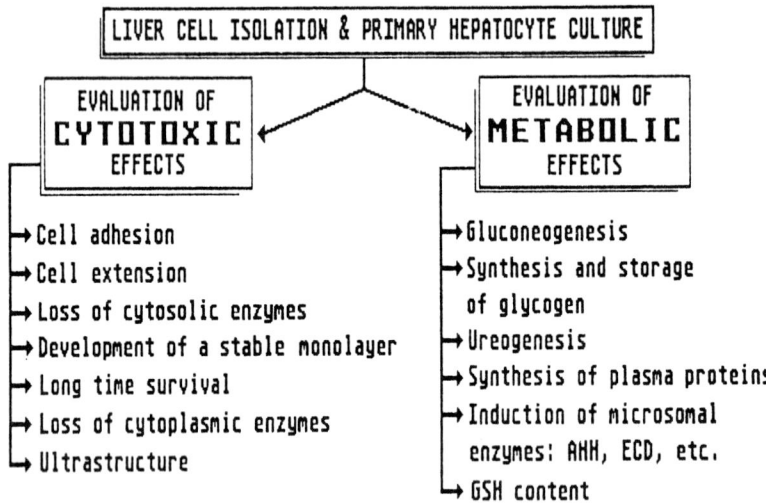

Cytotoxicity markers.

Cell viability was estimated by the dye exclusion test with 0.027% Trypan Blue. Cell attachment kinetics and the attachment index was measured in cultures exposed to xenobiotics at the time of seeding (Gómez-Lechón and Castell, 1983). Hepatocyte spreading on plates was evaluated in presence of the xenobiotics during the first 6 hours after cell plating, on micrographs obtained at set-time periods in an inverted phase contrast microscope. Leakage of the intracellular enzymes GOT and LDH, was measured in the medium of 6 or 24 hours cultures after treatment with the xenobiotic (Castell and Gómez-Lechón, 1987). The monolayers were periodically examined in phase contrast microscope. The ultrastructure was studied after 24, 48 and 72 hours of continous exposure to the xenobiotics following conventional fixation and embedding protocols (Castell et al. 1986).

Metabolic determinations.

The metabolic parameters were evaluated in 24 hour cultures after a variable pre-treatment with the xenobiotics. Normally, the xenobiotics were also present during the assay. The gluconeogenesis and the glycogen content of cells is measured after 6 h pretreatment as described (Castell et al. 1985). The rate of urea production after an ammonia load after 6 h pretreatment (Castell et al. 1985). The albumin synthesis rate is measured along 4 hours in the presence of the xenobiotic (Castell et al. 1985). RNA synthesis was studied by measuring the kinetics of uptake by cells and the incorporation into acid-insoluble material of ^{14}C orotic acid (10 µM, specific activity in the assay 30 µCi/ mol) as described (Castell et al. 1985).

RESULTS AND DISCUSSION

Comparison of cytotoxicity parameters to evaluate the effects of hepatotoxins on cultured hepatocytes.

Experiments on cytotoxicity are carried out during the first stages of the cell culture. Shortly after cell plating, hepatocytes enter into contact with the fibronectin coated plastic dishes and after an initial lag of about 10 min attach to the plates, showing sigmoid kinetics and reaching the maximum (65,000 cells/cm^2) after 1 hour incubation at 37ºC (Gómez-Lechón and Castell, 1983). This fibronectin-mediated attachment of hepatocytes is an active process that is highly selective for viable cells (Gómez-Lechón and Castell, 1983). It can be disturbed by direct alterations of the cell membrane (i.e. alteration of the functionality of the receptors for fibronectin), or indirectly, when a compound causes hepatocyte cell death. The Attachment Index although correlates well with the viability, is more sensitive. As shown in Fig 2A, considerable changes in cell attachment are observed for xenobiotics that apparently do not cause cell death.

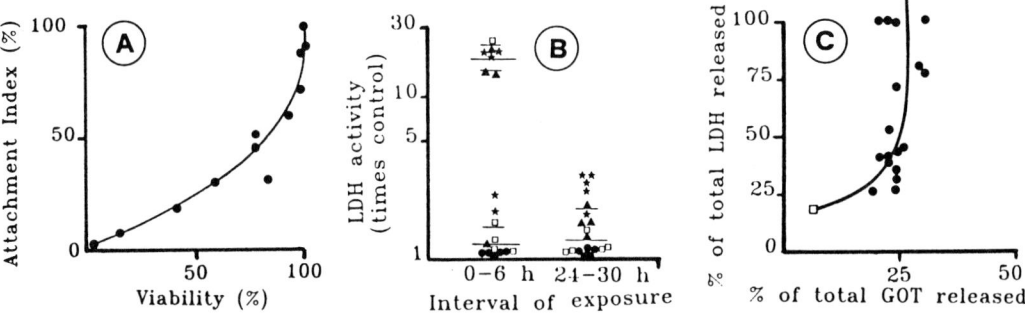

Fig. 2. A) Correlation between attachment index and viability of hepatocytes treated with several xenobiotics. B) Release of LDH to culture medium in cultures treated with (□) paraquat, (●) benorylate, (▲) butibufen, (✦) ibuprofen and (★) flurbiprofen. Compounds were added at the time of plating or at 24 hours of culture. Enzyme activity was assayed after 6 h exposure. C) Correlation between LDH and GOT leakage after 24 h treatment with different xenobiotics.

An important requirement for developing a stable hepatocyte monolayer in culture is the spreading of cells on the plates. Hepatocytes, once attached, are very restrictive in their environmental requirements for spreading because during approximately the first two hours, RNA and protein synthesis later followed by cytoskeleton rearrangement are involved in this process (Castell and Gómez-Lechón, 1987). Consequently, cell extension can be strongly influenced by the presence of xenobiotics as we have already shown (Castell and Gómez-Lechón, 1987). In fibronectin coated plates control hepatocytes begin to flatten out (by 2 hours in culture), until contact is made with neighbouring cells, resulting in confluent monolayers by 6-8 h. The effects of xenobiotics acting as RNA, protein synthesis or cytoskeleton rearrangement inhibitors will impair cell spreading if present during the first two hours of culture. When added later, cells are not so sensitive and spreading may apparently be accomplished by 8 h (Castell and Gómez-Lechón, 1987). The sensitivity of this parameter is similar to that of cell viability.

Cytotoxicity can be evaluated by the trypan blue dye exclusion test. This technique gives only a rough approximation of membrane damage because only seriously altered (i.e. dead) cells will not exclude the dye and stain. The release of cytosolic enzymes in the culture medium is a reliable parameter and has been widely used as an indicator of increased membrane permeability and, indirectly, as a marker of "in vitro" toxicity. In fact, this is also the case for hepatocytes. In addition enzyme leakage is more sensitive that cell viability. During the the first hours of culture cells are more susceptible to xenobiotics than after 24h. As shown in Fig 2B, when the same xenobiotics were added to the cultures at the time of cell plating, some of them caused important enzyme release. After 24 h, the addition of the same concentration of the xenobiotic produced only a moderate effect. The isozyme V of lactic dehydrogenase accounts for almost all the hepatic LDH activity. This isozyme is stable in the conditions of the culture medium. That means, the activity remains quite stable along the incubation time. When compared with other enzymes (i.e. GOT), LDH was a more sensitive parameter. As shown in Fig 2C, a 100% LDH release out of cell after exposure to a xenobiotic may be obtained when only 30-40% of total GOT is lost. That is, for a certain xenobiotic concentration, larger increases of LDH were measured in culture medium in comparison to GOT.

The ultrastructural study of hepatocytes reveals cellular damage in organelles by cytotoxic effects even when cells do not show any apparent morphological injury at the optical level. However, in spite of the work done by other authors in the evaluation of ultrastructural damage (Walton and Buckley, 1975), the quantification is still difficult to perform and subjectively evaluated, and remained, in our experience, as a useful but qualitative parameter (Castell et al. 1986).

Tabla 1. COMPARISON AMONG CYTOTOXIC AND METABOLIC INDICATORS OF HEPATOTOXICITY

Xenobiotic	LDH* mU/mg	Albumin synthesis µg/mgx h	Gluconeogenesis nmol /mgxmin	Glycogen nmol/mg	Ureogenesis nmol/mgxmin
Paraquat 10^{-4} M	6.5 % n.s.	91 %	86 %	-	88 %
Galactosamina 4 µM	5 % n.s.	90 %	-	70 %	-
Thioacetamide 230 µM	15 %	-	-	-	72 %
Chlorpromazine 10^{-5} M	5 % n.s.	80 %	-	-	-
Butibufen 0.4 mM	6 % n.s.	64 %	19 %	38 %	95 %
Control	8 %	100 %	100 %	100 %	100 %

* % of total intracellular enzyme content leakage. Enzyme was measured after the first 24 h exposure.

Metabolic effects of hepatotoxins on cultured hepatocytes.

Impairment of liver biochemical functions may occur at concentrations of xenobiotics having only moderate cytotoxic effects. We have studied in cells exposed to various xenobiotics several important metabolic functions and compared with LDH leakage, the most sensitive parameter for cytotoxicity. As shown in Table 1, several hepatotoxins showed clear metabolic effects at concentrations where the leakage of LDH was non significative in relation to the control. Metabolic parameters give a deeper insight on the hepatotoxicity than cytotoxic parameters.

Predictive value of the "in vitro" data.

To become of widespread use, an "in vitro" system must be sensitive enough to detect all potential hepatotoxins causing effects in vivo without false negatives and false positives. A first aspect of this problem is the sensitivity of each of the individual parameters used. A second aspect is the practical extrapolation of the in vitro results to in vivo. In our work we have approached this question in another way: How sensitive is the in vitro system in detecting the effects of well-known hepatotoxins?. Would our biological system be able to detect the hepatotoxicity of a compound in a blind test?. At what concentration in relation to the "in vivo" toxicity would a hepatotoxin be detected by the assay?, that is to say, how do the "in vitro" toxic concentrations correlate with the "in vivo" observed toxic doses. In an attempt to answer these questions, three well known hepatotoxins where studied in a blind test and handled as if they were unknown substances. The whole screening protocol was applied to each of them. The most sensitive cytotoxic and metabolic parameter together with the lower concentration showing a toxic effect has been tabulated (Table 2). In addition, representative values taken from literature for "in vivo" toxic concentrations of the compounds were considered. From this data and taking into account the pharmacokinetics of each compound (Castell and Gómez-Lechón, 1987; Tremery and Waring, 1983; Krainski et al. 1979; Marinozzi and Fiume, 1971), we estimated the "in vitro" equivalence of the "in vivo" toxic concentration and compared the limit of detection of the biological assay with the "in vivo" data. In the case of a-amanitin, a toxic that is largely taken up by the liver (Marinozzi and Fiume, 1971), it seemed reasonable to calculate the toxicity on the basis of liver weight/cell weight (Castell and Gómez-Lechón, 1987). The data obtained in our study shows that toxic effects were clearly observed at concentrations lower than those expected from theoretical calculations, which speaks in favour of the sensitivity of this biological assay.

Table 2. COMPARISON OF THE "IN VITRO" AND "IN VIVO" TOXICITY OF INDIRECT HEPATOTOXINS

Hepatotoxin	Concentration at which Cytotoxicity was first observed	Concentration at which Metabolic alterations were first observed	"In vivo" Toxicity mg/Kg b.w.	Estimated "In vitro" equivalence of "In vivo" toxicity
a- Amanitin	No effects at 1.5 ng/mg	Synthesis RNA 1.5 pg/mg	0.5-1 mg (11)	10 ng/mg cell prot.
D- Galactosamine	LDH * 40 μM	Glycogen synthesis 4 μM	200-375 mg (13)	1.85-3.5 mM
Thioacetamide	No effects at 230 μM	Ureogenesis 2.3 μM	50-200 mg (12)	1.33-5.32 mM

* Enzyme activity was measured after the first 24 h exposure.

The reversibility of the effects.

Another important aspect to more precisely interpret the in vitro data is the reversibility of the effects observed in vitro. The metabolic parameters are more accurate than the cytotoxic ones in detecting hepatotoxic effects on hepatocytes. However the relevance on this data needs further evaluation. Its clear that a transitory inhibition of albumin synthesis, for instance, although it indicates a toxic effect of the xenobiotic, may be not significant for in vivo toxicity, since the albumin pool of the organism is high and the half life is long. In contrast, an impairment of gluconeogenesis, even for few hours, could have important consequences in a fasted individual. In the experiment showed in Fig 3, the recovery time of hepatic gluconeogenesis has been followed after exposing hepatocytes to two times the therapeutical plasma concentration of 3 NSAID's. The results clearly shown that flurbiprofen not only impairs to a lesser extent the gluconeogenesis but also the recovery of the full metabolic capability of the cell is faster upon removal of the drug. One should therfore asume that this effect will probably be irrelevant in the whole animal.

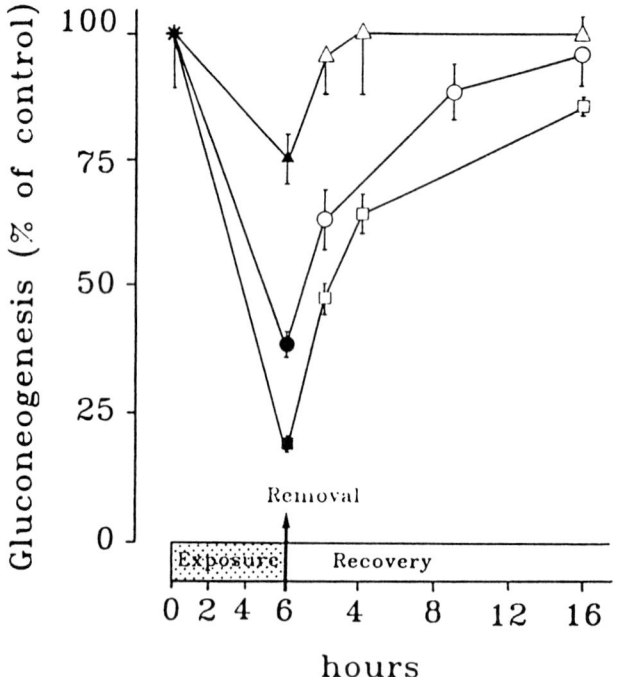

Fig. 3. Reversibility of the inhibitory effect on gluconeogenesis from 10 mM lactate of (■) butibufen, (●) ibuprofen and (▲) flurbiprofen. Cultures were exposed for 6 h to 2x the therapeutical plasma concentration. Then, the cultures were shifted to fresh medium.

REFERENCES

Acosta, D., Sorensen, E., Anuforo, D., Mitchell, D., Ramos, K., Santone, K., Smith, M. (1985): An in vitro approach to the study of target organ toxicity of drugs and chemicals. In Vitro 21, 495-504.

Castell, J.V., Gomez-Lechon, M.J., Coloma, J., Lopez, P. (1983): Preservation of the adult functionality of hepatocytes in serum-free cultures. In Hormonally defined media. A tool in cell biology. Eds. Fisher G., Wieser R.J. Springer-Verlag : Berlin West. pp. 333-336.

Castell, J.V., Montoya, A., Larrauri, A., Lopez, P., Gomez-Lechon, M.J. (1985): Effects of benorylate and impacine on the metabolism of cultured hepatocytes. Xenobiotica 15, 743-759.

Castell, J.V., Gomez-Lechon, M.J., Mayordomo, F. (1986a): Estudio sobre la potencial accion toxica del excipiente de la forma retard del dinitrato de isosorbica. Rev. Exp. Cardiologia 39, 220-226.

Castell, J.V., Gomez-Lechon, M.J., Miranda, M.A., Morera, M.I. (1987): Toxic effects of the photoproducts of chlorpromazine on cultured hepatocytes. Hepatology 7, 349-353.

Castell, J.V., Gomez-Lechon, M.J. (1987): The use of cultured hepatocytes to assess the hepatoxicity of xenobiotics. In Interaction between Drugs and Chemicals in Industrial Societies. Eds. G.L. Plaa, P. du Souich, S. Erill. Elsevier : Amsterdam, pp. 135-149.

Gomez-Lechon, M.J., Lopez, P., Castell, J.V. (1984): Biochemical functionality and recovery of hepatocytes after deep freezing storage. In Vitro 20, 826-832.

Gomez-Lechon, M.J., Castell, J.V. (1984): Phyllogenetically unrelated serum fibronectins mediate rat hepatocyte attachment and extension to culture dishes. Ciencia Biol. 8, 49-56.

Guillouzo, A. (1986): Use of isolated and cultured hepatocytes for xenobiotic metabolism and cytotoxicity studies. In Isolated and cultured hepatocytes. Ed. A. Guillouzo, C. Guguen-Guillouzo. Editions INSERM : Paris, John Libbey Eurotext : London. pp. 313-332.

Krainski, A., Sasse, D., Tsench H.F., Lesch, R. (1979): Histochemical studies on carbohydrate metabolism in rat liver after galactosamine administration. Virchow's Arch. B. Cell Pathol. 30, 131-142.

Marinozzi, V., Fiume, L. (1971): Effects of aminitin on mouse and rat liver cell nuclei. Exp. Cell Res. 67, 311-322.

Trennery, P.N., Waring, R.H. (1983): Early changes in thioacetamide-induced liver damage. Toxicol. Lett. 19, 299-307.

Walton, J.R., Buckely, I.K. (1975): Cell models in the study of mechanism of toxicity. Agents and Actions 5, 69-88.

Isolated and cultured rat hepatocytes as models for studying the cytotoxicity of two triterpenoid saponins

F. Braut-Boucher*, S. Achard-Ellouk*, H. Hoellinger*, D. Pauthe-Daide**, M. Henry**

* UDC CNRS-INSERM (UA 400), Faculté de Médecine, Université René Descartes, Paris, France. ** Laboratoire de Botanique, Faculté de Pharmacie, Toulouse, France

Key words : rat isolated hepatocytes, primary culture, triterpenoid saponins, cytotoxicity.

INTRODUCTION

Saponins are widely distributed in plant kingdom. Recently, a special attention has been given to triterpenoid saponins because of their anti-inflammatory, anti-molluscicid and anti-hepatotoxic activities (Oakenfull, 1981; Bezanger-Beauquesne et al. 1975). The hepatoprotective action concerned mainly triterpenoids of the oleanolic serie (Hikino et al. 1984; Kiso et al. 1984), but little attention gave on saponosides hepatocellular effects.

Isolated rat hepatocytes and primary monolayer foetal hepatocytes can provided useful informations about acute and chronic cytotoxicity (Kremers et al. 1983). Thus, using these models, and before investigation of eventual antihepatotoxic effects, we tested two new saponins : gypsoside and glucuronogypsogenin (Henry and Pauthe-Daide, 1985). Hepatocellular effects resulting from the action of saponins have been investigated by measure of metabolic, functional parameters and morphological changes.

MATERIAL AND METHODS

All chemicals were grade purity. Enzymes, coenzymes and substrates, for spectrophotometric assays, and collagenase were purchased from Boehringer (Manheim, WG). Bovine calf serum, Eagle's MEM medium, dexamethasone, penicillin, streptomycin, and trypsin were provided by Flow Laboratories (Herts, UK).

Gypsoside was obtained by purification of white saponin (Merck, Darmstadt, WG) on Fractogel TSK HW 40 column chromatography, eluted by 0.02% Na_2CO_3 in water. Glucuronogypsogenin was obtained after hydrolysis of gypsoside with 2N H_2SO_4 at reflux for one hour. These compounds were identified by NMR and GC-MS. The different oses were characterized by HPLC, and compared to standards (Henry and Pauthe-Daide, 1985).

GYPSOSIDE   GLUCURONOGYPSOGENIN

Preparation of isolated hepatocytes and primary culture of foetal hepatocytes

The animals used were male Wistar rats, weighing 200g 10. Freshly prepared hepatocytes (4×10^6 cells. ml^{-1}) were obtained with two steps collagenase perfusion technique according to Berry and Friend (1969).

Foetuses (18 days old) were removed from female Wistar rats and livers immediately excised in sterile conditions and washed with Dulbecco's medium before trypsination (0.25% trypsin for 15 min). Cell culture was performed according to Kremers et al. technique (1983). The cells were cultivated with dexamethasone (10^{-7} M) which maintained their specific functional activities. The media were removed 24 h after hepatocyte seeding and then replaced every day with treatment medium. Hepatocytes were placed in an incubator at 37°C under 5 % CO_2 in humidified air.

Treatment schedule

Hepatocytes suspension was distributed (3 ml) in gas-tight 25 ml Erlenmeyer flasks and incubated for 45 min with various concentrations of each saponin.

Gypsoside was solubilized in the incubation medium. Glucuronogypsogenin was dissolved in DMSO (1% v/v). Each compound was added in nutrient medium at the following concentrations : 10^{-6}, 5×10^{-6}, 10^{-4} and 5×10^{-4} M (treatment media). Controls received DMSO only. Assays were performed in triplicate.

Cell morphology and viability studies

Cell viability (90% for control) was calculated by trypan blue exclusion test (TBT). Cultured hepatocytes were examined daily under reverse phase contrast microscope, before and after hemalun eosin staining.

Biochemichal assays

Lactate dehydrogenase (LDH) (EC 1.1.1.2.) and transaminase (GOT) (EC 2.6.1.1.) were measured by standard enzymatic procedures (Cartier et al. 1967). Albumin was quantified by laser immunonephelometry according to Guguen-Guillouzo et al. (1983). Protein determination was carried out according to Lowry et al. (1951). Intracellular adenosine triphosphate (ATP) was assayed by enzyme spectrophotometric method (Buc et al. 1981). Cytochrome P-450 was measured in cells suspended in 50% glycerol phosphate buffer according to Omura and Sato (1964).

RESULTS

Cell morphology and viability

By TBT test, 50% decrease of cell viability was observed in isolated hepatocytes treated with 3×10^{-5} M gypsoside and 1.8×10^{-4} M glucuronogypsogenin. These concentrations carried away some cytoplasmic alterations such as vacuolization, retractation and disruption of the continous cell layer after 24 h of exposure.

Gypsoside effects on isolated or cultured rat hepatocytes

On isolated hepatocytes, gypsoside at the concentration of 3×10^{-5} M increased LDH and GOT leakages by 40% compared to control (Table 1A). With superior concentrations a strongly release of enzymes, albumin and a lost of ATP occured, revealing cellular lysis. No effect was registered on cytochrome P-450.

On cultured hepatocytes, an enhancement of LDH leakage (2 fold in comparison with control) was observed with 5×10^{-5} M gypsoside after 24 h of exposure. In these conditions protein level reached 40% of control and albumin secretion was slightly impaired.

Glucuronogypsogenin effects on isolated or cultured rat hepatocytes

On isolated hepatocytes glucuronogypsogenin at the concentration of 10^{-5} M had no apparent toxicity. With superior concentrations occured an increase of LDH and GOT values, and a depletion of ATP (until 50% of control at 1.8×10^{-4} M (Table 1B). No variation of cytochrome P-450 was noted.

On cultured hepatocytes, an important LDH release (3 fold compared to control) and decrease of protein and albumin levels (30% of control) were registered at the concentration of 5×10^{-4} M for 24 h.

DISCUSSION

The major aim of this present work was to determine the cytotoxic threshold of the new saponins.

On isolated hepatocytes the cytotoxic concentration for gypsoside was 3×10^{-5} M when it was 1.8×10^{-4} M for glucuronogypsogenin. Similar concentrations were obtained on cultured foetal hepatocytes. From these data could be determined the "highest tolerated doses" (HTD) (Riddell et al. 1986) which are 10^{-5} and 10^{-4} M for gypsoside and glucuronogypsogenin respectively. Thus, it appeared that the mono-glycosylated compound was less toxic than the poly-glycosylated aglycone. This difference of toxicity between both tested compounds could be explained by the glycosylation degree. This fact agrees with results presented by Hikino et al. (1984) studying the structure-activity relationship of Dianthus's saponins.

The most sensitive parameters to detect cytotoxicity, in our experimental conditions, are TBT test, LDH leakage, and ATP level. The variations of these criteria reflected the membrane injury. Consequently, it seems that the cellular membrane was the preferential target of the two tested compounds, as described for many other saponins by Oakenfull et al. (1981).

To define the cytotoxicity range, the isolated hepatocyte were a suitable model. But, to investigate the eventual hepatoprotective effect, the foetal hepatocytes in primary cultured were more adapted, because we can use weaker concentrations for longer time.

ACKNOWLEDGEMENTS : We are gratefull to the Metabolism Group of INSERM U-75, CHU NECKER, Paris, France, specially Dr. H. A Buc and A. Moncion.

TABLE 1 : EFFECTS OF GYPSOSIDE AND GLUCURONOGYPSOGENIN ON ISOLATED HEPATOCYTES

	CONCENTRATION x 10^{-5} M	TBT	ATP	LDH	GOT	ALBUMIN
A)						
	CONTROL	100	100	100	100	100
	1	80	101 ± 3	98	97	89 ± 7
	2	80	94 ± 7	111 ± 18	116 ± 24	–
GYPSOSIDE	3	50	91 ± 12	137 ± 6	145 ± 17	101 ± 8
	4	32	49 ± 14	224 ± 49	207 ± 6	–
	6	10	13 ± 5	343 ± 65	194 ± 10	144 ± 37
	9	10	10	412 ± 57	242 ± 53	157 ± 11
B)						
	CONTROL	100	100	100	100	100
	2	80	105 ± 5	96 ± 6	98 ± 3	111 ± 11
GLUCURONO-	4	67	112 ± 11	100 ± 1	101 ± 1	99 ± 4
GYPSOGENIN	10	60	96 ± 5	110 ± 14	120 ± 14	–
	18	40	61 ± 2	141 ± 23	144 ± 8	–
	24	20	28 ± 7	227 ± 3	252 ± 67	182 ± 21

Results are expressed in percentage of control. Three experiments were done. Control ATP value: 22.07 ± 34 nmoles. 10^{-6} cells; Control LDH value: 786 ± 30 nmoles. 10^{-6} cells; Control GOT value: 154 ± 45 nmoles. 10^{-6} cells; Control albumin value: 7.64 ± 0.32 ug. 10^{-6} cells.

REFERENCES

Berry, M.N., Friend, D.S. (1969) : High yield preparation of isolated rat liver parenchymal cells. A biochemical and fine structural study. J. Cell. Biol. 43, 29-43.

Bezanger-Beauquesne, L., Pinkas, M., Torck, M. (1975) : Les plantes dans la thérapeutique moderne. Maloine Ed. Paris.

Buc, H.A., Demaugre, F., Moncion, A. Leroux, J.P. (1981) : Metabolic consequences of pyruvate kinase inhibition by oxalate in intact rat hepatocytes. Biochimie. 63, 595-601.

Cartier, P., Leroux, J.P., Tempkine, H. (1967) : Techniques de dosages d'intermédiaires de la glycolyse dans les tissus. Ann. Biol. Clin. 25, 731-813.

Guguen-Guillouzo, C., Clement, B., Baffet, G., Beaumont, C., Morel-Chany, E., Glaise, D., Guillouzo, A. (1983) : Maintenance and reversibility of active albumin secretion by adult hepatocytes co-cultured with another liver epithelial cell type. Exp. Cell Res. 143, 47-54.

Henry, M., Pauthe-Daide, D. (1985) : Recherche de l'exploitation des capacités de glycosylation d'une suspension cellulaire de Saponaria L : Etude de la toxicité de la glucuronogypsogénine. 10ème colloque de la section de Microbiologie Industrielle et de Biotechnologie de la Société Française de Microbiologie, Lyon, 7-8 mars.

Hikino, H., Oshava, T., Kiso, Y., Oshima, Y. (1984) : Analgesic and antihepatotoxic actions of dianosides, triterpenoid saponins of Dianthus superbus var longicalcynus herbs, Planta Med. 44, 353-355.

Kiso, Y., Tohkin, M., Hikino, H., Hattori, M., Sakamoto, T., Namba, T. (1984) : Antihepatotoxic activity of glycyrrhizin I. Effects of free radical generation and lipid peroxidation. Planta Med. 44, 298-302.

Kremers, P., Letawe-Goujon, F., De Graeve, J, Duvivier, J., Gielen E. (1983) : The expression of different monooxygenases supported by cytochrome P-450 in neonatal rats and in primary foetal hepatocytes in culture. Eur. J. Biochem. 137, 603-608.

Lowry, O.W., Rosebrough, N.J., Randal, R.J. (1951) : Protein measurement with folin phenol reagent. J. Biol. Chem. 193, 265-275.

Oakenfull, D. (1981) : Saponins in food - a review. Food Chem. Toxicol. 6, 19-40.

Omura, T., Sato, R. (1964) : The carbon monoxide binding pigment of liver microsomes. J. Biol. Chem. 239, 2379-2385.

Riddell, R.J., Clothier, R.H., Balls, M. (1986) : An evaluation of the in vitro cytotoxicity assays. Food Chem. Toxicol. 24, 469-473.

Liver Cells and Drugs. Ed. A. Guillouzo. Colloque INSERM/John Libbey Eurotext Ltd. © 1988. Vol. 164, pp. 385-390.

Effects of ditercalinium in cultured rat hepatocyte : cytolocalization and ultrastructural mitochondrial damages

Robert Fellous[1], Marie-Ange Verjus[1], Dominique Coulaud[2], Alain Gouyette[1]

[(1)]Laboratoire de Pharmacologie Clinique et [(2)]Laboratoire de Microscopie Cellulaire et Moléculaire (UA 147 CNRS, INSERM U.140) Institut Gustave Roussy, 39, rue Camille Desmoulins, 94805 Villejuif Cedex, France

Key words : Ditercalinium, rat hepatocytes, cytoplasmic fluorescence and mitochondria.

INTRODUCTION

Ditercalinium (Fig. 1) is a DNA bisintercalating antitumor drug designed by Roques (1979). This dimer displays a large spectrum of antitumor activity through an original mechanism of action which differs from that of monointercalating compounds as described by Esnault (1984). In a phase I clinical trial, Le Chevalier (1986) reported an irreversible hepatotoxicity induced by ditercalinium when administrated as a 6 hour intravenous-infusion at a dose of 24 mg/m^2. An increase in alkaline phosphatase and γ glutamyl transpeptidase plasma levels, and a microvascular steatosis were described. The reinvestigation of ditercalinium disposition in rat using the tritium-labelled drug showed a fast distribution and a large accumulation in tissues, followed by a slow clearance. The thin sections of liver and kidneys exhibited ultrastructural mitochondrial changes (unpublished results). In the present report, we used rat hepatocyte cultures to study ditercalinium cytotoxicity assessed by ultrastructural modifications and by lactate dehydrogenase (LDH) leakage. Cytoplasmic localization of the drug was followed by its fluorescent properties. The labelled-drug, high-performance liquid chromatography (HPLC) and mass-spectrometry allowed the separation and the identification of the metabolites.

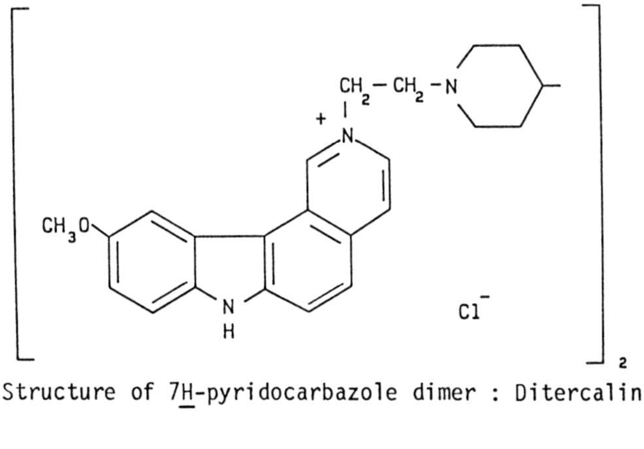

Fig. 1 : Structure of 7H-pyridocarbazole dimer : Ditercalinium

II - MATERIALS AND METHODS

1/ Isolation and culture of rat hepatocytes
Adult rat hepatocytes were isolated by Hepes-Collagenase infusion of liver Wistar rat and seeded in culture medium as described by Seglen (1976). Four hours later hydrocortisone hemisuccinate was added to the medium according to Baffet (1982). Cell monolayers were incubated with 1 µM of ditercalinium for various times.

2/ Preparation of cell for electron microscopy
Hepatocytes were fixed at room temperature by adding 1.5 % of glutaraldehyde to the culture medium. The cells were then scraped, centrifuged and resuspended in Sørensen fixative buffer. After washing with buffer, the slices were post-fixed for 1 h in 2 % osmium tetroxide, dehydrated and embedded in Epon.

3/ Fluorescence microscopy
Hepatocyte suspensions were seeded on glass coverslip and transferred to the culture chambers (5.3 cm^2 ; 2 ml). After 3 hours of exposure to ditercalinium, a fluorescent mitochondrial probe (diethyloxadicarbocyanine) was added to the culture medium for 5 min. After 3 washes with culture medium, hepatocytes were observed with a Olympus photomicroscope BH2 with high-pressure mercury lamp and filter combination BG12-0515 for ditercalinium, and in red long emission filter for diethyloxadicarbocyanine.

4/ LDH assay
LDH activity in cell free supernatant fraction was measured by recording the rate of change in absorbance at 340 nm due to NADH oxydation in the presence of pyruvate. The result was presented as percent of control.

5/ Separation and identification of metabolites
Supernatant of culture medium incubated for 24 or 48 hours with the drug was extracted with various solvents. For ditercalinium and SR95156B, the butanol extracted most of the metabolites. After evaporation, the residue was injected on a reverse-phase column (µ Bondapack-C18 Waters). The metabolites were separated using a mobile phase methanol/water (80/20), sodium formate 0.1 M and UV (254 nm) detection. The identification was made with the Fast Atom Bombardment Mass-Spectrometry (FAB MS) VG Instrument (Gouyette, 1987).

III - RESULTS AND DISCUSSION

1/ Cytoplasmic localization of ditercalinium using its fluorescent properties
Ditercalinium is a very slighty fluorescent compound, the quantum yield in water was 0.19 %. Wavelengths maxima of excitation and emission were 411 and 562 nm. (Fig 2a and b). In isopropanol, a polar hydrophobic media, the observed fluorescence is 30 times greater than in water.
The intracellular distribution of ditercalinium was studied by fluorescence microscopy. After 30 min, fluorescence was essentially located in the cytoplasm as filamentous fluorescence mitochondria. For the same exposure time, nuclei were not fluorescent. After four hours (Fig. 3), bright and granular fluorescence appeared around to the nuclei. Fluorescent granulations were probably altered mitochondria. To confirm mitochondrial localization of ditercalinium-induced fluorescence, we used 3,3'diethyloxadicarbocyanine, a fluorescent mitochondrial probe. A superposable fluorescent pattern was observed for both agents. Since these compounds are both biscationic and lipophilic, the concentration of ditercalinium in mitochondria probably results of the electric potential across mitochondrial membranes as described by Weiss (1987) for the dequalinium.

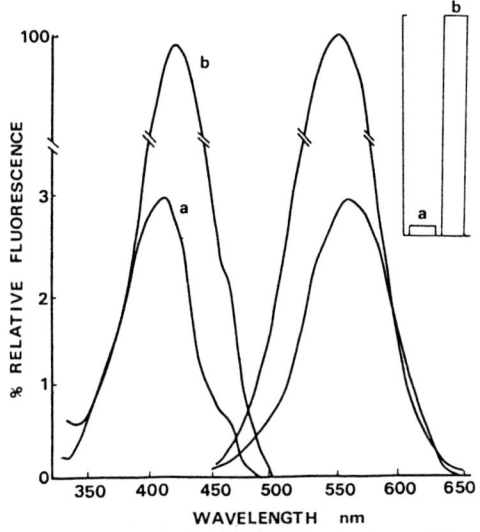

Fig. 2 : Fluorescence spectra of ditercalinium in water (a) and isopropanol (b). Maxima wavelengths of excitation and emission were 411 and 562 nm in water and 418, 550 nm in isopropanol. The relative fluorescence in water was only 3 % of that obtained in isopropanol.

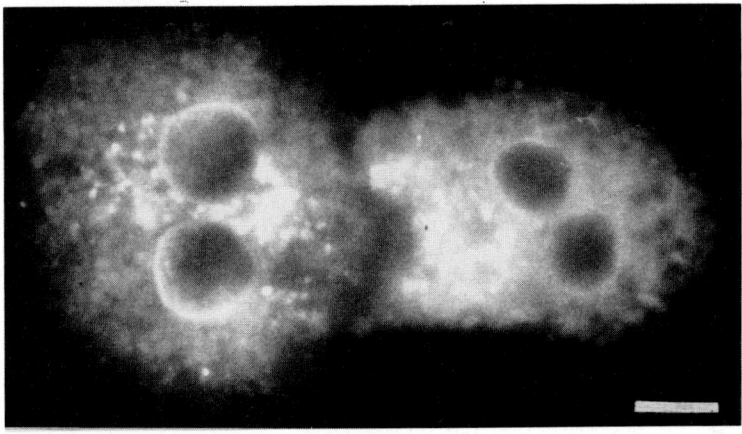

Fig. 3 : Intracellular fluorescence distribution of ditercalinium. Filamentous and granular fluorescences were observed. Scale bar equal 10 μm.

2/ Ditercalinium-induced ultrastructural changes in cultured rat hepatocytes

To further study mitochondrial alterations, electron microscopy experiments were made. Fig. 4a shows a control hepatocyte with numerous and rounded or oblong mitochondria. In electron dense matrix, many cristae were clearly observed. After four hours of ditercalinium exposure most of the mitochondria were swollen and their cristae were absent (Fig. 4b). Injury was more pronounced after 24 hours of ditercalinium incubation (Fig 4c). Many mitochondria were opened and membranous residues were enclosed in cavities. Nuclei and chromatin did not seem different from those in control hepatocytes. Other drugs such as methylglyoxal bis(guanylhydrazone) (Nass, 1984), ethidium bromide (Soslau, 1971) and paraquat (Ueda, 1985) induce similar damages.

3/ LDH Assay

The cytotoxicity of ditercalinium was assessed by measuring LDH leakage which evaluates the severity of cell injury.
Fig. 5 shows that ditercalinium-induced LDH leakage at 1 μM and 10 μM was both time- and dose-dependent. But at four hours of drug-incubation, the LDH leakage

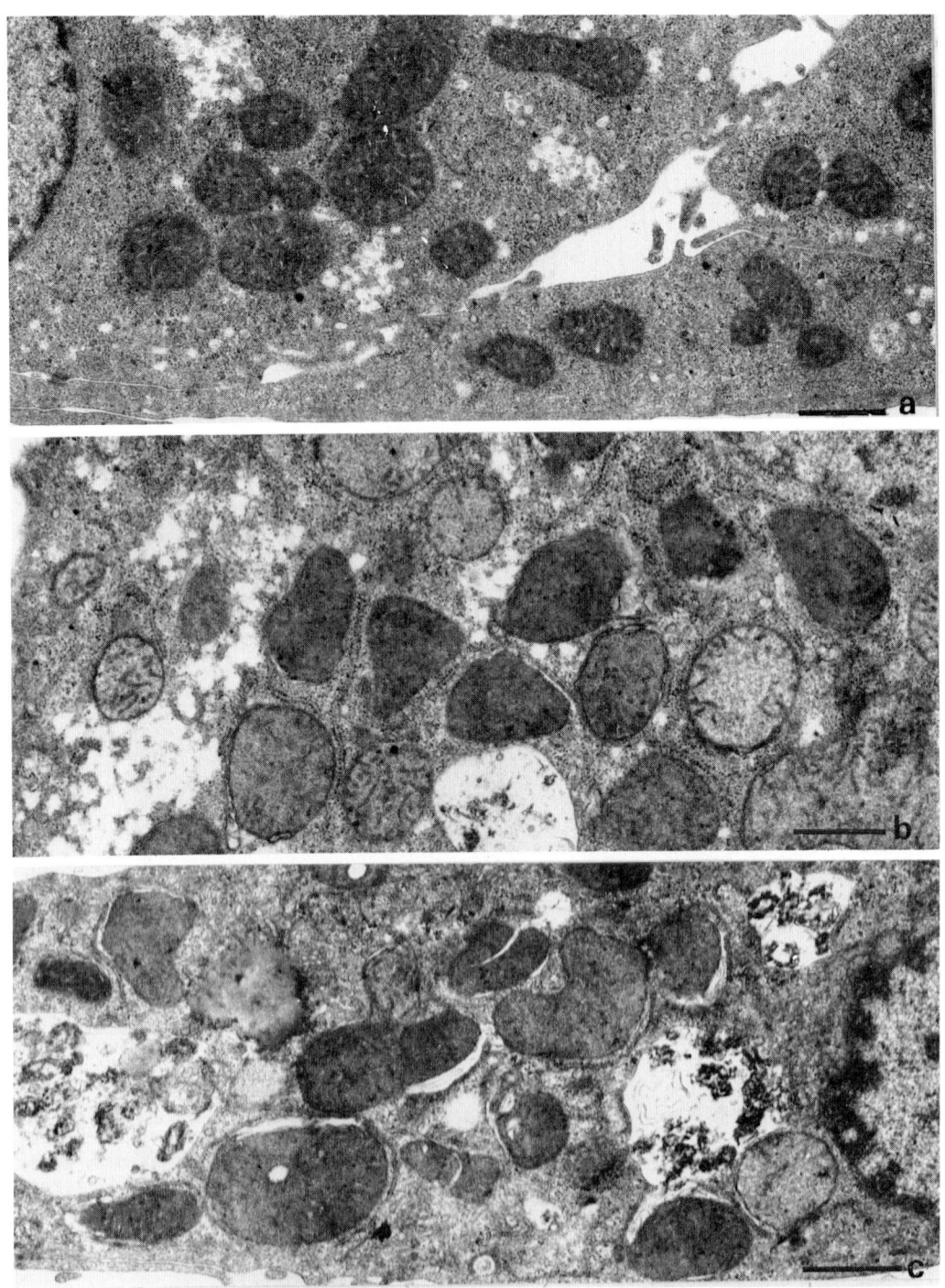

Fig. 4 : Electron microscopy of untreated hepatocytes (a) and treated hepatocytes (1 µM of ditercalinium) for 4 hours (b) and 24 hours (c). Mitochondria were considerably altered. Scale bars, 1 µm.

was not different of control while electron microscopy revealed mitochondrial damages as described above. Consequently, LDH leakage is not a good assay to evaluate early mitochondrial damages induced by the drug. More specific assays for mitochondrial alterations could be used e.g. in measuring ATP, respiratory complex activity or oxygen consumption.

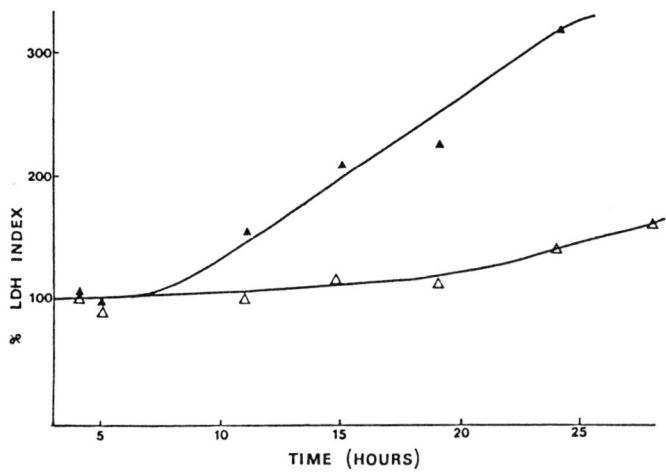

Fig. 5 : Kinetics of LDH leakage at 1 µM (Δ) and 10 µM (▲) of ditercalinium during 30 hours.

4/ Metabolism of antitumor drugs

Ditercalinium at 0.1 µM to 10 µM incubated with rat hepatocytes culture did not generate any metabolite. For comparison the same hepatocyte system was used with a derivative of ellipticine (SR 95156B). HPLC chromatogram of control supernatant hepatocytes is shown in Fig. 6a. Eight metabolites have been isolated (Fig. 6b) with SR 95156B and only 20 % of initial drug was unchanged after 24 hours of incubation. Structure identification of thees products is presently under investigation with FAB-MS.

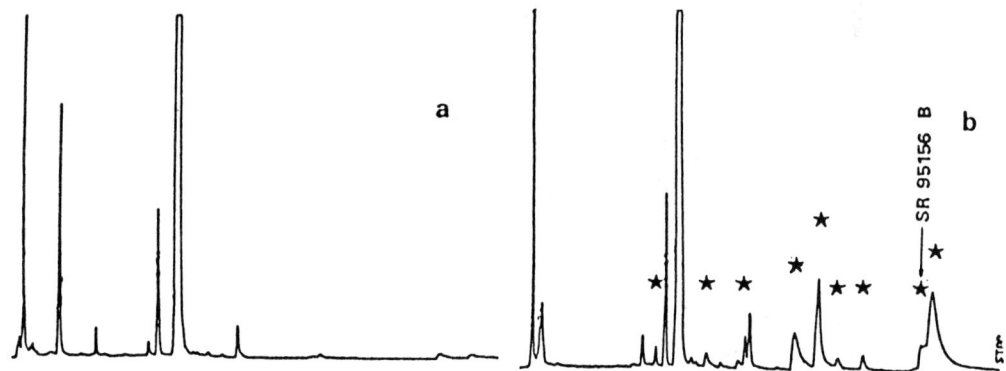

Fig. 6 : HPLC chromatogram of supernatant of the control hepatocytes (a) and hepatocyte treated with 10 µM of 1-[^{14}C] labelled-SR 95156 B. Eight metabolites (★) were isolated.

CONCLUSION

In this report, ditercalinium accumulation in mitochondria was studied in vitro, using rat hepatocytes in culture. The observed mitochondrial damages could play an important role in ditercalinium-induced hepatotoxicity reported in phase I clinical trial. We showed that cultured rat hepatocyte is an interesting tool to study or to confirm metabolism and/or toxicity.

ACKNOWLEDGMENTS

We thank Dr. G. Chabot for his help in editing the manuscript. This work was supported by funds from the Association pour la Recherche sur le Cancer (Villejuif).

REFERENCES

Baffet, G., Clement, B., Glaise, B., Guillouzo, A. and Guguen-Guillouzo, C. (1982) Hydrocortisone modulates the production of extracellular material and albumin in long-term cocultures of adult rat hepatocytes with other liver epithelial cells. Biochem. Biophys. Res. Commun., 109 : 507-512.

Esnault, C., Roques, B.P., Jacquemin-Sablon, A. and Le Pecq, J.B. (1984) Effects of new antitumor bifunctional intercalators derived from 7H-pyridocarbazole on sensitive and resistant L1210 cells. Cancer Res., 44 : 4355-4360.

Gouyette, A., Fellous, R., El Abed, I., Deniel, A., Auclair, C., Le Pecq, J.B. and Paoletti, C. (1987) FAB mass spectrometry during antitumor drug development. International Symposium on Applied Mass Spectrometry in the Health Sciences, Barcelone, September 28-30 , Abs. 156.

Le Chevalier, T.,Sevin, D., Sancho-Garnier, H., Spielman, M., Le Pecq, J.B. and Rouëssé, J. (1986) Phase I study of ditercalinium in adult patients with solid tumor. Fifth NCI EORTC Symposium, Amsterdam, October 22-24, Abstract 8-13.

Nass, M.M.K. (1984) Analysis of methyglyoxal bis (guanylhydrazone)-induced alteration of hamster tumor mitochondria by correlated studies of selective rhodamine binding, ultrastructural damage, DNA replication, and reversibility. Cancer Res., 44 : 2677-2688.

Roques, B.P., Pelaprat, D., Le Guen, I., Porcher, G., Gosse, C. and Le Pecq, J.B. (1979) DNA bifunctional intercalators : antileukemic activity of new pyridocarbazole dimers. Biochem. Pharmacol., 28 : 1811-1815.

Seglen, P.O. (1976) Preparation of isolated rat liver cells. Meth. Cell Biol., 13 : 29-83.

Soslau, G. and Nass, M.M.K. (1971) Effects of ethidium bromide on the cytochrome content and ultrastructure of L cell mitochondria. J. Cell. Biol., 51 : 514-524.

Ueda, T., Hirai, K.I. and Ogazaura, K. (1985) Effects of paraquat on mitochondrial structure and Ca-ATPase activity in rat hepatocytes. J. Electron Microsc., 34 : 85-91.

Weiss, M.J., Wong, J.R., Ha, C.S., Bleday, R., Salem, R.R., Steele, G.D. and Chen, L.B. (1987) Dequalinium, a topical antimicrobial agent, displays anticarcinoma activity based on selective mitochondrial accumulation. Proc. Natl. Acad. Sci. USA., 84 : 5444-5448.

Acute hepatocellular changes elicited by various antibiotics in the perfused liver and cultured hepatocytes from the rat

Roger G. Ulrich[1,*], Jeffrey W. Cox[2]

[1]Pathology and Toxicology Research and [2]Drug Metabolism Research, The Upjohn Company, Kalamazoo, Michigan 49001, USA
*Author to whom correspondence should be addressed

KEY WORDS

hepatocyte, antibiotics, gentamicin, amikacin, trospectomycin sulfate, spectinomycin, lamellar body

INTRODUCTION

The chronic administration of many antibiotics, including various erythromycins, aminoglycosides, and clindamycin, has the potential to produce lysosomal alterations (for reviews of drug-induced lysosomal alterations see Hruban, 1972, and Lullmann-Rauch, 1979). These alterations include the appearance of lamellar inclusion bodies, also referred to as myeloid bodies or whorled figures. Although often inferred, in no case has a cause-and-effect relationship been demonstrated between the appearance of lamellar bodies in the cytoplasm and cellular injury.

In preclinical drug safety evaluation studies, lamellar inclusion bodies were observed in the livers of dogs and various organs of rats given high, chronic doses of trospectomycin sulfate, a new aminocyclitol antibiotic, semi-synthetically derived from spectinomycin (White et al, 1983). The appearance of lamellar bodies was coincident with dose- and time-dependent increases in serum aspartate transaminase and alanine transaminase above control levels, but within normal ranges (data to be published). In the report presented here, we summarize various studies utilizing the perfused liver and isolated hepatocyte models designed to further investigate antibiotic-induced lysosomal alterations in rat liver and their role, if any, in cell injury. The antibiotics compared include the aminoglycosides gentamicin and amikacin, the macrolide erythromycin base, and the aminocylitols spectinomycin and trospectomycin sulfate.

MATERIALS AND METHODS

Antibiotics
The antibiotics used were trospectomycin sulfate (6'-propylspectinomycin hydrogen sulfate, lot #B1-0192-AS-006, The Upjohn Company), spectinomycin (spectinomycin dihydrochloride pentahydrate, lot #245AK, The Upjohn Company), erythromycin base (U.S.P. reference standard), gentamicin sulfate (lot #23F-0004, Sigma Chemical Company), and amikacin base (lot #74F1805, Bristol-Meyers). Dilutions used were all corrected for lot purity.

Liver Perfusion
In situ liver perfusions were performed as described by Cox et al (1985). Briefly, for each perfusion, a male Sprague-Dawley rat weighing 220-240 g was anesthetized with Metofane and the abdominal cavity was exposed with a U-shaped incision. The bile duct was canulated with PE-10 tubing and the portal vein was canulated with PE-240 tubing. The inferior vena cava was transected and the liver was flushed with heparinized saline (20 U/ml) by gravity flow. The thoracic vena cava was canulated and ligated, and the animal transferred to a temperature controlled chamber for normograde, recirculating liver perfusion. Livers were perfused at a constant portal venous pressure of 12 cm H_2O with 100 ml of medium consisting of 20% (v/v) freshly isolated rat erythrocytes, 0.1% (w/v) d-glucose, and 3% (w/v) bovine serum albumin in Krebs-Henseleit (K-H) buffer, equilibrated with 95% O_2/95% CO_2. Sodium taurocholate was infused at 38 micromol/h to stimulate bile production and the pH was maintained at 7.35 by the addition of $NaHCO_3$.

Following a 30 min equilibration period, antibiotics (gentamicin, trospectomycin sulfate, or erythromycin) were injected as bolus doses into the perfusate reservoir, yielding final concentrations of up to 1.8 mM. Viability was assessed by monitoring the liver perfusion rate, bile production rate, and rate of release of cytoplasmic lactate dehydrogenase (LDH, by method of Wacker et al, 1956) into the medium. Three hours after dosing, the livers were perfused in a single-pass mode with 100 ml K-H buffer followed by 60 ml of 3% glutaraldehyde in K-H buffer, then processed for transmission electron microscopy.

Cultured Hepatocytes
Male Sprague-Dawley rats, body weight 80-90 g, were used for isolation of hepatocytes. Rats were anesthetized with sodium pentabaritol, and livers were perfused with collagenase/hyaluronidase essentially as described by Elliget and Kolaja (1983). Monodispersed hepatocytes with a viability 97% were washed, then plated onto 35 mm^2 plastic dishes (Falcon Plastics) at a density of 10^5 cells/cm^2 in Leibovitz's L-15 medium prepared according to Elliget and Kolaja (1983) with 17% fetal bovine serum but without hydrocortisone. Cell monolayers were incubated at 37^0 C in an atmosphere of humidified 95% air/5% CO_2 for 24 h prior to drug treatment. The drugs were dissolved directly into medium at concentrations of 0.05, 0.10, and 0.50 mM. Cells were rinsed once with medium, then incubated with one ml of medium containing one of the five antibiotics. After 24 hours, media were removed from plates and assayed for LDH activity to assess plasma membrane injury (Jauregui et al, 1981). Activity was determined spectrophotometrically by monitoring the oxidation of NADH to NAD coupled to the reduction of pyruvate to lactate, as outlined in Sigma Chemical Company technical bulletin #340-UV (11-83). Monolayers were fixed with glutaraldehyde and processed for electron microscopy. Some plates were prepared for acid phosphatase cytochemistry using the method of Novikoff (1963), with lead nitrate as the capturing agent and B-glycerophosphate as the substrate.

RESULTS

Liver Perfusion

In control livers, bile production occurred at a rate of 1.4±0.2 ul/min/g wet weight, with a mean percent decrease of 22±4% over three hours (Fig. 1). Perfusion rate at a pressure of 12 inches of water was initially 2.45±0.35 ml/min/g liver wet weight, with a decrease of 11±2.5% over three hours (Fig. 2). LDH values were 2.08±0.28 (Table 1). Neither gentamicin nor trospectomycin sulfate significantly ($p<0.05$) affected bile production, perfusion rate or LDH levels at any concentration tested. By contrast, erythromycin significantly decreased bile production and increased LDH at the 0.1 mM concentration, and decreased perfusion rate at the 0.5 mM concentration.

Examination of perfused livers by electron microscopy revealed numerous cytoplasmic lamellar inclusion bodies in hepatocytes of livers perfused with 0.5 mM or greater trospectomycin sulfate (Fig. 3a). Erythromycin-treated samples showed areas of necrosis at higher concentrations, and secondary lysosomes were observed in all concentrations tested (Fig. 3b).

Hepatocyte Culture

The mean LDH value for media from control hepatocyte cultures was 91±34 (n=23). Of the antibiotic concentrations tested, only erythromycin at 0.50 mM showed a significant elevation above control levels ($p<0.05$; Fig. 4).

Light microscopic examination showed 0.50 mM erythromycin-treated cells to have a rounded morphology, with many cells detaching from the plates (not illustrated). Other cultures were indistinguishable from controls. Electron microscopic examination showed the 0.50 mM erythromycin-treated cells to be in various stages of degeneration. Cells at the 0.10 mM and 0.05 mM erythromycin levels had numerous cytoplasmic lamellar bodies and secondary lysosomes (Fig. 5a). Lamellar bodies were frequently observed in 0.50 mM trospectomycin sulfate (Fig. 5b), and less frequently observed at the 0.10 mM level. Similar structures were occasionally encountered in 0.50 mM gentamycin-treated cells. The lamellar bodies were positive for acid phosphatase activity (Fig. 6).

DISCUSSION

The potential of erythromycin to produce injury in the perfused liver over three hours is coincident with the appearance of secondary lysosomes, but not lamellar bodies. Longer exposure (24 hours) of hepatocytes in culture to erythromycin induced both secondary lysosomes and lamellar bodies, concurrent with membrane injury. The appearance of secondary lysosomes and lamellar bodies in our _in vitro_ experiments is consistent with _in vivo_ observations by Gray et al (1971), and cell injury data is similar to that obtained by Villa et al (1984, 1985). The ability of erythromycin to induce lamellar bodies in hepatocytes therefore appears to be secondary to cellular injury. Of the antibiotics tested, trospectomycin was the most potent inducer of lamellar bodies in both the perfused liver and the cultured hepatocyte models. In neither model, however, was this associated with cytotoxicity. The appearance of lamellar bodies, therefore, does not necessarily imply cellular injury.

The cellular origin of drug-induced lamellar bodies is thought to be the lysosome (Hruban, 1972; Lullmann-Rauch 1979), and acid phosphatase data from our experiments seem to support this hypothesis. Further experimentation is required, however, to determine if the lamellar body is formed from the lysosome, or if acid hydrolase activity is added after formation.

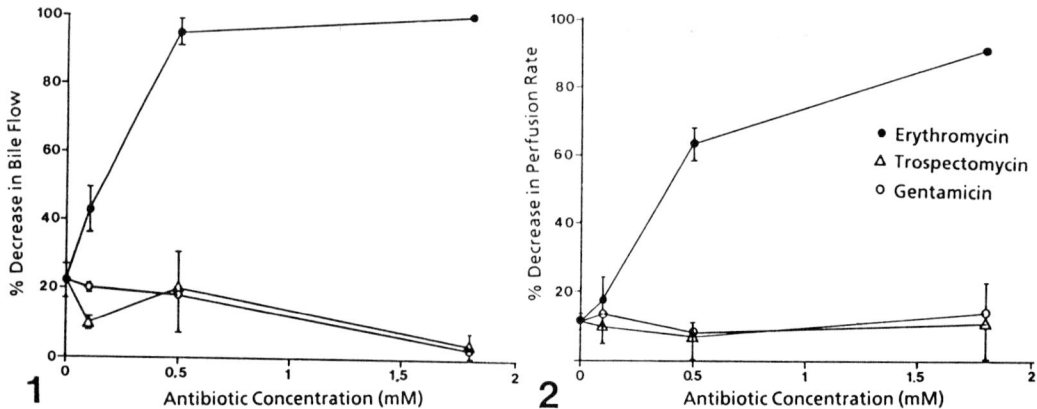

Figure 1. Percent decrease in production of bile in perfused livers after three hours as a function of antibiotic concentration. Brackets indicate range of 2-3 experiments.
Figure 2. Percent decrease in liver perfusion rate after three hours as a function of antibiotic concentration. Brackets indicate range of 2-3 experiments

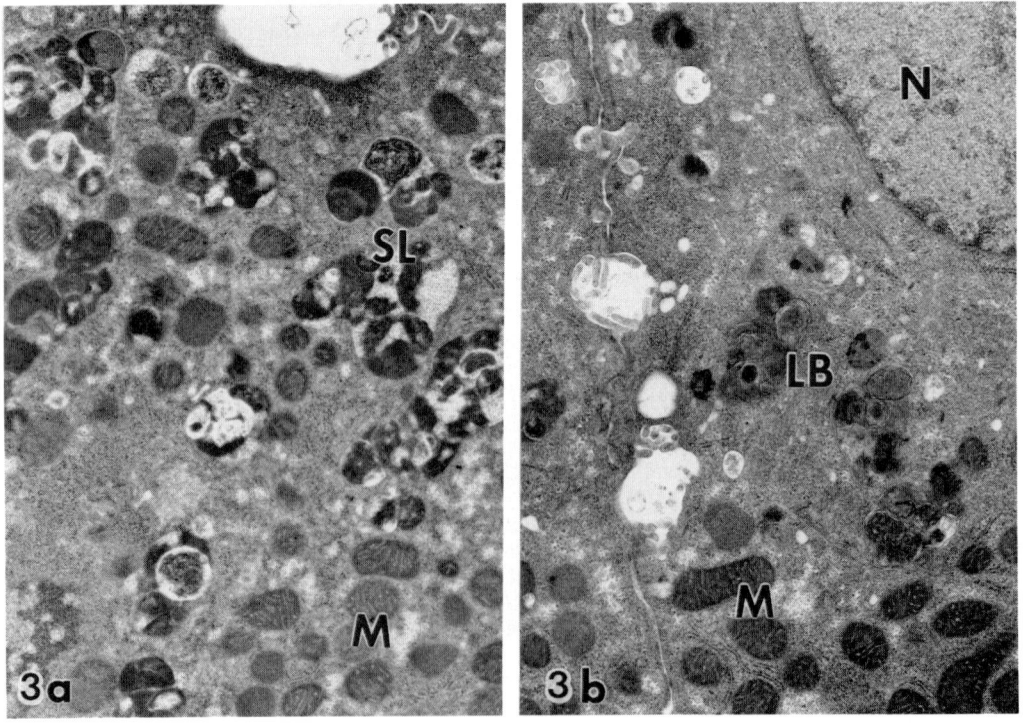

Figure 3. Transmission electron microscopy of (a) erythromycin (0.5 mM) and (b) trospectomycin sulfate (1.8 mM) perfused livers. LB=lamellar body, SL=secondary lysosome, N=nucleus, M=mitochondria.

Table 1. Effect of antibiotic treatment on the release of lactate dehydrogenase from the perfused rat liver.

Initial Antibiotic Concentration (mM)	LDH Release Rate (U/L/min)		
	Trospectomycin	Gentamicin	Erythromycin
0 (Control)		2.08 ± 0.28	
0.1	2.58 ± 1.26	2.17 ± 0.35	5.36 ± 1.51
0.5	3.10 ± 0.41	3.29 ± 0.64	25.9 ± * 1.1
1.8	1.81 ± 0.86	2.85 ± 0.76	53.1*

*Significantly different from the control value by Student's t-test ($P < 0.05$)

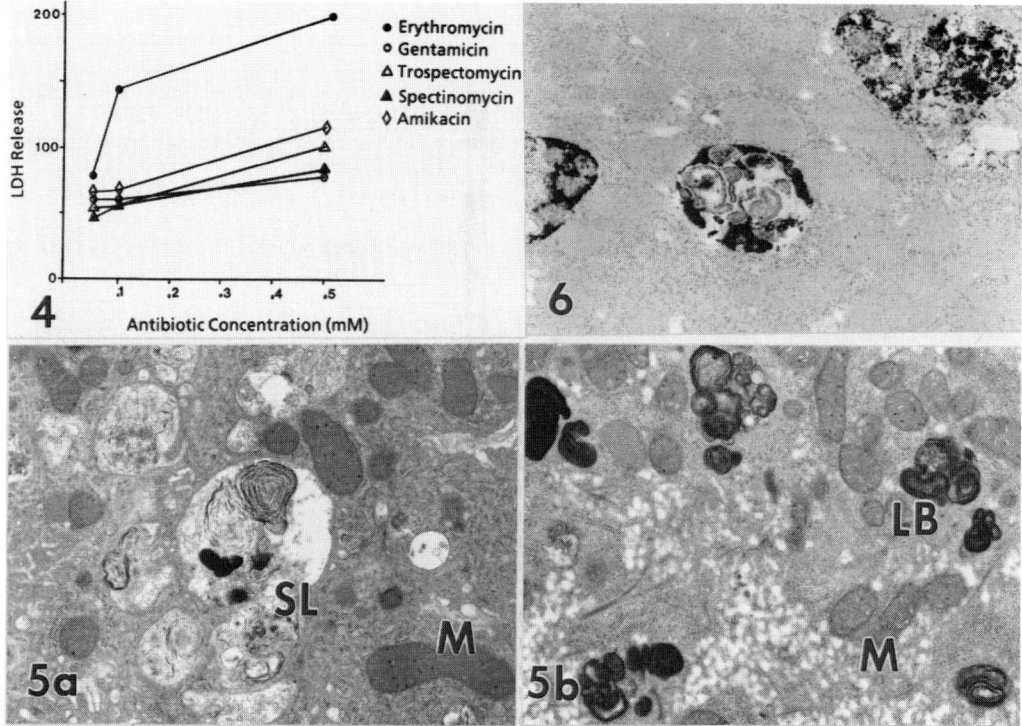

Figure 4. Mean media LDH Values from cultured hepatocytes after 24 hours as a function of concentration of the various antibiotics indicated.
Figure 5. Transmission electron microscopy of cultured hepatocytes treated for 24 hours with (a) 0.1 mM erythromycin or (b) 0.5 mM trospectomycin sulfate. LB=lamellar body, SL=secondary lysosome, N=Nucleus, M=mitochondria.
Figure 6. Transmission electron electron microscopy of Acid phosphatase cytochemistry shows the lamellar body to stain positive. Trospectomycin sulfate, 0.5 mM.

REFERENCES

Cox, J.W., S.R. Cox, G. VanGiessen and M.J. Ruwart. (1985): Ibuprofen stereoisomer hepatic clearance and distribution in normal and fatty in situ perfused rat liver. J. Pharmacol. Exp. Therap. 232, 636-643.

Elliget, K.A., and G.J. Kolaja. (1983): Preparation of primary cultures of rat hepatocytes suitable for in vitro toxicity testing. J. Tissue Cult. Methods 8, 1-6.

Gray, J.E., A. Purmalis, B. Purmalis and J. Mathews. (1971): Ultrastructural studies of the hepatic changes brought about by clindamycin and erythromycin in animals. Toxicol. Appl. Pharmacol. 19, 217-223.

Hruban, Z., A. Slesers and E. Hopkins. (1972): Drug induced and naturally occurring myeloid bodies. Lab. Invest. 27, 62-70.

Jauregui, H.O., N.T. Hayner, J.L. Driscoll, R.W. Holland, M.H. Lipski and P.M. Galletti. (1981): Trypan blue dye uptake and lactate dehydrogenase in adult rat hepatocytes - Freshly isolated cells, cell suspensions, and primary monolayer cultures. In Vitro 17, 1100-1110.

Lullmann-Rauch, R. (1979): Drug-induced lysosomal storage disorders. In Lysosomes in Applied Biology and Therapeutics, eds. Dingle, Jacques and Shaw, pp 49-130. New York: North-Holland Publishing Company.

Novikoff, A.B. (1963): Lysosomes in the physiology and pathology of cells: Contributions of staining methods. In Ciba Foundation Symposium on Lysosomes, eds. A.V.S. de Reuck and M.P. Cameron, pp 36-73. London: J. & A. Churchill, Ltd.

Villa, P., J.-M. Begue and A. Guillouzo. (1984): Effects of erythromycin derivatives on cultured rat hepatocytes. Biochem. Pharmacol. 33, 4098-4101.

Villa, P., J.-M. Begue and A. Guillouzo. (1985): Erythromycin toxicity in primary cultures of rat hepatocytes. Xenobiotica 15, 767-773.

Wacker, W., D. Ulmer and B. Vallee. (1956): Metalloenzymes and myocardial infarction, N. Engl. J. Med. 255, 449.

White, D.R., C. Maring and G. Cain, (1983): Synthesis and in vitro antibacterial properties of alkylspectinomycin analogs. J. Antibiotics 36, 339-342.

Effects of malotilate on human and rat hepatocytes in short-term and long-term primary culture

Bruno Clément, Jean-Maurice Dumont*, Damrong Ratanasavanh, Marie-France Latinier, Pierre Brissot, André Guillouzo.

*INSERM U.49, Unité de Recherches Hépatologiques, Rennes, France. *Zyma, Nyon, Suisse*

Keywords : hepatocytes, primary culture, human, rat, malotilate, collagen.

INTRODUCTION

Improvement of liver functions after acute induced hepatotoxicity or in various chronic liver diseases is a major concern of hepatologists. A number of substances have been proposed for their hepatoprotective effect but none of them has yet been found to have a wide efficient spectrum. Recently, several studies have suggested that malotilate (diiso propyl 1-3-dithiol-2-ylidenemalonate) may prevent acute experimental liver injury (Nakayama et al., 1978) as well as improve liver functions in chronic viral hepatitis and cirrhosis. The mechanism by which this compound acts is not clear. Prevention of hepatotoxicity by paracetamol has been related to an inhibition of the microsomal mixed function system (Younes and Siegers, 1985) but not the prevention of CCl_4-induced liver damage (Katoh et al., 1981 ; Katawa et al., 1982) and D-galactosamine liver injury, where metabolic activation does not take place (Dumont et al., 1987). Evidence has been provided that malotilate increased RNA and protein synthesis and augmented the nucleotide pool, particularly in injured liver (Imaizumi et al., 1982). Since this compound is efficient mainly when administered before the toxin in experimental models of acute liver injury, interest in it has been questioned. However, a semi-curative effect on liver functions and collagen accumulation has been demonstrated in rats already intoxicated by CCl_4 (Dumont et al., 1986) or egg yolk (Monna, 1986). In addition, malotilate has been reported to improve some liver functions and to decrease collagen deposition in chronic liver diseases (Igarashi et al., 1986) but this remains to be confirmed. To gain more information on the effects of malotilate on liver functions we decided to use both pure cultures and co-cultures of adult human and rat hepatocytes. These two model systems offer a unique opportunity to investigate malotilate effects since they represent culture conditions in which cell survival and liver functions are differently maintained (Guguen-Guillouzo et al., 1983 ; Clément et al., 1984).

MATERIAL AND METHODS

Cell isolation and culture.

Human hepatocytes were obtained from Kidney donors, aged from 20 to 30 years, most of whom died from traffic accidents and received little medication before kidney removal. No clinical pathology was observed in the liver of these donors. The cells were obtained by perfusion of the left hepatic lobe with collagenase, according to a method previously described (Guguen-Guillouzo et al., 1982). Freshly isolated hepatocytes were seeded at a density of 10^6 cells per 10 cm^2 plastic dish in 2 ml of Ham F_{12} containing 10 µg/ml bovine insulin, 0.2 % bovine serum albumin and 10 % fetal calf serum. The medium was renewed 6 to 12 h later. Co-cultures were set up by adding an equal density of rat liver epithelial cells (RLECs) in fresh medium (Clément et al., 1984). Cell confluency was reached within the following 24 h. After its first renewal the medium of both pure and co-culture was changed daily and supplemented with 7×10^{-5} M hydrocortisone hemisuccinate. Fetal calf serum was omitted.

Rat hepatocytes were isolated from 2-month-old male Sprague Dawley animals by perfusing the whole liver with collagenase (Guguen et al., 1975). Parenchymal cells were cultured in both pure and co-culture according to the conditions described for human hepatocytes. The first medium renewal occurred 4 h after hepatocyte seeding.

RLECs derived from 10-day-old Fisher rats by trypsinisation of the liver were co-cultured in Williams medium and used before transformation. These cells do not express specific liver functions (Morel-Chany et al., 1978).

Malotilate treatment.

Malotilate (MW : 288 daltons) was supplied by Zyma (Nyon, Switzerland). This compound was dissolved in 1,2 propanediol and added to the cultures in concentrations ranging from 5 to 200 µg/ml of medium (i.e. from 17.3 to 692 µM). The final concentration of the solvent did not exceed 1 %. The drug was added daily in serum-free medium either after 4 h (pure culture) or 48 h (co-culture) and every day thereafter.

Biochemical assays.

- Determination of lactate dehydrogenase leakage.

Lactate dehydrogenase (LDH) activity in the medium was determined by the method of Wroblevsky and Ladue (1965). Media were stored at -80°C until analysis.

- Measurement of albumin secretion rate.

Levels of secreted albumin were quantified by laser immunonephelometry as an index of specific liver function (Guguen-Guillouzo et al., 1983).

- ^3H-proline labeling.

Both collagen labeling and extraction were performed according to the procedure of Tseng et al. (1982) with slight modifications. At the beginning of the incubation time, the medium was renewed and supplemented with β-aminopropionitrile fumarate (100 µg/ml) and radiolabeled proline (1.6 µCi/ml of L-$[U-^{14}C]$ proline, 290 mCi/mmol, from Amersham U.K.). After 24 h, the medium was transferred at 4°C into a tube containing a protease inhibitor mixture (final concentrations : Tris 50 mM, pH 8, EDTA 20 mM ; phenylmethylsulfonyl fluoride (PMSF) 0.1 mM ; p-hydroxymercuribenzoate 1 mM ; N-ethylmaleimide 0.5 mM ; benzamidine 0.1 mM). The cell layer was washed with 1 ml of 0.1 M PBS containing 1 mM PMSF. The wash was added to the medium. The cell layer was washed twice again, then scraped in PBS-PMSF solution and centrifuged. Both medium and cell pellet were stored at -80°C until analysis.

Hydroxyproline content.

Cell pellets were suspended on ice in 1 ml of a solution containing 10 mM NaCl and 3 mM $MgCl_2$, then sonicated. Aliquots were stored at -20°C for total protein content determination. Trichloroacetic acid (TCA) and tannic acid were added to a final concentration of 5 % and 0.25 % respectively in both media and cell homogenates. Precipitates were collected by centrifugation and washed twice with 5 % TCA containing 1 mM cold proline. Pellets were dissolved in 0.5 N acetic acid containing pepstatin A (1 µg/ml) and vigourously stirred for 16 h at 4°C. After centrifugation, supernatants were collected and pellets were washed twice with 0.5 N acetic acid containing pepstatin A. Both washes and supernatants were combined into vials, lyophilized and dissolved in 6 N HCl. Samples were heated under vacuum at 110°C for 24 h. Hydrolysates were flushed with nitrogen, reconstitued with 1 ml of distilled water and filtered on 0.45 µm Millipore. Hydroxyproline and proline were eluted on a Dowex 50 W-X8 column as previously described (Cutroneo et al., 1972).

Assays of collagenase-sensitive proteins.
Media and homogenized cell layers were extensively dialyzed against 0.1 N acetic acid, then lyophilized and dissolved in 100 µl of 0.1 M Hepes pH 7.2 containing 2.5 mM N-ethylmaleimide and 0.5 mM $CaCl_2$. Fifty µl of each sample were incubated with purified bacterial collagenase (form III, Advanced Biofactures, Lynbrook, N.Y.) (Peterkofsky and Diegelmann, 1971).

RESULTS

Cell survival, morphology and albumin production.
Various concentrations of malotilate ranging from 10 to 100 µg/ml were tested on co-cultures of adult rat and human hepatocytes after confluency was reached. At 10 or 25 µg/ml, no obvious cell damage was visualized even after 3 weeks of daily treatment. Intracellular enlarged refringent spaces were observed within a few days and cell survival was not markedly different compared with controls. At 25 µg/ml, hepatocytes were less spread, they formed groups of more rounded cells. At 50 µg/ml, hepatocyte alterations were observed only after 3 or 4 days. At the concentration of 100 µg/ml, the drug was toxic within 24 h. Albumin production was not affected even after 2-3 weeks of daily treatment (Table I). In one experiment haptoglobin and hemopexin secretion rates were also determined in malotilate-treated rat hepatocyte co-cultures and found to be close to those found in control cultures (not shown).

TABLE I : SECRETION OF ALBUMIN BY HUMAN HEPATOCYTE CO-CULTURES WITHOUT OR WITH CONTINUOUS EXPOSURE TO MALOTILATE.

Treatment	Days of co-culture								
	3	4	7	9	10	11	13	14	15
None	6.8	11.2	22.2	19.0	20.4	11.0	14.0	16.4	12.2
Solvant	6.5	13.1	26.5	23.1	24.4	12.5	21.9	22.6	17.3
Malotilate (µg/ml) 5	5.5	9.3	21.8	18.1	24.4	18.5	16.6	21.1	15.7
10	6.9	21.2	24.9	21.3	29.2	17.6	21.1	25.0	21.6
25	5.3	12.8	16.9	17.6	21.0	13.5	16.3	18.5	13.8

The first drug addition was made 48 h after hepatocyte seeding. The values are expressed in µg albumin/ml of medium/24 h.

Protein synthesis.
Rat hepatocytes were incubated with labeled proline for 24 h, and formation of TCA precipitable radioactivity was measured in both culture medium and cell layer. No obvious effect of malotilate (25 µg/ml) on protein synthesis was observed in co-culture of rat hepatocytes, on days 3, 7 and 14 (Fig. 1). In contrast, in pure culture of both rat hepatocytes (day 3) and RLECs (day 7), secretion of labeled material was reduced by 25 % to 50 % in malotilate-treated cells, when compared with controls. The relative decrease of labeled proteins was identical in both media and cell layers.

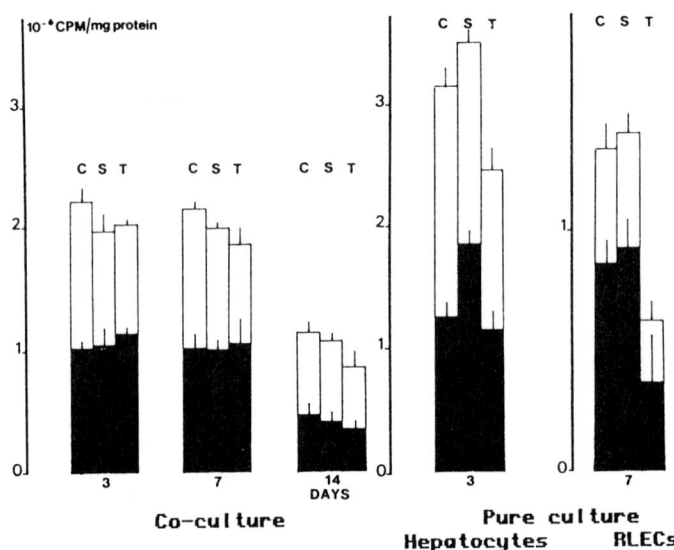

Figure 1 : Effect of malotilate on protein synthesis by rat hepatocytes and liver epithelial cells maintained in pure or in co-culture.
Media and cells were harvested after a 24 h incubation in the presence of ^{14}C-proline. The values of intracellular ■ and secreted ▢ proteins are expressed as cpm/mg cellular protein and are means of duplicate. (C : control culture ; S : solvent-treated culture ; T : malotilate-treated culture).

Collagen production
Collagen synthesis and secretion were estimated by formation of acetic-acid soluble material containing labeled hydroxyproline, and production of collagenase-sensitive labeled material in both pure and co-cultures of adult rat hepatocytes, in three independent experiments. Although quantitative differences were observed between each of them, the effect of 25 µg/ml malotilate was similar from one experiment to another. When compared to the values found in solvent-treated cells, malotilate slightly reduced hydroxyproline content in both media and cell layers from 3- and 7- days old co-culture. In 14 days old co-culture treated with malotilate this content was decreased by about 40 %. A comparable effect was found in 3 days old pure hepatocyte culture, while hydroxyproline content was 50 % reduced in 7 days old pure RLEC cultures treated with malotilate.

These results were confirmed by the determination of collagenase-sensitive material. Malotilate reduced collagenous material produced in co-culture, especially on day 3 and 7 (Table II). Its effect was enhanced in pure hepatocyte and RLEC cultures (not shown).

TABLE II: COLLAGENASE-SENSITIVE PROTEIN SYNTHESIS IN RAT HEPATOCYTE CO-CULTURES.

		Control	Solvent-treated cells	Malotilate-treated cells
Day 3	Medium	12666 ± 934	9933 ± 856	7759 ± 970
	Cell layer	1856 ± 642	1901 ± 430	1142 ± 263
	Total	14522 ± 1576	11834 ± 1286	8901 ± 1233
Day 7	Medium	6324 ± 749	5631 ± 873	3951 ± 732
	Cell layer	4005 ± 329	3412 ± 430	2631 ± 393
	Total	10329 ± 1078	9043 ± 1303	6582 ± 1125
Day 14	Medium	5027 ± 302	6128 ± 403	4997 ± 512
	Cell layer	2112 ± 124	2237 ± 226	2004 ± 129
	Total	7139 ± 426	8365 ± 629	7001 ± 641

Co-cultures of rat hepatocytes in 25 cm^2 flask were incubated with 4.8 µCi radiolabelled proline as described in the material section. Collagenase sensitive proteins were determined separately in both medium and cell layer according to the method of Peterkofsky and Diegelmann (1971). The data represent mean values ± SD of three individual cultures from a typical experiment.

DISCUSSION

The results reported here show that malotilate had no effect on both hepatocyte survival and plasma protein production. Since the same findings were observed whether this compound was added to hepatocyte cultures in the absence or presence of hydrocortisone which has been demonstrated to improve both cell survival and functions (not shown), the hepatoprotective effect of malotilate may be questioned. However, it must be taken into account that, in most cases, this drug showed the most convincing effects when administred before acute liver injury in experimental models (Katoh et al., 1981 ; Katawa et al., 1982).
A net decrease of protein synthesis demonstrated by incorporation of ^{14}C-proline was observed in pure cultures of both rat hepatocytes and liver epithelial cells. Since hydroxyproline content and collagenase-sensitive proteins were affected to a similar degree, it may be concluded that this inhibitory effect on protein synthesis concerned mainly collagenous proteins. This confirms studies by others with fibroblasts showing that malotilate inhibits collagen synthesis. Interestingly, no marked effect of malotilate was demonstrated in hepatocyte co-culture. It may be suggested that in this model the effect of malotilate on collagen production could be masked by the maintenance of active synthesis of specific hepatocyte proteins.

In summary, malotilate at a concentration which did not affect cell survival inhibits synthesis of collagenous proteins without benefit to specific liver functions.

REFERENCES.

Clément, B., Guguen-Guillouzo, C., Campion, J.P., Glaise, D., Bourel, M. and Guillouzo, A. (1984): Long-term co-cultures of adult human hepatocytes with rat liver epithelial cells : modulation of active albumin secretion and accumuulation of extracellular material. Hepatology 4, 373-380.

Cutroneo, K.R., Guzman, N.A. and Liebelt, G. (1972): Elevation of peptidylproline hydrolase activity and collagen synthesis in spontaneous primary mammary cancers of inbred mice. Cancer Res. 32, 2828-2833.

Dumont, J.M., Maignan, M.F., Janin, B., Herbage, D. and Perrissoud, D. (1986): Effect of malotilate on chronic liver injury induced by carbon tetrachloride in the rat. J. Hepatol. 3, 260-268.

Dumont, J.M., Maignan, M.F. and Perrissoud, D. Protective effect of malotilate against galactosamine intoxication in the rat. Arch. Int. Pharm. Ther., in press.

Guguen, C., Guillouzo, A., Boisnard, M., Le Cam, A. et Bourel, M. (1975): Etude ultrastructurale des hépatocytes de rat cultivés en monocouches en présence d'hémisuccinate d'hydrocortisone. Biol. Gastroenterol. 8, 223-231.

Guguen-Guillouzo, C., Campion, J.P., Brissot, P., Glaise, D., Launois, B., Bourel, M. and Guillouzo, A. (1982): High yield preparation of isolated human adult hepatocytes by enzymatic perfusion of the liver. Cell. Biol. Int. Rep. 6, 625-628.

Guguen-Guillouzo, C, Clément, B., Baffet, G., Beaumont, C., More-Chany, E., Glaise, D. and Guillouzo, A. (1983): Maintenance and reversibility of active albumin secretion by adult rat hepatocytes co-cultured with another liver epithelial cell type. Exp. Cell Res. 143, 147-54.

Igarashi, S., Hatahara, T., Nagai, Y., Hori, H., Sakakibara, K., Katoh, M., Sakai, A. and Sugimoto, T. (1986): Anti-fibrotic effect of malotilate on liver fibrosis induced by carbon tetrachloride in rats. Japan J. Exp. Med. 56, 235-245.

Imaizumi, Y., Katoh, M., Sugimoto, T. and Kasai, T. (1982): Effect of malotilate (diisopropyl 1,3-dithio-2-ylidenemalonate) on protein synthesis in rat liver. Japan J. Pharmacol. 32, 369-375.

Katawa, S., Sugiyama, T., Seki, K., Tarni, S., Okamoto, M. and Yamano, T. (1982): Stimulatory effect of cytochrome b_5 induced by p-nitroamisole and diisopropyl 1,3-dithio-2-ylidenemalonate on rat liver microsomal drug hydroxylations. J. Biochem. 92, 305-313.

Katoh, M., Kitada, M., Satoh, T., Kitagawa, H., Sugimoto, T. and Kasai, T. (1981): Further studies on the in vivo effect of diisopropyl 1,3-dithiol-2-ylidenemalonate (NKK-105) on the liver microsomal drug oxidation system in the rat. Biochem. Pharmacol. 30, 2759-2765.

Monna, T. (1983): Effect of malotilate on the experimental liver fibrosis (cirrhosis) induced by carbon tetrachloride or egg yolk sensitization. In Malotilate Proceedings of a symposium on Malotilate at the 7th World Congress of Gastroenterology. T. Ode and N. Tygstrup eds, pp. 44-53, Excerpta Medica, Amsterdam.

Morel-Chany, E, Guguen-Guillouzo, C., Trincal, G., Szajnert, M.F. (1978): Spontaneous neoplastic transformation in vitro of epithelial cell strains of rat liver : cytology, growth and enzymatic activities. Eur. J. Cancer 14, 1341-1352.

Nakayama, S., Kurimoto, M., Hajkamo, M., Kano, M. and Sakamoto, K. (1978): Pharmacological studies of diisopropyl 1,3-dithiol-2-ylidenemalonate (NKK-105), Report 2 : effects of NKK-105 on hepatic blood flow, bile flow and biliary components in dogs and rats. J. Med. Soc. Showa 38, 513-523.

Peterkofsky, B. and Diegelmann, R.F. (1971): Use of mixture of proteinase-free collagenases for the specific assay of radioactive collagen in the presence of other proteins. Biochemistry 10, 988-994.

Poeschl, A., Rehn, D., Dumont, J.M., Mueller, P.K. and Hennings, G. (1987): Malotilate reduces collagen synthesis and cell migration activity of fibroblasts in vitro. Biochem. Pharmacol. (in press).

Tseng, S.C.G., Lee, P.C, Ells, P.F., Bissell, D.M., Smuckler, E.A. and Stern, R. (1982): Collagen synthesis by rat hepatocytes and sinusoïdal cells in primary monolayer culture. Hepatology 2, 13-18.

Wroblevski, F. and Ladue, J.C. (1955): Lactic dehydrogenase in blood. Proc. Soc. Exp. Biol. 90, 210-214.

Younes, M. and Siegers, C.P.(1985): Effect of malotilate on paracetamol-induced hepatotoxicity. Toxicol. Lett. 25, 143-146.

Effect of DMSO on microsomal monooxygenase activities in cultured rat hepatocytes

Pia Villa*, Amalia Guaitani

Experimental Liver Toxicology Unit. Istituto di Ricerche Farmacologiche Mario Negri, Via Eritrea 62, 20157 Milan, Italy
*Scientist of the CNR (National Research Council) Center of cytopharmacology.

KEY-WORDS

DMSO, cultured rat hepatocytes, ethoxycoumarin deethylase, differentiation.

INTRODUCTION

Dimethylsulphoxide (DMSO) is a dipolar, aprotic, organic solvent which is active in biological systems (de la Torre, 1983). Addition of 1-2% (v/v) DMSO to the culture medium induces differentiation in rodent and human tumor cells (Friend et al.,1971; Collins et al.,1978), suppresses radiation-induced transformation in vitro (Kennedy and Symons,1987) and maintains differentiation in cultured rat hepatocytes (Isom et al.,1985). Induction of haem synthesis by DMSO in Friend virus-induced murine erythroleukemia cells (Beaumont et al.,1984) and hepatoma cells (Galbraith et al.,1986) has also been described. From previous work with rat hepatocytes the main problem is that with unsupplemented media the microsomal monooxygenase (MMO) activities decline rapidly in culture. It seems likely that under simple culture conditions requirements for specific regulation of MMO system or for preserving the normal differentiated state of hepatocytes are lacking. To date, the loss of cytochrome P-450-dependent MMO activities has been temporarily prevented by addition of a variety of compounds, such as hormones, ligands, haem precursors or by co-culture with another liver cell type (Guillouzo,1986).
The present study was undertaken to investigate the effect of DMSO on the MMO system in rat hepatocytes maintained for up to 3 days in primary culture. Ethoxycoumarin is a substrate oxidized by different species of cytochrome P-450, therefore its deethylation in intact cells was used as a convenient and sensitive assay of drug-metabolizing activity (Edwards et al.,1984).

MATERIALS and METHODS

Liver cell culture
Hepatocytes (0.85×10^6), prepared from male Crl:CD (SD)BR rats by perfusing the liver with a collagenase solution, were seeded in 1.5 ml medium (75% minimum essential medium and 25% medium 199 supplemented with 0.2% w/v bovine serum albumin, 0.1 mg/100 ml insulin and 5% foetal calf serum (F.C.S.) and buffered at pH 7.4 with bicarbonate). The medium, without F.C.S. and with 7×10^{-5} M hydrocortisone hemisuccinate, was renewed 3h, 24h and 48h after hepatocyte seeding.

Hydrocortisone was omitted 24h and 48h after plating when the cells were assayed for tyrosine aminotransferase induction.

Treatments
DMSO was added to the cells in concentrations ranging from 0.5% (0.07 M) to 2% (0.28 M) after 3h, 24h or 48h of culture and every 24h after the first treatment.

Assays
a) 7-Ethoxycoumarin deethylase (ECD) activity: the cells were incubated with Krebs-Henseleit buffer containing 7-ethoxycoumarin (7-EC) (final concentration 300 µM) for 30 min at 37°C. The enzymatic reaction was stopped by freezing cells plus supernatant medium. Thawed samples were homogenized for 30 sec with an Ultraturrax homogenizer, hydrolysed by β-glucuronidase/sulphatase treatment for 1h and the hydroxycoumarin produced was extracted with chloroform (Edwards et al., 1984). ECD assay was not affected by the presence of DMSO during the culture;
b) Tyrosine aminotransferase activity was assayed according to Granner and Tomkins (1970);
c) Protein synthesis: 72h after seeding, control and DMSO-treated cells were allowed to incorporate L-[U-^{14}C]leucine for 3h and trichloroacetic acid-insoluble material was prepared from the cells and the medium and its radioactivity was determined.
Statistical significance of the results was analyzed by Dunnett's test (1955).

RESULTS

Three days after plating, hepatocytes, fed a chemically defined medium with no F.C.S. and supplemented with 2% (v/v) DMSO, formed a monolayer with improved morphology (well defined borders and clearer clefts between adjacent hepatocytes) compared with untreated cells, as already described by Isom et al. (1985).
A well-accepted expression of differentiated liver cell function is the ability of hepatocytes to induce liver specific enzymes such as tyrosine aminotransferase (TAT) in response to hormones. In agreement with previous reports (Miyazaki et al., 1985), the basal intracellular level of TAT activity and its induction rate by glucocorticoids declined with time in culture (Table 1). Addition of 2% DMSO kept the initial basal TAT activity after 3 days of culture and it was synergistic with dexamethasone in induction of this enzyme (Table 1).

Table 1. Effect of DMSO on the induction of tyrosine aminotransferase (TAT) in cultured rat hepatocytes.

Treatment	Time in culture (hours)	TAT activity (mU/mg protein)	(%)[d]
None	0	15.39 ± 0.99	
None	24	10.16 ± 0.65°	100
Dexamethasone 10^{-7} M [a]	24	46.91 ± 1.29°	462
None	72	8.57 ± 0.56°	100
DMSO 2% [c]	72	16.23 ± 0.52	189
Dexamethasone 10^{-7} M [b]	72	22.58 ± 1.45°	263
DMSO 2% [c] + Dexamethasone 10^{-7} M [b]	72	57.31 ± 0.52°	669

[a,b] Dexamethasone was added 3h (a) and 48h (b) after hepatocyte seeding.
[c] DMSO was added 24h and 48h after hepatocyte seeding.
[d] Enzyme activity is expressed as a percentage of that in untreated cells at the same times of culture.
° $p<0.01$ vs. fresh isolated cells.

The effects of different concentrations of DMSO on MMO activities were evaluated
during 3 days of culture (Fig. 1). In untreated cells ECD activity declined during
culture and 72h after seeding only 30% of the initial activity remained, in
agreement with previous results (Guillouzo, 1986). The concentration of 0.5% DMSO,
added 3 or 24h after seeding and every 24h after the first treatment, maintained
the initial ECD activity throughout culture. Higher concentrations of DMSO were
also added 3, 24 or 48h after hepatocyte plating. Immediately after attachment,
monolayers were relatively unresponsive during the first 24h of exposure to DMSO,
as already shown for other inducers (Edwards et al.,1984). Repeated treatment with
1 and 2% DMSO induced 2-3 times more 72h-ECD compared with the initial activity
($p<0.01$) (Fig. 1).

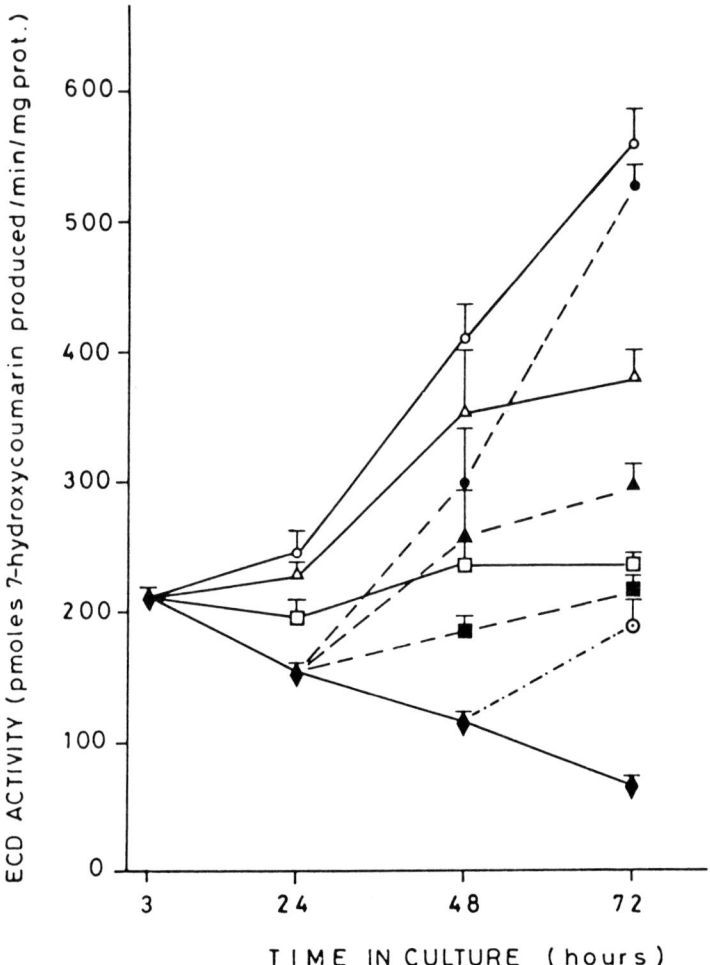

Fig. 1: Time- and dose-dependent effects of DMSO on ECD activity in cultured rat
hepatocytes. DMSO was added to the cells at different concentrations
(0.5%□—□,■- -■; 1%△—△,▲--▲; 2%O—O,●--●,O-·-O) after 3h (□—□,
△—△, O—O), 24h (■- -■,▲--▲,●--●) and 48h (O-·-O) of culture and
every 24h after the first treatment.
◆—◆ECD activity in untreated cells.
The results are means ± S.E. of 4-5 different hepatocyte preparations.

The increased ECD activity and the higher TAT induction did not reflect a more general effect of DMSO on protein synthesis because the incorporation of $[^{14}C]$-leucine into total cellular protein was the same in DMSO-treated as in control cells after 3 days of culture (data not shown). DMSO-mediated increase in ECD activity required de novo protein synthesis: incubation of 24h-cultured rat hepatocytes with DMSO and cycloheximide, at a concentration which inhibited general protein synthesis by 90%, abolished the response to DMSO (Table 2).

Table 2. Effect of cycloheximide on ethoxycoumarin deethylase (ECD) activity in control and DMSO-treated rat hepatocytes in primary culture.

Treatment	Time in culture (hours)	ECD activity (pmoles hydroxycoumarin/min/mg prot.)
None	24	156 ± 5
None	48	103 ± 6 +
Cycloheximide 2.5 µM	48	90 ± 3°
DMSO 1%	48	263 ± 23°
DMSO 1% + Cycloheximide 2.5 µM	48	177 ± 6

+ $p < 0.05$ and ° $p < 0.01$ vs. untreated hepatocytes after 24h of culture.

Different cytochromes P-450 have been described and the two main forms are those induced by barbiturates (e.g. phenobarbital -PB) and polycyclic aromatic hydrocarbons (e.g. 3-methylcholanthrene -3-MC) (Fry et al.,1980). Inhibitors selective for either PB-inducible (metyrapone -MET) or 3-MC-inducible (diphenyloxazole -PPO) haemoproteins were then used to study the characteristics of the MMO activities induced by DMSO (Fig. 2).

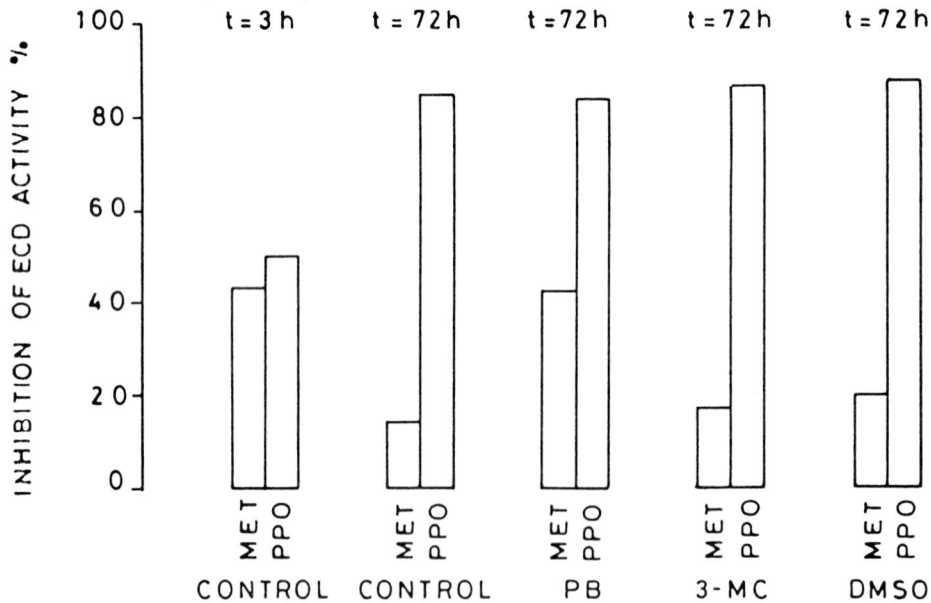

Fig. 2: Effects of two inhibitors on ECD activity in control and induced cultured hepatocytes. The cells were assayed for ECD activity in the absence and presence of the inhibitors MET or PPO as described by Fry et al. (1980). The inducers (2mM PB, 3µM 3-MC and 2% DMSO) were added 24 and 48h after seeding. The results are means of 3 different experiments.

In agreement with previous results (Fry et al.,1980) throughout the first 3 days of culture there is a gradual shift in the types of haemoprotein present. At the beginning of the culture PB- and 3-MC-inducible cytochromes P-450 are present in approximately equal catalytic amounts, but during the culture period there is a decrease in the PB-P-450 with a concomitant increase in the 3-MC-P-450 form, confirming different in vitro stability of cytochrome P-450 subspecies (Guillouzo, 1986). PB-treatment induced the normal P-450 even against a high background of the 3-MC P-450 form and treatment with 2% DMSO induced the P-450 form comparable to that induced by 3-MC, which in culture appears to be the most stable and most easily inducible cytochrome P-450 subspecies (Fig. 2).

DISCUSSION

A broad spectrum of effects induced by DMSO in biological systems has been described (Friend and Freedman,1978) but how the multiple properties of this chemical affect differentiation must yet be explained (Kennedy and Symons,1987). Our data extend previous results on the maintenance of differentiated cultured rat hepatocytes (Isom et al.,1985): a liver-specific function, such as TAT induction by dexamethasone, is well maintained by 2 days' exposure to DMSO and the monooxygenase activities, which decline rapidly in culture, are maintained and induced depending on DMSO concentration. It must still be determined whether DMSO's effect on the MMO system reflects a greater differentiation of the hepatocytes or a specific activity of DMSO on haem synthesis. Some monooxygenase inducers, like PB, have also been described as supporting long-term survival of functional hepatocytes in primary culture while others, like 3-MC, were ineffective (Miyazaki et al.,1985). Therefore it seems unlikely that intracellular increases of detoxifying enzymes in hepatocytes enable them to survive longer in culture. The interaction with cell membrane function seems a very important factor in the maintenance or induction of differentiation by PB (Miyazaki et al.,1985) and especially by DMSO which affects ion fluxes and membrane permeability and fluidity (Friend and Freedman,1978). DMSO is also a powerful scavenger of hydroxyl radicals (Cederbaum et al.,1977) and this may be an additional property contributing to its effect on the MMO system; the use of other substances with a different ability to scavenge free radicals could shed further light on the matter.
In conclusion these preliminary data suggest that DMSO, by regulating drug-metabolizing activities, could be a useful new tool for studying the regulatory factors of cytochrome P-450 maintenance in cultured rat hepatocytes.

ACKNOWLEDGMENTS

We thank Patrizia Arioli for her technical assistance.
This work was supported by the CNR (National Research Council, Rome, Italy), Special Project Oncology No. 86.02681.44.

REFERENCES

Beaumont, C., Deybach J.C, Grandchamp B., Da Silva V., De Verneuil H., Nordmann Y. (1984): Effects of succinylacetone on dimethylsulfoxide-mediated induction of heme pathway enzymes in mouse Friend virus-transformed erythroleukemia cells. Expl. Cell Res. 154, 474-484.
Cederbaum, A.I., Dicker E., Rubin E., Cohen G. (1977): The effect of dimethyl-sulfoxide and other hydroxyl radical scavengers on the oxidation of ethanol by rat liver microsomes. Bioch. biophys. Res. Comm. 78, 1254-1262.
Collins, S.J., Ruscetti F.W., Gallagher R.E., Gallo R.C. (1978): Terminal differentiation of human promyelocytic leukemia cells induced by dimethyl sulfoxide and other polar compounds. Proc. natn. Acad. Sci. USA. 75, 2458-62.

de la Torre, J.C., ed. (1983): Biological actions and medical applications of dimethyl sulfoxide. Ann. N. Y. Acad. Sci. 411, 1-404.

Dunnett, C.W. (1955): A multiple comparison procedure for comparing several treatments with control. J. Am. statist. Assoc. 50, 1096-1121.

Edwards, A.M., Glistak M.L., Lucas C.M., Wilson P.A. (1984): 7-Ethoxycoumarin deethylase activity as a convenient measure of liver drug metabolizing enzymes: regulation in cultured rat hepatocytes. Biochem. Pharmac. 33, 1537-1546.

Friend, C, Scher W., Holland J.C., Sato T. (1971): Hemoglobin synthesis in murine virus-induced leukemic cells in vitro: Stimulation of erythroid differentiation by dimethyl sulfoxide. Proc. natn. Acad. Sci. U.S.A. 68, 378-382.

Friend, C., Freedman H.A. (1978): Effects and possible mechanism of action of dimethylsulfoxide on Friend cell differentiation. Biochem. Pharmac. 27, 1309-1313.

Fry, J.R., Wiebkin P., Bridges J.W. (1980): 7-Ethoxycoumarin O-deethylase induction by phenobarbitone and 1,2-benzanthracene in primary maintenance cultures of adult rat hepatocytes. Biochem. Pharmac. 29, 577-581.

Galbraith, R.A., Sassa S., Kappas A. (1986): Induction of haem synthesis in Hep G2 human hepatoma cells by dimethyl sulphoxide. A transcriptionally activated event. Biochem. J. 237, 597-600.

Granner, D.K., Tomkins G.M. (1970): Tyrosine aminotransferase (rat liver). Meth. Enzym. 7A, 633-637.

Guillouzo, A. (1986): Use of isolated and cultured hepatocytes for xenobiotic metabolism and cytotoxicity studies. In Isolated and cultured hepatocytes, eds. A. Guillouzo & C. Guguen-Guillouzo, pp. 313-332. London, Libbey Eurotext.

Isom, H.C., Secott T., Georgoff I., Woodworth C., Mummaw J. (1985): Maintenance of differentiated rat hepatocytes in primary culture. Proc. natn. Acad. Sci. U.S.A. 82, 3252-3256.

Kennedy, A.R., Symons M.C.R. (1987): 'Water Structure' versus 'Radical Scavenger' theories as explanations for the suppressive effects of DMSO and related compounds on radiation-induced transformation in vitro. Carcinogenesis 8, 683-688.

Miyazaki, M., Handa Y., Oda M., Yabe T., Miyano K., Sato J. (1985): Long-term survival of functional hepatocytes from adult rat in the presence of phenobarbital in primary culture. Expl. Cell Res. 159, 176-190.

The influence of polycyclic aromatic hydrocarbons on the morphology and the cytochrome P-450 enzyme expression in cultured hepatocytes

Dieter Müller-Enoch, Gianna Vergani*, Thomas Nagenrauft

*Departments of Physiol. Chemistry and *Anatomy, University of Ulm, D-7900 Ulm, FRG*

KEYWORDS

Liver parenchymal cells, normal rat liver, hepatoma cells, morphology, P-450 levels.

INTRODUCTION

Primary culture of liver parenchymal cells has become important in studying the biotransformation, cytotoxicity, and genotoxicity of xenobiotics. Therefore we studied the influence of the polycyclic aromatic hydrocarbons, 3-MC and BP on the morphology and on the P-450 enzyme pattern in cell cultures grown as monolayers of normal rat liver parenchymal cells and in the well differentiated rat hepatoma clonal strain MH_1C_1, originally derived from the 7795 Morris hepatoma.

MATERIALS AND METHODS

<u>Chemicals:</u> Chemicals and biochemicals of the highest purity available were usually obtained from E. Merck (Darmstadt, FRG) and Boehringer Mannheim (Mannheim, FRG). 3-Methylcholanthrene (3-MC) and benzo(a)pyrene (BP) were purchased from Sigma Chemie (München, FRG). Dimethylsulphoxide (DMSO) were from E. Merck (Darmstadt, FRG).

<u>Primary Monolayer Cultures of liver parenchymal cells:</u> Rat liver parenchymal cells were prepared from a twenty days old SIV 50 Rat (SAVO Kisslegg, FRG) according to Vergani <u>et al</u>. (1979). The MH_1C_1 hepatoma cell line used in this study were purchased from the Flow Laboratories (Irvine, Scotland, UK).

All cells were cultured in Ham's F-10 medium (Biochrom, West Berlin) supplemented with 10 % fetal calf serum in a CO_2-incubator in NUNC Flasks (NUNC, Roskilde, DK) at 37°C. The medium was changed every two days.

The morphology of the cells were examined by scanning electron microscopy (SEM). Cells grown on cover slids were rinsed with warmed PBS (Phosphate buffered saline after Dulbecco) under microscopical control, to remove the culture medium. Fixation was carried out at 37°C for 0.5 to 2 hours in a 3.5 % glutaraldehyde dissolved in 0.1 M phosphate buffer with 2 % sucrose, pH 7.3. After a brief rinse of double destilled water, the cells were dehydrated in a Peters exchange apparatus (Hert, München, FRG) and transferred to dimethoxipropane according to Muller and Jacks (1975). After the critical-point-drying in CO_2, the cells were spattered with 10 nm gold and examined in a Philips PSEM 500 according to Vergani and Frösch (1987).

Cell treatment with 3-methylcholanthrene, benzo(a)pyrene and dimethylsulfoxide: Cells after eight days of culture were treated with 3-MC dissolved in DMSO, with BP dissolved in DMSO or with DMSO alone, the final concentrations of 3-MC and BP were 10 µM and for DMSO 0.25 % (v/v). The effect of the compounds used, on the morphology of the cells was evaluated after 24 h.

P-450 enzymes and antibodies: All materials used for the purification procedure of P-450 enzymes and all other reagents for gel electrophoresis and immunoquantification of the P-450 forms were performed by Western Blots as described by Guengerich et al. (1982) and Müller-Enoch et al. (1985). The cytochrome $P-450_{BNF-B}$, $P-450_{ISF-G}$, $P-450_{UT-A}$ and $P-450_{PB/PCN-E}$ enzymes were isolated from mal Sprague-Dawley rats. Antibodies to thes P-450 enzymes were raised in female New Zealand White Rabbits. These antibodies were used to characterize and to quantitate the P-450 enzymes in the cells after separation on SDS-Page and blotting on nitrocellulose.

RESULTS AND DISCUSSION

The morphology of the cells were examined by SEM. Figure 1 shows the SEM-picture of cells from normal rats without treatment. These cells have a polygonal shape, epithelial-like form, microvilli and filopodia. After 24 h culture with DMSO, the cells lose their contact with neighborning cells and have more microvilli and less filopodia (Fig. 2). Figure 3 shows the SEM-picture of the same cells, treated with benzo(a)pyrene for 24 hours. The cells have very few microvilli, sparely filopodia and are greater than the untreated cells.

Figure 1a shows the SEM-picture of the MH_1C_1 cells as control, they have epithelial-like form, microvilli and filopodia and are comparable to the isolated liver epithelial cells of normal rats (Fig. 1). After 24 h culture with DMSO the cells show blebs, long filopodia (Fig. 2a) and Morris cells treated with 3-MC for 24 h exhibit more blebs and are smaller compared to control and to DMSO-treated MH_1C_1. It should be noted here, that the Morris cells are very fragile.

SDS-polyacrylamid gel electrophoresis of solubilized cells of normal rats and of MH_1C_1 hepatoma cells grown as monolayers for eight day, and treated with BP and DMSO for six more days, show only faint protein bands at about M_r = 50.000 Dalton for normal cells. But with MH_1C_1-cells which are exposed to 3-MC under the same conditions used for the normal cells, a pattern of protein bands with apparent monomeric molecular weights from 49000-55000 Dalton are well detectable.

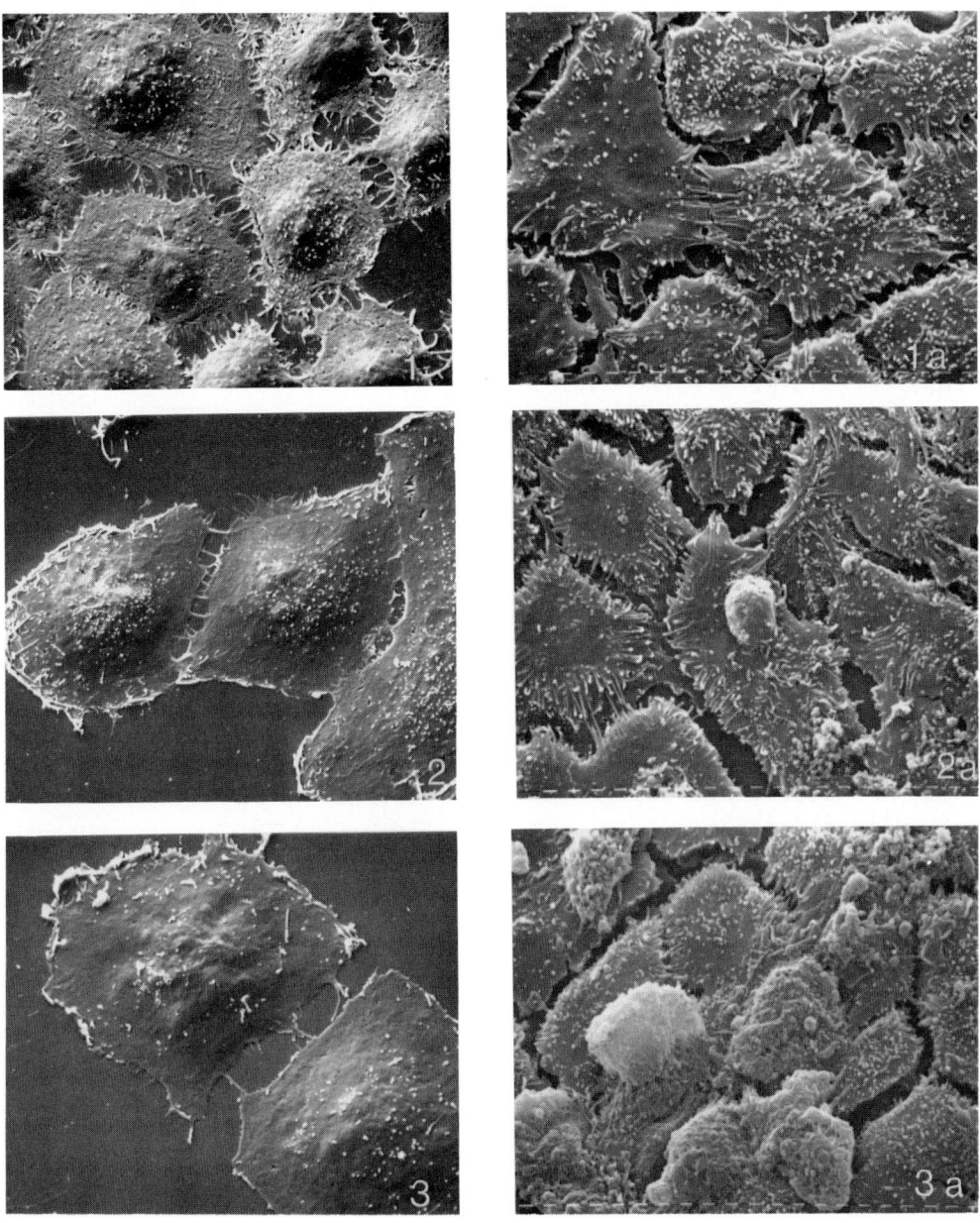

Fig. 1-3 show SEM-pictures of normal rat parenchymal cells. x 1750
Fig. 1 control medium, Fig. 2 medium with DMSO
Fig. 3 medium with 3-MC
Fig. 1a-3a show SEM-pictures of Morris cells. x 3500
Fig. 1a control medium, Fig. 2a medium with DMSO
Fig. 3 medium with 3-MC

Table 1. Immunochemical quantitation of P-450 enzymes in Liver Parenchymal Cell Cultures of Normal and of Morris Hepatoma (MH_1C_1) rats.

Cell Cultures	Treatment	spec. content of pmol P-450/mg Protein	
		$P-450_{BNF-B}$	$P-450_{ISF-G}$, $P-450_{UT-A}$, $P-450_{PB/PCN-E}$
Normal	-	-	-
Normal	DMSO	<5	-
Normal	3-MC	7	-
Normal	BP	6	-
MH_1C_1	-	12	-
MH_1C_1	DMSO	15	-
MH_1C_1	3-MC	105	-
MH_1C_1	BP	70	-

Electrophoresis, transfer, staining, and densitometry of P-450 enzymes were carried out with 40 µg of rat liver cell protein or 0.5-4 pmol of purified P-450 per well. All values represent of at least two determinations. A standard curve was prepared on each nitrocellulose sheet.
Abbreviations: ßNF, ß-naphthoflavone; ISF, isosafrole; UT, untreated; PB, phenobarbital; PCN, pregnenolone-16α-carbonitrile.

The characterisation of the individual P-450 enzymes in the cells (normal and MH_1C_1) was performe by Western Blots, which show no immunochemical detection of the P-450 enzymes $P-450_{UT-A}$, and $P-450_{PB/PCN-E}$, which are the major P-450 forms in liver microsomal fractions of untreated rats. But in normal and Morris cells, which were exposed to 3-MC and BP, the $P-450_{BNF-B}$ enzyme was well detectable.

The quantitation of individual P-450 forms in the cells can be done by immunoblot techniques of electrophoretically separated cellular proteins. The measurement of the amount of a given form of P-450 is performed by comparing the staining intensities of an unknown sample to a standard curve developed with known quantities of the purified P-450 proteins (Guengerich et al. 1982, Müller-Enoch et al. 1985). Table 1 shows the results of the immunochemical quantitation of the P-450 enzymes. There are no detectable amounts of $P-450_{ISF-G}$, $P-450_{UT-A}$ or $P-450_{PB/PCN-E}$, but there are 100 and 70 pmol/mg protein of $P-450_{BNF-B}$ in the Morris MH_1C_1 cells, treated with 3-MC or BP, respectively.

The results presented here show, that 3-MC- or BP-treatment of rat liver parenchymal cells, have an influence on the morphology of the cells and of the expression of the P-450$_{\beta NF-B}$, which is enhanced up to 15-fold in 3-MC- treated MH$_1$C$_1$ hepatoma cells compared to 3-MC-treated parenchymal cells of normal rats.

REFERENCES

Guengerich, F.P., Wang, P., and Davidson, N.K. (1982): Estimation of multiple forms of microsomal cytochrome P-450 in rats, rabbits, and humans using immunochemical staining coupled with sodium dodecyl sulfate-polyacrylamide gel electrophoresis. Biochemistry, 21: 1698-1706.

Muller, L.L., Jacks, T.J. (1975). Rapid chemical dehydration of samples for electron microscopic examination. J. Histochem. Cytochem. 23: 107-110.

Müller-Enoch, D., Dannan, G.A., Rudolf, B., and Friedl, H.-P. (1985): Induction of cytochrome P-450 isozymes in liver microsomes of rats treated with the cardiotonic agent sulmazole. Arzneim.-Forsch./Drug Res. 35: 698-703.

Vergani, G., Pentz, S., and Herrmann, M. (1979): Effects of sera from scalded rats on epithelial liver cells in vitro. Virchows Arch. B Cell Path. 31, 31-35, 1979.

Vergani, G., Frösch, D. (1987): Morphologie epitheloider Rattenleberzellen in Kultur. Verh. Anat. Ges., in press.

Expression of glutathione S-transferase isoenzymes in cultured and co-cultured rat hepatocytes

Yves Vandenberghe, Veerle Seneca, Antoine Vercruysse, André Guillouzo*, Brian Ketterer**

Dept. Toxicology, Free University Brussels, Brussels, Belgium.
*INSERM U.49, Rennes, France. **Courtauld Institute of Biochemistry, University of London, London, UK

KEYWORDS

Rat hepatocytes, culture, glutathione S-transferase, isoenzymes, subunit separation.

INTRODUCTION

In order to evaluate the use of cultured hepatocytes as an in vitro model for pharmaco-toxicological studies, phase I oxidation-reduction reactions have been widely studied in culture under different conditions. (Guzelian, 1977; Dickins, 1980; Edwards, 1984). Much less, however, is known about the behaviour of phase II reactions such as glutathione conjugation, in cultured hepatocytes.

Glutathione S-transferase (GST) plays an important role in the protection of cells against toxic and carcinogenic substances. In rat, 7 homodimers and 4 heterodimers have been identified and characterized (Ketterer, 1986a). For the liver, until now, 9 isoenzymes have been described, all having a different activity towards known substrates, of which 1-chloro-2,4-dinitrobenzene (CDNB) is the most commonly used (Ketterer, 1986a).

In previous work, the GST activity has been measured in rat hepatocytes cultured under different conditions (Vandenberghe, 1987). The changes observed suggest variations in GST content as well as changes in the isoenzymic composition. In order to detect these variations, we have purified and separated GST isoenzymes from conventional and co-cultured rat hepatocytes, from whole liver and from freshly isolated cells. These results are presented here.

MATERIALS AND METHODS
Cell isolation and culture
Adult hepatocytes were isolated from 2-month-old Sprague-Dawley rats as described previously (Vandenberghe, 1987). They were seeded at a density of 10×10^6 cells for 175 cm^2 flasks. The cell culture medium consisted of 75% minimal essential medium and 25% medium 199, containing 200 µg/ml bovine serum albumin, 10 µg/ml bovine insulin and 10% foetal calf serum (standard medium). 4 hours after seeding, the medium was renewed and 7×10^{-5}M hydrocortisone hemisuccinate was

added to the medium during the whole culture period. Two modifications of the standard medium (St.) were tested : foetal calf serum-free standard medium (St-FCS) and foetal calf serum-free standard medium containing 25 mM nicotinamide (St-FCS + Nic.). Co-cultures were set up as previously described (Vandenberghe, 1987). Cells were harvested after 4 days of culture. The pellets were stored at -80°C until analysis.

GST assay
GST activity was determined spectrophotometrically according to Habig (1974).

Purification of GST isoenzymes and HPLC analysis
For the purification of GST isoenzymes, cells were homogenized in 22 mM phosphate buffer pH 7.0 containing 1.15% KCl, 1 mM ethylenediaminetetra acetic acid and 0.25 mM phenylmethylsulfonylfluoride. The homogenized suspension was centrifuged for 1 hour at 105.000 g. The supernatant was loaded on a GSH affinity column packed with epoxy activated sepharose 6B reacted with glutathione. The GST fraction was eluted with a solution containing 5 mM glutathione and 50 mM Tris (pH 9.1 at room temperature). The collected samples were used for HPLC analysis.

The HPLC was carried out using a 10 x 0.8 cm waters µ Bondapak C-18 reversed phase column in a Z module. The solvents were water (A) and 0.1% trifluoro acetic acid in acetonitrile (B). The samples were injected at 35% B. During a run a linear gradient was used from 35% to 55% B over 60 min. with a flow rate of 15 ml min^{-1}. Detection was carried out at 214 nm.

GST subunits, separated by HPLC, were identified by comparing their retention time with those from purified GST.

Proteins were determined using the Bio-Rad protein assay with bovine serum albumin as a standard.

RESULTS

1. GST activity of cenventional and co-cultured rat hepatocytes towards CDNB
Figs. 1 and 2 show the GST activity of conventional and co-cultured rat hepatocytes respectively. The values for whole liver and freshly isolated hepatocytes

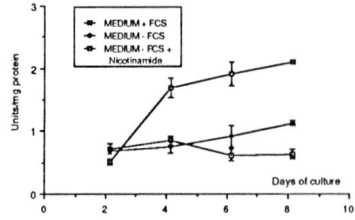
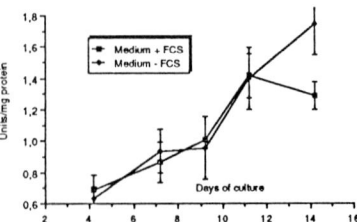

Fig. 1. Conventional culture   Fig. 2. Co-culture
GST activities towards CDNB
FCS : foetal calf serum; each point represents the mean ± S.E. of three to five independent experiments in duplicate or triplicate.

are 1.08 ± 0.046 and 1.05 ± 0.05 Units . mg protein^{-1} respectively. Epithelial cells used for co-culture have an activity of 0.17 to 0.28 Units . mg protein^{-1}.

2. GST subunit composition

The subunit composition of whole liver (Fig. 3A) and freshly isolated hepatocytes (Fig. 3B) show only slight differences. Once in culture, changes occur. In general, under all culture conditions studied here (Figs. 4A, 4B, 4C, 5A and 5B) the amounts of subunits 1 and 2 decrease and 4, but especially 3 increase. New is the expression of subunit 7.

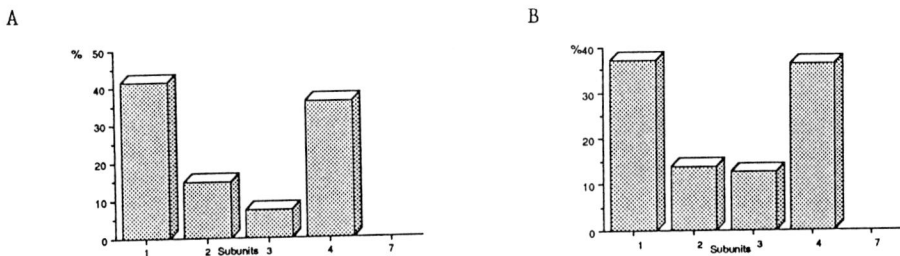

Fig. 3. GST subunit composition of whole liver (A) and freshly isolated hepatocytes (B) after HPLC separation. Results are expressed in % of total amount.

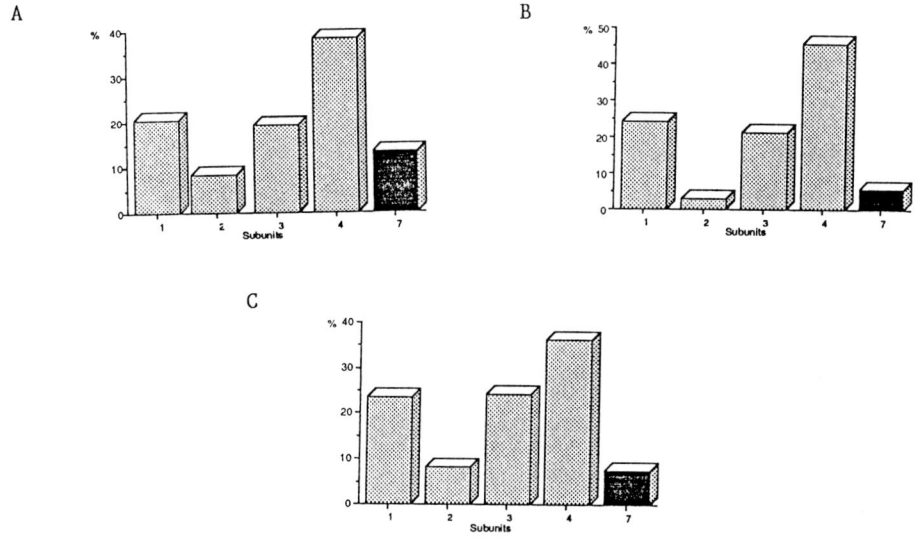

Fig. 4. GST subunit composition of 4 days conventional cultured rat hepatocytes in standard medium (A) and foetal calf serum free standard medium (B) and foetal calf serum free standard medium with nicotinamide (C).
Each point represents a mixture of 10 dishes of 10 x 10^6 hepatocytes.
Results are expressed in % of total amount.

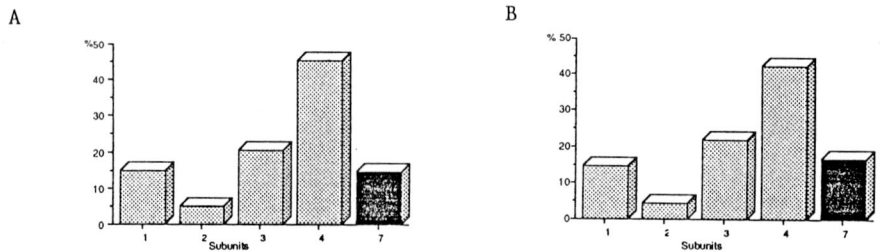

Fig. 5. GST subunit composition of 4 days co-cultured rat hepatocytes in standard medium (A) and foetal calf serum free standard medium (B). Each point represents a mixture of 10 dishes of 10×10^6 hepatocytes. Results are expressed in % of total amount.

DISCUSSION

The GST activity measurement, with CDNB as substrate, in cultured rat hepatocytes are characterized by an initial decrease during the first days of culture. This could be explained by the loss of subunits 1 and 2. The expression of subunit 7, probably isoenzyme 7-7, gives only a small compensation as far as the activity measurements are concerned, since isoenzyme 7-7 is less active towards CDNB than are 1-1 and 2-2 (Ketterer, 1986b).

The higher activity observed for hepatocytes cultured in the presence of nicotinamide could be due to the better maintenance of subunit 1 and the increase of subunit 3.

The major finding of this study is the expression of subunit 7 in culture. Its presence has, so far, never been described in mature liver. It is a known marker of kidney and primary hepatoma (Ketterer, 1986b), but it is completely absent in fetal liver. Since a primary hepatoma is also marked by low amounts of isoenzymes 1-1, 1-2 and 2-2 (Ketterer, 1986b), our findings could mean that cultured rat hepatocytes evolute, in terms of GST, rather to a primary hepatoma than to a fetal-like state.

REFERENCES

Dickins, M. and Peterson, R.E. (1980) : Effects of a hormone-supplemented medium on cytochrome P-450 content and mono-oxygenase activities of rat hepatocytes in primary culture. Biochemical Pharmacology 29, 1231-1238.

Edwards, A.M., Glistak, M.L., Lucas, C.M. and Wilson, P.A. (1984) : 7-ethoxycoumarin deethylase activity as a convenient measure of liver drug metabolizing enzymes : regulation in cultured rat hepatocytes. Biochemical Pharmacology 33, 1537-1546.

Guzelian, P.S., Bissell, D.M. and Meyer, U.A. (1977) : Drug metabolism in adult rat hepatocytes in primary monolayer culture. Gastroenterology 72, 1232-1239.

Habig, W.H., Pabst, M.J. and Jakoby, W.B. (1974) : Glutathione S-transferase. The Journal of Biological Chemistry 249, 7130-7139.

Ketterer, B. (1986a) : Detoxication reactions of glutathione and glutathione transferase. Xenobiotica 16, 957-973.

Ketterer, B., Meyer, D.J., Coles, B., Taylor, J.B. and Pemble, S. (1986b) : Glutathione transferase and carcinogenesis. In : Antimutagenesis and anticarcinogenesis mechanisms, eds. Shankel D.M., Hartman P.E., Kada T. and Hollaender A., pp. 103-126. Plenum Publishers Corporation.

Vandenberghe Y., Ratanasavanh., D., Glaise, D. and Guillouzo, A. (1987) : Influence of medium composition and culture conditions on glutathione S-transferase activity in adult rat hepatocytes during culture. In vitro (in press).

Effect of ethanol on the synthesis and secretion of proteins in cultured adult rat hepatocytes

Jesus Pazo-Carrera*, Georges Baffet**, Maryvonne Rissel, André Guillouzo

INSERM U.49, Unité de Recherches Hépatologiques, Hôpital de Pontchaillou, 35033 Rennes Cedex, France.
Present address : *Department of Animal Physiology, University of Santiago de Compostela, Spain
**Corresponding author

Keywords : Ethanol, rat hepatocytes, primary cultures, protein synthesis, enzyme activities.

INTRODUCTION

Conflicting reports exist on the effect of ethanol on hepatic protein synthesis measured by the incorporation of radioactive aminoacids in vivo. Many studies have demonstrated that administration of ethanol resulted in an inhibitory effect (Morland and Sjetnam, 1976 ; Smith-Kielland and Morland, 1981) but an increase (Baraona et al., 1977) or no effect (Baraona and Lieber, 1970 ; Cerdan et al., 1980) have also been reported. By contrast, most studies on in vitro systems, including rat liver slices (Perin et al., 1974 ; Tuma and Sorrel, 1981), isolated perfused liver (Kirsch et al., 1973) and freshly isolated hepatocytes (Morland and Bessesen, 1977 ; Bengtsson et al., 1984) have evidenced an inhibition of protein synthesis. However, since alcohol treatment of these in vitro liver preparations was limited to a few hours it may be questioned as to whether this reflects the in vivo chronic ethanol exposure. To gain further informations on longer effect of ethanol on hepatocytes we have treated rat hepatocytes in primary culture for 1-5 twenty-four hour periods. The results reported here show that such an ethanol exposure resulted in a dose-dependent inhibition of protein synthesis in the presence of concentrations ranging between 20 and 135 mM.

MATERIAL AND METHODS

Adult normal hepatocytes were obtained by perfusing rat liver (Sprague-Dawley ; 150-200 g) with 0.025 % collagenase (Worthington) buffered with 0.1 M Hepes [4-(2-hydroxyethyl)-1 piperazine ethane sulfonic acid)], pH 7.4, according to the method previously described (Guguen et al., 1975)
Hepatocytes were placed at the density of 1 x 10^6 cells in Petri dishes of 3 cm in diameter in Ham's F_{12} medium supplemented with 10 % fetal calf serum containing per ml penicillin (100 IU), streptomycin sulfate (100 µg), insulin (10 µg) and bovine serum albumin (1 mg). The medium supplemented with 7 x 10^{-5} M hydrocortisone hemisuccinate, was renewed 4 h later and every day thereafter. Ethanol was added at various concentrations ranging between 20 and 135 mM, 4 h after cell seeding and renewed or not every day for 5 days. Hepatocyte cultures were examined daily under phase-contrast microscopy.

Enzyme activities.
The following enzyme activities were analysed : lactic dehydrogenase(LDH) (Weisshaar et al., 1975), aspartate aminotransferase (ASAT) (Schmidt and Schmidt, 1963), alanine aminotransferase(ALAT) (Wroblewski and Ladue, 1956) and gamma-glutamyltransferase (GGT) (Persign and Van der Slik, 1976).

Protein synthesis
Protein synthetic activity was measured by the incorporation of ^{35}S-methionine. Cells were rinsed with 0.1 M Hepes buffer and incubated in methione-free Eagle medium containing 10 µCi ^{35}S-methionine (Amersham, 800 mCi/mmol) and supplemented with 1 mg/ml albumin, 10 µg/ml insulin and hydrocortisone hemisuccinate.
After incubation, media and cell monolayers were collected separately. Proteins were precipitated with trichloroacetic acid at final concentration of 10 %, washed 3 times and radioactivity in the samples was determined by liquid scintillation counting.
Samples were analyzed by one dimensional gel electrophoresis. One dimensional slab gel electrophoresis was performed according to Laemmli (1970) using a 7.5-15 % linear gradient. The proteins were solubilized in SDS sample buffer containing mercaptoethanol (1 mM) and heated at 95°C for 2 min.
In addition, albumin was quantified in culture media by laser immunonephelometry (Eckman et coll., 1970).

RESULTS AND DISCUSSION

At concentrations ranging between 20 and 135 M ethanol had little effect on cell morphology, even after a 5 days exposure. At 45 mM ethanol reduced cell spreading and the highest concentration induced accumulation of lipid droplets in the cytoplasm of hepatocytes (Fig. 1) suggesting an alteration of lipid metabolism as previously found in vivo and with in vitro liver systems (Baraona et al., 1977 ; Edmonson, 1980 ; Bengtsson et al., 1984).

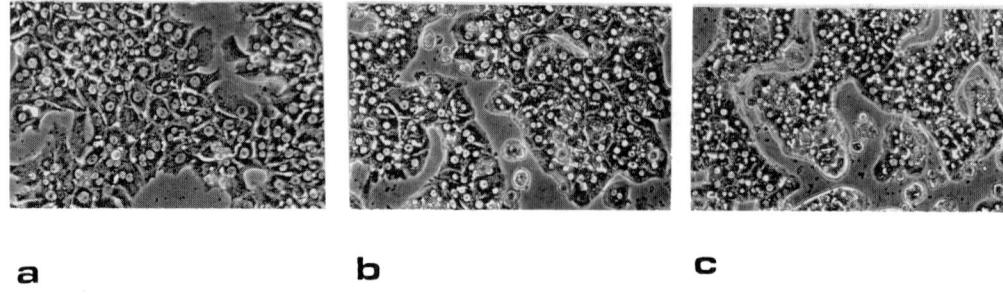

a   b   c

Figure 1 : Cell morphology of alcohol-treated cultured hepatocytes (72h). Ethanol was added at the concentration of 45 mM (b) or 135 mM (c). Control untreated culture (a). (x 180).

Cytosolic enzyme activities (LDH, GPT, GOT) which are often used as indexes of hepatotoxicity were decreased in both the cells and media whatever the concentration of ethanol. At the highest concentration the lowest enzyme activity was found (Figs. 2A and 2B). Similar results were obtained with LDH and transferases (results not shown). These decreased activities could reflect an inhibition in their synthetic rate and perhaps also a reduced leakage related to a stabilizing effect of ethanol on the plasma membrane.

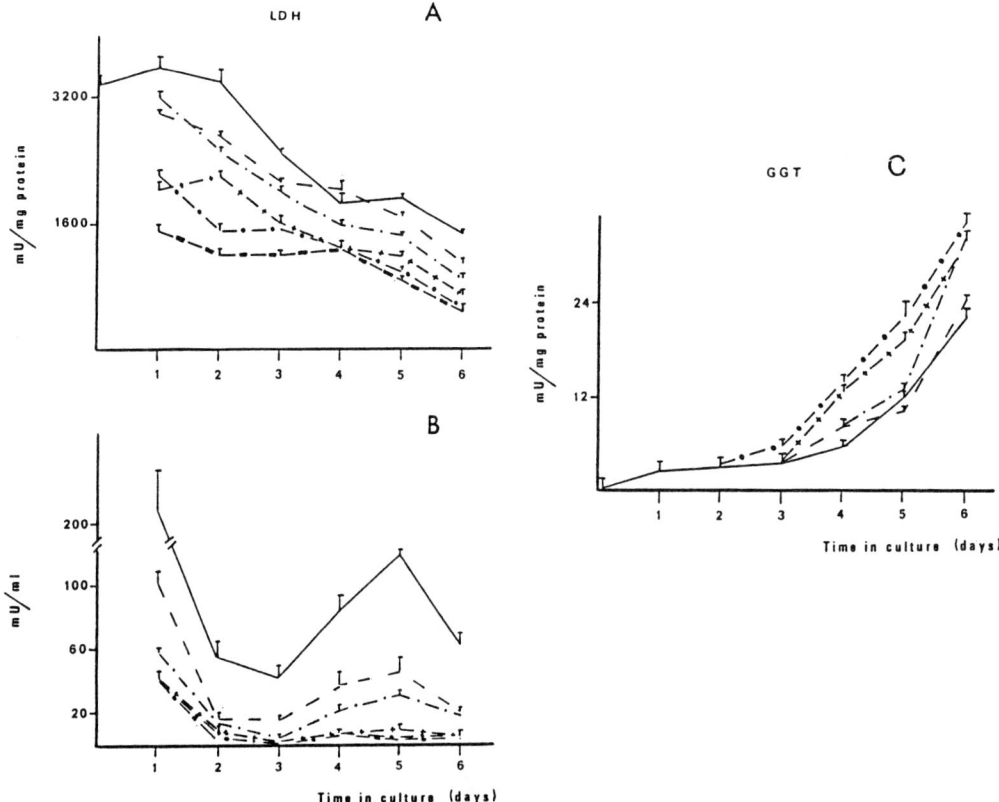

Figure 2 : Lacticdehydrogenase (LDH) and gamma-glutamyltransferase activity in alcohol-treated hepatocyte cultures.
LDH activity was measured in both the medium (A) and cells (B), gamma-glutamyltransferase in the cells (C). Ethanol was added at various concentrations : 20 mM (– – –) ; 45 mM (– · –) ; 90 mM (—+—) ; 135 mM (—•—) ; 180 mM (—■—). (———) control, untreated culture. The values are means± SE.

By contrast, GGT activity was increased in both control and ethanol-treated cultures after 3 days. A dose-dependent effect of ethanol was noticed. After 5 daily treatment with 135 mM ethanol a two-fold increase was demonstrated compared to untreated cultures (Fig. 2C). This observation is consistent with previous findings showing that serum GGT is increased in man and rat after ethanol intoxication (Petrides et Teschke, 1980 ; Nishimvra et al., 1981 ; Barouki et al., 1983).

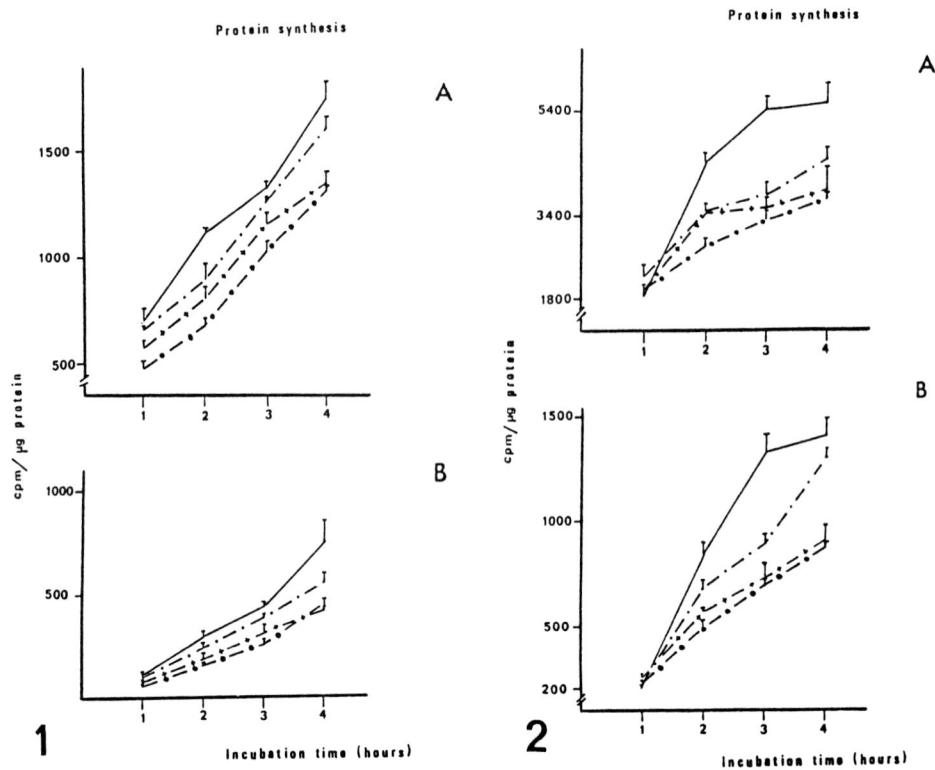

Figure 3 : Effect of ethanol on neosynthetized secreted (A) and intracellular (B) proteins after 4 h (1) or 24 h (2) of culture.
Cells were incubated in methionine-free medium containing 10 µCi ^{35}S-methionine during 1, 2, 3 or 4 hours.
For legend see Fig. 2.

	ETHANOL CONCENTRATION (mM)			
	0	45	90	135
CELLS	11312 ± 147	8996 ± 419	9674 ± 503	7726 ± 268
MEDIUM	4622 ± 416	4461 ± 437	4179 ± 316	3569 ± 313

TABLE I : Levels of ^{35}S-methionine incorporation into secreted and intracellular proteins of adult rat hepatocytes cultured for 3 days in the presence or absence of ethanol.
The results are expressed as cpm/µg intracellular protein ; the values are means± S.E.

Determination of neosynthetized secreted and intracellular proteins by incorporation of ^{35}S-methionine in 4h, 24h and 72h cultures revealed an inhibitory effect of ethanol which raised about 30 % (Fig. 3). A 72 h exposure of alcohol has the same inhibitory effect as an acute treatment (4 h) (Table I). A dose-response was evidenced. There was a highly decrease in protein synthesis with 135 mM ethanol. Similarly, albumin secretion rate was decreased in a dose-dependent manner in alcohol-treated cultures (Fig. 4).

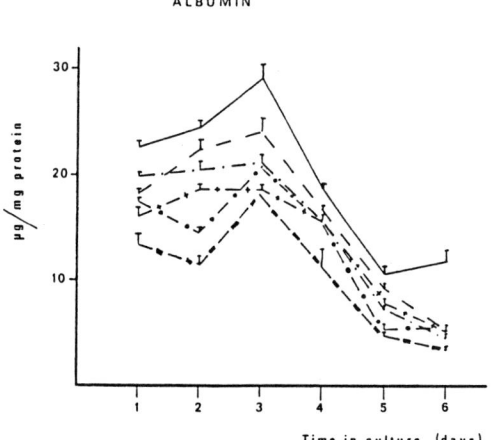

Figure 4 : Effect of ethanol on albumin secretion in cultured rat hepatocytes. For legend see Fig. 2.

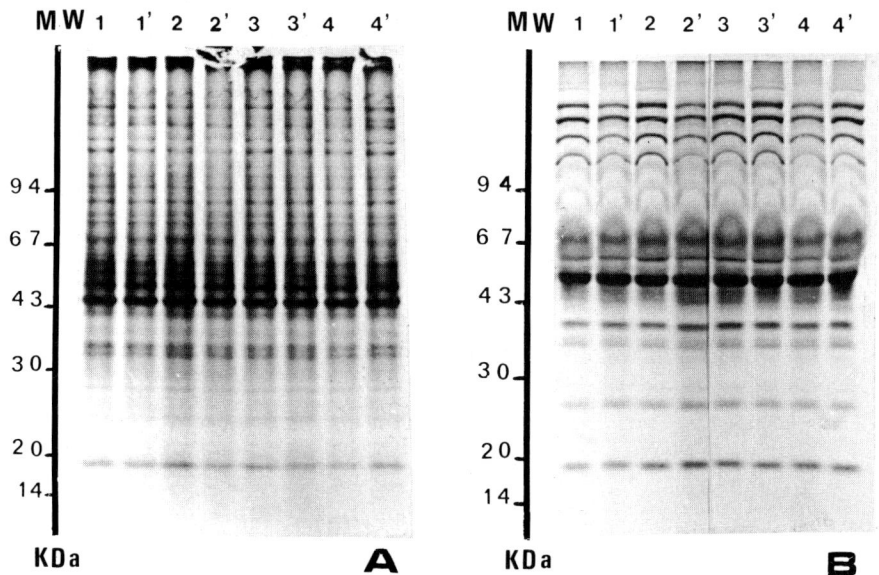

Figure 5 : Gel electrophoretic analysis of total neosynthetized proteins in the presence (2 : 45 mM ; 3 : 90 mM ; 4 : 135 mM) or absence of ethanol (1).
Intracellular proteins (A) and secreted proteins (B). Experiments were carried out on duplicate (1, 1'- 2, 2' - 3, 3' - 4, 4').

In order to determine whether the inhibitory effect of ethanol affected all or most of the proteins or only some specific ones, proteins of both treated and untreated cultures were analysed on SDS polyacrylamide gels. As shown in figure 5, no marked qualitative differences could be visualized between either secreted or intracellular proteins of alcohol-treated and untreated cultures. Princen et al. (1981) came to the same conclusion by analysing the products synthesised by membrane-bound polyribosomes purified from control and ethanol-intoxicated rat livers on SDS polyacrylamide gels.

The decline in the amount of secreted albumin and whole proteins levels could be the reflect of a decrease in the synthesis and/or secretion rate. Since the inhibition effect of ethanol was similar on both intracellular and secreted proteins and no qualitative changes were found by monodimensional gel electrophoresis it may be postulated that the drug affected mainly protein synthesis in our culture model.

ACKNOWLEDGMENTS

Jesus Pazo Carrera was supported by a fellowship from the french government. We thank A. Vannier for typing this manuscript

REFERENCES

Baraona, E. and Lieber, C.S. (1970): Effect of chronic ethanol feeding on serum lipoprotein metabolism in the rat. J. Clin. Invest. 49, 769-778.

Baraona, E., Leo, H.A., Borowsky, S.A. and Lieber, C.S. (1977): Pathogenesis of alcohol-reduced accumulation of protein in the liver. J. Clin. Invest. 60, 546-554.

Barouki, R., Chobert, M.N., Finidori, J., Bilson, M.C. and Hanoune, J. (1983): The hormonal induction of gamma-glutamyltransferase in rat liver and in a hepatoma cell line. Mol. Cell. Biochem. 53/54, 77-88.

Bengtsson, G., Smith-Kielland, A. and Morland, J. (1984): Ethanol effects on protein synthesis in non parenchymal liver cells, hepatocytes, and density populations of hepatocytes. Exp. Mol. Pathol. 41, 44-57.

Cerdan, S., Robels, S.S., Martin-Requero, A., Ayuso, M.S. and Parrilla, R. (1982): Acute effects of ethanol on the rate of hepatic protein synthesis in the rat in vivo. Int. J. Biochem. 14, 615-620.

Eckman, Z., Robbins, J.B., Van Der Hamer, C.J.A., Lentz, O. and Scheinber, I.H. (1970): Automation of quantitative immunochemical microanalysis of human serum transferrin : a model system. Clin. Chem. 16, 558-561.

Edmonson H.A. (1980): Pathology of alcoholism. Am. J. Clin. 74, 725-742.

Guguen, C., Guillouzo, A., Boisnard, M., Le Cam, A. and Bourel, M. (1975): Etude ultrastructurale de monocouches d'hépatocytes de rat adulte cultivés en présence d'hémisuccinate d'hydrocortisone. Biol. Gastroentérol. 8, 223-231.

Kirsch, R.E., Frith, L.O'.C., Stead, R.H. and Saunders, S.J. (1973):Effect of alcohol on albumin synthesis by the isolated perfused rat liver. Am. J. Clin. Nutr. 26, 1191-1194.

Laemmli, U.K. (1970): Cleavage of strutural proteins during the assembly of the head of bacteriophage T4. Nature 227, 680-685.

Morland, J. and Bessesen, A. (1977): Inhibition of protein synthesis by ethanol in isolated rat liver parenchymal cells. Biochim. Biophys. Acta 474, 312-320.

Morland, J. and Sjetnan, A. (1976): Effect of ethanol intake on the incorporation of labelled amino acids into liver proteins. Biochem. Pharmacol. 25, 2125-2130.

Nishimura, M., Stein, H., Berges, W. and Teschke, R. (1981): Gamma-glutamyltransferase activity of liver plasma membrane : induction following chronic alcohol consumption. Biochem. Biophys. Res. Commun. 99, 142-148.

Perin A., Scalabrino, G., Sessa, A. and Arnaboldi, A. (1974): In vitro inhibition of protein synthesis in rat liver as consequences of ethanol metabolism. Biochim. Biophys. Acta 366, 101-108.

Persijn, J.P. and Van Der Slik (1976): A new method for the determination of gamma-glutamyltransferase in serum. J. Clin. Chem. Clin. Biochem. 14, 421-428.

Petrides A.S. and Teschke R. (1980): Hepatic gamma-glutamyltransferase (γ-GT) : its increase in activity due to chronic alcohol consumption and its mechanism. Rev. Franç. Gastroenterol. 159, 22-30.

Princen, J.M.G., Mol-Backx, G.P.B.M. and Yap, S.H. (1981): Acute effects of ethanol intake on albumin and total protein synthesis in free and membrane-bound polyribosomes of rat liver. Biochim. Biophys. Acta 655, 119-127.

Schmidt, E. and Schmidt, F.W. (1963): Enzyme-bestimmungen in serum bei leber-erkrakungen. Funktions-muster als hilfsmittel der diagnose. Enzym. Biol. Clin. 3, 1-52.

Smith-Kielland, A. and Morland, J. (1981): Reduced hepatic protein synthesis after long-term ethanol treatment in fasted rats. Dependence on animal handling before measurement. Biochem. Pharmacol. 30, 2377-2379.

Tuma, D.J. and Sorrel, M.R. (1981): Effects of ethanol on the secretion of glycoproteins by rat liver slices. Gastroenterology 80-82.

Weisshaar, D., Gossrau, E. and Faderl, B. (1975): Normbereiche von alpha-HBDH, LDH, AP und LAP bei messungt mit substrat-optimierten testasaätzen. Med. Wel. 26, 387-391.

Wroblewski, F. and Ladue, J.S. (1956): Serum-glutamic pyruvic transaminases in cardiac and hepatic disease. Proc. Soc. Exp. Biol. Med. 91, 569-571.

Effects of ornithine alpha-ketoglutarate on albumin secretion by adult rat hepatocyte co-cultures

Gérard Lescoat, Béatrice Desvergne, Nicole Pasdeloup, Denise Glaise, Jean-Pierre Gazeau*, Robert Molimard*, Yves Deugnier, Pierre Brissot, Michel Bourel

*Unité de Recherche Hépatologique, INSERM U.49, Hôpital de Pontchaillou, 35033 Rennes Cedex, France. *Laboratoires J. Logeais, Issy-Les-Moulineaux, France*

Keywords : Ornithine alpha-ketoglutarate, albumin, adult rat hepatocyte.

INTRODUCTION

Ornithine alpha-ketoglutarate (OKG), or ornicetil^R is the salt complex of L(+) ornithine and alpha-ketoglutarate in a respective molar ratio 2/1. This drug has been proposed in the treatment of hypercatabolic states observed during different kinds of trauma. Among the characteristic alterations of the hypercatabolic states, enhanced energy demand and augmented protein breakdown can be noted (Kinney, 1976 a, b) ; the final result being a loss of weight and a negative nitrogen balance. To modify this hypercatabolic state, one way could be to favor metabolism processes by using hormones and/or by providing a supply of energetic substrate by the treatment with OKG. It has been demonstrated that OKG improved nitrogen economy (Cynober et al., 1984a, b ; Leander et al., 1985) by decreasing urea and ammonia formation (Leander et al., 1985), but also by stimulating insulin (Krassowski et al., 1981) and growth hormone release (Donnadieu et al., 1971 ; Elalouf et al., 1980) which promoted intracellular amino acid transport and protein synthesis. Therefore, the combined effects of reduced urea and ammonia formation correlated to an enhanced protein synthesis could explain the observed nitrogen economy following OKG administration (Cynober et al., 1984 a, b ; Leander et al., 1985).
The purpose of the present data was first to demonstrate that OKG was able to stimulate protein hepatocyte secretion without the necessity of an hormonal intermediate and second to identify the respective roles of the two molecule components while considering also the metabolites of L-ornithine. For this purpose, adult rat hepatocyte co-cultures were used and their albumin (ALB) secretion was measured in the medium.
Our results demonstrate that hepatocyte ALB secretion can be stimulated directly in vitro by OKG ; the component implicated in the phenomenon appears to be L-ornithine. Moreover, in our co-culture model, the polyamine pathway seems likely to be the primordial way of action of OKG.

MATERIAL AND METHODS

Cell culture
Adult rat hepatocytes were isolated from 2-month-old Sprague-Dawley rats by canulating the portal vein and perfusing the liver with a collagenase solution.

Hepatocytes were collected and suspended in a mixture of 75 % Eagle minimum essential medium and 25 % medium 199 with Hanks' salts, supplemented with 10 % fetal calf serum and containing, per ml : kanamycin (50 µg), streptomycin (50 µg), penicillin (90 IU), bovine insulin (5 µg), bovine serum albumin (1 mg) and $NaHCO_3$ (22 mg). Usually 2.5×10^6 hepatocytes were suspended in 4 ml of medium in 25 cm^2 Nunclon flasks. The medium was changed 3-4 h later and for co-culture about 2.5×10^6 rat liver epithelial cells (RLEC) were seeded per flask in order to reach confluence within 24 h. RLEC were originally isolated by trypsinization of 10 day-old rat livers according to the William's procedure described elsewhere (Morel-Chany et al., 1978) and maintained by serial subculture in William's medium supplemented with 10 % fetal calf serum. In the present study, the co-culture model was used because we demonstrated previously that it confered a long-term differentiated state to hepatocytes (Guguen-Guillouzo et al., 1983 ; Fraslin et al., 1985). For experimental purpose the control cultures were maintained in an Eagle arginine-free medium supplemented with 10^{-7} M dexamethasone and 10 % fetal calf serum. For the treated cultures, the same medium supplemented with 0.03 mM OKG (Laboratoires J. Logeais, Issy-Les-Moulineaux/France) 0.03 mM alpha-ketoglutaric acid, 0.06 mM L-ornithine, 0.03 mM L-arginine, 0.06 mM putrescine or 0.03 mM spermine (Sigma Chemical Company, St Louis, MO/USA) was used. These different concentrations were evaluated in order to add to the culture medium the same amount of nitrogen.

Albumin assay
Culture media were collected every two days and stored at -20°C. ALB was quantified by laser immunonephelometry (Ritchie, 1975). Standard rat albumin and incubation media were mixed in appropriate dilutions of anti-rat albumin antiserum in NaCl 0.9 % containing 4 % polyethylene glycol. Light scatter was measured after 1 h incubation at room temperature. Standard rat albumin and antiserum were from Cappell Laboratories, Division of Biological Corporation, Cochranville/U.S.A. The limit of sensitivity of the assay was 2 µg/ml. Inter-and intra- assay variations did not exceed 10 %.

Statistics.
Experimental values are means $\pm$ SEM of triplicate cultures ; experiments were repeated two or three times. Significance was assessed using student's t-test at the level of 0.05 (NS : not significant ; * $p < 0.05$; ** $p < 0.01$; *** $p < 0.001$).

RESULTS

1 - Co-culture morphology.

Supplementation of an arginine-free medium with 0.03 mM OKG appeared to improve the morphology of the co-cultures. In the absence of OKG (Fig. 1a), bile canaliculus formations gradually disappeared. On the opposite, in the presence of 0.03 mM OKG, the hepatocytes maintained their regular specific organization while remaining well spread (Fig. 1b).

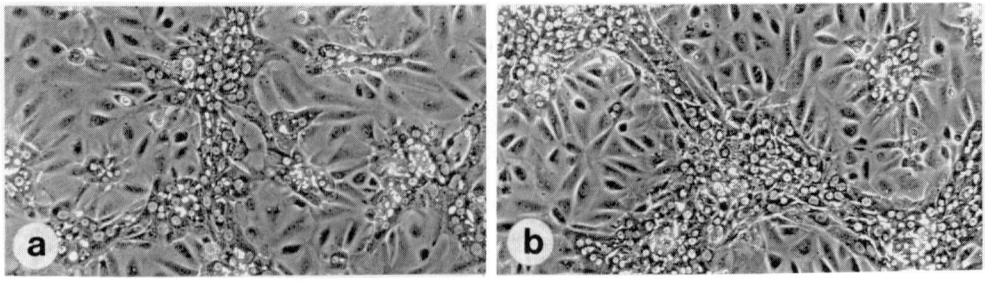

Figure 1 : Phase-contrast micrographs of adult rat hepatocyte co-cultures maintained in the absence (a) or presence (b) of 0.03 mM OKG. Day 5 of co-culture (170 x).

2 - Hepatocyte albumin secretion.

a) - In the presence of 0.03 mM OKG in the culture medium, hepatocyte ALB secretion was increased (Table 1).

Days of culture	ALB secretion (µg/ml)		
	Control	p	OKG
1	35 ± 1	NS	34 ± 1
3	45 ± 2	NS	42 ± 1
5	26 ± 2	***	33 ± 2
7	25 ± 1	***	34 ± 2

TABLE 1 : Effect of 0.03 mM OKG on hepatocyte ALB secretion.

b) - What are the respective roles of the two molecule components of OKG ? We observed that the addition of 0.03 mM alpha-ketoglutaric acid to the culture medium was without effect on ALB secretion (Table 2). However, the OKG effect was reproduced by the presence of 0.06 mM L-ornithine (Table 3) ; thus this amino acid appeared to be the component implicated in the phenomenon.

Days of culture	ALB secretion (µg/ml)		
	Control	p	Alpha-ketoglutaric acid
1	80 ± 4	NS	76 ± 4
3	70 ± 3	NS	59 ± 8
5	34 ± 3	NS	35 ± 2
7	24 ± 2	NS	26 ± 3

TABLE 2 : Effect of 0.03 mM alpha-ketoglutaric acid on hepatocyte ALB secretion.

Days of culture	ALB secretion (µg/ml)		
	Control	p	L-ornithine
1	35 ± 1	NS	36 ± 1
3	45 ± 2	NS	44 ± 2
5	26 ± 2	***	34 ± 1
7	25 ± 1	***	34 ± 1

TABLE 3 : Effect of 0.06 mM L-ornithine on hepatocyte ALB secretion.

c) - In our co-culture model, the stimulatory effect of L-ornithine on ALB secretion could be mediated by two possible ways : the production of arginine in the urea cycle and the polyamine synthesis. Indeed, we observed that the addition of 0.03 mM L-arginine (Table 4), 0.06 mM putrescine (Table 5) or 0.03 mM spermine (Table 6) stimulated ALB synthesis. Therefore, in our model, arginine as well as polyamines appeared to be potent stimulators of albumin secretion.

Days of culture	Control	p	ALB secretion (µg/ml) L-arginine
1	80 ± 3	NS	83 ± 4
3	70 ± 3	NS	76 ± 2
5	34 ± 3	***	49 ± 2
7	23 ± 2	***	50 ± 2

TABLE 4 : Effect of 0.03 mM L-arginine on hepatocyte ALB secretion.

Days of culture	Control	p	ALB secretion (µg/ml) Putrescine
1	30 ± 1	NS	28 ± 1
3	34 ± 3	NS	40 ± 2
5	21 ± 1	*	29 ± 2
7	14 ± 1	**	20 ± 2

TABLE 5 : Effect of 0.06 mM putrescine on hepatocyte ALB secretion.

Days of culture	Control	p	ALB secretion (µg/ml) Spermine
1	35 ± 1	NS	38 ± 2
3	45 ± 2	NS	44 ± 1
5	26 ± 2	***	36 ± 1
7	24 ± 1	***	33 ± 1

TABLE 6 : Effect of 0.03 mM spermine on hepatocyte ALB secretion.

d) - To discriminate between the arginine and the polyamine pathway, we blocked the biosynthesis of polyamines by the use of a potent inhibitor of ornithine decarboxylase : alpha-methyl ornithine (MO). Added to the culture medium of the control cultures, MO (1 or 3 mM) was without incidence on ALB secretion (Table 7) ; however, the dose 3 mM abolished the effect of 0.18 mM OKG as soon as day 5 of culture (Table 7). This result suggested that stimulation of ALB synthesis by OKG was rather mediated by polyamine synthesis.

Days of culture	OKG	p	ALB secretion (µg/ml) Control	p	OKG + MO
1	14 ± 1	NS	14 ± 1	NS	14 ± 0.5
3	14 ± 0.5	***	6 ± 0.5	***	15 ± 0.5
5	20 ± 1	***	8 ± 0.5	NS	9.5 ± 0.5
7	20 ± 1	***	7 ± 0.5	NS	8 ± 0.5

TABLE 7 : Effect of 3 mM alpha-methyl ornithine on ALB secretion of hepatocytes maintained in the presence of 0.18 mM OKG.

DISCUSSION

The present studies concerned the in vitro effects of OKG on adult rat hepatocytes. They provided evidence that this drug favoured hepatocyte survival and increased greatly their ALB secretion. Moreover, the OKG component implicated in the phenomenon appeared to be L-ornithine. Therefore, our data demonstrated that the presence of L-ornithine in an arginine-deprived culture medium of adult hepatocytes stimulated their ALB secretion. This result confirmed first our previous observations concerning fetal rat and human hepatocyte cultures (Lescoat et al., 1987) and second the results of Oratz et al. (1983) showing that the addition of 10 mM L-ornithine to the perfusate of a rabbit liver resulted in stimulation of ALB secretion. Moreover, as in our experimental conditions, the same authors demonstrated also that L-arginine was as effective as L-ornithine in stimulating the synthesis of this protein in the rabbit. However, by inhibiting ornithine decarboxylase with alpha-methyl ornithine, the increase in ALB secretion observed in the presence of OKG disappeared. This observation suggested that if the ornithine to polyamine pathway was blocked, ornithine did not stimulate ALB synthesis and offered support to the concept that in our co-culture OKG stimulation of ALB production was mediated by polyamine synthesis. A comparable result has been obtained by Oratz et al. (1983) using a perfused rabbit liver.

In conclusion, these data emphasize that ALB secretion can be stimulated directly by OKG ; the component implicated in the phenomenon is L-ornithine. Moreover, in our co-culture model, the polyamine pathway seems likely to be the primordial way of action of OKG. Experiments are now in progress, first to confirm these results in human co-cultures and second to clarify the OKG mechanism of action.

ACKNOWLEDGMENTS

We thank Merrel Dow Research Institute, Strasbourg Research Center (France) for the generous gift of alpha-methyl ornithine and Mrs A. Vannier for typing the manuscript.

REFERENCES

Cynober, L., Vaubourdolle, M., Dore A. and Giboudeau J (1984a): Kinetics and metabolic effects of orally administered ornithine α-ketoglutarate in healthy subjects fed with a standardized regimen. Am. J. Clin. Nutr. 39, 514-519.

Cynober, L., Saizy, R., Nguyen Dinh, F., Lioret, N. and Giboudeau, J. (1984b): Effects of enterally administered ornithine alpha-ketoglutarate on plasma and urinary amino acid levels after burn injury. J. Trauma, 24, 590-596.

Donnadieu, M., Combouriou, M. and Schimpff, R.M. (1971): Comparaison de différentes épreuves de stimulation utilisées pour l'étude de la fonction somatotrope chez l'enfant. Path. Biol. 19, 293-301.

Elalouf, M., Mizrahi, R., Zannetti, A., Vigneron, B., Leclere, J. and Hartemann, P. (1980): Test d'exploration de la fonction somatotrope par l'ornithine chez l'adulte. Rev. Franc. Endocrinol. Clin. 21, 357-360.

Fraslin, J.M., Kneip, B., Vaulont, S., Glaise, D., Munnich, A. and Guguen-Guillouzo, C. (1985): Dependence of hepatocyte-specific gene expression on cell-cell interactions in primary culture. Embo J. 4, 2487-2491.

Guguen-Guillouzo, C., Clément, B., Baffet, G., Beaumont, C., Morel-Chany, E., Glaise, D. and Guillouzo, A. (1983): Maintenance and reversibility of active albumin secretion by adult rat hepatocytes co-cultured with another liver epithelial cell type. Exp. Cell Res. 143, 47-54.

Kinney, J.M. (1976a): Surgical hypermetabolism and nitrogen metabolism. In Metabolism and response to injury, eds. A.W. Wilkinson and D.P. Cuthbertson, pp. 121-134, Pitman Medical, Kent.

Kinney, J.M. (1976b): Surgical diagnosis, patterns of energy, weight and tissue change. In Metabolism and response to injury, eds. A.W. Wilkinson and D.P. Cuthbertson D.P., pp. 237-252, Pitman Medical, Kent.

Krassowski, J., Rousselle, J., Maeder, E. and Febber, J.P. (1981): The effect of ornithine alpha-ketoglutarate on insulin and glucagon secretion in normal subjects. Acta Endocrinol. 98, 252-255.

Leander, U., Furst, P., Vesterberg, K. and Vinnars, E. (1985): Nitrogen sparing effect of ornicetil in the immediate postoperative state clinical biochemistry and nitrogen balance. Cl. Nutri. 4, 43-51.

Lescoat, G., Thézé, N., Fraslin, J.M., Pasdeloup, N., Kneip, B. and Guguen-Guillouzo, C. (1987): Influence of ornithine on albumin synthesis by fetal and neonatal hepatocytes maintained in culture. Cell Dif. 21, 21-29.

Morel-Chany, E., Guillouzo, C., Tringal, G. and Szajnert, M.F. (1978): "Spontaneous" neoplastic transformation in vitro of epithelial cell strains of rat liver : cytology, growth and enzymatic activities. Eur. J. Cancer 14, 1341-1352.

Oratz, M., Rothschild, A., Schreiber, S.S., Burks, A., Mongelli, J. and Matarese, B. (1983): The role of the urea cycle and polyamine in albumin synthesis. Hepatology 3, 567-571.

Ritchie R.F. (1975) : Automated immunoprecipitation analysis of serum proteins. In The plasma proteins : Structure, Function and Genetic Control, ed. F.W. Putman, Vol. II, pp. 375-425, Academic Press : New York.

Studies of the toxic activity of ricin on Zajdela's hepatoma cells

M. Decastel, G. Haentjens, M. Aubery, Y. Goussault

CNRS UA 71, INSERM U.180, 45 rue des Saint-Pères, 75006 Paris Cedex 06, France

KEYWORDS

Ricin, protein synthesis inhibition, internalization, tumour cells.

INTRODUCTION

Ricin is a plant toxin, which is composed of an A and a B chain connected by a disulphide bond. The toxin binds to cell surface receptors through the B-chain. Once the ricin has entered the cell, the A-chain specifically inhibits protein synthesis by decreasing the affinity of the 60 S ribosomal subunit for the elongation factors (Olsnes & Sandvig, 1983). Since the entry of a few A-chain molecules inhibits cellular protein synthesis within a few hours, the most reliable and sensitive way to measure entry into the cytosol is to monitor inhibition of protein synthesis. We used this method to study the uptake of ricin in cells issued from an experimental tumour ascite induced in rats, the Zajdela's hepatoma cells. Ricin is more potent on tumour cells than on normal cells (Lin & al., 1970). The mechanism of this sensitivity is still unknown and could be related to the mode of entry of ricin in tumour cells. Two pathways have been found for ricin uptake, the neutral one (Moya & al., 1985; Simmons & al., 1986) and the acidic one (Simmons & al., 1986). In the present work, these two pathways were characterized with respect to their sensitivities to lactose and/or mannan, ammonium chloride (NH_4Cl) and after intracellular potassium (K^+) depletion. The obtained data suggested that ricin was taken up via a neutral pathway (by binding to galactose receptors), and that Zajdela's hepatoma cells have lost the acidic pathway.

MATERIALS AND METHODS

The toxin. Ricin was prepared from *R. communis* seeds (var. *sanguineus*) according to the procedure of Nicolson & Blaustein (1972). Ricin was homogeneous as shown by polyacrylamide gel electrophoresis, immunoelectrophoresis and analytical ultracentrifugation.

The tumour cells. Zajdela hepatoma ascite cells were originally produced by dimethylaminoazobenzene injection into Sprague Dawley rats and maintained in the ascite form by intra-peritoneal transplantation (2.5×10^7 cells/0.25 ml/animal) in 8-week-old Sprague Dawley rats, 250 g in weight (Charles River, France). Tumour cells in suspension were harvested 7 days following transplantation and washed twice in minimum essential medium (MEM)[1], twice in 50 mM sodium Hepes[2], pH 7.4, 150 mM NaCl and 1 mM $CaCl_2$ (buffer A), and then resuspended in buffer A or in buffer A supplemented with 1 mM KCl (buffer B).

Measurement of cell protein synthesis inhibition. Cells were dispensed into sterile plastic culture tubes, and the toxin to be tested was added at the indicated concentration. At the end of the experiments, the medium was removed. The cells were then washed twice with buffer A and 0.5 ml of a leucine-free medium that contained 0.1 µCi of [^{14}C]leucine was added in each tube. Following 90 min of incubation, 0.5 ml of 20% TCA was added. After 25 min at room temperature, the precipitated material was washed with 10% TCA, and then dissolved in 0.5ml of 0.1 M NaOH. Each solubilized precipitate was transferred into counting vials, 4ml of ACS were added and the radioactivity was counted in a β counter.

Intracellular K^+ depletion of cells. Cells were hypotonically shocked for 5 min by incubation in MEM[1]/water (1:1), followed by incubation for 25 min in isotonic K^+-free medium (buffer A supplemented with 5 µg/ml insulin and 20 µg/ml transferrin (buffer C)).

Abbreviations used in this paper: MEM[1], Minimum essential medium; Hepes[2], N-2-Hydroxyethylpiperazine-N'-2-Ethanesulfonic Acid.

RESULTS AND COMMENTS.

Effect of specific ligands on ricin cytotoxicity.

Ricin is able to bind to the galactose residues of cell surface glycoconjugates (Nicolson & Blaustein, 1972; Olsnes & al., 1974) or to be recognized through its saccharide residues by the mannose receptor-mediated uptake (Simmons & al., 1986; Skilleter & al., 1986). To characterize the receptors involved in the uptake of ricin in Zajdela's hepatoma cells, we measured the toxic activity of ricin in the presence and absence of a saturating amount of lactose (150 mM) and/or yeast mannan (1 mg/ml), which act as competitive inhibitors of their respective receptors. As illustrated in "Fig. 1", the inhibitory effect of ricin was suppressed, in the same order of magnitude, when either lactose or lactose plus yeast mannan were added in the medium. On the other hand, its toxic activity was enhanced when yeast mannan was present. The IC_{50} (concentration of ricin resulting in a 50 per cent inhibition of [^{14}C]leucine incorporation into cellular protein), calculated in our inhibition system, decreased. It was equal to 1.5×10^{-9} M in absence of mannan and became equal to 9×10^{-10} M in its presence. Lactose alone was able to inhibit ricin uptake (ricin cytotoxicity), and mannan alone was able to activate the uptake (by favouring the binding of a greater number of ricin molecules to the galactose receptors). These results suggested that, exclusively the receptors with galactose residues are involved in the internalization, though these receptors and the mannose receptors are both able to bind ricin.

Characterization of the pathway taken by ricin to enter these cells.

Ricin has been shown to move inside the cells through neutral (Moya & al., 1985; Simmons & al., 1986) or acidic (Simmons & al., 1986; Skilleter & al., 1986) endocytic compartments, following binding to the cell receptors. To define the nature of these compartments (the pathway used), we measured the toxic activity of ricin after treatment of the tumour cells with NH_4Cl, which raises the pH of acidic vesicles (Maxfield, 1982) and after intracellular K^+ depletion, which inhibits formation of coated pits (Larking & al., 1983). There were no changes in the capacity of ricin to inhibit protein synthesis whether the cells were preincubated with 10 mM NH_4Cl, added 25 min prior to addition of ricin, "Fig. 2", or after 25 min of intracellular K^+ depletion, "Fig. 3". The IC_{50} remained unchanged and were equals to 1.5×10^{-9} M. These results suggested that, to move in the cytosol of the tumour cells, ricin uses compartments with neutral pH instead of coated pits, coated vesicles or endosomes usually encountered in the acidic route. Ricin, in these tumour cells, would be taken up via exclusively the neutral route, contrary to macrophages (Simmons & al., 1986). The acidic route would have disappeared in the Zajdela's hepatoma cells. This feature might be related to the pathological behaviour of these cells. Indeed, by using electronic microscopy, Flaig (1984) showed that coated pits, coated vesicles and endosomes are not visible in Zajdela's hepatoma cells.

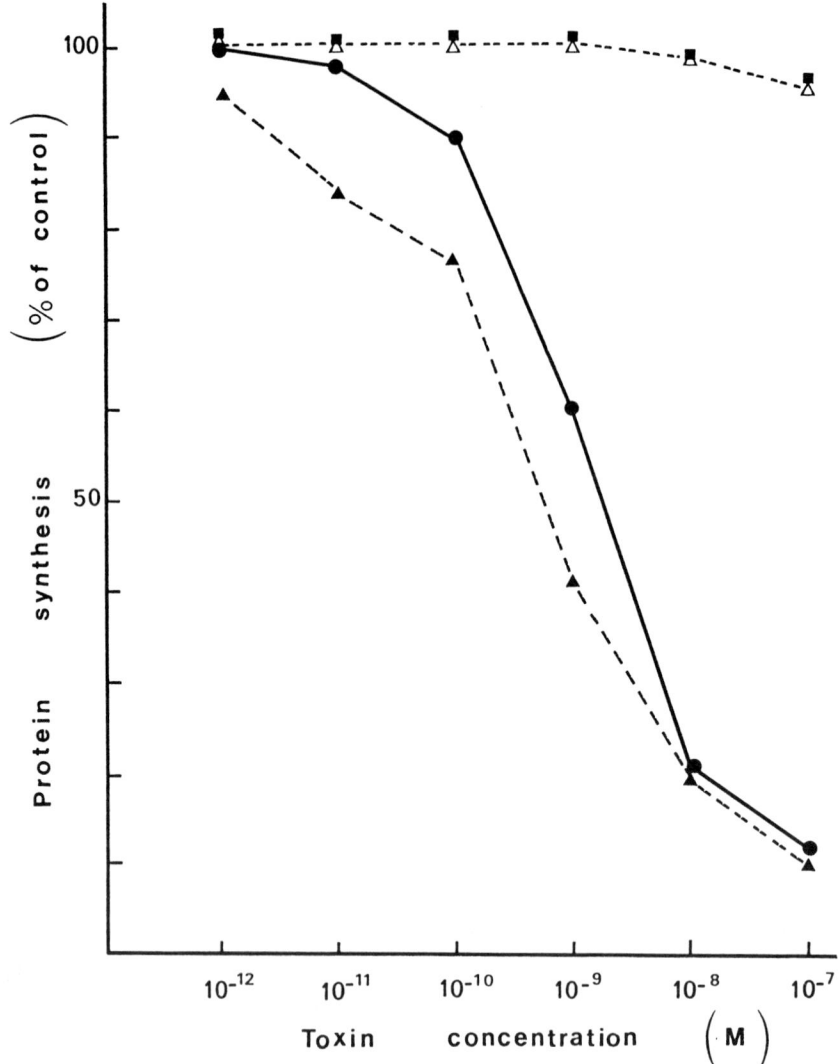

Fig. 1. Effect of saccharides on the cytoxicity of ricin in Zajdela's hepatoma cells. Cells (2.0 x 10⁶) were incubated with the toxin in buffer A, containing either no inhibitor (●——●), 0.15 M lactose to block B-chain binding (△-----△), 1 mg/ml yeast mannan to block mannose receptor-mediated binding (▲--▲) or lactose + yeast mannan (■-----■). Protein synthesis was assayed by incorporation of [^{14}C]leucine, as described in Materials and Methods.

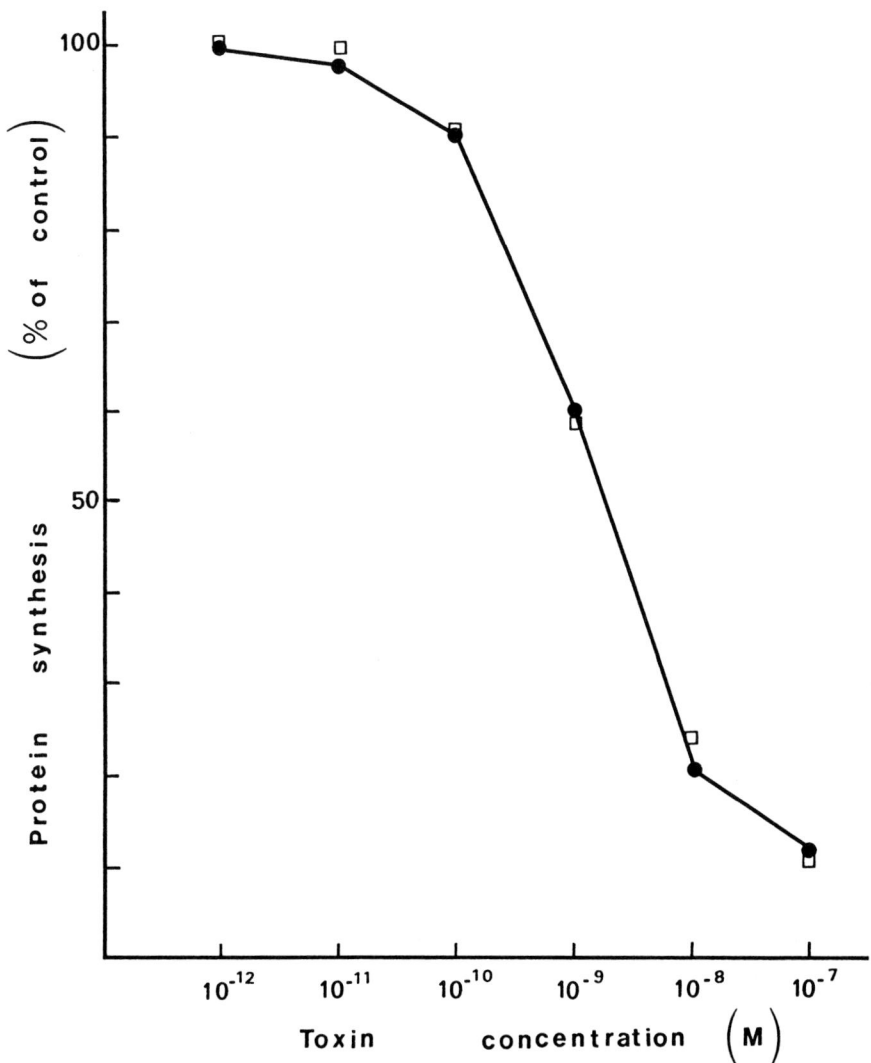

Fig. 2. Effect of ammonium chloride on the cytotoxicity of ricin in Zajdela's hepatoma cells. (●——●) no ammonium chloride. (□——□) 10 mM ammonium chloride. Cells were then assayed for inhibition of [^{14}C]leucine incorporation as described in materials and methods.

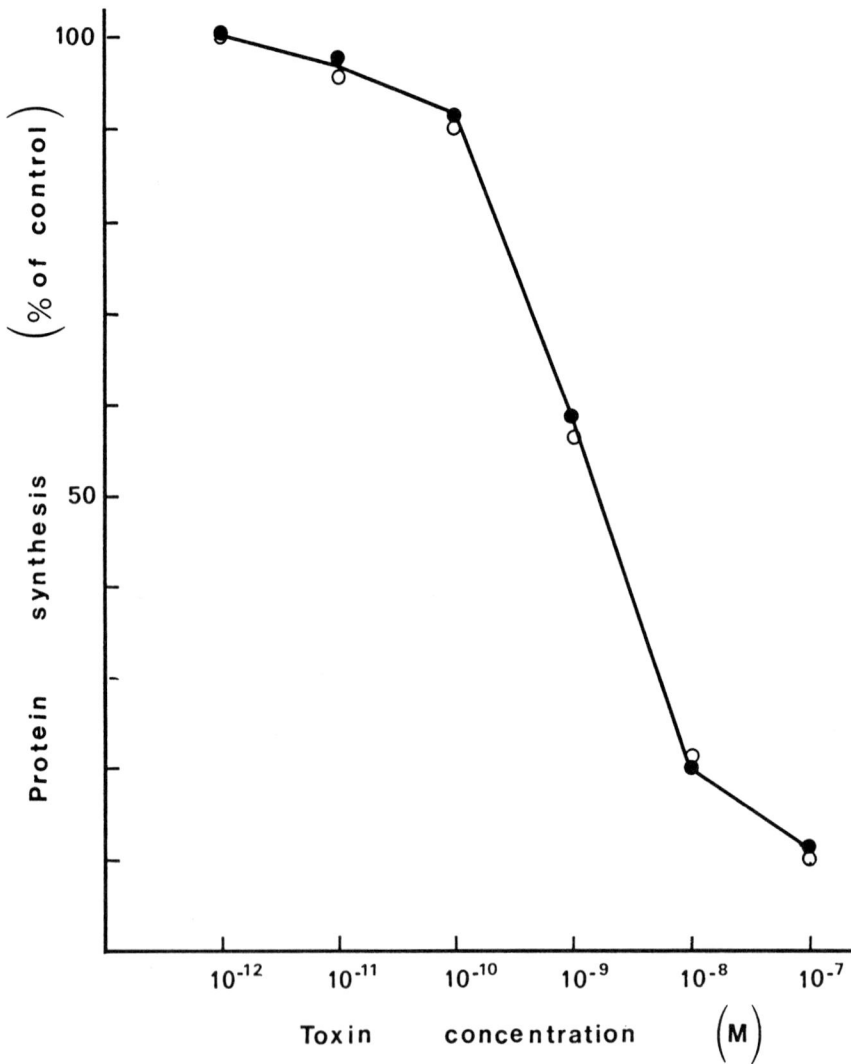

Fig. 3. Effect of ricin on protein synthesis of Zajdela's hepatoma cells after intracellular K^+ depletion. Experiments were performed as described in materials and methods. (●—●) with K^+, (○—○) without K^+.

REFERENCES

Flaig-Staedel, C. (1984): Resurgence de fonctions differenciées dans des cellules d'hépatome en culture. Thèse de Doctorat d'Etat.

Larking, J.M., Brown, M.S., Goldstein, J.L. & Anderson, R.G. (1983): Depletion of intracellular potassium arrests coated pit formation and receptor mediated endocytosis in fibroblasts. Cell. 33, 273-285.

Lin, J.Y., Tserng, K.Y., Chen, C.C., Lin, L.T. & Tung, T.C. (1970): Abrin and ricin : New anti-tumour substances. Nature 227, 292-293.

Maxfield, F.R. (1982): Weak bases and ionophores rapidly and reversibly raise the pH of endocytic vesicles in cultured mouse fibroblasts. J. Cell. Biol. 95, 676-681

Moya, M., Dautry-Varsat, A., Goud, B., Louvard, D. & Boquet, P. (1985): Inhibition of coated pit formation in Hep_2 cells blocks the cytotoxicity of dyphtheria toxin but not that of ricin toxin. J. Cell. Biol. 101, 548-559.

Nicolson, G.L. & Blaustein, J. (1972): The interaction of ricinus agglutinin with normal and tumour cell surfaces. Biochim. Biophys. Acta 266, 113-557.

Olsnes, S. & Sandvig, K. (1983): Receptor Mediated Endocytosis. Recept. Recognit. Ser. B. 15, 188-236.

Olsnes, S., Saltvedt, E. & Pihl, A. (1974): Isolation of galactose binding lectins from *Abrus precatorius* and *Ricinus communis*. J. Biol. Chem. 249, 803-810.

Simmons, B.M., Stahl, P.D. & Russell, J.H. (1986): Mannose receptors-mediated uptake of ricin toxin and ricin A-chain by macrophages. J. Biol. Chem. 261, 7912-7920.

Skilleter, D.N. & Foxwell, B.M.J. (1986): Selective uptake of ricin A-chain by hepatic non-parenchymal cells in vitro. FEBS lett. 196, 344-348.

Phenobarbital induces cytochrome P-450 mRNAs and enhances aflatoxin B1 toxicity in rat hepatoma cells

Laurent Corcos, Jean-Pierre Rousset

Unité de Génétique de la Différenciation, Département de Biologie Moléculaire, Institut Pasteur, 25 rue du Dr Roux, 75724 Paris Cedex 15, France

KEY WORDS

Cytochrome P450, Phenobarbital induction, Aflatoxin B1, Hepatoma cells, Northern blots.

INTRODUCTION

Differentiated rat hepatoma cells derived from the clonal line H4IIEC3 express the specifically hepatic cytochrome P450 genes (Wiebel et al., 1980 and 1984). Cytochromes P450 belong to a superfamily of inducible enzymes involved in the metabolism of endogenous substrates and in the detoxification of many drugs as well as in the activation of procarcinogens (Adesnik & Atchison, 1985). Aflatoxin B1 (AFB1), a mycotoxin produced by some strains of Aspergillus, is involved in the etiology of liver cancer (Wogan & Butler, 1969). AFB1 is not toxic per se, but undergoes metabolic activation via cytochromes P450 (Gurtoo et al., 1978 ; Metcalfe et al., 1981). Differentiated rat hepatoma cells, which express phenobarbital (PB) inducible cytochromes P450, have been shown to be more sensitive to AFB1 than dedifferentiated cells which fail to produce these enzymes (Lambiotte & Thierry, 1978 ; Loquet & Wiebel, 1982). We report here that the increase in specific cytochrome P450 enzyme activities after PB treatment (see Wiebel et al., 1980, 1984 for published values) can be accounted for by an increase in the accumulation of specific cytochrome P450 mRNAs. Moreover, the sensitivity of differentiated cells to AFB1 is greatly enhanced after a PB pretreatment of the cultures. Hence, PB inducible cytochrome P450 enzymes must be involved in the activation of AFB1 to toxic metabolites in differentiated rat hepatoma cells.

MATERIALS AND METHODS

1. Cells

Fao cells are differentiated derivatives of clonal line H4IIEC3 (Deschatrette & Weiss, 1974). RAB1-4 cells were isolated from cultures of Fao cells treated by 10 µM AFB1 for 24 hours (Corcos et al., 1987). They are stably resistant to AFB1 and lack PB inducible cytochrome P450 enzymes. C2-neo cells derive from a dedifferentiated subclone of Fao, and carry the dominant selectable neo marker which allows growth in the presence of 400 µg/ml geneticin G418 sulfate ; hereafter these cells will be referred to as C2 (Corcos et al., 1987). They lack both basal and induced cytochrome P450 enzymes. Cell culture conditions were as described previously (Corcos et al., 1987).

2. PB treatment
PB in ethanol was added to the culture medium at a final concentration of 1.6 mM, and renewed each day for 3 days. Cells were then treated by AFB1 or harvested for RNA preparation. ACI male rats (from which hepatoma cell lines were initially derived) were given daily intraperitoneal injections of PB (100 mg/kg), for three days ; the last injection (coincident with food withdrawal) was 16 hours prior to sacrifice. Livers were used for preparation of total RNA (see below).

3. AFB1 treatment
Dishes were inoculated 16 hours prior to treatment. AFB1 dissolved in dimethylsulfoxide or the corresponding volume of the solvent was added to the culture medium and the cells incubated for 24 hours. The final concentration of AFB1 was 10 µM. Cultures were rinsed, fed with fresh medium, and fixed for colony counting 12 to 20 days later.

4. cDNA probes
a. PB inducible cytochrome P450 genes
The R17 cDNA clone isolated by M. Adesnik et al. from liver mRNA of PB treated rats, contains a 1100 bp insert homologous to the P450b and P450e mRNAs which share 98% homology (Adesnik & Atchison, 1985). The ptF2 cDNA clone isolated by T. Friedberg et al. from liver mRNA of PB treated rats contains a 409 bp insert homologous to P450 PB1 mRNA (Friedberg, 1986).

b. PAH*inducible cytochrome P450 genes
The C6 cDNA clone isolated by M. Affolter et al. from liver mRNA of Arocolor treated rats contains an insert homologous to the P450c and P450d mRNAs which share more than 70% homology (Affolter et al., 1986).

5. RNA preparation and hybridization
Preparation of total RNA, electrophoresis, blotting and hybridization were done as described (Corcos et al., 1987).

RESULTS

1. Phenobarbital induces distinct cytochrome P450 mRNAs in rat hepatoma cells
a. P450b/e
In rat liver, the genes coding for cytochromes P450b and P450e are highly inducible by PB (Adesnik & Atchison, 1986). The R17 cDNA probe reveals the accumulation of both P450b and P450e mRNAs. The figure shows that the intensity of the hybridization signal found with R17 is about five times higher for the mRNA of Fao rat hepatoma cells than for rat liver. In contrast, PB induces this specific mRNA only two to three fold in Fao, but more than 60 fold in liver. Aldrin epoxidase (AE) activity is a faithful indicator of PB inducible cytochrome P450 liver enzyme activities (Wolff et al., 1980) and undergoes a three fold increase after PB induction in Fao (Wiebel et al., 1984). The increase in mRNA for P450b/e must account for most of the increase in AE activity.

b. P450 PB1
In liver, cytochrome P450 PB1 mRNA is found at a high level in untreated animals, and is only slightly inducible by PB (Adesnik & Atchison, 1985). In contrast, the basal level of this mRNA is very low in Fao cells, but is highly inducible by PB, such that the induced level in Fao is comparable to the basal level in liver (see figure). The increase in mRNA for P450 PB1 in Fao cells could account for some of the increase in AE activity following PB treatment.

*PAH = polycyclic aromatic hydrocarbon

c. P450c/d

These genes are the major members of the PAH inducible family. The C6 cDNA probe reveals the accumulation of both cytochrome P450c and P450d mRNAs. In liver, comparable amounts of P450c and P450d mRNAs are found (see figure), and they are not increased by PB treatment. The situation is different in Fao cells : only P450c mRNA is present, and unexpectedly it undergoes a great increase after PB treatment (see figure). The increase of the P450c mRNA content of Fao cells is likely to account for most of the aryl hydrocarbon hydroxylase (AHH) activity found in PB treated cells (unpublished results) because AHH activity has been shown to be correlated with the expression of the P450c gene both in vivo and in vitro (Israel & Whitlock, 1983).

2. Phenobarbital treatment enhances the killing of hepatoma cells by AFB1

Table I gives the sensitivity to AFB1 of two hepatoma lines that have been treated or not with PB. The differentiated line Fao is highly sensitive to AFB1, and the proportion of cells killed is increased at least 50 fold following PB induction. This result is consistent with the fact that Fao cells produce PB inducible AE (Wiebel et al., 1984). As a control, cells of line RAB1-4 were tested under the same conditions ; it will be recalled that these cells were selected for their resistance to AFB1, and that they contain no P450b/e or P450 PB1 mRNA (Corcos et al., 1987). As expected, the RAB1-4 cells are highly resistant to AFB1 ; the decrease in resistance to AFB1 following PB treatment is slight and its basis will be investigated.

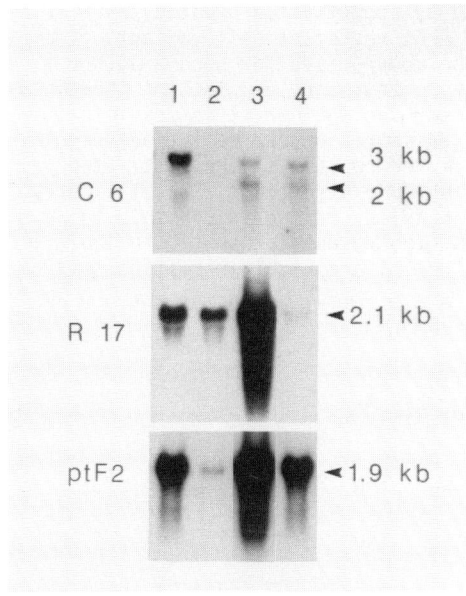

Northern blot of P450 RNAs in Fao and rat liver.
For each slot, 15 μg of total RNA were used. The hybridization probe used is indicated. The mRNA for P450c and P450d are of 3 and 2 kb, respectively. Lane 1, Fao + PB ; 2, Fao - PB ; 3, PB treated liver ; 4, untreated liver.

Table I
Sensitivity of rat hepatoma cells to AFB1

Rat hepatoma cell lines

	Fao		RAB1-4	
	-PB	+PB	-PB	+PB
Frequency of resistant colonies	$7.5 \; 10^{-5}$	$1.5 \; 10^{-6}$	$4.6 \; 10^{-1}$	$8 \; 10^{-2}$
-PB/+PB	50		6	

3. AFB1 resistant cells can be recovered from mixed cultures treated by AFB1, and following PB induction

It has been shown by others that fibroblasts lacking cytochrome P450 enzymes can be mutagenized by the AFB1 metabolites secreted by cocultivated hepatocytes (Langenbach et al., 1978). Attempts to isolate AFB1 resistant cell variants from a population of sensitive cells could thereby be compromised for such a poison effect would result in the elimination of truly resistant cells, lacking inducible cytochrome P450 enzyme activity. In order to determine whether it is possible to isolate cell lines deficient in the pathway of PB induction, C2 cells, deficient in PB inducible cytochrome P450 enzymes (unpublished results), were cultivated with Fao cells, and incubated with AFB1 following PB pretreatment. C2 cells carry the dominant selectable neo marker absent in Fao cells, making it possible to distinguish C2 from Fao cells in mixed cultures. The results presented in Table II show that C2 cells, even in coculture with Fao cells, are highly resistant to AFB1 under both basal and induced conditions.

Table II
Recovery of C2 cells
cocultivated with Fao cells*

	-AFB1		+AFB1	
	-PB	+PB	-PB	+PB
Number of colonies	419	212	376	140

*C2 cells were cocultivated with Fao cells, treated by PB and AFB1 three days before G418 was added to the culture medium.

DISCUSSION

1. We have demonstrated that the induction of cytochrome P450 enzymes by PB in rat hepatoma cells is paralleled by an increase in the content of specific cytochrome P450 mRNAs. The induction properties of cytochromes P450 by PB in Fao cells are different from those of rat liver for each of the three mRNAs examined. In particular, P450c mRNA is induced by PB although this has never been observed in vivo. However, PB has previously been shown to induce the accumulation of P450c mRNA in other hepatoma cell lines (Mc Manus et al., 1986), and this unusual response could be a consequence of the tumor phenotype.

2. The fact that C2 cells are rescued with high efficiency from mixed cultures treated by AFB1, under both basal and induced conditions, shows that cells with a low content of PB inducible cytochrome P450 enzymes are not killed at high frequency in a population of AFB1 treated sensitive cells. Hence, AFB1 treatment following PB induction of cells with a high content of PB inducible cytochrome P450 enzymes could lead to the isolation of cells deficient in specific steps of the pathway of PB induction.

3. We show here that killing of Fao cells by AFB1 is increased after PB treatment. Thus, only one cell in nearly a million rather than one in ten thousand, is able to survive ; the enhancement in killing is 50 fold. However, the activity probably responsible for AFB1 activation to toxic metabolites, P450b/e (see below), is only induced two to three fold by PB. Nevertheless, this small induction is not incompatible with the enhancement in killing observed, for the exact relationship between enzyme activity and degree of damage by AFB1 is unknown. In addition, the less than 0.01% cells affected represents such a small minority of the population that an average induction factor may be irrelevant to them. That P450b/e, and not P450 PB1 or P450c is involved in the metabolic activation of AFB1 by hepatoma

cells comes from the observation that highly resistant cells never have activity of the former, while the presence of the latter enzymes is sometimes observed (Corcos et al., 1987).

ACKNOWLEDGMENTS

We are especially grateful to M. Weiss for encouragement during the progress of this work, and for help in the preparation of the manuscript. We thank M. Adesnik and A. Anderson for their gifts of the cDNA probes used and F.J. Wiebel for helpful suggestions. This work was supported by grants from the Association pour la Recherche sur le Cancer and a contract of the Biotechnology Action Program of the Commission of the European Community. L.C is a fellow of the Ligue Nationale Française contre le Cancer.

REFERENCES

Adesnik, M. & Atchison, M. (1985) : Cytochrome P450 genes and their regulation. C.R.C. Critical Reviews in Biochemistry 19, 247-305.
Affolter, M. et al. (1986) : cDNA clones for liver cytochrome P450s from individual Arocolor-treated rats : Constitutive expression of a new P450 gene related to phenobarbital-inducible forms. DNA 5, 209-218.
Corcos, L. et al. (1987) : Selection of aflatoxin B1 resistant cell variants from differentiated rat hepatoma cells : Expression of cytochromes P450. Manuscript submitted for publication.
Deschatrette, J. & Weiss, M.C. (1974) : Characterization of differentiated and dedifferentiated clones from a rat hepatoma. Biochimie 56, 1603-1611.
Friedberg, J. et al. (1978) : Isolation and characterization of cDNA clones for cytochromes P450 immunochemically related to rat hepatic P450 form PB1. Biochemistry 25, 7975-7983.
Gurtoo, H.L. et al. (1978) : Association and dissociation of the Ah locus with the metabolic activation of aflatoxin B1 by mouse liver. J. Biol. Chem. 253, 3952-3961.
Israel, D.I. & Whitlock J.P. (1983) : Induction of mRNA specific for cytochrome P1-450 in wild type and variant mouse hepatoma cells. J. Biol. Chem. 258, 10390-10394.
Lambiotte, M. & Thierry, N. (1979) : Enhancement of aflatoxin B1 cytotoxicity in differentiated rat hepatoma cultures by a prior glucocorticoid treatment of the monolayer. Biochem. Biophys. Res. Commun. 89, 933-942.
Langenbach, R. et al. (1978) : Cell specificity in metabolic activation of aflatoxin B1 and benzo(a)pyrene to mutagens for mammalian cells. Nature 276, 277-280.
Loquet, C. & Wiebel, F.J. (1982) : Geno- and cytotoxicity of nitrosamines, aflatoxin B1 and benzo(a)pyrene in continuous cultures of rat hepatoma cells. Carcinogenesis 3, 1213-1218.
Mc Manus, M.E. et al. (1986) : Induction by phenobarbital in McA-RH7777 rat hepatoma cells of a polycyclic hydrocarbon inducible cytochrome P450. Biochem. Biophys. Res. Commun. 137, 120-127.
Metcalfe, S.A. et al. (1981) : A comparison of the effects of pretreatment with phenobarbitone and 3-methylcholanthrene on the metabolism of aflatoxin B1 by rat liver microsomes and isolated hepatocytes *in vitro*. Chem. Biol. Interactions 35, 145-157.
Wiebel, F.J. et al. (1980) : Presence of cytochrome P450 and cytochrome P448 dependent monooxygenase functions in hepatoma cell lines. Biochem. Biophys. Res. Commun. 94, 466-472.
Wiebel, F.J. et al. (1984) : Phenobarbital induces cytochrome P450 and cytochrome P448 dependent monooxygenases in rat hepatoma cells. Chem. Biol. Interactions 52, 151-162.
Wogan, P.M. & Butler, W.H. (1967) : Dose-response characteristics of aflatoxin B1 carcinogenesis in the rat. Cancer research 27, 2370-2376.

Effects of ethanol on gamma-glutamyltransferase of a rat hepatoma cell line

Michèle Levy[1], Denyse Bagrel[1], Nicole Sabolovic[1], Marie-Madeleine Galteau[1], Marie Wellman[1], Sylvie Rolin[2], Gérard Siest[1]

[1]Centre du Médicament, UA CNRS 597, 30 Rue Lionnois, 54000 Nancy, France. [2]Université Libre de Bruxelles, Département de Biologie Moléculaire, 67 Rue des Cheveaux, 1640 Rhode-St-Genese, Belgique

KEY WORDS

Gamma-glutamyltransferase, ethanol, enzyme induction, hepatoma cells

INTRODUCTION

Gamma-glutamyltransferase (GGT, EC 2.3.2.2.) has been widely investigated these last years. It has been proposed as an indirect index of enzyme induction in man where its plasma activity is enhanced by alcohol or by different drugs (oral contraceptives, antiepileptic drugs ...) (Bagrel et al., 1979). Some inducers of cytochrome P-450 dependent monooxygenases increase hepatic GGT synthesis and consequently its plasma activity in experimental animals (Galteau et al., 1980). However, the measurement of GGT remains a non very specific index of induction of liver drug metabolizing enzymes, undergoing numerous metabolic controls (Siest et al., 1987a). For example, the rise of GGT activity provoked by ethanol in vivo has been suspected to be a consequence of the increase in circulating glucocorticoid hormones (Cobb et al., 1981).
However, the mechanism by which ethanol stimulates the activity of this enzyme is not well understood. It was then logical to study this phenomenon in an in vitro model which could allow the determination of the direct action of a xenobiotic without any environmental regulations.

Hepatoma cell line cultures are very convenient systems for such experiments. Two cell lines issued from Reuber H35 hepatoma cells have already been proposed for studying GGT induction by dexamethasone or ethanol (Barouki et al., 1982, 1983). However, the lines these authors used i.e. Fao and C2 expressed a very low GGT activity. We were interested in performing this work in a Reuber H35 (Pitot et al., 1964) derived hepatoma cell line, H 5-6 (Sperling et al. 1980), a subclone of H 5 (Deschatrette et al., 1974 ; Rogier et al., 1986), Moreover, preliminary experiments had shown that this cell line intensely expressed GGT (Siest et al., 1987b).

MATERIEL AND METHODS

Cell Cultures
Hepatoma cells H 5-6 have been cloned from H4IIEC3 line (Pitot et al., 1964) which is a descendant of Reuber H35 hepatoma cells (Reuber, 1961). They were pro-

vided by Pr. O. HANKINSON (Laboratory of Biomedical and Environmental Sciences, Los Angeles).
Cells were grown in Dulbecco's Minimum Essential Medium (Gibco) containing 10 % Nu-serum (Sochibo), 100 units/ml penicillin, 100 µg/ml streptomycin and 0.25 µg/ml fungizone (Gibco), at 37°C, in an atmosphere of 95 % air and 5 % CO_2.

Treatment of cells
Cells (1 - 1.5x10^6) where seeded in 100 mm plastic dishes in order to perform experiments during the exponential phase of growth. Medium was changed 48 hr after seeding and replaced by fresh medium containing or not ethanol (final concentrations: 150 or 300 mM). This medium was removed after 72 hr.
After various times of treatment (6 hr to 120 hr), the culture medium was collected, centrifuged at 300 g for 10 mn and frozen at -20°C.
Cells were washed twice by phosphate-buffered saline (PBS) (Eurobio), pH 7.4, scrapped and resuspended in PBS. After a 10 mn centrifugation at 300 g, cells were stored at - 80°C.

Cells viability
Cell viability has been checked by using trypan blue exclusion test.

Biochemical assays
Cellular proteins were determined by the method of Lowry et al. (1951) using bovine serum albumin as standard. Gamma-glutamyltransferase activity was measured according to the method of Szasz (1969) using gamma-L-glutamyl-3-carboxy-4-nitroanilide and glycylglycine as substrates. Lactate-dehydrogenase activity (LDH, EC 1.1.1.27) was determined according to Mathieu et al. (1982). To quantify the immunoreactive GGT, an ELISA method (sandwich type) has been developed in our laboratory. The same procedure that described by Taniguchi et al. (1983) was used but with the following modifications: horseradish peroxidase was used as enzyme for labeling of polyclonal anti-rat-GGT kidney GGT IgG.

Histochemical detection of GGT
GGT activity was detected by the method of Rutenburg et al. (1969) slightly modified by Manson et al. (1981), using N-(L-gamma-glutamyl)-4-methoxy-2-naphthylamide as substrate.

Two-dimensional electrophoresis
Two-dimensional electrophoresis was performed as described previously (Antoine et al., 1987). 300 µg of cell proteins solubilized in a mixture containing urea (2 M), 2-mercaptoethanol (5 %), Nonidet P-40 (3 %), sodium deoxycholate (0.5 %) were loaded on each gel. After electrophoresis the gels were silver stained by the method of Oakley slightly modified in our laboratory (Galteau et al., 1986).

RESULTS

Effects of ethanol on cellular gamma-glutamyltransferase
H 5-6 cells express a high basal activity of GGT: 100-150 mU/mg proteins. These values are about 100 times more important than those of rat adult hepatocytes. This activity is relatively stable during 120 hours upon culturing (Fig. 1).
The effect of ethanol is dose-dependent. When cells are treated with ethanol 150 mM for 48 h, a slight increase (about 70 %) of cellular GGT activity can be detected. A treatment with ethanol 300 mM for 48 h provokes a shift of about 160 % in enzyme activity.
Moreover, ethanol effect on GGT activity needs a delay: no GGT induction can be detected after a 12 hr-treatment, but the increase of activity is optimal after 48 hr of treatment and is maintained if ethanol is kept into culture medium.

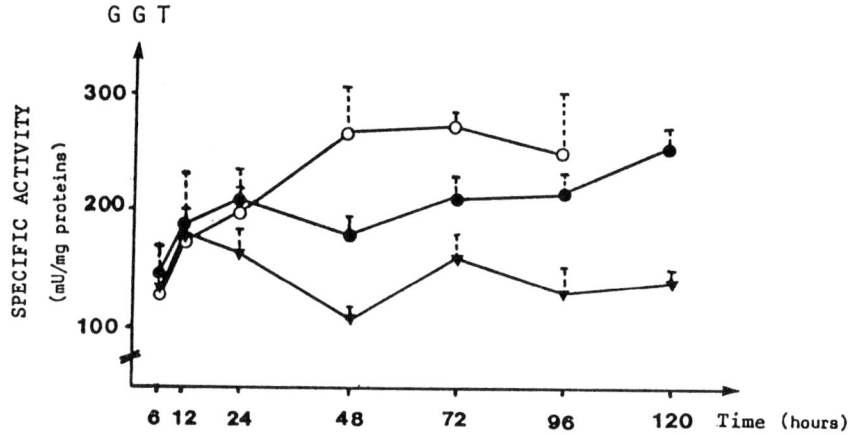

Fig. 1: Ethanol effect on gamma-glutamyltransferase activity in H 5-6 hepatoma cells. Cells in exponential phase of growth are treated with ethanol 150 mM (●), 300 mM (○), or not treated (▲). Values represent means ± SE of at least 3 values obtained from 3 different experiments.

The induction of GGT in H 5-6 cells has been corroborated by histoenzymatic assay. GGT is easily detected in H 5-6 control cultures in which all cells present an evident activity, as aggregates not homogeneously distributed on the membrane. When these cells are treated with ethanol, the staining is highly enhanced demonstrating an increasing activity (Fig. 2).

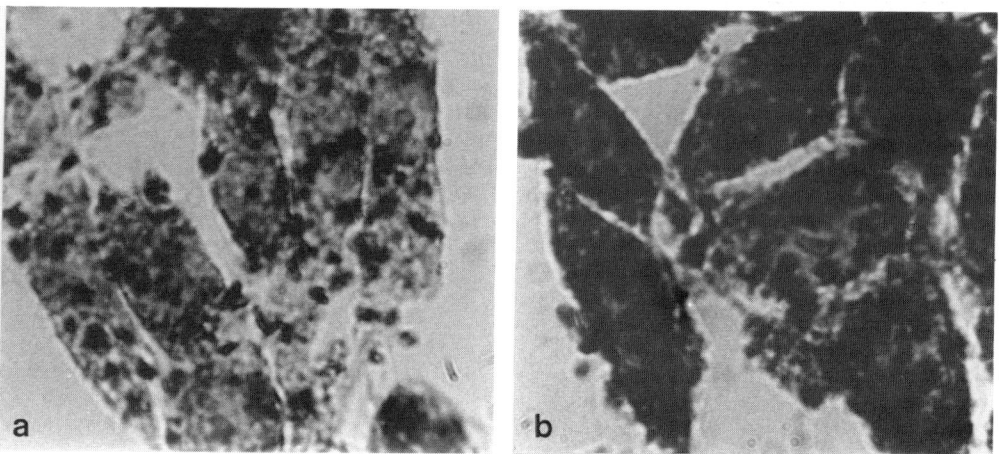

Fig. 2: Histochemical demonstration of GGT activity in H 5-6 cells cultured for 48 h. a) Control cells. b) Cells treated with ethanol 150 mM.

In order to differentiate an eventual increase of GGT synthesis from a modification of its catalytic properties, the measurement of immunoreactive GGT protein by an ELISA method has been realized.

Table I shows that H 5-6 cells present a basal concentration of 60 to 100 ng of GGT per mg of total cellular proteins. These values are comparable with the data obtained by Taniguchi (1983) for azodye induced hepatoma. When the cells were treated by 150 mM ethanol, we observed that after 24 and 72 hours the concentration of GGT protein increased about 1.5 times. Specific activity varying from 2.3 to 1.5 mU per ng of immunoreactive GGT for 24 and 72 hours controls respectively. It seems that ethanol treatment increases the level of the GGT protein without modification of its specific activity.

Table 1 : Determination of GGT levels in H 5-6 cells by enzyme immunoassay and by enzyme specific activity

	N	ng/mg cell proteins* m (s)	mU/mg cell proteins m (s)	mU/ng proteins GGT m (s)
Control				
24 h	5	73.1 (20.7)	157.6 (18.0)	2.26 (0.57)
72 h	3	106.3 (27.7)	151.7 (2.5)	1.48 (0.39)
Ethanol 150 mM				
24 h	4	120.5 (5.3)	244.6 (20.1)	2.47 (1.3)
72 h	3	157.3 (45.7)	255.0 (20.0)	1.71 (0.44)

*Cell content in GGT protein (expressed in ng of GGT per mg of total proteins) has been measured by immunoenzymatic method (type ELISA) as described in Materials and Methods.

Toxic effects of ethanol

During our induction experiments, we used relatively high ethanol concentrations and we verified its eventual toxic effect.
Comparison of control and treated cell growth is depicted in Fig. 3. Cell multiplication is reduced by ethanol and this effect is dose-dependent. When cells are exposed to ethanol 300 mM longer than 48 h, phase contrast microscopy reveals some cellular mortality. However, Fig. 3 shows that cell growth is not inhibited, but only diminished.

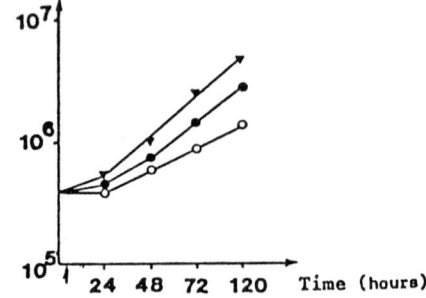

Fig. 3: Growth curve of control (▲) or ethanol-treated (150 mM ● and 300 mM ○) H 5-6 cells. Each point represents the mean of 3 experiments (two identical dishes are used for each counting).

Toxic effect can be evaluated by LDH release (Aguiar et al., 1985). We verified that the release of LDH in the medium at both ethanol concentrations was negligible (less than 2 % of cell content).
Lastly, we checked the effect of ethanol on extracellular release of GGT.
Table 2 shows that ethanol increases GGT activity in culture medium. However, this rise reflects the total (cells + medium) increase of activity, the ratio of released to total GGT being the same in control and treated cells.

Table 2: Effect of ethanol on extracellular release of GGT

Time of exposure	Cells	N	Control m (s)	Ethanol 150 mM m (s)	Ethanol 300 mM m (s)
6 h	*GGT_t **$\frac{GGT_r}{GGT_t}$ x 100	7 7	244.4 (10.1) 21,8 (7.0)	188.9 (26.8) 20.1 (7.6)	167.0 (23.7) 19.2 (5.6)
24 h	GGT_t $\frac{GGT_r}{GGT_t}$ x 100	5 5	181.9 (16.5) 52.6 (8.1)	293.5 (22.9) 50.1 (4.1)	382.5 (17.4) 57.4 (7.1)
48 h	GGT_t $\frac{GGT_r}{GGT_t}$ x 100	5 5	218.5 (27.8) 51.3 (6.2)	362.0 (39.6) 59.2 (11.2)	554.5 (60.5) 59.0 (10.9)

*GGT_t: total GGT (cells + medium) expressed as mU/mg cells proteins
**GGT_r: GGT released in culture medium

Effect of ethanol on cellular proteins

Most of the spots revealed by two-dimensional electrophoresis are located in the central region (pH: 4.5-7.5, Mw: 28-66 Kd). Profiles of homogenates prepared from control or ethanol treated (48 h, 150 mM) cells are similar (Fig. 4). Ethanol exposure is responsible for two kinds of modifications. On one hand, many spots are increased after treatment. They generally correspond to relative molecular weights lower than 45 KD. On the other hand, some peptides are reduced by treatment. In this case, they present a high apparent Mw (66 KD) or a low one (Mw < 21 KD). Such modifications were also observed in rat after a phenobarbital treatment (Antoine et al., 1987).

CONCLUSION

Study of GGT induction in cultured cells has been carried out in our laboratory on rat, mouse or human hepatoma cells (unpublished results).
Reuber H35 derivative H 5-6 cells seemed to be an interesting model for exploration of in vitro effects of ethanol on GGT activity.
This cell line has been selected because of its high basal GGT activity. Although this enzyme has been shown to be a useful diagnostic marker for hepatocellular carcinomas and other tumors (Braun et al., 1987), very few cultured hepatoma cell lines exhibit so high activity (100-150 mU/mg proteins). This expression level facilitates the measurement of the activity of intracellular GGT and of GGT released in the culture medium as measurement of the immunoreactive protein itself.
Ethanol concentrations used in these experiments are not dramatically cytotoxic: cells growth is slowed but not inhibited and cell death percentages are low. Moreover, no extracellular release of LDH, was observed. In the same way, the

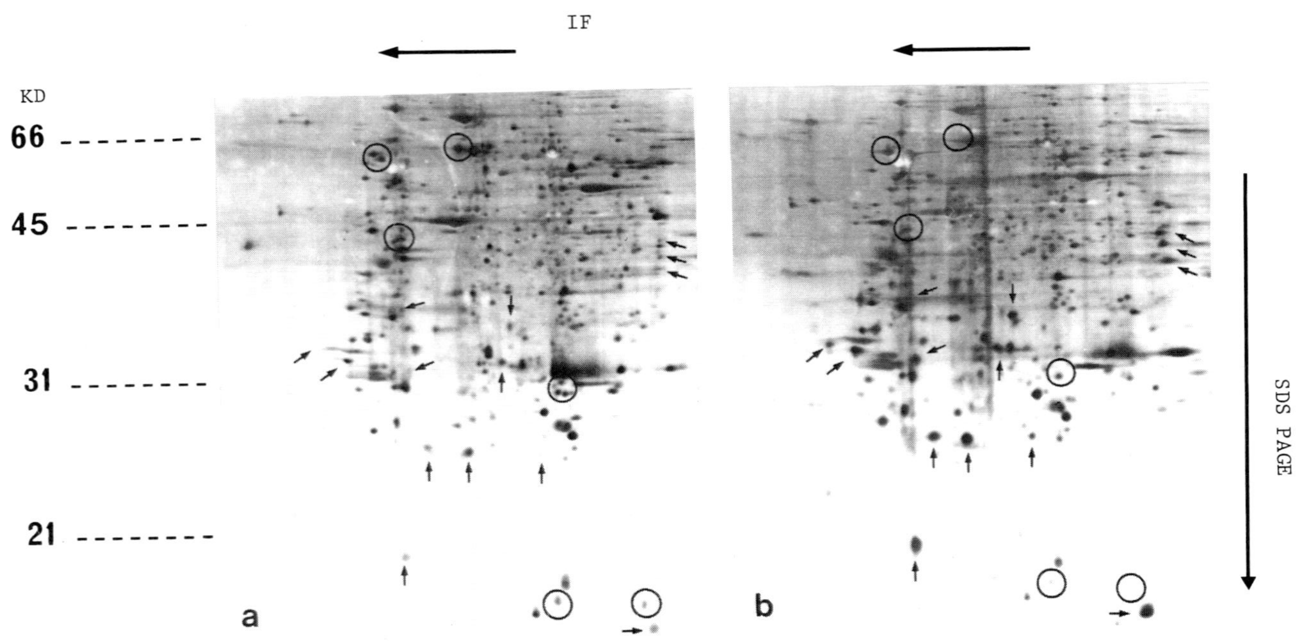

Fig. 4: Two dimensional electrophoretic patterns of rat hepatoma H5-6
a: control cells
b: cells treated 48 h by ethanol 150 mM. Arrows point to the polypeptides which appear or are intensified; circles indicate the location of missing polypeptides
IF: isoelectric focusing
KD: molecular weight marker in kilodalton
SDS: sodium dodecylsulfate - PAGE: polyacrylamide gel electrophoresis

ratio of GGT released in the culture medium is not enhanced by ethanol. These results let suppose that these treatments did not alter plasma membranes. It appears that the increase in cellular H 5-6 GGT after ethanol exposure is not due to activation of this enzyme but to the increase in its biosynthesis as proved by determination of immunoreactive GGT. This induction needs a 24 hours delay, is optimal after a 48 hour-treatment and depends on the ethanol dosage. Induction factor we obtained is consistent with those found by Barouki et al. (1983) in C_2 cells, a descendant of Reuber H 35 hepatoma cells too.
Two-dimensional electrophoresis experiments have shown ethanol induced proteic modifications. Further investigations using immunologic revelation will allow identification of some of these modified peptides. Modifications of enzyme activities will be related with qualitative or quantitative variations of the corresponding peptides.

Cultures H 5-6 cells represent an excellent system for the study of in vitro effects of ethanol on GGT expression. Further investigations will allow to define this action at molecular level.

ACKNOWLEDGMENTS

This work has been supported by grants from the "Comité Lorraine de la Fondation pour la Recherche Médicale" and from the "Haut Comité d'Etude et d'Information sur l'Alcoolisme" (Decision N°2497).

BIBLIOGRAPHY

AGUIAR, K., GALTEAU, M.M., SIEST, G., FOURNEL, S., MAGDALOU, J. (1985): Comparative effect of a series of hypolipidemic compounds on the release of enzymes from isolated hepatocytes. Biochem. Pharmacol. 34, 379-380.
ANTOINE, B., RAHIMI-POUR, A., SIEST, G., MAGDALOU, J., GALTEAU, M.M. (1987): Differential Time-Course of Induction of Rat Liver Gamma-Glutamyltransferase and Drug-Metabolizing Enzymes in the Endoplasmic Reticulum, Golgi and Plasma Membranes after a Single Phenobarbital Injection. Evaluation of Protein Variations by Two-Dimensional Electrophoresis. Cell. Biochem. Functions, 5, 217-231.
BAGREL, D., SIEST, G., GALTEAU, M.M. (1979): Interprétation des variations de l'activité de la GGT. Etude de l'effet des médicaments. In: Mises au point de Biochimie Pharmacologique, ed. G. SIEST, C. HEUSGHEM, pp. 236-268, Paris : Masson.
BAROUKI, R., CHOBERT, M.N., BILLON, M.C., FINIDORI, J., TSAPIS, R., HANOUNE, J. (1982): Glucocorticoid hormones increase the activity of -glutamyltransferase in a highly differentiated hepatoma cell line. Biochim. Biophys. Acta, 721, 11-21.
BAROUKI, R., CHOBERT, M.N., FINIDORI, J., AGGERBECK, M., NALPAS, B., HANOUNE, J. (1983): Ethanol effect in a rat hepatoma cell line: induction of -glutamyltransferase. Hepatology, 3, 323-329.
BRAUN, J.P., SIEST, G., RICO, A.G. (1987): Uses of gamma-glutamyltransferase in experimental toxicology. Adv. Vet. Sci. Comp. Med., 31, 151-172.
COBB, C.F., VAN THIEL, D.M., GAVALER, J.S. et al. (1981): Effects of ethanol and acetaldehyde on the rat adrenal. Metabolism, 30, 537-543.
DESCHATRETTE, J., WEISS, M.C. (1974): Characterization of differentiated and dedifferenciated clones from a rat hepatoma. Biochimie, 56, 1603-1611.
GALTEAU, M.M., SIEST, G., RATANASAVANH, D. (1980): Effects of phenobarbital on the distribution of gamma-glutamyltransferase between hepatocytes and non parenchymal cells in the rat. Cell. Mol. Biol., 26, 267-273.

GALTEAU, M.M., RAHIMI-POUR, A., CAUDIE, C., QUINCY, C., SIEST, G. (1986): La coloration argentique pour l'étude des protéines séparées par électrophorèse bidimensionnelle en gel de polyacrylamide. In: Progrès Récents en Electrophorèse Bidimensionnelle, ed. M.M. GALTEAU, G. SIEST, pp. 53-68, Nancy : Presses Universitaires.
LOWRY, O.H., ROSEBROUGH, N.J., FARR, A.L., RANDALL, R.J. (1951): Protein measurement with the folin phenol reagent. J. Biol. Chem., 193, 265-275.
MANSON, M.M., LEGG, R.F., WATSON, J.V., GREEN, J.A., NEAL, G.E. (1981): An examination of the relative resistances to Aflatoxin B1 and susceptibilities to ɣ-glutamyl p-phenylene diamine mustard to -glutamyltransferase negative and positive cell lines. Carcinogenesis, 2, 661-670.
MATHIEU, M.M., ARTUR, Y., AUBRY, C. et les membres de la Commission Enzymologie de la Société Française de Biologie Clinique (1982): Recommandations pour la mesure de la concentration catalytique de la lactate-déshydrogénase dans le sérum humain à 30°C. Ann. Biol. Clin., 40, 123-125.
PITOT, H.C., PERAINO, C., MORSE, P.A., POTTER, V.R. (1964): Hepatomas in tissue culture compared with adapting liver in vivo. Natl. Cancer. Inst. Monographs, 13, 229-241.
REUBER, M.D. (1961): A transplantable bile-secreting hepatocellular carcinoma in the rat. J. Natl. Cancer. Inst., 26, 891-897.
ROGIER, E., CASSIO, D., WEISS, M.C., FELDMANN, G. (1986): An ultrastructural study of rat hepatoma cells in culture, their variants and revertants. Differentiation, 30, 229-236.
RUTENBURG, A.M., KIM, H., FISCHBEIN, J.W., HANKER, J.S., WASSERKRUG, H.L., SELIGMAN, A.M. (1969): Histochemical and ultrastructural demonstration of gamma-glutamyltranspeptidase activity. J. Histochem. Cytochem., 17, 517-526.
SIEST, G., BATT, A.M., FOURNEL-GIGLEUX, S., GALTEAU, M.M., WELLMAN-BEDNAWSKA, M., MINN, A., AMAR-COSTESEC, A. (1987a): Induction of plasma and tissue enzymes by drugs: significance in toxicological studies. Xenobiotica (accepté sous presse).
SIEST, G., BAGREL, D., LEVY, M., FEBVRE, N., FOURNEL-GIGLEUX, S., ROLIN, S., SABOLOVIC, N., WELLMAN-BEDNAWSKA, M., GALTEAU, M.M., TOYODA, Y. (1987b): The use of hepatoma cells in culture as an alternative to the study of drug metabolizing enzymes. In: Proceedings of the ISSX 2nd European Meeting, 29 March - 3 April, Frankfurt (RFA), ed. TAYLOR and FRANCIS Ltd (accepté sous presse).
SPERLING, L., TARDIEU, A., WEISS, M.C. (1980): Chromatin repeat length in sonatic hybrids. Proc. Natl. Acad. Sci. USA, 77, 5, 2716-2720.
SZASZ, G. (1969): A kinetic photometric method for serum gamma-glutamyltranspeptidase. Clin. Chem., 19, 124-136.
TANIGUCHI, N, YOKOSAWA, N., IIZUKA, S., SAHO, F., TSUKADA, Y., SATOH, M., DEMPO, K. (1983): ɣ-glutamyltranspeptidase of rat liver and hepatoma tissues: an enzyme immunoassay and immunostaining studies. Ann. NY Acad. Sci., 417, 203-212.

An *in vivo-in vitro* model to study the cellular transformation elicited by liver tumor promoters : application to phenobarbital, butylated hydroxytoluene and butylated hydroxyanisole

Paule Martel, Catherine Chaumontet, Valérie François, Khalid Ben Reddad, Gérard Pascal

Laboratoire des Sciences de la Consommation, INRA-CRJ, Domaine de Vilvert 78350 Jouy-en-Josas, France

KEYWORDS

In vivo-in vitro model, tumor promoters, liver epithelial cells, phenobarbital, butylated hydroxytoluene, butylated hydroxyanisole.

INTRODUCTION

The existence of substances acting as tumor promoters on experimental hepatocarcinogenesis has been first demonstrated by Peraino et al. (1971), with acetylaminofluorene (AAF) and phenobarbital (PB) as initiator and tumor promoter, respectively. Other *in vivo* models have been proposed (Solt and Farber, 1976 ; Pitot et al., 1978) that give results only after quite long experiments. Later, Kitagawa et al. (1980) have described an *in vivo-in vitro* model where each of the two steps, initiation and promotion lasted about twelve weeks.

Recently, we have developed a shorter *in vivo-in vitro* procedure which could be very useful to study the effects and the mechanisms of action of liver tumor promoters. Thus, in order to shorten the first stage, we chose to carry out initiation on newborn animals by a single injection of the hepatocarcinogen, according to Peraino et al. (1981). Then, one week later, liver epithelial cells could be isolated and then submitted to the *in vitro* action of liver tumor promoters. Furthermore, this model would present the advantage to work on epithelial cells which are known to be at the origin of the majority of human tumors, i.e. adenocarcinomas and hepatocellular carcinomas (Weinstein et al., 1975; Montesano et al., 1980).

Butylated hydroxytoluene (BHT) and butylated hydroxyanisole (BHA), two antioxidants commonly used as food additives, have been shown to exert tumor promoting actions in various organs and tissues of rodents, *in vivo* (Ito et al., 1986). In particular, there is good evidence that they could be liver tumor promoters : an enhancing effect of BHT on hepatic tumorigenesis in rats previously fed AAF for a brief period, has been reported by Peraino et al. (1977). Likewise, the incidence of nitrosodiethylamine (DEN)-initiated neoplastic liver lesions, in $B_6C_3F_1$ mice, has been shown to be increased by oral exposure to BHA (Hagiwara, Diwan and Ward, 1986).

The present work studies the effects of BHT, BHA and PB on the transformation of liver cells in our model, PB being the tumor promoter of reference.

MATERIALS AND METHODS

Initiation
Within 1 day after birth, 10 newborn Wistar rats were injected i.p., with a single dose of hepatocarcinogen (AAF 30 mg/kg).

Isolation of liver
One week later, liver cells were isolated by a fractional trypsinization of the pooled livers essentially as described by Chessebeuf et al. (1974).

Selection of liver epithelial cells
Liver epithelial cells were separated from contaminant fibroblasts by means of a serum-free medium, composed of Ham's F_{10} basal medium supplemented with free fatty acids adsorbed on bovine albumin, according to Chessebeuf and Padieu (1984). This method gave successful rise to primary cultures and then to long term cell lines that could be easily cultivated in serum-supplemented medium (10 % fetal calf serum).

First characterization of the cell line
Before the tumor promotion assay, the cell line was cultured in the absence of any treatment, for about twenty weeks. The cellular transformation was assessed by the ability of the cells to grow in soft agar (Montagnier and Gruest, 1979) and by the induction of the γ-glutamyl-transpeptidase activity, γ-GT (Rutenburg et al., 1969). Aliquots of the cell line at early stages were maintained in liquid nitrogen, and could be subcultured and used for subsequent tumor promotion assay.

In vitro tumor promotion
The cell transformation elicited by PB, BHT and BHA was followed by the two previous criteria : growth in soft agar and γ-GT activity. The main stages of the experimental in vivo-in vitro procedure are illustrated in Fig. 1.

The growth behaviour of the cells in culture was studied by counting, in a Coulter Counter, the number of the cells in two dishes of each treatment, over two weeks after plating. The modification of the binding of ^{125}I-epidermal growth factor (^{125}I-EGF) was evaluated on confluent cells after a 4 hour incubation. EGF was iodinated by the chloramine T method to the activity of 30-60 µCi/µg.

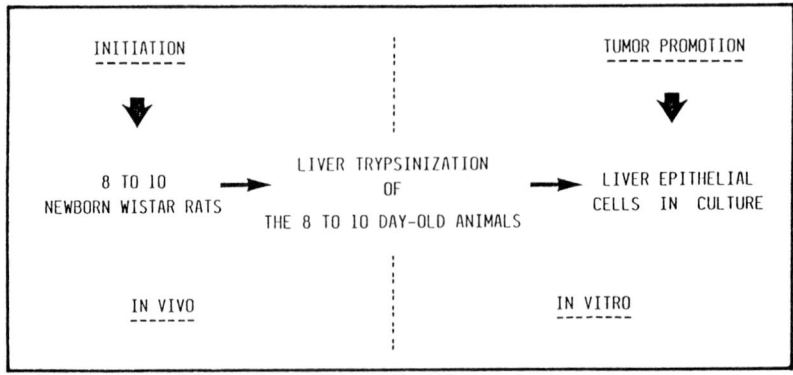

Fig. 1. The in vivo-in vitro procedure proposed to study the effects of liver tumor-promoters.

RESULTS

Characterization of the 27E cell line

The 27E cell line was obtained from AAF-initiated rats (30 mg/kg). These liver epithelial cells were selected after a 2 week culture in the serum-free medium. After about 20 passages of culture in the serum-supplemented medium, in absence of tumor promoters, these cells remained untransformed according to the two criteria that have been followed (not shown). Therefore, the 27E cell line has provided untransformed cells from initiated animals, that could be submitted to the transforming action of tumor promoters.

Long-term incubation with tumor promoters was started with 27E cells at the 8th passage (noted $27E_8$). Cells were fed the complete medium containing or not PB, BHT or BHA, at 3 non cytotoxic concentrations (cf. Table 1).

1	CONTROL	(DMSO 1%)
2	PB	10^{-3} M
3	PB	$3\ 10^{-4}$ M
4	PB	10^{-4} M
5	BHT	$3\ 10^{-5}$ M
6	BHT	10^{-5} M
7	BHT	$3\ 10^{-6}$ M
8	BHA	10^{-4} M
9	BHA	$3\ 10^{-5}$ M
10	BHA	10^{-5} M

Table 1. Nature of the treatments applied to 27E cells.

Growth in soft agar

After a 13 week treatment with PB, BHT or BHA, the 27E cells did not show the ability to grow in soft agar (results not shown).

γ-GT activity

The induction of the γ-GT activity has been determined at 2 stages of the experimentation. After 6 weeks of incubation, only BHA 10^{-4}M strongly induced the γ-GT activity. When tested after 15 weeks of culture, the γ-GT activity was still unchanged in the control, but significantly stimulated by the 3 substances in a dose-response manner (cf. Fig. 2).

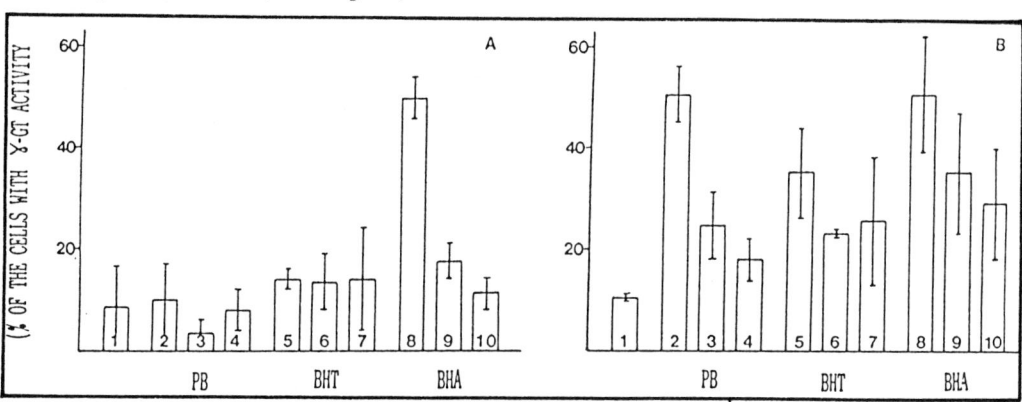

Fig. 2. Induction of the γ-GT activity by PB, BHT or BHA. A : in $27E_{13}$ cells (after 6 weeks of incubation) ; B : in $27E_{22}$ cells (after 15 weeks of incubation). Each point represents the mean ± SEM of 2 independent experiments.

Proliferative activity
During a 2 week study, no modification of the proliferative velocity was observed, except for PB and BHA at the highest concentration. The number of cells per plate at confluence (10 days after plating) was about the same with the different treatments. However, the stability of the confluent population was readily increased with PB 1-3 10^{-4}M and BHT 0,3-3 10^{-5}M (cf. Fig. 3).

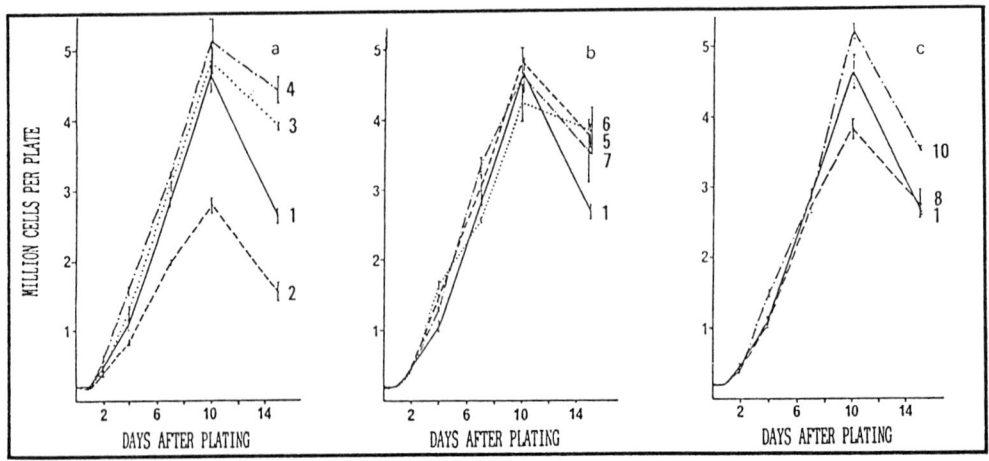

Fig. 3. Proliferative activity of 27E$_{26}$ cells in the presence of PB(a), BHT(b) and BHA(c).

EGF binding
The modification of the capacity of the cells to bind EGF has been investigated with confluent 27E$_{23}$ cells. Fig. 4 shows that EGF binding was reduced with the highest concentrations of PB and BHA, whereas it was increased with PB 10^{-4}M and BHT 0,3-3 10^{-5}M.

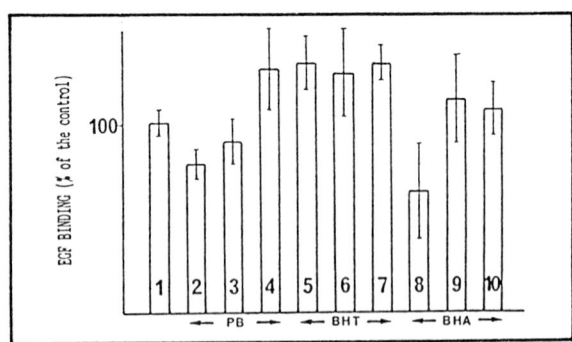

Fig. 4. EGF binding to confluent 27E$_{23}$ cells. The results, expressed as the percentage of the control, are the mean ± SEM of 2 independent experiments.

DISCUSSION

In the model described here, the exposition to the hepatocarcinogen is carried out *in vivo*, under the influence of the whole organism. The fact that it is performed on newborn animals does not prevent the initiation to occur since newborn rats appear more susceptible than older animals to chemically induced hepatocarcinogenesis (Peraino et al, 1981).

This mode of initiation not only shortens the first stage of the procedure, but also enables liver epithelial cells to be isolated at the most favorable period : one week after birth. In absence of promoting treatment, the 27E cells remained untransformed at least during 20 weeks of culture, and provided an interesting cellular material to study the effects of liver tumor promoters, *in vitro*.

With this system, PB and BHA did not confer on the cells the ability to grow in soft agar after 13 weeks of culture. An other experiment, with a longer incubation time, will be necessary to confirm the total absence of effects of the 3 substances and to consider the validity of this marker of the transformation of liver epithelial cells. In other respects, the γ-GT activity was rapidly induced by BHA and then by PB and BHT, in a response-dose manner. The induction of γ-GT activity has been considered to be a good marker of the transformation of liver epithelial cells to malignant tumors (Montesano et al., 1980 ; Sulakhe and Lautt, 1987). However, Preat et al. (1986) observed an induction of γ-GT activity by BHT, in absence of development of liver cancers, in the model of Solt and Farber (1976) with DEN as initiator. In order to validate our observations, the cells which have been cultured with PB, BHT or BHA will be soon injected to syngenic rats to detect the development of tumors.

Two of the most efficient treatments in the induction of γ-GT activity, PB 10^{-3}M and BHA 10^{-4}M, reduced the proliferation velocity of 27E cells. This effect was not due to a general cytotoxic action of these drugs, since they did not interfere with the incorporation of Leucine (results not shown). It should be more likely related to the reduction of EGF binding and of thymidine incorporation (not shown). Therefore, if the induction of γ-GT activity is really a good marker of cellular transformation, the stimulation of the proliferative activity does not appear to be a necessary or at least synchronous event. In other respects, the increase in the stability of the cells at confluence, observed with PB and BHT, indicates an enhancement of their resistance to a high cell density. A scanning electron microscopy study, to detect the ability of cells to pile up, is still in progress.

This model appears to be very useful to study the cellular transformation elicited by BHT and BHA, on liver cells. It will contribute to the evaluation of their eventual tumor promoting action when used as food additives or therapeutic agents. It may be helpful to detect other liver tumor promoters.

This work was supported by PIREN-CNRS and INRA.

REFERENCES

- Chessebeuf, M., Olsson, A., Bournot, P., Desgres, J., Guiguet, M., Maume, G., Maume, B.F., Perissel, B., Padieu, P. (1974) : Long term cell culture of rat liver epithelial cells retaining some hepatic functions. Biochimie. 56, 1365-1379.
- Chessebeuf, M., Padieu, P. (1984) : Rat liver epithelial cell cultures in a serum-free medium : primary cultures and derived cell lines expressing differentiated functions. In vitro. 20, 780-795.
- Hagiwara, A., Diwan, B.A., Ward, J.M. (1986) : Modifying effects of butylated hydroxyanisole, di(2-ethylexyl)phtalate or indomethacin on mouse hepatocarcinogenesis initiated by N-nitrosodiethylamine. Jpn. J. Cancer Res. 77, 1215-1221.
- Ito, N., Hirose, M., Fukushima, S., Tsuda, H., Shirai, T., Tatematsu, M. (1986) : Studies on antioxidants : their carcinogenic and modifying effects on chemical carcinogenesis. Fd. Chem. Toxic. 11, 1071-1082.
- Kitagawa, T., Watanabe, R., Kayano, T., Sugano, H. (1980) : In vitro carcinogenesis of hepatocytes obtained from acetylaminofluorene-treated rat liver and promotion of their growth by phenobarbital. Gann. 71, 747-754.

.Montagnier, L., Gruest, J. (1979) : Cell-density-dependence for growth in agarose of two human lymphoma lines and its decrease after Epstein-Barr virus conversion. Int. J. Cancer, 23, 71-75.

.Montesano, R., Bannikov, G., Drevon, C., Kuroki, T., Saint Vincent, L., Tomatis, L. (1980) : Neoplastic transformation of rat liver epithelial cells in culture. Ann. N.Y. Acad. Sci. 349, 323-331.

.Peraino, C., Fry, R.J.M., Staffeldt, E. (1971) : Reduction and enhancement by phenobarbital of hepatocarcinogenesis induced in the rat by 2-acetylaminofluorene. Cancer Res. 31, 1506-1512.

.Peraino, C., Fry, R.J.M., Staffeldt, E., Christopher, J.P. (1977) : Enhancing effects of phenobarbitone and BHT on 2-acetylaminofluorene induced hepatic tumorigenesis in the rat. Fd. Cosmet. Toxicol. 15, 93-96.

.Peraino, C., Staffeldt, E.F., Ludeman, V.A. (1981) : Early appearance of histochemically altered hepatocyte foci and liver tumors in female rats treated with carcinogens one day after birth. Carcinogenesis. 2, 463-465.

.Pitot, H., Barsness, L., Goldsworthy, T., Kitagawa, T. (1978) : Biochemical characterization of stages of hepatocarcinogenesis after a single dose of diethylnitrosamine. Nature. 271, 456-458.

.Preat, V., De Gerlache, J., Lans, M., Taper H., Roberfroid, M. (1986) : Comparative analysis of the effect of phenobarbital, dichlorodiphenyltrichloroethane, butylated hydroxytoluene and nafenopin on rat hepatocarcinogenesis. Carcinogenesis. 7, 1025-1028.

.Rutenburg, A.M., Rim, H., Fischbein, J., Hauker, J., Wasserkrug, H., Selignan, A. (1969) : Histochemical and ultrastructural demonstration of γ-glutamyl transpeptidase activity. J. Histochem. Cytochem. 17, 517-526.

.Solt, D.B., Farber, E. (1976) : New principle for the analysis of chemical carcinogenesis. Nature. 263, 702-703.

.Sulakhe, S.J., Lautt, W.W. (1987) : A characterization of γ-glutamyltranspeptidase in normal perinatal, premalignant and malignant rat liver. Int. J. Biochem. 19, 23-32.

.Weinstein, I.B., Orenstein, J.M., Gebert, R., Kaighn, E., Stadler, U.C. (1975) : Growth and structural properties of epithelial cell cultures established from normal rat liver and chemically induced hepatomas. Cancer Res. 35, 253-263.

Liver Cells and Drugs. Ed. A. Guillouzo. Colloque INSERM/John Libbey Eurotext Ltd. © 1988. Vol. 164, pp. 465-471.

Expression of *Ki-ras, myc* and *fos* protooncogenes during progression of spontaneous malignant transformation of epithelial rat liver cells in culture

Christiane Lafarge-Frayssinet*, Marylene Garcette**, Rodica Emanoil-Ravier**, Edith Morel-Chany*, Charles Frayssinet*

Laboratoire de Pathologie Cellulaire de l'ER 304, IRSC, BP 8, 94802 Villejuif, France.
**INSERM, U.107, Hôpital Saint-Louis, 75010 Paris, France*

Key words : protooncogenes, progression of malignancy, rat liver cells, cell culture.

INTRODUCTION

From normal rat liver we have established epithelial cell lines which generally did not degenerate but presented after a certain number of subcultures evidence of neoplastic transformation. The conversion of these cells to malignant state was accompanied by changes in their differentiation characteristics. Morphological changes and modification of their enzymatic pattern have been previously reported (Morel-Chany et al., 1978 and 1985).

Although we do not know the cause of this spontaneous malignant transformation some similar observations have been made for rat epithelial liver cells by Sato et al. (1968); Oshiro et al. (1972). Viruses have been incriminated as causal agent and Weinstein et al. (1975) reported viral particles in their cultures, however neither viral nor PPLO particles were observed in our cells after ultrastructural examination. In this work, we have studied the progression of the spontaneous malignant transformation occuring in our cells using parameters such as morphological changes, growth in soft agar and gamma glutamyl transpeptidase (γGT) expression which are more often considered as markers of the neoplastic transformation.

The recent developments in cancer research have shown that the increase and/or changed activity of certain genes collectively termed as cellular or protooncogenes can lead to neoplastic development alone or together with other factors. Consequently in relation with the others parameters we have studied the expression of three protooncogenes involved in hepatic tumorigenesis : Ki-ras, myc and fos.

For the whole study the strongly malignant LF hepatoma cell line established in our laboratory was used as reference.

MATERIALS AND METHODS

- Cell line and medium
. Epithelial cell lines, fibroblasts free, were initiated from the liver of 10 day-old Fischer rats according to Williams et al. (1971). They were grown in William's medium (Eurobio, France) supplemented with 10% foetal calf serum (Flow, England), glutamine and antibiotics. The cells were usually plated at 5×10^4 cells/ml medium in plastic flasks incubated at 37°C in a humidified incubator with 5% CO_2 atmosphere and subcultured weekly.

LF hepatoma cell line was established in the laboratory from a transplantable Wistar rat hepatoma originated from a chemically induced hepatoma. It was grown in a minimal essential medium (MEM Eurobio) supplemented as for the liver cell lines. These cells were routinely subcultured like the others. All lines were periodically screened for mycoplasma contamination.

- Histology

To follow their morphological development, the cells were seeded on slides in petri dishes. They were fixed in Boin's solution and stained in hemalun-eosin according to the technique described by Ganter and Jolles (1970).

- Ability to grow in soft agar

Malignant cells in vitro unlike normal cells grow when suspended in a semi solid substrate. The ability to form colonies in soft agar was screened according to the technique of Montagnier and Mc Pherson (1964). To prove the validity of this technique in our system, the LF hepatoma cells which always give rise to colonies in soft agar were always included as controls in each series.

- Determination of gamma glutamyl transpeptidase (γ GT) activity

γGT activity was assayed by 1/ the histochemical procedure of Rutenberg et al. (1969) using γ-glutamyl-4-methoxy-2-naphthylamide (Sigma) as substrate. Fast blue BBN (Sigma) as diazonium coupling reagent and glycyl-glycine (Sigma) as acceptor. The cultures were then observed under a light microscope ; the red positively stained cells were those that contained γ GT. 2/ According to the biochemical method of Orlowski and Meister (1963) using γ-glutamyl-p-nitroso-anilide as substrate.

- Expression of oncogenes

Total RNA was isolated from fresh cultures or frozen (liquid nitrogen) cultures stored at - 80°C using the lithium chlorure-urea procedure of Auffray et al. (1980) or the guanidine thiocynate method of Chirgwin et al. (1979). The total RNA was spotted directly on 20xSSC treated nitrocellulose filters or nylon membranes. ^{32}P labelled probes were prepared by nick translation of the following oncogenes clones : **Myc** - the 1.5 Kb sac 1 fragment containing the second exon from a human c myc kindly provided by Dr D. Stehelin (Lille). **Ki-ras** - the 1 Kb Eco RI fragment from the clone Hi Hi 3 of Kirsten murine sarcoma virus kindly provided by Dr E. Sclolnick (USA). **Fos** - the 3.1 Kb Xhol-Ucol DNA fragment of the human fos gene provided by Amersham. The filters were incubated for 48 h at 42°C. After hybridization the filters were washed and autoradiographs were prepared. The autoradiographs were quantified by scanning in a recording spectrophotometer (Vernon, France).

RESULTS

- Morphological changes (Fig. I)

During the first passages (Ia) the non transformed cells presented a flattened epithelial shape growing in a mosaic like pattern. The cells had a very high adhesion to the substrate on which they grew and to their neighboring. The cells underwent neoplastic transformation after a certain number of transfers (30-40) and gradual morphological changes might be observed: Loss of contact inhibition and overlapping in the cultures (Ib); appearance of large cells at about 90th transfer (Ic); increased loss of contact inhibition with piling up and appearance of giant cells (Id).

Figure I. Progressive morphological transformation in cell cultures with time.

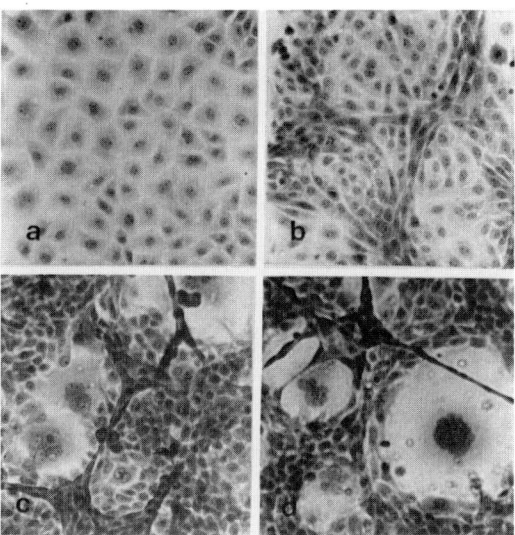

Magnification (x 140). a (16th passage) ; b,c,d; (50th to 230th passages).

Figure II. Gradual increase with the number of subcultures in the size of cell colonies formed in soft agar.

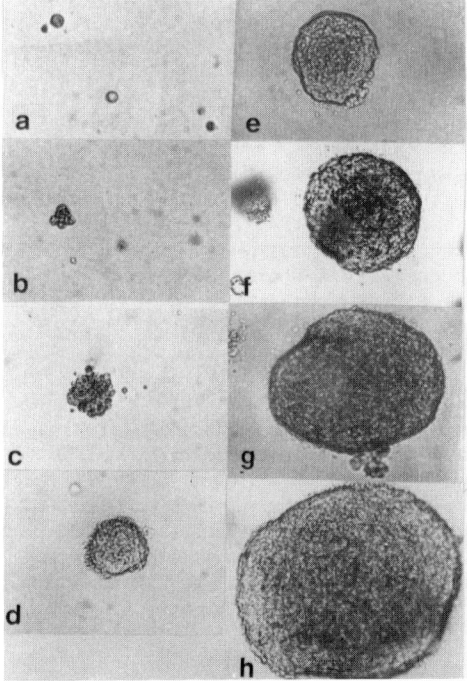

Passages studied between the 35th and 200th passages. Bar = 0,1 mm.

- Growth in soft agar (Fig. II)
The acquisition of anchorage independence was detected by the agar test. The ability for the cells to give colonies in agar appeared between 30 and 40th transfers. A progressive improvement in plating efficiency in soft agar was observed and the colonies became more numerous and larger with the number of subcultures.

γ GT activity (Table 1)
γGT is considered as a marker for early changes in hepatocytes following exposure to chemical carcinogens (see Vanderlaan and Phares, 1981 for review) as well as after virally neoplastic transformation (Lafarge-Frayssinet et al., 1984). We observed that γGT activity appeared relatively late during the process of spontaneous neoplastic transformation. Only some cells were positively stained at approximatively the 40th transfer. The activity expressed by only little groups of cells became detectable after about 60 transfers. After the 120th transfer all the cells were positively stained and the γ GT activity was almost as important as for LF hepatoma cells.

Table 1. Progressive increase of γGT activity in liver cells in culture.

Passage number	γGT activity	
	Histochemical detection*	Biochemical detection**
8	0	UD***
10	0	NM****
23	0	UD
32	+ (some cells)	UD
35	+	UD
42	+	NM
57	++ (some groups of cells)	5
79	+++ (almost all the cells)	11
120	++++ (all the cells)	17
LF hepatoma	++++	25

*Both the number and the size of positively stained group of cells were appreciated. ** γ GT activity was expressed as $mU/10^6$ cells.
***UD : undetectable ****NM : non measured.

- Oncogenes expression (Fig. III and IV)
Our results showed the increase of c fos, c myc and c ki-ras expression all along the progression of malignant transformation of the cells : weak for the early passages, the oncogenes expression increases as soon as the cells became malignant. An overexpression is observed in LF hepatoma cells and also when the number of subcultures increases; the amount of the transcripts evaluated by the densitometric scanning was about 200 fold for c ki-ras, 150 fold for c fos and 40 fold for c myc. Although the expression was more important for c ki-ras and c fos than for c myc there was a good correlation among the three oncogenes.

Figure III. Expression of c fos during progression of malignant transformation of epithelial rat liver cell lines.

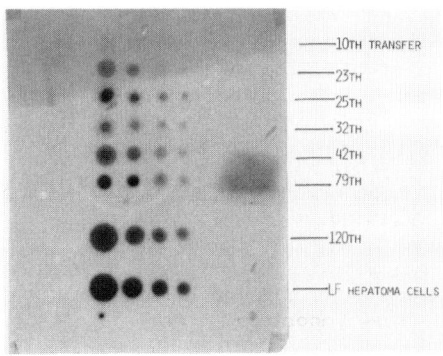

Fig. IV. Expression of c ki-ras and c myc during progression of malignant transformation of epithelial rat liver cell lines.

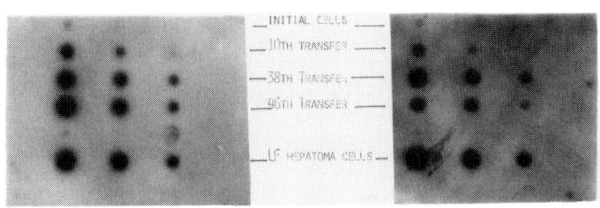

c Ki-Ras   c myc

DISCUSSION

We have observed a spontaneous transformation in our epithelial liver cell lines. Although the origin of this transformation remains unknown, this phenomenon has been regularly detected. The changes that we observed were first the loss of strong adhesiveness to the support then gradual morphological modifications which were correlated with the loss of contact inhibition and finally the capacity to grow in soft agar. γGT activity is only reexpressed at a late state after the cells are able to grow in soft agar. As several oncogenes have been involved in liver carcinogenesis, the progression of normal to malignant state can now be defined in molecular terms. We have shown that in correlation with the parameters previously studied there is an increase of expresion of three cellular oncogenes. The amounts of transcripts of c ki-ras, c fos and c myc are weak in the liver cells of 10 day-old rats (initial cells); these results are in agreement with those of Yaswen et al. (1985); the expression remain low during the first subcultures, then increase progressively to attain 200 fold the initial amount for c ki-ras, 150 fold for c fos and 40 fold for c myc. Nevertheless the expression of the three oncogenes in the late subcultures is always lower than in LF hepatoma cells. Oncogene expression has been described during progression of mouse mammary tumor cells by Sonnenberg et al. (1987) as well as in liver cells in culture during chemical carcinogenesis

469

(Corral et al., 1985 ; Kruijer et al., 1986); but up to now nothing had been done during the progression of spontaneous transformation in liver cells in culture.

In conclusion the spontaneous progression of normal to malignant state for liver cells is a slow process which requires many subcultures for the manifestation of a strong malignancy. It is not known whether this progression is due to an increase of the proportion of neoplastic cells as suggested by the increasing number of colonies observed in soft agar or whether it is due to a tumorogenic potency of all the cells which is progressively enhanced as suggested by the increasing size of colonies. The second case would suggest that the degree of transformation of the cells and particularly the expression of oncogenes may be for a long time sensible to external stimuli. In this eventuality, positive or negative modulation might be possible: positive modulation with tumor promotors for example or negative modulation with non cytotoxic chemotherapeutic agents.

REFERENCES

Auffray, C., Rougeon, F. (1980) : Purification of mouse immunoglobulin heavy chain messenger RNAs from total myeloma tumor RNA. Eur. J. Biochem. 107, 303-314.

Chirgwin, J.M., Przybyla, A.E., Mc Donald, R.J., Rutter, W.J. (1979) : Isolation of biologically active ribonucleic acid from sources enriched in ribonuclease. Biochemistry 18, 5294-5299.

Corral, M., Tichonicky, L., Guguen-Guillouzo, C., Corcos, D., Raymondjean, M., Paris, B., Kruh, J., Defer, N. (1985) : Expression of c fos oncogene during hepatocarcinogenesis, liver regeneration and in synchronized HTC cells. Expt. Cell Res. 160, 427-434.

Ganter, P., Jolles, G. (1970) : Histochimie normale et pathologique Vol. 2, p. 1418, Paris: Gauthier-Villars.

Kruijer, W., Skelly, H., Botteri, F., Van der Putter, H., Barber, J.R., Verma, I.M., Leffert, H.L. (1986) : Proto-oncogenes expression in regenerating liver is stimulated in cultures of primary adult rat hepatocytes. J. Biol. Chem. 17, 7929-7933.

Lafarge-Frayssinet, C., Estrade, S., Rosa-Loridon, B., Frayssinet, C., Cassingena, R. (1984) : Expression of gamma glutamyltranspeptidase in adult rat liver cells after transformation with SV40. Cancer Let. 22, 31-39.

Montagnier, L., Mac Pherson, I. (1964) : Croissance sélective en gélose de cellules de hamster transformées par le virus de polyome. C.R. Acad. Sci. 258, 4171-4173.

Morel-Chany, E., Guillouzo, C., Trincal, G., Szajnert, M.F. (1978) : "Spontaneous" neoplastic transformation In vitro of epithelial cell strains of rat liver : cytology, growth and enzymatic activities. Europ. J. Cancer 14, 1341-1352.

Morel-Chany, E., Lafarge-Frayssinet, C., Trincal, G. (1985) : Progression of"spontaneous" malignant transformation of epithelial rat liver cell lines. Cell Biol. Tox. 1, 11-22.

Orlowski, M., Meister, A. (1963) : γ-glutamyl-p-nitroanilide : A new convenient substrate for determination and study of L- and D-γ-glutamyl-transpeptidase activities. Biochim. Biophys. Acta 73, 679-681.

Oshiro, Y., Gerschenson, L.E., Di-Paolo, J.A. (1972) : Carcinoma from rat liver cells transformed spontaneously in culture. Cancer Res. 32, 877-879.

Rutenberg, A.M., Kim, H., Fischbein, J.W., Hanker, J.S., Wassenkrug, H.L., Seligman, A.M. (1969) : Histochemical and ultrastructural demonstration of glutamyltranspeptidase activity. J.Histochem. Cytochem. 17, 517-526.

Sato, J., Namba, M., Usdui, K., Nagano, D. (1968) : Carcinogenesis in tissue culture. VIII. "Spontaneous" malignant transformation of rat liver in long-term culture. Jap. J. Exp. Med. 38, 105-108.

Sonnenberg, A., Van Balen, P., Hilgers, J., Schuuring, E. Nusse, R. (1987): Oncogenes expression during progression of mouse tumor cells; activity of a proviral enhancer and the resulting expression of int-2 is influenced by the state of differentiation. Embo J. 6, 121-125.

Vanderlaan, M., Phares, W. (1981) : γ-glutamyltranspeptidase : a tumor cell marker with a pharmacological function. Histochem. J. 13, 865-877.

Wenstein, B., Orenstein, J.M., Gebert, R., Kaighn, M.E., Stadier, U.C. (1975) : Growth and structural properties of epithelial cell cultures established from normal rat liver and chemicaly induced hepatomas. Cancer Res. 35, 253-266.

Williams, G.M., Weisburger, E.K., Weisburger, J.H. (1971) : Isolation and long term culture of epithelial-like cells from rat liver. Exp. Cell Res. 69, 106-112.

Yaswen, P., Goyette, M., Shauk, P.R., Fausto, N. (1985) : Expression of c ki-ras, c ha-ras, and c myc in specific cell types during hepatocarcinogenesis. Mol. Cell Biol. 5, 780-786.

Nephrotoxicity

Néphrotoxicité

Stimulation of renal ammoniagenesis by the antiepileptic drug : sodium valproate. *In vivo* and *in vitro* studies

Guy Martin, Jean Besson, Bernard Ferrier, Christian Michoudet, Mireille Martin, Daniel Durozard, Gabriel Baverel

INSERM U.80 et CNRS UA 1177, Laboratoire de Physiologie Rénale et Métabolique, Faculté de Médecine Alexis Carrel, 69008 Lyon, France

KEYWORDS : Valproate - Hyperammonemia - Kidney - Ammoniagenesis - Antiepileptic drug - Adverse effect.

INTRODUCTION

Sodium valproate, a widely used antiepileptic drug (Simon and Penry, 1975), has been reported to induce hyperammonemia with extremely rare clinical manifestations (Coulter and Allen, 1981 ; Marescaux et al., 1984). This adverse effect has been attributed to an inhibition by valproate of the urea synthesis in the liver (Coudé et al., 1983). Recent arterio-venous measurements across the human and rat kidney (Warter et al., 1983, 1984) have suggested that this hyperammonemia may also be due to an increased release of ammonia into the renal vein secondary to an increased renal production of ammonia from circulating glutamine. However, the latter studies cannot be taken as proof for an increased renal venous release of ammonia because the renal blood flow was not measured.

In an attempt to clarify this question, we have precisely quantified the renal blood flow and the release of ammonia into the renal vein in the rat in vivo. We have also investigated the possible mechanisms whereby valproate stimulates ammonia production by using isolated rat and dog kidney-cortex tubules.

MATERIALS AND METHODS.

Male Wistar rats (180-300 g.) obtained from Iffa -Credo (St Germain -sur-l'Arbresle, France) and mongrel dogs (10-20 kg.) of either sex were used in our experiments . For the in vivo experiments designed to measure the renal venous release of ammonia in rats, the surgical preparation was as reported in a previous publication (Ferrier et al., 1985). A control clearance period of 25 min. was secured in the absence of valproate. At the end of the control period, 200mg./kg. body wt. of sodium valproate in 0.9% NaCl were injected intravenously. A second 25 min. clearance period started 15 min. after valproate injection. In each experiment, para-aminohippurate (PAH) was infused through the left jugular vein to get a constant plasma concentration of PAH. Each clearance period was bracketted by two arterial blood samples to measure blood ammmonia and plasma PAH concentrations, the mean values for ammonia and PAH being used for the calculations. At the middle of the clearance periods, 1 ml sample of renal venous blood was obtained by puncturing the left renal vein with a collecting glass pipette connected to a syringe. Ammonia and PAH concentrations were determined on deproteinized and neutralized samples by the method of Kun and Kearney (1974) and of Smith et al. (1945), respectively. Renal blood flow was estimated from the renal clearance and extraction of PAH by applying the Fick principle and renal blood flow was calculated from the renal plasma flow and hematocrit.

Rat and dog kidney-cortex tubules were prepared by collagenase treatment of renal cortical slices and incubated in 4 ml of Krebs-Henselheit buffer for 60 min. as described previously (Baverel et al., 1978). L-glutamine (5 mM) or L-glutamate (5 mM) were used as substrate in the absence or the presence of valproate. Incubations were terminated by adding perchloric acid (final concentration 2%). In all experiments, zero-time flasks were prepared with and without substrates by adding perchloric acid before the tubules. After removal of the denaturated proteins by centrifugation, the supernatant was neutralized with 20% (w/v) KOH for metabolite determination. Glutamine, glutamate, ammonia, glucose, and also the dry wt. of the amount of tubules added to the flasks were determined as decribed previously (Baverel et al., 1978). Net substrate utilization and product formation were calculated as the difference between the total flask contents (tissue + medium) at the start of the experiment and after the period of incubation. The metabolic rates are expressed in μmol of substances removed, or produced, per g. dry weight of tubules per hour. Values are given as means ± SEM.

RESULTS AND DISCUSSION.

Table 1 shows the effects of valproate on the concentration of ammonia in arterial and renal venous blood as well as on the renal venous release of ammonia in rats. Confirming previous findings by Warter et al. (1983), valproate administration was followed by a significant hyperammonemia . It is important to note that valproate injection did not alter renal blood flow. Table 1 also shows that valproate administration caused a large increase in the renal venous release of ammonia. Thus, these results clearly indicate that the kidneys might contribute to the systemic hyperammonemia observed after valproate administration.

Table 1. Effect of valproate on the renal venous release of ammonia in rats.

	Period 1 (control)	Period 2 (valproate)	Statistical significance
Arterial ammonia concentration (mM)	0.059 ± 0.015	0.097 ± 0.015	$P < 0.001$
Renal venous ammonia concentration (mM)	0.127 ± 0.012	0.238 ± 0.017	$P < 0.01$
Renal blood flow (ml/kg × min)	36.48 ± 3.73	33.54 ± 3.00	NS
Renal venous release of ammonia (nanomol/kg × min)	4540 ± 48.5	8022 ± 931	$P < 0.01$

Values are means ± SEM for 4 experiments. Statistical difference was measured by the paired Student's t test against the control period without valproate.

Table 2. Effect of valproate on the metabolism of 5 mM L-glutamine in rat and dog kidney tubules.

Species	Experimental condition	Metabolite removal (−) or production (+):			
		Glutamine	Glutamate	Ammonia	Glucose
Rat	Glutamine (5 mM)	−661.1 ±61.8	+128.5 ±13.4	+1128.2 ±52.8	+119.3 ±5.5
Rat	Glutamine (5 mM) + Valproate (10^{-4}M)	−845.9 ±62.2 $P < 0.001$	+174.0 ±18.4 $P < 0.01$	+1502.7 ±68.3 $P < 0.001$	+151.7 ±8.6 $P < 0.01$
Dog	Glutamine (5 mM)	−481.0 ±30.2	+121.8 ±17.5	+866.3 ±49.7	+74.1 ±4.3
Dog	Glutamine (5 mM) + Valproate (10^{-4}M)	−826.5 ±63.9 $P < 0.01$	+148.2 ±24.2 $P < 0.05$	+1381.8 ±157.5 $P < 0.02$	+122.5 ±10.7 $P < 0.02$

Each flask contained 12.0 ± 5.1 and 22.5 ± 3.5 mg dry wt. of tubules prepared from renal cortex of 5 rats and 4 dogs, respectively. Statistical difference was measured by the paired Student's t test against the control without valproate.

Table 2 shows that, in both rat and dog kidney tubules, valproate stimulated glutamine utilization. This effect, which was more pronounced in dog than in rat kidney tubules, was accompanied by a 33.2 and 59.5% increase in ammonia formation in rat and dog kidney tubules, respectively. It should be noted that increased removal of glutamine via glutaminase occurred despite an augmented accumulation of glutamate, a well known end-product inhibitor of glutaminase (Goldstein, 1966). This observation strongly suggests that valproate primarily stimulated renal glutaminase, the enzyme responsible for the release as ammonia of the amide nitrogen of glutamine. The fact that the increase in the production of ammonia caused by valproate was greater than the increase in glutamine removal implies that flux through glutamate dehydrogenase, the enzyme responsible for the release as ammonia of the amino nitrogen of glutamine, was also augmented. This may explain why valproate also stimulated glucose formation (Table 2).

Table 3. Effect of valproate on the metabolism of 5 mM L-glutamate in rat and dog kidney tubules.

Species	Experimental condition	Metabolite removal (−) or production (+):			
		Glutamate	Ammonia	Glutamine	Glucose
Rat	Glutamate (5 mM)	−517.1 ±26.6	+340.0 ±46.6	+102.7 ±12.6	+81.5 ±6.1
Rat	Glutamate (5 mM) + Valproate (10^{-4}M)	−557.8 ±70.2 NS	+458.9 ±61.2 $P<0.01$	+51.1 ±18.8 $P<0.01$	+82.3 ±8.8 NS
Dog	Glutamate (5 mM)	−284.9 ±15.5	+361.2 ±8.6	—	+66.1 ±2.5
Dog	Glutamate (5 mM) + Valproate (10^{-4}M)	−292.5 ±14.1 NS	+344.3 ±7.0 NS	—	+58.8 ±2.4 $P<0.01$

Each flask contained 25.4 ± 0.9 and 23.3 ± 1.3 mg dry wt. of tubules prepared from renal cortex of 5 rats and 4 dogs, respectively. Statistical difference was measured by the paired Student's t test against the control without valproate.

Table 3 shows that, in both rat and dog kidney tubules, valproate did not alter glutamate utilization. Ammonia formation (by glutamate dehydrogenase) also remained unchanged in the presence of valproate in dog kidney tubules which did not synthezise glutamine because glutamine synthetase is absent from the dog kidney (Lemieux et al.,1976). In contrast, valproate addition significantly increased ammonia formation in rat kidney tubules ; this effect was clearly due to the large inhibition of glutamine synthesis caused by valproate. Flux through glutamate dehydrogenase calculated as the sum of the ammonia and the glutamine found did not significantly changed in the presence of valproate; this means that, with glutamine as substrate, the increase in the flux through glutamate dehydrogenase observed in the presence of valproate was secondary to the increase in flux through glutaminase (see Table 2).

Although our data clearly demonstrate that valproate stimulated flux through rat and dog renal glutaminase and inhibited flux through rat glutamine synthetase, no direct effect of valproate on assayed activities of these enzymes could be demonstrated (results not shown). This suggests that valproate exerted its effects on both enzymes by some indirect mechanism which remains to be elucidated. In this respect, it should be pointed out that valproate has been shown to be metabolized by rat kidney tubules (D. Durozard and G. Baverel, 1987).

ACKNOWLEDGEMENTS

This study was supported by grants from M.R.T. (84-C-1155) and SANOFI RECHERCHE (Centre de Recherches CLIN-MIDY, Service de Toxicologie). Excellent technical assistance was provided by Véronique Pélamatti.

REFERENCES

Baverel, G., Bonnard, M., d'Armagnac de Castanet, E., Pellet, M. (1978) : Lactate and pyruvate metabolism in isolated renal tubules of normal dogs. Kidney Int. 14, 567-575.

Coudé, F.X., Grimber, G., Parvy, P., Rabier, D., Petit, F. (1983) : Inhibition of ureagenesis by valproate in rat hepatocytes. Role of N-acetylglutamate and acetyl-CoA. Biochem. J. 216, 233-236.

Coulter, D.L., Allen, R.J. (1981) : Hyperammonemia with valproic acid therapy. J. Pediatr. 99, 317-319.

Durozard, D., Baverel, G. (1987) : Gas chromatographic method for the measurement of sodium valproate utilization by kidney tubules. J. Chromatogr. 414, 460-464.

Ferrier, B., Martin, M., Baverel, G. (1985) : Reabsorption and secretion of α-ketoglutarate along the rat nephron. A micropuncture study. Am. J. Physiol. 248, F404-F412.

Goldstein, L. (1966) : Relation of glutamate to ammonia production in the rat kidney. Am. J. Physiol. 210, 661-666.

Kun, E., Kearney, E.B. (1974) : Ammonia. In : Methods of Enzymatic Analysis, ed. H.U. Bergmeyer, pp 1802-1806, New York : Academic Press.

Lemieux, G., Baverel, G., Vinay, P., Wadoux, P. (1976) : Glutamine synthetase and glutamyl transferase in the kidney of man, dog and rat. Am. J. Physiol. 231, 1068-1073.

Marescaux, C., Warter, J.M., Rumbach, L., Micheletti, G., Chabrier, G., Imler,M. (1984) : Valproate-induced hyperammonemia : Role of diet. Wld. Rev. Nutr. Diet. 43,174-178.

Simon, D., Penry, J.K. (1975) : Sodium di-n-propylacetate in the treatment of epilepsy : a review. Epilepsia, 16, 549-573.

Smith, H.W., Finkelstein, N., Aliminosa, L., Crawford, B., Graber, M. (1945) : The renal clearances of substituted hippuric acid derivatives and other aromatic acids in dog and man. J. Clin. Invest. 24, 388-404.

Warter, J.M., Imler, M., Marescaux, C., Chabrier, G., Rumbach, L., Micheletti, G., Krieger, J. (1983) : Sodium valproate-induced hyperammonemia in the rat : role of the kidney. Eur. J. Pharmacol. 87, 177-182.

Warter, J.M., Marescaux, C., Chabrier, G., Rumbach, L., Micheletti, B., Imler, M. (1984) Métabolisme rénal de la glutamine chez l'homme au cours des traitements par le valproate de sodium. Rev. Neurol. (Paris), 140, 370-371.

Chronobiological approach of mercury-induced toxicity and of the protective effect of high dilutions of mercury against mercury-induced nephrotoxicity

Jean-Charles Cal, Francis Larue, Catherine Dorian, Joël Guillemain, Pierre Dorfman, Jean Cambar

Groupe d'Etude de Physiologie et Physiopathologie Rénales, Faculté de Pharmacie, 91, rue Leyteire, 33000 Bordeaux, France

KEY-WORDS: chronotoxicology, nephrotoxicity, mercury, high dilutions, homoeopathy.

INTRODUCTION

Heavy metals, as mercury, cadmium or lead are largely used in many chemical industries. Directly released into the atmosphere, they present some risks for human health, inducing particularly occupational pathologies or dramatic environmental catastrophes, as in Minamata in Japan.

The toxicity of these different metals, especially mercuric compounds, has been extensively explored for a long time both in animals and in men. Their administration or inhalation produces a rapidly developing and reproducible injury particularly in nervous and renal systems. If heavy metal-induced nephrotoxicity has been well established, the influence of the time of testing has been to date rarely investigated.

Chronotoxicology has been well documented for some decades after the first observations with nikethamide (CARLSON and SERIN, 1950), as it was reported in recent reviews (SCHEVING et al., 1974 - CAMBAR and CAL, 1985). All these studies have shown a biorythmicity in living organisms and have pointed out that the time of testing is a major determinant of toxicity. Such an evidence of circadian and circannual variations in toxic and pharmacological effects of drugs highlights a new aspect of experimental and clinical medicine and can explain in part the well known variability in experimental results between different toxicologic investigations.

Chronotoxicological approach of heavy metals, recently undertaken, has been particularly focused on mercury, cadmium or platinum in rodents (review in CAL et al., 1986) and in man (LEVI, 1987). More recently similar data have been reported with other nephrotoxicants, from the antibiotics group (review in DORIAN, 1988). In the present paper, the circadian and circannual variations in mercuric-chloride induced mortality in mice are described.

Many investigations have been conducted in an attempt to reduce mercury-induced toxicity. Several drugs have been used including organic compounds rich in thiols or increasing metallothionein synthesis or even other metals in pretreatment. In view of these previous findings, pretreatment with high dilutions of metals - the so-called homoeopathic dilutions - have been tested and recognized as protective against metal-induced toxicity (CAMBAR et al, 1983). In the second part of this paper, are reported the experiments designed to demonstrate the protective effect of high mercuric dilutions against the toxic effect of mercuric chloride in mice and to test, for the first time, the influence of timing in the calendar scale on the provided protection.

A - CHRONOTOXICOLOGY OF MERCURIC CHLORIDE

1) Circadian approach

700 female Swiss mice (18-20g) were standardized for ten days to temperature and humidity-controlled quarters ($24 \pm 1°C$; 50%) on a LD 12:12 illumination schedule (light from 0800 hr to 2000 hr) and allowed food (Laboratory U.A.R. chow) and tap water ad libitum. Mice were housed 10 per cage (first test in February) and 15 per cage (second test in March); they received an IP injection of 0.5 ml of mercuric chloride at 4 different clock hours i.e. 0200, 0800, 1400 or 2000. Lethal acute renal failure was induced in mice by injection of 4, 5 or 6 mg Hg/kg and the total number of dead mice was recorded 10 days after drug administration. A classical statistical analysis (frequency comparison tests), was performed on the data.

The results indicate that mercuric chloride-dependent toxicity, as indexed by percent mortality, varies considerably as a function of administration time since mortality rates for a same hour of injection, irrespective of the dose ranged from 42.5% at 0200hr to 70% at 2000hr ($p<0.001$). Thus a circadian rhythm in mercuric chloride induced lethality was exhibited in mice with highest mortality occurring at 2000hr and lowest at 0200hr.

The findings of this study have shown that murine response to mercuric chloride is circadian stage dependent. Indeed, mercury induced lethality has exhibited a prominent circadian periodicity since LD50 reached 5.54 ± 0.18 mg Hg/kg at 0200 hr, the time of lowest mortality in the middle of the nocturnal span, and fell to 4.14 ± 0.47 mg Hg/kg at 2000 hr, the time of greatest susceptibility, coinciding with the end of the daily span of rodent inactivity. Data pertaining to survival time following intoxication support those for survival rate. Indeed when mice were injected with mercuric chloride at 0800, 1400 or 2000, the average time-to-death was short (6 days) whereas it was greatly increased when the animals were dosed at 0200 (9 days).

2) Circannual approach

Under the same experimental conditions, in order to assess the tolerance of mice to mercury along the circannual time scale in the absence of any protective treatment, 1170 animals were given a single IP injection of 0.5 ml of mercuric chloride (4, 5 or 6 mg Hg/kg) at one of 4 equispaced circadian stages (02.00, 08.00, 14.00 or 20.00 hrs) and at one of 6 months: january, february, april, june, september and november. The total number of dead mice was also recorded ten days after drug administration.

The results indicate that mercuric chloride-dependent toxicity, as indexed by percent mortality, varies greatly as a function of administration time. It ranged, for instance, for 5 mg Hg/kg from 53.33 (trough) to 86.67% (peak) in September, from 53.33 to 93.33% in June, from 60 to 100% in January and from 66.67 to 93.33% in February, April and November. Thus, regardless of dose and time of day, along the circannual time scale, tolerance to mercury appeared higher in winter with a peak in February (mortality rate: 68.9%) and lower in autumn with a statistically significant trough in November (mortality rate: 81.7% - p<0.01). The analysis of data by single cosinor method highlighted a statistically significant circahemiannual rhythm (period equal to six months - p<0.001) in mercuric chloride-induced toxicity in mice with highest mortality occurring in spring and autumn. It is noticeable that the cosine curve representative of the rhythm is exceptionally well fitted to the experimental data.

In conclusion, the purpose of this study was not to demonstrate the widely described mortality or acute renal failure induced by mercuric chloride in mice, but to evidence a time dependent toxicity of this heavy metal. Such results demonstrate indeed circadian as well as seasonal variations in mice tolerance to lethal dosages of mercury. A better knowledge of the biochemical and cellular mechanisms determining this time-dependent response of mice to mercury should open the way to further investigations so as to optimize the clinical use of nephrotoxic drugs acting as well at the proximal tubular level.

B - CHRONOBIOLOGICAL VARIATIONS IN THE PROTECTIVE EFFECT OF HIGH MERCURY DILUTIONS AGAINST MERCURY-INDUCED LETHALITY

1) Protective effect of high mercury dilutions against mercury-induced lethality

In order to study the effect of a pretreatment with high mercury dilutions against mercuric chloride toxicity, female Swiss mice received a daily IP injection of 0.5 ml of the homoeopathic dilution or of 0.5 ml of succussed distilled water (control animals) throughout a 7-day period, and on the 7th day, one hour after the last administration of the pretreatment, a single IP injection of 5, 6 or 7 mg Hg/kg of mercuric chloride. Mortality was recorded ten days after intoxication. The homoeopathic drug was prepared by Dolisos laboratories from a mother solution (1g Hg/l in distilled water) - the so-called "Mercurius corrosivus 3d" - diluted 1:9 to get Mercurius corrosivus 2c (0.1g Hg/l) and then potentized to Mercurius corrosivus 9c (10^{-15} pg/l) and to Mercurius corrosivus 15c (theoretical concentration: 10^{-15} pg Hg/l) by serial centesimal dilutions 1:99 and automated succussion (100 impacts) at each step of dilution.

- In non pretreated mice given 5, 6, or 7 mg Hg/kg, mortality rates were respectively 73.4%, 78.5% and 93.3%.
- When mice were pretreated with Mercurius corrosivus 9c, the mortality induced by the same mercuric chloride doses were respectively 50%. 66.7% and 73.4%.
- When mice were pretreated with Mercurius corrosivus 15c, the mortality induced by the same mercuric chloride doses decreased respectively to 26.7%, 35.7% and 78.5%.

Thus, no mather at which level of dilution Mercurius corrosivus was administered mercury-induced mortality in pretreated mice, was statistically decreased (p<0.001). This was especially true when the animals were challenged with 5 mg Hg/kg since mortality rates were 26.7% in Mercurius corrosivus 15c pretreated mice, 50% in 9c pretreated ones and 73.4% in control mice.

2) Circannual approach of the effectiveness of high mercury dilutions

Another series of experiments were conducted so as to assess the influence of timing in the circannual time scale on the effectiveness of high mercury dilutions against mercuric chloride-induced mortality in mice. Under the same experimental conditions than previously, the animals were pretreated only with Mercurius corrosivus 15c or distilled water and challenged with 5 mg Hg/kg. Such a protocol was repeated at 5 months of the year: October, December, February, April and May. A statistical analysis was performed on the data by means of classical frequency comparison tests and by the single cosinor rhythmometric procedure with a special program designed by J.C Cal for the Apple III microcomputer.

Mortality incidence over the 10-day period after administration of 5 mg Hg/kg of mercuric chloride was regularly higher in control mice than in pretreated ones but the effectiveness of Mercurius corrosivus varied considerably as a function of the time of year. Indeed, for example, a statistically significant protection was highlighted in December since 93.1% of control animals died, whereas only 73.4% of the pretreated ones died at the same time ($p<0.01$); in contrast, this protective effect was not significant in February.

The ratio of the difference in mortality rates between pretreated and control groups to control mortality rate - the so-called "protection index" - appeared as a function of calendar time. A circannual rhythm in this index was detected by the analysis by the single cosinor method ($p<0.0113$). Thus the protective effect of Mercurius corrosivus assessed by the protection index exhibited circannual variations with a computative acrophase in August and a mesor equal to about 58%. In such instances, it may be apt to apply the term of chronoeffectiveness of the homoeopathic drug.

CONCLUSION

In conclusion, if many authors have already reported that some substances, particularly heavy metals, can reduce mercury-induced toxicity, the present study demonstrates for the first time that very high dilutions (Mercurius corrosivus 15c) of this metal can largely reduce this lethality. Moreover, if similar protective effects of metal dilutions against metal have been already reviewed (WURMSER, 1985), evidence that such a protective effect can be detected at different times in the year and even presents statistically significant circannual variations, as often described for other pharmacological or toxicological effects, shows the reproducibility of experimental homoeopathic data.

This report demonstrates thus that mercury toxicity can be reduced by high mercury dilutions given at well choosen times in the day or in the year. Finally, after further investigations, such a research may benefit the patient by leading to drug administration and especially to the clinical use of high dilutions, timed according to tolerance rhythms in order to take advantage of predictable states having improved toxic-therapeutic ratios.

ACKNOWLEDGEMENTS

The present paper is the summary of the results gained in fulfilment of a research project entitled "Chronobiological Approach of Nephrotoxicants" for which the authors gratefully acknowledge the financial support (Grant n°84.C.1156) from the Ministère de la Recherche et de l'Enseignement Supérieur. The main findings have been presented at this congress.

REFERENCES

Cal, J.C., Dorian, C. and Cambar, J.(1986): Circadian and circannual changes in nephrotoxic effects of heavy metals and antibiotics. Ann. Rev. Chronopharm. 2 , 143-176.

Cambar, J., Desmouliere, A., Cal, J.C. and Guillemain, J.(1983): Mise en évidence de l'effet protecteur de dilutions homéompathiques de Mercurius corrosivus vis à vis de la mortalité au chlorure mercurique chez la souris. Ann. Homéo. Franç. 25 , 6-12.

Cambar, J. and Cal, J.C.(1985): Rythmes biologiques et toxicité des agents physiques, chimiques et médicamenteux. Le Pharmacien Biologiste 73 , 259-269.

Carlson, A. and Serin, F.(1950): Time of day as a factor influencing the toxicity of nikethamide. Acta Pharmacol. Toxicol. (Kbh) 6 , 181-186.

Dorian, C., Catroux, P. and Cambar, J.(1988): Chronobiological approach of aminoglycosides. In press in Arch. Toxicol.

Levi, F.(1987): Chronobiologie et cancers. Path. Biol. 35 , 960-968.

Levi, F., Hrushesky, W.J.M., Blomquist, J., Lakatua, D., Haus, E., Halberg, F. and Kennedy, B.J.(1982): Reduction of cis-diammine-dichloroplatinum nephrotoxicity in rats by optimal circadian drug timing. Cancer Res. 42 , 950-955.

Scheving, L., von Mayersbach, H. and Pauly, J.E.(1974): An overview of chronopharmacology. J. Eur. Toxicol. 7 , 203-227.

Wurmser, L.(1985): La raison et l'intuition. Homéopathie française 73 , 313-317.

Author Index
Index des auteurs

Achard-Ellouk, S.	379
Acosta, D.	221
Agheli N.	181
Albrecht, R.	185
Amar, C.	175
Antignac, E.	197
Atteba, S.	186
Aubert, R.	181
Aubery, M.	437
Baffet, G.	423
Bagrel, D.	451
Baradat, M.	325
Barthel, A.M.	321
Baverel, G.	475
Bayliss, M.K.	281
Beaune, Ph.	31, 103, 175
Bégué, J.M.	235, 293, 309, 357, 365
Bell, J.A.	281
Belpaire, F.M.	315
Benchekroun, Y.	269
Benhamou, J.-P.	3
Ben Reddad, K.	459
Bernadou, J.	43
Berthault-Peres, P.	301
Berthou, F.	287
Besson, J.	475
Blaauboer, B.J.	351
Boelsterli, U.A.	335
Bogaert, M.G.	315
Boisset, M.	185
Bon, M.	259
Bonfils, C.	41
Boré, P.	301
Bories G.F.	325
Bork, R.W.	31
Bouis, P.	335
Bourel, M.	431
Bradbury, A.	281
Braut-Boucher, F.	279
Brazier, J.L.	269
Brissot, P.	397, 431
Bromet, N.	111, 293, 357
Bruckner, J.V.	221
Cabanac, S.	259
Cal, J.C.	481
Callaerts, A.	329
Cambar, J.	481
Cano, J.P.	301
Cariou, Y.	103
Cassand, P.	197
Castell, J.V.	374
Chanussot, F.	99
Chaumontet, C.	459
Chautan, M.	99
Chedeville, A.	95
Chesné, C.	235, 343
Chevanne, F.	309
Chevreau, P.	113
Chiapetta, P.V.	117
Chindavijak, B.	315
Claeyssens, S.	95
Clair, P.	41
Claude, J.R.	181
Clément, B.	397
Coles, B.	69
Colin, C.	197
Collignon, F.	253
Connelly, J.C.	191
Connolly, A.K.	191
Corcos, L.	445
Cosson, C.	203
Coulange, C.	301
Coulaud, D.	385
Cox, J.W.	391
Cresteil, T.	51
Dalet, C.	41
Danan, G.	23
Dannan, G.A.	31
Dansette, P.M.	175
Daujat, M.	41
Decastel, M.	437
Defrance, R.	293
Delbos, J.M.	111
Désage, M.	269
De Smet, F.	315
Desvergne, B.	431
De Sousa, G.	301
Deugnier, Y.	431
Dock, L.	275
Dorfman, P.	481
Donato, T.	371
Donatsch, P.	335
Dorian, C.	481

Ducros, M.	301
Dumont, J.M.	397
Durozard, D.	475
Eisen, H.J.	51
Emanoil-Ravier, R.	465
Esnault, C.	99
Fabre, G.	301
Fabre, I.	301
Fellous, R.	385
Ferrier, B.	475
Fraeyman, N.	315
François, V.	459
Frayssinet, C.	465
Gaillot, J.	253
Galteau, M.M.	451
Garcette, M.	465
Gazeau, J.P.	431
Ged, C.	31
Gelé, P.	111, 293
Génissel, P.	357
Gibassier, D.	321
Gires, P.	253
Glaise, D.	431
Gomez-Lechon, M.J.	371
Goussault, Y.	437
Gouy, D.	181
Gouyette, A.	385
Greischel, A.	85
Gripon, P.	343
Grislain, L.	111, 293, 357
Groen, K.	123
Guaitani, A.	405
Guédes, Y.	365
Guengerich, F.P.	31, 89
Guguen-Guillouzo, C.	235
Guillemain, J.	481
Guillouzo, A.	235, 287, 293, 309, 321 343, 357, 365, 397, 417, 423
Haentjens, G.	437
Haque, S.J.	59
Hauton, J.	99
Henry, M.	371
Hinton, R.H.	191
Hoellinger, H.	371
Homberg, J.C.	175
James, O.F.W.	13
Jernström, B.	275
Jonsson, M.	275
Kenna, J.G.	161
Kernaleguen, D.	365

Ketterer, B.	69, 417
Kiechel, J.R.	211
Kiffel, L.	175
Kremers, P.	245
Lacarelle, B.	301
Lafarge-Frayssinet, C.	465
Lafont, H.	99
Larrauri, A.	371
Larrey, D.	129, 143
Larue, F.	481
Laruelle, C.	99
Latinier, M.F.	397
Lavoinne, A.	95
Le Bigot, J.F.	211
Le Bot, M.A.	365
Le Corre, P.	321
Leroux, J.P.	175, 263
Lescoat, G.	431
Le Verge, R.	309, 321
Levy, M.	451
Lloyd, R.S.	31
Lopez, P.	371
Mackenzie, P.I.	59
Malet-Martino, M.C.	113, 259
Mansuy, D.	175
Martel, P.	459
Martin, G.	475
Martin, M.	475
Martin, M.V.	31
Martin, S.	253
Martinez, M.	275
Martino, R.	113, 259
Matray, F.	95
Maurel, P.	41
Mennes, W.C.	351
Meunier, B.	235
Meyer, D.J.	69
Michoudet, C.	475
Moatti, N.	203
Mocaër, E.	111, 293
Mocquard, M.T.	357
Molimard, R.	431
Montoya, A.	371
Morel-Chany, E.	465
Müller-Enoch, D.	81, 85, 89, 411
Muto, T.	31
Myara, I.	203
Nagenrauft, T.	81, 411
Narbonne, J.F.	197
Neuberger, J.	161
Nicol M.	103

Pascal, G.	459
Pasdeloup, N.	431
Pauthe-Daide, D.	371
Pazo-Carrera, J.	103, 423
Peleran J.C.	325
Pelissier, M.A.	185
Peret, J.	95
Pessayre, D.	129, 143
Pichard, L.	41
Piguet, V.	253
Pineau, T.	41
Placidi, M.	301
Plouin, P.F.	203
Prescott, L.F.	153
Price, S.C.	191
Rahmani, R.	301
Rampal, M.	301
Raquillet, L.	357
Ratanasavanh, D.	103, 235, 287, 293, 321, 357, 365, 397
Rawlins, M.D.	13
Renton, K.W.	117
Ribon, B.	269
Richard, B.	301
Riché, C.	287, 365
Riou, J.P.	269
Rissel, M.	423
Robert, J.	365
Rogiers, V.	329
Rolin, S.	451
Rolland, A.	309
Rouer, E.	263
Rouet, P.	263
Rousset, J.P.	445

Sabolovic, N.	451
Sado, P.	321
Santak, J.	81
Santone, K.S.	221
Seneca, V.	417
Shinriki, N.	31
Siest, G.	451
Sonck, W.	329
Stavchansky, S.A.	221
Stevenson, D	191
Sutra J.F.	325
Taylor, J.B.	69
Trommelen, G.J.J.M.	123
Ulrich, R.G.	391
Umbenhauer, D.R.	31
Van Bezooijen, K.F.A.	123
Vandenberghe, Y.	417
Van Holsteijn, C.W.M.	351
Vedrine, Y.	253
Vercruysse, A.	329, 417
Vergani, G.	411
Verjus, M.A.	385
Vialanex, J.P.	259
Vic, P.	181
Villa, P.	305
Vignaud (du), P.	111, 293, 357
Warnet, J.M.	181
Wellman, M.	451
Wilson, K.	281
Woodhouse, K.W.	13
Wynne, H.	13

Subject Index
Index des mots-clés

Acetaldehyde 134
Acetaminophen 130, 131, 135, 144, 149
Acetone 154
Acetylation 143-149, 325
Acetylamino fluorene 71, 218
N-Acetyl-cysteine 156
Acid phosphatase 393
Acute cytolytic hepatitis 25
Adriamycin 74
Adverse drug reactions 13-18, 23-27
Aflatoxin B$_1$ 71-218, 239, 445-449
Age 48, 155
Ageing 13-18, 123-125
Ajmaline 8, 10, 136
Albumin 239, 347, 359, 374, 375, 399, 427, 431-435
Alcohol 14, 167
Alcoholism 6
Aldrin epoxidase 247, 263-266, 446
Aldrin epoxidation 14
Alkaline phosphatase 7, 9, 385
Alpha-bromoisovaleryl urea 72, 73
Alpha-methyldopa 9, 135, 136, 167
Alpha-methyl ornithine 434
Alpha-naphtylisothiocyanate 191-196
Amanitin 375
Amikacin 391-395
Amineptine 111-112, 130, 136, 293-300
2-Amino-3-methylimidazo [4,5-f] quinoline 325-328
Aminopyrine 14
Aminotransferases 7, 9
Amiodarone 9, 181-183
Amitriptyline 293, 296
Ammoniagenesis 475-479
Amodiaquine 7, 130, 145
Androsterone 60
Aniline 351-354
Anthracyclines 365-370
Antibiotics 391-395
Antipyrine 16, 315-319
Arginine 433
Ascorbate 185-188
ATP 222, 226, 229, 381
Auto-antibodies 26, 136, 162, 167, 175-179

Barbiturates 6
Benorylate 373

Benoxaprofen 18
Benzanthracene 52, 53, 247
Benzo(a)pyrene 51, 55, 72, 197-200 275-278, 412
Benzo(a)pyrene hydroxylase 52, 53, 246, 249
Benzodiazepines 6
Betanaphthoflavone 42, 164, 176, 249
Bile 326
Bile acids 60, 335-340
Bile duct lining cell 191-196
Bilirubin 60, 64
Bleomycin 74
Brain 62
Bufuralol 90
Butibufen 373, 374, 376
Butylated hydroxyanisole 459-463
Butylated hydroxytoluene 459-463

Cadmium 481
Caffeine 14, 269-274, 287-291
Calcium 134, 221-230
Cannabinol 248
Captopril 203-208
Carbamazepine 8, 117-121
Carbon disulphide 154
Carbon tetrachloride 131, 137, 221-230
Carboxymethyl-cystein 145
Carcinogens 70, 72
Catalase 144
Chloramphenicol 60, 62
Chlorpromazine 6, 8, 10, 136, 145, 374
Cholestasis 3, 136, 144, 191-196
Cholesterol 99
Cholic acid 337
Chronotoxicology 481-484
Ciclosporin A (see cyclosporin)
Cimetidine 143, 154, 156
Clofibrate 42, 60
Clometacin 7, 9
Cobaltous chloride 154
Co-culture 235-241, 297, 359, 397-402, 417-420, 431-435
Collagen 203-208, 397-402
Collagenase 401
Converting enzyme inhibitors 203-208
Cryopreservation 343-348
Cycloheximide 408

Cyclosporin 42, 213, 335-340
Cyproheptadine 10, 136
Cytochrome P-450 .... 31-36, 41-48, 51-56
    71, 81, 85, 89, 103-108, 123-125, 132
    137, 144, 175-179, 237, 245-250, 263
                     353, 411-415, 445-449

Dantrium 239
Daunorubicin 365-370
N-Dealkylation 281-285, 322
Debrisoquine 9, 144
Debrisoquine hydroxylation 31-36, 89
Demethylation 238
Development 74
Dexamethasone 42, 45, 53, 64, 246
                                247, 406, 409
Dextromethorphan 137, 145
Diabetic rat 263-266
Diastereoisomers 295
Diethylnitrosamine 218
3,3'Diethyloxadicarbocyanine 386
Dihydralazine 7, 177
Dihydroergotamine 217
N-dimethyl-4-aminoazobenzene 71
Disopyramide 321-324
Ditercalinium 385-390
Dithiocarb 154
Dimethylsulphoxide 240, 405-409
DNA glycosylase 73
DNA ligase 73
DNA polymerase 73
Dog   111-112, 281-285, 353, 391, 475, 477
Doxorubicin 309-312, 365-370
Drug-induced hepatitis 3-8
Drug related antibodies 161-170

Enalapril 203
Enantiomers 321-324
Epirubicin 365-370
Epoxide hydrolase 5, 132, 143-149
                                197, 265
Erythrocytes 146, 147
Erythromycin .. 42, 45, 117-121, 135, 136
                         217, 237, 391, 393

Estradiol 60
Estrogens 8
Ethane 74
Ethanol 35, 42, 135, 154, 156
                         423-428, 451-457
Ether 154
Ethoxycoumarin deethylase 249, 405-409
7-Ethoxycoumarin 0-deethylation 14
Etiocholanolone 60

Fasting 135
Fatty acids 181-183
Fenofibrate 99-102
Fetal hepatocytes 245-250
Fibroblasts 146
Fluoropyrimidines 113-116
Fluorouracil 113-116, 162, 259-261
Fluperlapine 216, 238
Flurbiprofen 373, 375, 376
Fœtus 48

Galactose 14
Galactosamine 374, 375
Gamma-glutamyl-transferase 7, 385
                     425, 451-457, 461, 465, 468
Gentamicin 391-395
Glucagon 263-266
Glucocorticoïds 45, 144, 406
Gluconeogenesis 374, 376
Glucose-6-phospatase 226, 230
Glucuronidation 60, 238, 303, 330
Glucuronylation 281-285
Glucuronogypsogenin 379, 381
Glucuronosyltransferases 59-65
Glutamate dehydrogenase 477
Glutamine 477
Glutaminase 477
Glutathione 5, 95-98, 132, 133, 134
    135, 143-149, 153-157, 197-202, 275-278
Glutathione peroxidase 69-76, 132
Glutathione reductase 132
Glutathione synthetase 143-149
Glutathione transferases .. 69-76, 103-108
                     132, 238, 276, 417-420
Glycogen 374
Granulocytes 147
Guinea pig 73, 154, 191
Gypsoside 379, 381

Halothane 6, 7, 18, 131, 136, 143
                             148, 161-170, 175
Hamster 154, 155, 353
Haptoglobin 400
Hemopexin 400
Hepatocarcinogenesis 75
Hepatoma cells 52, 165, 218, 411-415
                     437-442, 445-449, 451-457
Hepatotoxicity 3-10, 143-149, 153-157
                             161, 222, 293
HMG (hydroxymethylglutaryl-) coenzyme
A reductase 99-102
Humans 111-112, 134, 135, 137, 475
Human liver 51-56
Human hepatocytes 216, 218, 237

287-291, 293-300, 301-307, 353-363, 365-370
397-402
5-Hydroperoxymethyl uracil 73
Hydroproline 400
6 β-Hydroxycortisol 34
Hyperammonemia 475-479

Ibuprofen 373, 376
Idiosyncrasy 5, 134, 162, 165
Imidazole 64
Imipramine 136
Indocyanin green 15
Inflammation 315-319
Iproniazid 26, 136, 143
Isaxonine.. 7, 136
Isosulmazole 6, 7, 135, 136, 143
144, 145, 81

Josamycin' 137

Ketoconazole 7, 143
Ketotifen 215, 216, 237
Kidney 62, 131, 175, 475-479

Labetolol 16
Lactalbumin 95-98
Lactate dehydrogenase 225, 229, 239,
248, 297, 322, 339, 359, 374, 381, 389,
425, 455
Lamellar body 393
Laminin 240
Lead 481
Leucocyte 163
Lidocaine 315-319
Lignocaine 16
Liver epithelial cells 235, 347, 360,
400, 412, 459-463, 465-470
Loxtidine 281-285
Lung 62, 70
Lymphocyte 146, 147, 148, 163, 164
167, 168
Lysosome 130, 297, 360, 391, 393

Malotilate 397-402
Man 73, 99, 155, 162, 163, 165,
169, 295, 353, 481
Mebendazole 249
Mephenytoin 89, 145, 148
Mephenytoin hydroxylase 52, 53
Mephenytoin hydroxylation 31-36
Mercury 481-484
Methotrexate 9
Methoxsalen 137
3-Methylcholanthrene 42, 47, 52, 63
64, 75, 86, 154

Methylpyrazole 64
Metronidazole 147
Metyrapone 154
Mevinoline 99-102
Microsomes 148, 175, 185-188, 222,
247, 253-257, 263-266
Midazolam 301-397
Midecamycin 136, 137
Mitochondrion 385-390
Mitoxantrone 301-307
Monkey 217, 353
Monoamine oxidase inhibitors 7
Monooxygenase 245-250, 287-291, 405-409
Morphine 62
Mouse 52, 70, 135, 137, 154, 155
191, 259, 481
Mutagenesis 197-202

1-Naphthol 62
Navelbine 304
Nephrotoxicity 481-484
Nifedipine 145, 237
Nifedipine oxidation 31-36, 69
4-Nitroanisole demethylase 53
Nitrofurantoin 17, 147
4-Nitrophenol 60, 62
Nikethamide 481
Nuclear magnetic resonance 113-116
259-261

Ornithine alpha-ketoglutarate 431-435
Oxidation 143-149, 238, 303
β-Oxidation 295
Oxiphenisatin 9

Papaverine 7, 9
Paracetamol 6, 72, 73, 143, 153-157
164, 238, 347
Paraquat 373, 374
Pefloxacin 253-257
Penicillin 143
Perfused liver 253-257, 259-261
Perhexiline maleate 9, 130, 137, 145
Perindopril 203
Perindoprilate 203
Peroxidation 5, 132, 133, 144, 146, 185-188
Pharmacogenetic 143-149
Phenacemide 148
Phenacetin 145
Phenacetin O-deethylation 31-36
Phenobarbital 36, 42, 53, 63, 64, 75,
86, 148, 154, 164, 176, 193, 237, 246,
247, 408, 445-449, 455, 459-463
Phenobarbitone (see phenobarbital)
Phenylindanedione 8

Phenytoin 6, 145, 148, 149
Phospholipase A_2 .... 62, 73
Phosphilase C 230
Phospholipidosis 181-183
Pimobendan 81
Pindolol 216, 238
Piperonyl butoxide 154
Pirprofen 130
Placenta 70
Platinum 481
Polyamine 433
Polycyclic aromatic hydrocarbons 36,
    42, 51, 60, 246, 249, 408, 411-415, 446
Polymethacrylic nanospheres 309-312
Polymorphonuclear cell 146
Pregnenolone-16α-carbonitrile   42, 45, 64
Probenecid 156
Prolidases 203-208
Propranolol 315-319
Protein synthesis .. 400, 423-428, 437-442
Protooncogene 465-470
Pyrazole 64

Quinidine 89-92

Rabbit 41-48, 154, 163, 165, 169,
                                  216, 237, 253
Ramipril 203
Ramiprilate 203
Red blood cell 70
Renal cell 146
Ricin 437-442
Rifampicin   6, 32, 42, 45, 47, 64, 137, 144
mRNA 41-48, 445-449

S-3341 357-363
Saponins 379-382
Scoparone O-demethylation   81, 82, 85-88
Sex 48, 74
Sheep 353
SKF 525A 316
Small intestinal mucosa 62
Spectinomycin 391-395
Spiramycin 136, 137
Stereoselectivity 321-324
Streptozotocin 265

Sulfation 238
Sulfonamide 146, 148, 149
Sulmazole 81
Suloctidil 8, 9
Sulphinpyrazone 156

Taurocholate 337
Testis 62
Testoterone 60
Tetrachlorodibenzo-p-dioxin 52, 53, 55
Theophylline 123-125
Thioacetamide 374, 375
Thymine 73
Tienilic acid 7, 9, 136, 175-179
Ticlopidine 8
Ticrynafen 26
Tolbutamide 32, 145
Transaminases 162, 374, 381, 391, 425
Transferrin 347
Triacetyloleandomycin 8, 117
Triazolam 16
Trichloroethylene 132
Tricyclic antidepressants 8, 10
Trioxsalen 137
Tripelennamine 218
Troleandomycin 10, 45, 48, 135,
                                       136, 144, 217
Trospectomycin sulfate 391-395
Turpentine 316
Tyrosine aminotransferase 406

UDP glucuronosyltransferases
    (see Glucuronosyltransferase)
Urea 475
Ureogenesis 374
Urine 326

Valproate 329-333, 475-479
Valproic acid 7
Vinca alkaloids 301-307
Vindesine 304
Vinyl chloride 132
Vitamin A 103-108, 185-188, 197
Vitamin C 132, 198
Vitamin E 132, 144, 185-188, 198

Wealing rat 95-98

Reproduction photomécanique
IMPRIMERIE LOUIS-JEAN
BP 87 — 05002 GAP
Tél. : 92.51.35.23
Dépôt légal : 730 — Octobre 1989
Imprimé en France